IAP Recent Advances in
PEDIATRICS

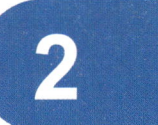

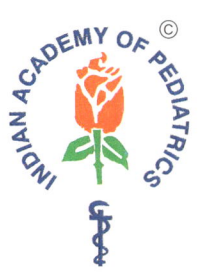

IAP Recent Advances in PEDIATRICS

2

Editor-in-Chief
PSN Menon
MD MNANS FIAP FIMSA
Consultant and Head
Department of Pediatrics
Jaber Al-Ahmed Armed Forces Hospital
Kuwait
Former Professor of Pediatrics
All India Institute of Medical Sciences
New Delhi, India

Executive Editor
Alok Gupta
MD FIAP
Pediatrician, Counselor and Environmentalist
Pediatric Specialties Clinic, Jaipur
Former Assistant Professor in
Pediatric Medicine
Mahatma Gandhi Medical
College and Hospital
Jaipur, Rajasthan, India

Academic Editors
Piyush Gupta
MD FAMS FIAP
Professor and Head
Department of Pediatrics
University College of Medical Sciences
New Delhi, India

P Ramachandran
MD DNB
Professor of Pediatrics and
Associate Dean (PG studies)
Sri Ramachandra Medical College and Research Institute
Sri Ramachandra Institute of Higher Education and Research (SRIHER)
Chennai, Tamil Nadu, India

Forewords
Remesh Kumar R
Bakul Jayant Parekh
Upendra Kinjawadekar

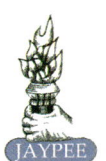

JAYPEE BROTHERS MEDICAL PUBLISHERS
The Health Sciences Publisher
New Delhi | London

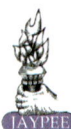 **Jaypee Brothers Medical Publishers (P) Ltd**

Headquarters
Jaypee Brothers Medical Publishers (P) Ltd
EMCA House, 23/23-B
Ansari Road, Daryaganj
New Delhi 110 002, India
Landline: +91-11-23272143, +91-11-23272703
+91-11-23282021, +91-11-23245672
Email: jaypee@jaypeebrothers.com

Corporate Office
Jaypee Brothers Medical Publishers (P) Ltd
4838/24, Ansari Road, Daryaganj
New Delhi 110 002, India
Phone: +91-11-43574357
Fax: +91-11-43574314
Email: jaypee@jaypeebrothers.com

Overseas Office
JP Medical Ltd.
83 Victoria Street, London
SW1H 0HW (UK)
Phone: +44 20 3170 8910
Fax: +44 (0)20 3008 6180
Email: info@jpmedpub.com

Website: www.jaypeebrothers.com
Website: www.jaypeedigital.com

© 2022, Indian Academy of Pediatrics

The views and opinions expressed in this book are solely those of the original contributor(s)/author(s) and do not necessarily represent those of editor(s) of the book.

All rights reserved. No part of this publication may be reproduced, stored or transmitted in any form or by any means, electronic, mechanical, photocopying, recording or otherwise, without the prior permission in writing of the publishers.

All brand names and product names used in this book are trade names, service marks, trademarks or registered trademarks of their respective owners. The publisher is not associated with any product or vendor mentioned in this book.

Medical knowledge and practice change constantly. This book is designed to provide accurate, authoritative information about the subject matter in question. However, readers are advised to check the most current information available on procedures included and check information from the manufacturer of each product to be administered, to verify the recommended dose, formula, method and duration of administration, adverse effects and contraindications. It is the responsibility of the practitioner to take all appropriate safety precautions. Neither the publisher nor the author(s)/editor(s) assume any liability for any injury and/or damage to persons or property arising from or related to use of material in this book.

This book is sold on the understanding that the publisher is not engaged in providing professional medical services. If such advice or services are required, the services of a competent medical professional should be sought.

Every effort has been made where necessary to contact holders of copyright to obtain permission to reproduce copyright material. If any have been inadvertently overlooked, the publisher will be pleased to make the necessary arrangements at the first opportunity. The **CD/DVD-ROM** (if any) provided in the sealed envelope with this book is complimentary and free of cost. **Not meant for sale.**

Inquiries for bulk sales may be solicited at: jaypee@jaypeebrothers.com

IAP Recent Advances in Pediatrics

Volume 1: 2020
Volume 2: **2022**

ISBN: 978-93-5465-613-2

Printed at: Samrat Offset Pvt. Ltd.

In Dedication and Fond Memories

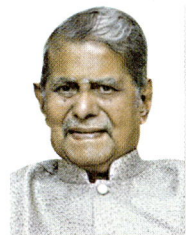

Prof Alagirisamy Parthasarathy
MD DCH FIAP
DSc (Honoris Causa): The Tamil Nadu Dr MGR Medical University
Chennai, India
National President 1997, Indian Academy of Pediatrics
Emeritus Professor of Pediatrics
The Tamil Nadu Dr MGR Medical University
Chennai, Tamil Nadu, India
(August 08, 1938–May 15, 2021)

Prof Alagirisamy Parthasarathy, National President 1997, Indian Academy of Pediatrics (IAP), was a multi-faceted person. Fondly called "Partha sir" by both his contemporaries and juniors and just "Dear Partha" by his seniors, he had an endearing quality that made him lovable to all. Like the "PARTHASARATHY" to Arjun, he motivated and helped many academicians to come up and shine in their chosen fields.

Prof Parthasarathy graduated from the prestigious Madras Medical College, Chennai, Tamil Nadu, in the year 1964. He completed his postgraduate diploma (DCH) course in the year 1973 and degree (MD Pediatrics) in 1976 from Madras Medical College and Institute of Child Health, Chennai. He was also trained in Clinical Epidemiology at Christian Medical College, Vellore, Tamil Nadu, India.

He started taking keen interest in the activities of IAP and soon occupied various important positions to serve the organization. He was awarded the fellowship of IAP (FIAP) in 1989 for carrying out many flagship programs. He gained all-India recognition in IAP by his visionary ideas and successful implementation of many projects. He was elected as National President, IAP in the year 1997. He took up many path-breaking programs during his tenure and beyond in the field of vaccines and immunization. He served as the Regional Adviser, Association of Pediatric Societies of South-East Asia Region for three years (1997–1999).

Prof Parthasarathy worked in Tamil Nadu Health services in various positions. He retired as Senior Clinical Professor of Pediatrics, Madras Medical College, Chennai, and Deputy Superintendent, Institute of Child Health and Hospital for Children, Chennai, Tamil Nadu, India. His seminal contribution was in the field of immunization services, and he was a pioneer in many successful programs in collaboration with the state health services and international organizations including UNICEF. He brought out many manuals for the healthcare workers involved in immunization activities.

Right from 90's, Prof Parthasarathy found his passion of bringing out textbooks. He was the Founder Editor-in-Chief of Indian Journal of Practical Pediatrics (IJPP), which was launched under the banner of IAP in 1993. He held this post for two years and nurtured the journal from gestation to its toddlerhood. During his presidentship, he conceptualized and brought out the IAP Textbook of Pediatrics which proved a boon to pediatric students and practitioners. The next three decades saw a flurry of publications from IAP under his editorship in the form of IAP Guidebook on Immunizations, IAP Immunization Card, IAP Color Atlas of Pediatrics (2011), Atlas of Pediatric Infectious Diseases (2012), Textbook of Pediatric Infectious Diseases (2012), IAP Textbook of Vaccines (2014), IAP Algorithms for Common Pediatric Illnesses (2015) and many more.

Besides IAP, in the past 20 years, under the banner of Partha's Series of Books for Pediatric and Adolescent Practitioners, he brought out eight books—Case Scenarios, Frequently Asked Questions, Management Protocols, 101 Clinical Pearls, Management Algorithms, Investigations and Interpretations, Comprehensive Manual, and Current Trends in Diagnosis and Management.

He was the Founder Editor-in-Chief of Partha's Immunization Digest (First Edition 2005 to Fourth Edition 2020), Handbook on Adolescent and Adult Immunization (2014), Fundamentals of Pediatrics, Selected Topics in Pediatrics for Practitioners, and Associate Editor of Atlas of Tropical Pediatrics (American Academy of Pediatrics, 2009). Colleagues had to be up on toes to keep up with his speed of work and meticulousness for details.

Prof Parthasarathy was bestowed with numerous awards and orations in his lifetime. Indian Academy of Pediatrics proudly conferred him with Lifetime Achievement Award of IAP in 2021.

Prof Parthasarathy had the unique gift of drafting in an elegant, but simple language and was prompt in communication. He showed great affection towards his colleagues, junior and senior alike. He always appreciated and encouraged the initiative by any colleague towards child health activities. He had a great command of Tamil as well and had written many beautiful Tamil poems. He wrote his autobiography in Tamil titled "Kanne Pappa" ("Dear Child") and this was released during the Chennai Book Exhibition, 2020.

Prof Parthasarathy was fortunate to have a very loving family. His wife, Mrs Nirmala Parthasarathy, is a gentle and kindhearted lady. Partha sir's children Mr Balaji and Dr (Mrs) Prathiba doted on their father. He was blessed with four grandchildren.

It was his brainchild to bring out a biennial treatise on "Recent Advances in Pediatrics" under IAP. We deem it a great honor to dedicate this second volume titled "IAP Recent Advances in Pediatrics, Volume 2" to this great soul. Thousands of us pediatricians, will always remember him day in and day out. Prof Parthasarathy was a very pious person, and we are sure he is blessing all of us to continue his good work in the service of children.

Contributors

Abhishek Somasekhara Aradhya
MD DM
Consultant Neonatologist
Department of Pediatrics
Ovum Woman and Child Specialty Hospital
Bengaluru, Karnataka, India

Ajeitha Loganathan MD
Fellow in Pediatric Hemato-oncology
Consultant, Pediatric Hemato-oncology
G Kuppuswamy Naidu Memorial Hospital
Coimbatore, Tamil Nadu, India

Alec Reginald Errol Correa MD DM
Assistant Professor
Institute of Liver and Biliary Sciences
New Delhi, India

Alok Gupta MD FIAP
Pediatrician, Counselor and
Environmentalist
Pediatric Specialties Clinic, Jaipur
Former Assistant Professor in
Pediatric Medicine
Mahatma Gandhi Medical
College and Hospital
Jaipur, Rajasthan, India

Arvind Bagga MD
Professor of Pediatrics
Division of Pediatric Nephrology
All India Institute of Medical Sciences
New Delhi, India

Ashish Kumar Simalti MD FNB
Department of Pediatrics
Military Hospital
Dehradun, Uttarakhand, India

Bala Ramachandran
AB (Ped) AB (Ped Crit Care) FCCM
Head, Department of Intensive Care and
Emergency Medicine
Kanchi Kamakoti CHILDS
Trust Hospital
Chennai, Tamil Nadu, India

Balu Vaidyanathan MD DM
Clinical Professor
Department of Pediatric Cardiology
Head, Fetal Cardiology Division
Amrita Institute of Medical Sciences and
Research Institute
Kochi, Kerala, India

Deepak Bansal MD DNB FAMS FIAP
Professor
Pediatric Hematology and Oncology Unit
Advanced Pediatrics Centre
Postgraduate Institute of
Medical Education and Research
Chandigarh, India

Dheeraj Shah MD DNB MNAMS
Director Professor
Department of Pediatrics
University College of Medical Sciences
New Delhi, India

Dhiren Gupta MD
Deputy Director
Pediatric Intensive Care,
Pulmonology and Allergy
Institute of Child Health
Sir Ganga Ram Hospital
New Delhi, India

Gouri Rao Passi MD DNB
Consultant and Head
Department of Pediatrics
Choithram Hospital and Research Centre
Indore, Madhya Pradesh, India

Jagatshreya Satapathy MD
Senior Resident
Department of Pediatrics
All India Institute of Medical Sciences
New Delhi, India

John Matthai MD FAB FIAP FRCPCH
Professor
Consultant Pediatric Gastroenterologist
Masonic Medical Centre for Children
Coimbatore, Tamil Nadu, India

Contributors

Julius Xavier Scott MD DCH DNB FPHO
Professor and Head
Pediatric Hemato-oncology
Sri Ramachandra Medical College and
Research Institute
Chennai, Tamil Nadu, India

K Ravikumar MD FNB
Associate Consultant
Pediatric Intensive Care Unit
Kanchi Kamakoti CHILDS Trust Hospital
Chennai, Tamil Nadu, India

Madhulika Kabra MD
Professor
Division of Genetics
Department of Pediatrics
All India Institute of Medical Sciences
New Delhi, India

Mahesh Babu Ramamurthy
MD FRCPCH
Senior Consultant and Head
Division of Pediatric
Pulmonology and Sleep
Assistant Professor
Department of Pediatrics, KTPNUCMI
National University Hospital, Singapore

Mani Ram Krishna DNB FNB
Fellow in Pediatric Cardiology
Clinical Assistant Professor
Department of Pediatric Cardiology
Amrita Institute of Medical Sciences and
Research Institute
Kochi, Kerala, India

Nandita Chattopadhyay
DCH DNB PGDDN FNNF FIAP
Professor and Head of Pediatrics
MGM Medical College
Kishanganj, Bihar, India
Director, UDBHAAS Child
Development Centre
Kolkata, West Bengal, India

Narendra Bagri MD
Associate Professor
Division of Pediatric Rheumatology
Department of Pediatrics
All India Institute of Medical Sciences
New Delhi, India

Naveen Sankhyan DM
Professor and In-charge
Pediatric Neurology Unit
Advanced Pediatrics Centre
Postgraduate Institute of
Medical Education and Research
Chandigarh, India

Nidhi Bedi MD
Associate Professor
Department of Pediatrics
SGT Medical College, Hospital and
Research Institute
Gurugram, Haryana, India

Nitin Dhochak DM
Senior Research Associate
Department of Pediatrics
All India Institute of Medical Sciences
New Delhi, India

Piyush Gupta MD FAMS FIAP
Professor and Head
Department of Pediatrics
University College of Medical Sciences
New Delhi, India

Praveen Mathur MS MCh FMAS
Commonwealth Fellow in Pediatric
Laparoscopy
Senior Professor and Head
Department of Pediatric Surgery
Additional Principal,
SMS Medical College and Attached
Hospitals
Jaipur, Rajasthan, India

Priyanka Khandelwal MD DM
Senior Research Associate
Division of Pediatric Nephrology
Department of Pediatrics
All India Institute of Medical Sciences
New Delhi, India

Priyanka Mittal MS MCh
Assistant Professor
Department of Pediatric Surgery
SMS Medical College and
Attached Hospitals
Jaipur, Rajasthan, India

Rajendra Nath Srivastava
FRCP FIAP FAMS
Consultant Pediatric Nephrologist
Indraprastha Apollo Hospitals
New Delhi, India

Rashmi Sarkar MD MNAMS
Professor of Dermatology
Lady Hardinge Medical
College and Hospital
New Delhi, India

Rashna Dass Hazarika
MD Fellow PID MECS Dip Management
Senior Consultant in Pediatrics and
Neonatology
Nemcare Superspeciality Hospital
RIGPA Children's Clinic
Guwahati, Assam, India

Renu Suthar MD DM
Associate Professor
Pediatric Neurology Unit
Advanced Pediatrics Centre
Postgraduate Institute of
Medical Education and Research
Chandigarh, India

Richa Jain MD DM
Associate Professor
Pediatric Hematology and
Oncology Unit
Advanced Pediatrics Centre
Postgraduate Institute of
Medical Education and Research
Chandigarh, India

Sapna Nayak MD
Senior Resident
Department of Endocrinology
Sanjay Gandhi Postgraduate Institute of
Medical Sciences
Lucknow, Uttar Pradesh, India

Shiv Sajan Saini MD DM
Associate Professor
Advanced Pediatrics Centre
Postgraduate Institute of
Medical Education and Research
Chandigarh, India

Siddharth Mahesh
MBChB BMed Sci
Pediatric ST1 Trainee
West Midlands Deanery
United Kingdom

Soonu Udani
MD FICCCM
Medical Director and Head
Critical Care and Emergency Services
SRCC Children's Hospital
Narayana Health
Mumbai, Maharashtra, India

Srinivas G Kasi MD DCH
Consultant Pediatrician
Kasi Clinic
Bengaluru, Karnataka, India

Suhani Shah MD
Fellow
Department of Pediatric Neurology
SRCC Children's Hospital
Narayana Health
Mumbai, Maharashtra, India

Sumaira Khalil
DNB MNAMS
Assistant Professor
Department of Pediatrics
University College of Medical Sciences
New Delhi, India

Sushil Kumar Kabra MD
Professor
Department of Pediatrics
All India Institute of Medical Sciences
New Delhi, India

Contributors

Udhay Preet Sidhu MD DVL
United Medical Center and
Skinglo Clinic
Bengaluru, Karnataka, India

Vidya Krishna MD MRCPCH
Fellow, Infectious Diseases and
Infection Control
Specialist Registrar
Department of BMT, Immunology and
Infectious Diseases
Great Ormond Street Hospital
London, UK

Vijayalakshmi Bhatia MD
Professor
Department of Endocrinology
Sanjay Gandhi Postgraduate Institute of
Medical Sciences
Lucknow, Uttar Pradesh, India

Yogesh Waikar MD DNB MNAMS
Fellow in Pediatric
Gastroenterology and Liver Transplant
Pediatric Gastroenterologist,
Hepatologist and Endoscopist
Superspeciality GI Kids Clinics and
Imaging Centre
Nagpur, Maharashtra, India

Reviewers

Amar Jeet Chitkara MD DNB
Director and Head
Department of Pediatrics
Max Super Specialty Hospital
New Delhi, India

Amita Mahajan MD MRCPCH CCST
Senior Consultant
Pediatric Hematology and Oncology
Indraprastha Apollo Hospital
New Delhi, India

Aspi Irani MD DCH
Consultant Pediatrician
Nanavati Max Super Specialty Hospital
Mumbai, Maharashtra, India

Baldev S Prajapati
MD DPed FIAP MNAMS
Professor and Head
Department of Pediatrics
GCS Medical College
Hospital and Research Centre
Ahmedabad, Gujarat, India

Bharat Agarwal MD DCH DNB MNAMS
Prof Emeritus and Former Head
Department of Pediatric Hematology
and Oncology
BJ Wadia Hospital for Children
Mumbai, Maharashtra, India

C Leema Pauline MD DM
Professor of Neurology
Institute of Child Health and
Hospital for Children
Madras Medical College
Chennai, Tamil Nadu, India

Ebor Jacob James DCH DNB FIAP FICCM
Professor
Pediatric Critical Care
Christian Medical College
Vellore, Tamil Nadu, India

Elizabeth KE PhD MD DCH FIAP FRCPCH
Professor and HOD Pediatrics
Sree Mookambika Institute of
Medical Sciences
Kulasekharam, Tamil Nadu, India

Jaydeep Choudhary DNB MNAMS FIAP
Professor
Department of Pediatrics
Institute of Child Health
Kolkata, West Bengal, India

Jeeson Unni MD DCH FIAP
Senior Consultant
Department of Child and
Adolescent Health
Aster Medcity
Kochi, Kerala, India

Ketan Parikh MS MCh
Consultant Pediatric Surgeon and
Laparoscopist
Jaslok Hospital, Seven Hills Hospital and
LH Hiranandani Memorial Hospital
Mumbai, Maharashtra, India

Meenu Singh MD FCCP FIAP
Professor of Pediatrics
In-charge, Pediatric Pulmonology,
Asthma and Allergy Clinics
Advanced Pediatrics Centre
Postgraduate Institute of
Medical Education and Research
Chandigarh, India

MKC Nair DSc PhD MD M.Med.Sc MBA MA
(Phil) MA (MC&J) FNNF FIAP FIACAM FAMS
Formerly Vice Chancellor and
Professor Emeritus-Research, KUHS
Founder Director, CDC and Emeritus
Professor in Child Adolescent and
Behavioural Pediatrics, CDC
Director, NIMS-SPECTRUM-Child
Development Research Centre
NIMS Medicity
Neyyattinkara
Thiruvananthapuram, Kerala, India

Reviewers

Preeti Galagali MD PGDAP FIAP
Director and Consultant
Adolescent Health Specialist
Bangalore Adolescent Care and
Counseling Centre
Bengaluru, Karnataka, India

Ram Gulati MD MRCPCH
Consultant Dermatologist
Dr Gulati's Clinic
Jaipur, Rajasthan, India

Sadagopan Srinivasan MD DCH
Adjunct Professor
Department of Pediatrics
Dr Mehta Multispeciality Hospital
Chennai, Tamil Nadu, India

Sathish Kumar MD DCH
Consultant Pediatric Rheumatologist
Professor of Pediatrics
Christian Medical College
Vellore, Tamil Nadu, India

Sheffali Gulati MD FIAP FIMSA MNAMS
Professor and Chief
Child Neurology Division
Department of Pediatrics
All India Institute of Medical Sciences
New Delhi, India

Shubha R Phadke MD DM
Professor and Head
Department of Medical Genetics
Sanjay Gandhi Postgraduate
Institute of Medical Sciences
Lucknow, Uttar Pradesh, India

Suhas V Prabhu MD DCH MNAMS
Consultant Pediatrician
PD Hinduja Hospital
Mumbai, Maharashtra, India

Susan Uthup MD DNB DM DNB FISN
Professor and Head
Department of Pediatric Nephrology
SAT Hospital, Government Medical College
Thiruvananthapuram, Kerala, India

Sutapa Ganguly MD
Professor
Department of Pediatrics
KPC Medical College
Kolkata, West Bengal, India

Vinod H Ratageri MD DCEH
Professor
Department of Pediatrics
Karnataka Institute Medical Sciences
Hubli, Karnataka, India

Foreword

I am delighted to write the foreword for "*IAP Recent Advances in Pediatrics, Volume 2 (IAPRAP2)*", which is modeled on the lines of IAPRAP1 and is considered to be its first sibling. This is an outstanding project and a worthy tribute to the memory of the doyen of Pediatrics, the Late Dr A Parthasarathy, who had initially conceived it and inspired the present team to strive hard to make it a reality. I congratulate all colleagues involved in designing and compiling this volume, which is certainly the product of a Herculean effort.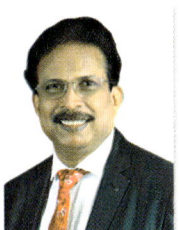

One of the chief impediments that we experience as doctors is the scattered nature of our knowledge resources. Ready reference materials regarding the latest academic advances as well as clinical updates are to be found in a sea of publications. A busy clinician will certainly be hard pressed to keep track of the different subjects, authors or publishers or to wade through the tomes in the bookshelves to find something that is urgently needed. Hence this project addresses the urgent need for a comprehensive source of authentic updated information on the multitude of subjects that govern clinical practice.

The books in this series are designed to serve like a "pediatric digest" spanning almost 510 pages and covering the most recent reviews in all major subspecialties. Furthermore the inputs provided by both academicians and clinicians are curated and peer-reviewed by reputed subject experts in the respective fields. Updated editions will be published every two years, giving this project a much needed encyclopedic feel, or a "go-to book", quite reminiscent of the erstwhile Encyclopedia Britannica. I am sure the entire pediatric community of India will be grateful to the project leaders and the contributors for making their life easier along with the great difference it can make to patient care.

I am proud that this book is being released on the occasion of Pedicon 2022 at Noida and will perhaps be the first major publication to reach the hands of the readers during my Presidential term. I am proud to welcome this new baby into our fold, fathered by no less a visionary than the Late Dr A Parthasarathy and nurtured with befitting care and affection by the Editor-in-Chief, Dr PSN Menon, the Chief Academic Editors, Dr Piyush Gupta and Dr P Ramachandran and the Executive Editor, Dr Alok Gupta. The list of those who have contributed their efforts to this volume reads like a "Who's Who" of the world of Indian pediatrics. Their painstaking involvement in this project makes it all the more appreciable. I am elated to present this book to the readers and wish you a highly satisfactory outcome in treating this as your treasured reference resource at all times.

Remesh Kumar R
National President 2022
Indian Academy of Pediatrics

Foreword

Dear friends,

Greetings from Indian Academy of Pediatrics!

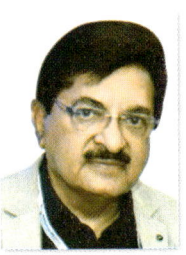

Another year has gone by and the Covid situation still looms large on our head. It was the first time that the world unitedly fought against this invisible threat. Covid has brought about a new way to think and process information. A need was felt to educate our members about the various subspecialty topics in Pediatrics. This was simply due to issues faced by several common pediatricians to diagnose diseases related to the subspecialties, in time. Not catching the disease at an early stage can lead to complications many a time. Keeping these thoughts in mind, IAPRAP was conceived. Basically, IAPRAP was a book that was launched with the latest data from the pediatric subspecialties under the IAP's umbrella. This task was conceptualized by our mentor and guru – late Dr A Parthasarathy – and was very well received. After all, to have all the data compiled in such a concise and lucid, easy-to-understand manner was nothing short of a miracle. Hats off to the team who could manage this with such ease and aplomb!

This book was supposed to be released every 2 years. Unfortunately, due to the pandemic situation, I thought that the second issue might be delayed. After all, such coordination and data gathering are not for the ones with faint heart. But, lo and behold, I was pleasantly surprised when I got a mail requesting for my message in this ambitious project. Seeing the contents of the book, I was astounded to realize that the team has not left any corners unturned in their endeavor for excellency in getting this book published. It is much more polished and better in every sense. I am truly proud of the team who has conquered this challenging task and seen it to completion without compromising on quality of the knowledge delivered. Not only is it probably one of the best books for a common pediatrician who wants to gain some of the knowledge in the subspecialty, but also for students who might be confused about which subspecialty field to take up post the completion of their graduation.

I would like to take this opportunity to thank the team who have truly burnt the midnight oil to bring about this gem of a masterpiece in your hands. Not only was it challenging to bring about the content of this book together, but also to have it peer-reviewed within the time frame given to them. Not to forget the pandemic situation prevailing throughout the world and I am certain that you will better understand and appreciate the efforts taken by them to complete this herculean task.

Given the myriad of topics discussed, I am certain that this book will find its place in all the pediatricians' bookshelves. A hearty congratulation to one and all on achieving this milestone.

Bakul Jayant Parekh
National President 2020
Indian Academy of Pediatrics
President, IPA Congress 2023
Secretary General, SAPA
Global Academic Convenor, GAPIO

Foreword

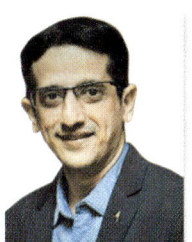

I'm delighted to be writing a foreword for this wonderful book on *"IAP Recent Advances in Pediatrics, Volume 2 (IAPRAP2)"*.

For every pediatrician – be it someone working in a PHC of a low-resource, rural part of the country, or one who serves at a tertiary hospital in a metro city – staying updated on various advances in the field is undeniably crucial. This book is perfectly curated to cater to pediatricians across the board. The topics are chosen with care, to be relevant to as wide an audience as possible. We must accept the fact that topics such as noise-induced hearing loss, rising rates of junk food consumption and hyperconsumption of audio-visual media have become extremely relevant in contemporary times, but are rarely discussed in any standard textbooks of pediatrics. Additionally, social phenomena of child neglect/abuse and child labor gravely affect the mental and physical development of children, and pediatricians should be amongst the first to recognize such instances. Most medical professionals have less than adequate exposure to such topics, and I am glad this book attempts to address this gap in our knowledge.

We are in the midst of an unprecedented COVID-19 pandemic. It was natural for this book to include two chapters related to SARS-CoV-2 infection and the vaccines. The advances in the field of medical genetics, role of biologicals and tumor markers and NAFLD are providing an insight into what lies in the future of medicine. An evidence-based review of these not commonly discussed topics is a great value addition to this book.

I would strongly recommend this book to any postgraduate/pediatrician who wants to keep themselves up to date. Similar to IAPRAP1, it should be an essential addition to every departmental and hospital library.

Upendra Kinjawadekar
National President Elect 2022
Indian Academy of Pediatrics

Preface

The book "IAP Recent Advances in Pediatrics, Volume 2 (IAPRAP2)", the biennial treatise, once again brings to the readers, the recent scientific advances in the field of pediatrics across different spheres.

The idea conceptualized by Late Professor A Parthasarathy, a doyen of Pediatrics, was solemnized in 2020 with the release of the first volume. The IAP National President 2021, Prof Piyush Gupta, and the Central IAP Team 2021, approved to publish the second volume in 2022.

The second volume is being brought out as per the vision of team IAP to constantly update all the readers. Advances in the various fields of pediatrics starting from neonatology and extending to development, nutrition, immunization, infectious diseases, adolescence, critical care, and different organ systems are presented with scientific evidence from recent publications. Newer insights in the fields of environment (noise pollution), child rights, genetics, and SARS-CoV-2 vaccines are some additional highlights of this volume. The second volume includes 27 chapters with at least one topic covered under each subspecialty. The chapters have been carefully prepared by eminent pediatricians across the country as well as from abroad and peer-reviewed by equally illustrious colleagues.

This compendium is aimed to update the knowledge of pediatricians across a wide spectrum, from pediatric residents to senior faculty, researchers, and consultants.

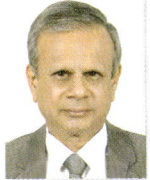 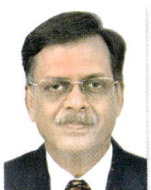 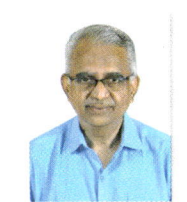 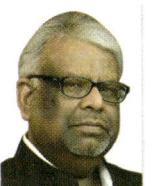

PSN Menon   **Alok Gupta**   **P Ramachandran**   **Piyush Gupta**

Acknowledgments

The second volume of the book, "*IAP Recent Advances in Pediatrics, Volume 2 (IAPRAP2)*" is now in your hands, after being released during PEDICON-2022, Noida, Uttar Pradesh, India.

We very sincerely thank all the authors and the reviewers for their contributions to IAPRAP2, without which this book would not have seen the light of the day.

The book is being published by M/s Jaypee Brothers Medical Publishers, New Delhi, India. We thank Shri Jitendar P Vij (Group Chairman), Mr Ankit Vij (Managing Director), Mr MS Mani (Group President), Ms Chetna Malhotra Vohra (Associate Director–Content Strategy), Ms Pooja Bhandari (Production Head), Dr Rajul Jain (Senior Development Editor) and team of M/s Jaypee Brothers Medical Publishers, for burning the midnight oil in bringing out this tome in a very timely manner.

We are grateful to Indian Pediatrics as well as Central IAP for granting permissions to reproduce material for the Chapter 26 on "Child Abuse, Neglect and Exploitation" by Dr Rajendra Nath Srivastava, Chapter 21 on "Junk and Ultra-processed Foods" by Dr Sumaira Khalil and Dr Dheeraj Shah besides IAP consensus reports used in Chapter 11 "Cow's Milk Protein Allerby" by Dr John Matthai and Chapter 21 "Media Use" by Dr Nidhi Bedi and Piyush Gupta.

We are thankful to the office bearers and the executive board members of Central IAP for the continuous support and encouragement at all stages in bringing out this volume.

The editorial services of Shri Shaji Jacob Ninan to the Editor-in-Chief is gratefully acknowledged.

We request all the readers to please give your feedback to enable us to plan future editions.

Contents

NEONATOLOGY

1. **Neonatal Shock** 1
   Shiv Sajan Saini, Abhishek Somasekhara Aradhya

NUTRITION

2. **Junk and Ultra-processed Foods** 19
   Sumaira Khalil, Dheeraj Shah

INFECTIOUS DISEASES

3. **SARS-CoV-2 Infection** 40
   Dhiren Gupta, Ashish Kumar Simalti

4. **Systemic Antifungal Therapy** 56
   Vidya Krishna

5. **Meningococcal Disease** 79
   Rashna Dass Hazarika

IMMUNIZATIONS

6. **SARS-CoV-2 Vaccines** 101
   Srinivas G Kasi

NEUROLOGY

7. **Autoimmune Encephalitis** 138
   Naveen Sankhyan, Renu Suthar

8. **Infantile Spasms** 161
   Gouri Rao Passi

CARDIOLOGY

9. **Cardiac Arrhythmias** 169
   Mani Ram Krishna, Balu Vaidyanathan

PULMONOLOGY

10. **Cystic Fibrosis: An Emerging Illness in India** 190
    Nitin Dhochak, Sushil Kumar Kabra

GASTROENTEROLOGY

11. Cow's Milk Protein Allergy 215
    John Matthai

HEPATOLOGY

12. Nonalcoholic Fatty Liver Disease 230
    Yogesh Waikar

NEPHROLOGY

13. Renal Tubular Disorders 243
    Priyanka Khandelwal, Arvind Bagga

ENDOCRINOLOGY

14. Ambulatory Management of Type 1 Diabetes Mellitus 264
    Sapna Nayak, Vijayalakshmi Bhatia

PEDIATRIC HEMATOLOGY

15. Autoimmune Hemolytic Anemia 289
    Richa Jain, Deepak Bansal

ONCOLOGY

16. Tumor Markers 307
    Julius Xavier Scott, Ajeitha Loganathan

RHEUMATOLOGY

17. Biologicals and Other Targeted Therapies in Rheumatology 324
    Jagatshreya Satapathy, Narendra Bagri

GENETICS

18. Recent Advances in the Diagnosis and Treatment of
    Genetic Disorders 343
    Alec Reginald Errol Correa, Madhulika Kabra

OTORHINOLARYNGOLOGY

19. Obstrutive Sleep Apnea 361
    Siddharth Mahesh, Mahesh Babu Ramamurthy

DEVELOPMENTAL PEDIATRICS

20. Nurturing Care for Early Childhood Development 376
    Nandita Chattopadhyay

ADOLESCENT PEDIATRICS

21. Media Use 396
    Nidhi Bedi, Piyush Gupta

ENVIRONMENTAL MEDICINE

22. Noise-induced Hearing Loss 411
    Alok Gupta

CRITICAL CARE

23. Management of Burns 428
    K Ravikumar, Bala Ramachandran
24. Refractory Status Epilepticus 442
    Soonu Udani, Suhani Shah

PEDIATRIC SURGERY

25. Intussusception 460
    Praveen Mathur, Priyanka Mittal

CHILD RIGHTS, ABUSE AND EXPLOITATION

26. Child Neglect, Abuse and Exploitation 477
    Rajendra Nath Srivastava

DERMATOLOGY

27. Skin Care of the Newborn 499
    Rashmi Sarkar, Udhay Preet Sidhu

Index *511*

Neonatology

Neonatal Shock

Shiv Sajan Saini, Abhishek Somasekhara Aradhya

■ INTRODUCTION

Shock is a clinical syndrome of acute circulatory dysfunction, resulting in insufficient delivery of oxygen, and vital nutrients to the body tissues relative to their metabolic demand. The resultant ischemic conditions lead to anaerobic metabolism, increased production of lactic, and inorganic acids. Progressively worsening cellular hypoxemic and acidotic conditions lead to deterioration in the functioning of various organ system(s) including cardiorespiratory, neurological, metabolic, hematological, renal, and endocrine functions. Continued worsening culminates in multiorgan failure and eventually death. The case fatality rates in neonatal shock are very high. Therefore, early recognition and appropriate intervention are the key for improved survival and better neurodevelopmental outcomes.[1,2]

■ INCIDENCE

There is extremely limited data published on the incidence and spectrum of neonatal shock. The incidence of shock in neonatal intensive care units (NICUs) is variable and depends on the population characteristics and study setting. The incidence of hypotension is inversely proportional to the gestational age. Almost 50% of very low birth weight (VLBW) neonates experience at least one episode of hypotension in NICU. The incidence of shock varies between 3 and 10% of NICU admissions. The incidence increases to 10–28% in extremely preterm neonates and is around 4% in those born at <36 weeks gestation.[3] A study published from the British Columbia Children's Hospital (Vancouver, Canada) found 15% incidence (249 episodes in 1,641 admissions) of neonatal shock among full-term neonates.[4] A recent study from a tertiary care referral hospital from north India reported 12.0% incidence (95% confidence interval: 10.9–13.2%) of shock among 3,271 admissions over 2-year time period.[5] While the cardiogenic shock is likely to be more common the developed countries among term neonates, septic shock is the most common form of shock in term and preterm neonates on developing countries setting.[4,5]

■ PATHOPHYSIOLOGY

Inadequate tissue perfusion in a state of shock leads to reduced oxygen and nutrients delivery, increased oxygen consumption, and inadequate oxygen utilization.[6] In the initial stages of shock, there is redistribution of blood in various organ systems of the body. The circulation to vital organs, i.e., brain, heart, and adrenals is maintained at the cost of nonvital organs such as skin, muscles, gut, lungs, etc.[2] This phenomenon is known as "diving reflex". In the early stages of shock, the compromised tissue perfusion clinically manifests as a change in the color of the skin (pale or off-colored skin), decreased skin temperature (cold peripheries), reduced pulse volume (thready pulses), delayed capillary refill time (CRT), and decreased urine output. The blood pressure (BP) is usually maintained at this stage. This physiological state is commonly referred to as peripheral circulatory failure or compensated shock. Later with the involvement of vital organs, myocardial performance decreases, and adrenal dysfunction sets in. The BP drops (hypotension) at this stage, which is referred to as decompensated shock. Although the terms "shock" and "hypotension" are loosely used interchangeably, it is important to realize that hypotension is a late manifestation of shock.[7] As the neonate transitions from compensated to decompensated shock, the outcome worsens, and risk of mortality increases.

Shock happens due to derangement in one or more of three important contributors of circulation, i.e., preload, myocardial conductivity, and afterload. Decreased preload leads to improper filling of heart, thereby reducing the myocardial output. Preload is decreased in hypovolemic shock and tension pneumothorax. Contrastingly preload can be increased in some etiologies of shock involving poor myocardial contractility such as asphyxia and transitional circulation. Generally myocardial contractility is decreased in shock such as asphyxia, arrhythmias, and transitional circulation. However, myocardial contractility is increased in hyperdynamic circulation such as hemodynamically significant patent ductus arteriosus (hs-PDA) and in early stages of septic shock. In late stages of shock, myocardial contractility is universally decreased. Changes in afterload depends upon the state of shock. Afterload is increased to variable extent in early stages (except distributive shock namely septic and anaphylactic) owing to increased sympathetic activity as body's compensatory response. However, afterload is decreased with the onset of the decompensated shock. **Table 1.1** presents the summary of pathophysiology of different etiologies of shock in neonates.

■ ETIOLOGY

Various etiologies can cause shock in neonates.[8-10] These include (but are not limited to) perinatal asphyxia, circulatory maladaptation during transition from fetal to neonatal life (especially in extreme preterm neonates),

TABLE 1.1: Pathophysiology of neonatal shock in different etiologies.

Clinical scenario	Preload	Myocardial contractility	Afterload	Main mechanism
Hypovolemia, e.g., fetomaternal bleed, intracranial bleed, etc.	Decreased as intravascular volume is reduced	Not affected	Not affected and may slightly increase initially	Predominantly decreased preload
Septic shock	Relative hypovolemia due to venodilation	Initially hyperdynamic but later depressed myocardial functions	Decreased vasomotor tone	Mainly vasomotor dysregulation but all sectors affected
Asphyxia	Increases	Depressed due to myocardial injury	Increases initially, at later stages decreases	Predominantly myocardial dysfunction
Intracardiac shunts e.g., PDA	Increases	Increased myocardial work due to hyperdynamic circulation, not able to meet demands of body	Decreased due to systemic to pulmonary shunts	Predominantly myocardial dysfunction and decreased afterload
Transitional circulation in ELBW neonates	Increases	Depressed (suddenly increased LV afterload after birth)	Increases in early stages; decreases later	Predominantly myocardial dysfunction
Adrenal insufficiency	Variable	Depressed	Decreased	Combination of decreased afterload and myocardial dysfunction
Raised intrathoracic pressure, e.g., pneumothorax and high pressures on ventilator, etc.	Decreased (poor venous return)	Not affected primarily, however, low output due to poor myocardial capacity to distend	Increases as intrathoracic pressure compresses vessels	Mainly-decreased preload and poor cardiac filling

(ELBW: extremely low birth weight; LV: left ventricle; PDA: patent ductus arteriosus) intracardiac shunts, sepsis, fluid loss, adrenal insufficiency, arrhythmias, and raised intrathoracic pressure. There is extremely limited data regarding the etiological spectrum of shock in neonates. Only one study from a tertiary care referral NICU of a developed country has defined the spectrum of etiologies of neonatal shock.[4] These authors found cardiogenic shock as a most typical cause of shock among term neonates. On the contrary, septic shock is the main type of shock in the developing countries especially in preterm neonates. A prospective observational study done in a tertiary care set up showed that three most common reasons of shock in neonates include septic shock, severe birth asphyxia, and hemodynamically significant PDA.[11]

■ CLINICAL FEATURES

Shock at the bedside is commonly assessed by macrohemodynamic parameters which include heart rate, pulse volume, temperature (core and peripheral), BP, CRT, color, and urine output. As hypotension is a late sign of shock, signs of the peripheral circulatory failure (i.e., compensated stage) should be recognized at an earlier stage to achieve better outcomes. The clinical manifestations of shock are detailed below.

Heart Rate Abnormalities

Tachycardia (heart rate > 160/min) is a nonspecific finding commonly seen in shock. Tachycardia indicates compensatory mechanisms of the neonate to increase cardiac output as neonatal heart has a limited ability to increase stroke volume.[11] Bradycardia is a preterminal finding. There are numerous other common causes of tachycardia in newborn especially dehydration, pain, PDA, drug effect (caffeine), sepsis, etc. Therefore, tachycardia is nonspecific and should be combined with other clinical features for the diagnosis of shock.

Hypotension

Hypotension refers to BP below fifth centile for the gestational and postnatal age. **Table 1.2** depicts BP thresholds at fifth centile as per gestational age (modified from McNamara et al.).[12] Traditionally, BP is used to measure adequacy of the systemic circulation. However, BP has following caveats for assessment of hemodynamic stability in neonates:
- It is well known that low BP is a late marker of shock.
- Blood pressure is a product of cardiac output and systemic vascular resistance (SVR). Decreased cardiac output may be masked if SVR is elevated. However, tissue perfusion decreases if cardiac output is decreased. Thus, despite BP being stable during shock, the tissue perfusion may be seriously compromised.

TABLE 1.2: Blood pressure (BP) thresholds at fifth centile as per gestational age.

	Fifth centile (mm Hg)		
Gestation (weeks)	Systolic	MAP	Diastolic
<30	42	30	20
31	45	30	20
32	46	30	21
33	47	30	22
34	48	31	23
35	49	32	24
36	50	32	25

(MAP: mean arterial pressure)

- Blood pressure obtained by noninvasive methods such as oscillometry and invasive methods have a wide range of confidence limits of agreement. In hypotensive neonates, BP obtained by noninvasive methods is higher than invasive methods. On the contrary, noninvasive BP is lower than invasive BP in hypertensive neonates. Thus, there is a poor agreement between noninvasive and invasive BPs under pathological conditions.[1,9,10,13] BP by noninvasive methods measure mean arterial pressure (MAP) and estimate systolic and diastolic BP by mathematical algorithms. Hence, MAP should be given more importance than systolic or diastolic BP, when measured by noninvasive methods.
- Furthermore, "normal" range of BP is not clear for various gestational ages and postnatal ages. The available charts give statistical cutoffs of data obtained from limited number of neonates at a particular gestation age and postnatal age. The statistical cut-off does not necessarily translate into abnormal circulation.
- Another challenge with BP is that it correlates poorly with systemic blood flow especially in extreme prematurity. Sometimes in borderline low BP situations, subjects can have adequate perfusion as they have adequate cardiac output. In these situations, signs of peripheral circulations are normal and metabolic status is maintained. Thus, BP needs to be interpreted cautiously in neonates by assessing the range of clinical signs of perfusion.[14]

Apart from hemodynamic assessment, BP measurement helps to identify ductal dependent systemic circulation, where BP in lower limbs may be lower than right upper limb.

Delayed Capillary Refill Time

Capillary refill time is assessed over bony surface like sternum or forehead. Delayed CRT beyond 4 seconds in presence of hypotension and/or tachycardia or other signs indicate shock. Contrasting "flash" refill (along with bounding pulses and low BP) is seen in conditions of decreased SVR and indicates shock (warm shock).

Other Signs of Hemodynamic Monitoring

Low pulse volume or thready pulses, core-peripheral temperature difference of >3°C (mainly for term neonates), and pale color indicate inadequate perfusion.

Signs of Other Organs Involvement due to Poor Perfusion

Neurologic Signs

Nonspecific signs such as lethargy, irritability, poor tone, and poor neonatal reflexes can be present. Decreased cerebral perfusion can also cause periodic breathing or apnea.

Respiratory Signs

Tachypnea is a common finding either due to lung involvement by sepsis or as a compensatory response to metabolic acidosis.

Renal Signs

There is a good correlation between reduced urine output and hypotension. However, there is a significant time lag between oliguria and hypotension.

Though there are many clinical signs of hemodynamic assessment, these signs have some limitations. While some of the signs of peripheral circulation are nonspecific, e.g., heart rate; some others are subjective, e.g., feeble pulses. Individually CRT and core-periphery temperature difference correlate poorly with organ perfusion.[13,15] BP measurements also have many caveats. It is clear from the above discussion that no single parameter in isolation can accurately detect shock especially in early stages. Therefore, combined information of all parameters [heart rate, CRT, color, urine output, temperature (core and peripheral temperature), and BP] should be utilized for assessment of circulation.[16]

Due to the subjective nature of many of the signs of hemodynamic assessment, a requirement of objective definition of shock was felt. An objective definition of *septic shock* was proposed by International Pediatric Sepsis Consensus Conference.[17] Septic shock is defined as presence of cardiovascular dysfunction in presence of sepsis. Cardiovascular dysfunction is defined, if neonate has either of following criteria despite administration of isotonic intravenous (IV) fluid ≥ 40 mL/kg in 1 hour:

- Decrease in BP (hypotension) < fifth percentile for age or systolic BP <2 SD (Standard deviation) below normal for age, OR
- Need for vasoactive drug to maintain BP in normal range (dopamine > 5 µg/kg/min or dobutamine, epinephrine, or norepinephrine at any dose), OR

- *Two of the following:* Unexplained metabolic acidosis: base deficit > 5.0 mEq/L; increased arterial lactate > 2 times upper limit of normal; oliguria: urine output <0.5 mL/kg/hr; prolonged capillary refill: >5 sec; and core to peripheral temperature gap > 3°C.

However, this definition is applicable only for term neonates. Wynn and Wong proposed a modified definition for preterm neonates.[10] The salient differences in definition for preterm neonates (from International Pediatric Sepsis Consensus Definition) are: fluid administration limit is >10 mL/kg in infants < 32 weeks, systolic BP < 2 SD, or MAP < 30 mm Hg with CRT > 4 seconds. Although this definition is given for the diagnosis of neonatal septic shock, it may be used for the diagnosis of other types of shock.

■ INVESTIGATIONS

Shock is a clinical diagnosis. Laboratory investigations aid in categorizing severity and etiology of shock. The laboratory evaluation includes metabolic, biochemical, hematological, and microbiological workup.

The correctable metabolic/biochemical derangements should be screened and managed upfront in all cases, which include blood glucose levels, serum electrolytes, and serum calcium. Hypoglycemia and electrolyte disturbances (especially hypocalcemia and hyperkalemia) should be treated aggressively.

Blood gas analysis is a useful means to get information about metabolic status as well as respiratory gas exchange. Modern blood gas machines are also capable of measuring serum electrolytes including ionized calcium levels, hematocrit, blood glucose as well as serum lactate levels. Elevated lactate (>4 mmol/L) and mixed venous saturation are not good markers of shock in neonates.[1,10] Apart from systemic hypoperfusion states, lactate is also produced in local ischemic conditions and even in neonatal sepsis without shock. Furthermore, its levels may increase in the presence of liver dysfunction as it causes decreased metabolism of lactate. After initiation of management of shock, lactate levels can transiently rise with improvement in circulatory status as the lactate from under-perfused tissue beds shifts to central circulation. Nevertheless, standalone lactate levels can be used along with other hemodynamic variables and blood gas values to define shock. Moreover, serial lactate values will be helpful in monitoring the response to therapy.

Hematological workup includes assessment of hematocrit, complete blood count (CBC), and platelet levels. In sepsis, leukocyte counts may be either elevated or low (predominantly leukopenia in neonates). In addition, absolute neutrophil count can be low and immature to total neutrophil ratio (ITR) can be elevated (>0.2).

Microbiological investigations must be performed whenever septic shock is considered. Blood culture should be obtained before giving the first dose of antibiotics. Culture of cerebrospinal fluid (CSF) should be sent in all cases of sepsis once the neonate is stabilized. Site-specific infective focus (aspirates, swabs, etc.) should be cultured, wherever indicated. If viral infections (especially *Herpes simplex* virus or enteroviruses) are suspected, appropriate serological, or polymerase chain reaction (PCR) tests should be performed to identify causative organisms.[18]

Functional Echocardiography

Functional echocardiography has gained importance for hemodynamic assessment in the last few years.[19]

For *preload assessment*, inferior vena cava (IVC) collapsibility is proposed. There is currently not enough literature in neonates to support its use in preload assessment. Nevertheless, presence of collapsing IVC during inspiration, and narrower left ventricular cavity (opposite papillary muscles encountering each other during systole, *i.e., kissing sign*) suggests depleted intravascular volume status. These echocardiographic markers should be used along with body weight, urine output, serum sodium, and osmolality to assess preload status.

Assessment of cardiac systolic functions is done with the help of ejection fraction, fractional shortening, rate-corrected velocity of myocardial fiber shortening, etc.

Assessment of diastolic functions is done with the help of early to atrial peak systolic velocity ratio, isovolumetric relaxation time, etc.

There is no parameter to directly measure SVR. SVR is indirectly estimated by the following formula:

$$\text{Cardiac output (CO): BP} = \text{CO} \times \text{SVR}$$

Functional echocardiography can be a useful supplement to the clinical examination especially in preterm neonates. Additionally, functional echocardiography can help to exclude common mimickers of sepsis like hemodynamically significant PDA, duct dependent systemic circulation such as hypoplastic left heart, coarctation of aorta, etc. Details of functional echocardiography are beyond the scope of the current text which is available in published reviews on this topic.[19]

Measurement of Tissue Hypoxia

Central venous pressure, mixed venous oxygen saturation (SvO_2), and arteriovenous difference have been used to assess tissue hypoxia. Although useful, their widespread use is limited due to the invasive nature of the measurement and technical challenges in neonates. There is limited experience for assessing microcirculatory parameters (e.g., near infrared spectroscopy [NIRS], plethysmographic signal of pulse oximeter-perfusion index, and visible light technology) in the management of neonatal shock.[20]

The hemodynamic parameters get affected variably in the different form of neonatal shock. **Table 1.3** shows the alteration in hemodynamic parameters among four main categories of neonatal shock.

TABLE 1.3: Hemodynamic parameters in main categories of neonatal shock.

Shock type		Preload		Myocardial		Afterload	
		Central venous pressure	Left atrial pressure	Contractility	Cardiac output	Systemic vascular resistance	Blood pressure (BP)
Hypovolemic		↓↓↓	↓↓↓	↔ or ↑	↓	↑	↔ or ↓
Cardiogenic	Systolic	↑↑	↑↑	↓↓↓	↓↓	↑↑	↔ or ↓
	Diastolic	↑	↑↑	↔	↔ or ↓	↑↑	↔ or ↓
Obstructive		↑↑	↑↑	↓	↓	↑	↔ or ↓
Septic	Early	↓	↓	↔ or ↑	↑↑↑	↓↓↓	↔ or ↓
	Late	↔ or ↑	↑	↓	↓↓	↓↓	↓↓

Note: Adapted from Nelson Textbook of Pediatrics, 21st edition.

■ APPROACH TO MANAGEMENT

The management of shock can be divided into stabilization of the neonate and definitive therapy. It is important to know the cause of shock to plan the definitive therapy. The management begins with the stabilization of the neonate which is dealt in the next section. The following **Table 1.4** depicts the history, clinical clues, and investigative parameters to find the etiology of shock.

■ TREATMENT

Initial stabilization involves maintenance of TABC (temperature, airway, breathing, and circulation).

- As with all emergencies in neonates, the management of shock starts with provision of a thermoneutral environment.
- The airway is stabilized followed by breathing support either with CPAP or mechanical ventilation depending on the severity of respiratory distress and hemodynamic compromise. Although CPAP can be tried in early stages of shock (e.g., compensated shock), it may be preferable to intubate and start elective positive pressure ventilation in presence of hypotension or requirement of more than one vasoactive agent.
- An IV line is required for fluid/vasoactive drugs administration. With initiation of vasoactive agents, enteral feeds should be stopped, and IV fluids should be started. Central venous access [umbilical venous on first day of life or peripherally inserted central catheter (PICC) line] is preferable for reliable delivery of vasoactive drugs. Vasopressors should preferably be given through central line.

The management of neonatal shock is presented in **Flowchart 1.1**.

Neonatal Shock

TABLE 1.4: Etiologies of various forms of neonatal shock.

Types of shock	Etiologies of shock	History	Clinical clues	Investigative parameters*
Hypovolemic	Loss of body fluids (blood and water/electrolyte)	Concealed or revealed hemorrhage, diarrhea, and polyuria	Clinical signs of dehydration may be present	• Serum sodium and osmolality may be raised • Functional echocardiography can help in doubtful situations
Cardiogenic	• Birth asphyxia, congenital heart diseases cardiomyopathies, arrhythmias • *Electrolyte abnormalities*: Hypocalcemia, severe anemia, and drugs, e.g., opioids and magnesium sulfate	• Birth asphyxia • Antenatal-diagnosed congenital heart diseases • Interrupted feeding/perspiration during feeding, history of maternal/neonatal drug use • Maternal diabetes and antenatal scans	• Signs of congestive cardiac failure • Murmurs • Hydrops • Severe pallor	• Biomarkers (CK-MB) • Serum electrolytes • ECG abnormalities • Echocardiography
Obstructive	• *Increased intrathoracic pressure*: Tension pneumothorax, increased intrathoracic ventilator pressure • *Ventricular outflow obstruction*: Ductal dependent CHDs and pulmonary embolism • Pericardial tamponade	• Resuscitation details • Positive pressure ventilation • Antenatal scans • Known congenital heart diseases	• Asymmetric chest rise/auscultatory findings • Feeble femoral pulses • Presence of central lines	• Chest X-ray • Blood gas analysis • Upper and lower limb BP • Echocardiography
Distributive/septic	• Early septic shock with decreased afterload (bacterial, viral, or fungal) • Anaphylaxis • Loss of sympathetic vascular tone secondary to spinal cord or brainstem injury • Drugs, e.g., β₂ agonists	• Maternal or postnatal risk factors of infection • Drug administration	• Signs of SIRS • Multiple organ involvement	• Sepsis markers • Culture of sterile body fluids (especially blood and CSF) • Organ specific investigations

(CHD: congenital heart disease; CK-MB: creatine kinase-muscle brain; CSF: cerebrospinal fluid; ECG: electrocardiography; SIRS: systemic inflammatory response syndrome)

Note: *This list is representative and not comprehensive.

Flowchart 1.1: Algorithm for stepwise and time sensitive management of shock.

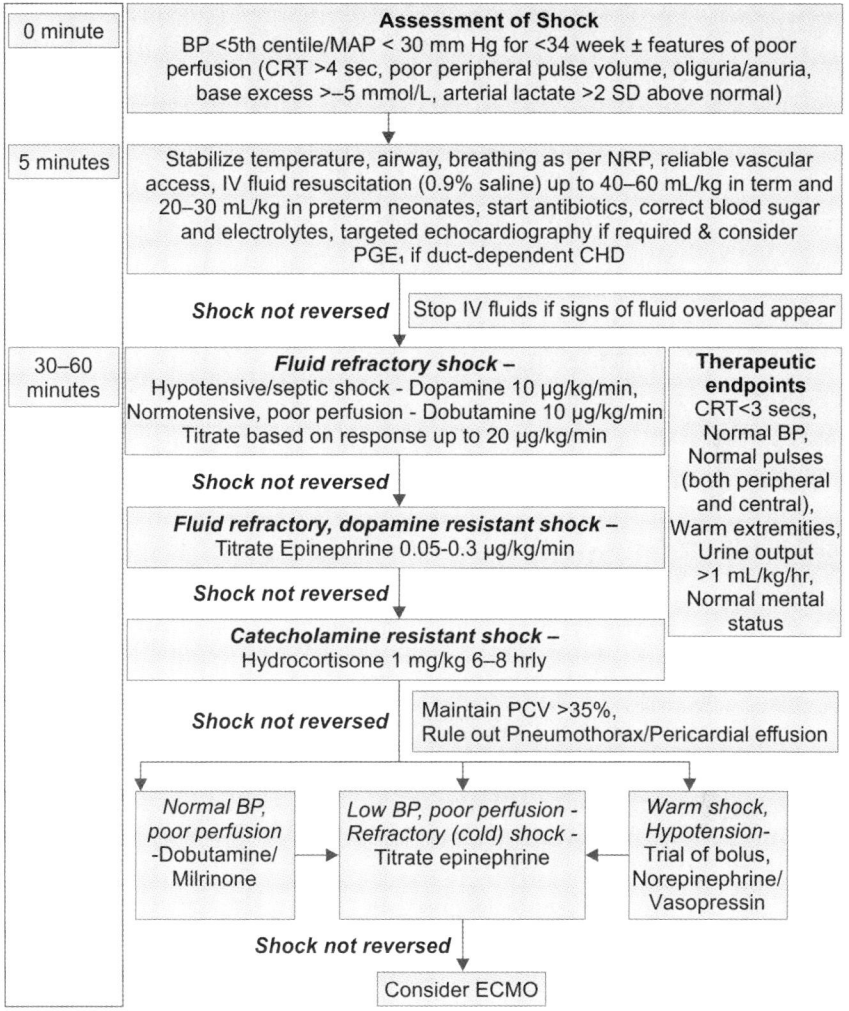

Source: Modified from Davis et al.[32]
(BP: Blood pressure; CHD: congenital heart disease; CRT: capillary refill time; ECMO: extracorporeal membrane oxygenation; IV: intravenous; MAP: mean arterial pressure; NRP: Neonatal resuscitation program; PCV: packed cell volume; PGE: prostaglandin E1; PT: preterm; SD: standard deviation)

Volume Resuscitation

Volume resuscitation is the first line of therapy in neonatal shock. Crystalloids (normal saline) are preferred over 5% albumin as they are associated with lower risk of fluid overload. Further albumin is associated with increased risk of infection and impaired gas exchange.[15] Initial fluid bolus of 10 mL/kg (irrespective of gestational age) is infused over 15–30 minutes [longer duration for extremely low birth weight (ELBW) neonates]. Up to 40–60 mL/kg is advised for term neonates and 20–30 mL/kg for preterm neonates.[1,10,16] The conservative fluid resuscitation in preterm neonates is advised due to increased risk of fluid overload, opening of PDA, and intraventricular hemorrhage. Currently, there is no gold standard measure for preload optimization. Therefore, fluid resuscitation is guided by response to fluid bolus(es) and signs of fluid overload.[18,19] Functional echocardiography may offer additional clues as discussed previously. It is important to realize that absolute hypovolemia is unlikely, except in conditions of blood loss or gastrointestinal (GI) losses. Thus, fluid should be used cautiously in the management of cardiogenic shock secondary to asphyxia, PDA, and transitional circulation where myocardial contractility is impaired.

Pharmacologic Therapy

The mainstay of pharmacologic therapy are three classes of drugs—inotropes, vasopressors, and lusitropes.[8] Inotropes primarily increase myocardial contractility and hence are suitable for conditions in which myocardial dysfunction is primary problem, e.g., birth asphyxia or transitional circulation, etc. Vasopressors improve BP through increase in vascular tone and are thus suitable for conditions with decreased afterload, e.g., septic shock and/or in presence of hypotension. Lusitropes improve myocardial relaxation, increase systemic blood flow, and are thus useful for conditions with diastolic dysfunction. Appropriate vasoactive agents should be chosen based on the underlying pathophysiology and intended effect. A single drug can have either inotropic or vasopressor effect depending on its infusion rate. Commonly used agents in neonates, their doses, and their predominant actions are summarized in **Table 1.5**.[1,8,10,15,21]

Generally, inotropes are advised in peripheral circulatory failure with normal BP. Vasopressors are used in hypotension. Depending on the underlying pathophysiological mechanism, the initial choice of vasoactive agents may vary. The choice of vasoactive agents in different clinical scenarios is discussed below.

Shock in Transitional Circulation

Although usually practiced, fluid resuscitation should be cautiously used as generally there is no setting of volume loss. Inotropes (dopamine 5–10 µg/kg/min or dobutamine 5–20 µg/kg/min) should be started initially to support poor myocardial performance. If there is hypotension, vasopressors are required. However, vasopressors should be carefully used as they can markedly increase SVR, thereby decreasing cardiac output further. A stepwise titration of low to moderate dose dopamine and epinephrine is advised in hypotensive neonates to achieve mean BP 3–6 mm Hg higher than that for the gestational age.[22,23]

TABLE 1.5: Vasoactive drugs, dose, and important actions.

Agent	Dose	Action	Special features
Dopamine	5–9 µg/kg/min, mainly on β-receptors 10–20 µg/kg/min (vasopressor), additionally on α-receptors	↑ HR and ↑ myocardial contractility ↑ BP by increasing systemic vascular resistance (SVR)	• 5% dextrose is preferred for dilution. Preferable to change infusions every 12 hours rather than 24 hours[22] • Acts by releasing stored norepinephrine; the stores might exhaust with continuing shock • Thyroid screening to be postponed till 12 hours after the drug is stopped
Dobutamine	5–20 µg/kg/min	↑ contractility, cardiac output, and ↓ SVR	Direct actions on β-receptors. Effective in presence of myocardial dysfunction
Epinephrine	0.1–0.2 µg/kg/min (inotropy) ≥0.3–1 µg/kg/min (vasopressor)	↑ contractility and HR ↑ SVR	• Direct actions on adrenergic receptors • Caution beyond 0.5 µg/kg/min as arrhythmias may happen • Adverse effect includes ↑ HR, serum lactate, and hyperglycemia
Milrinone	Loading: 50–75 µg/kg IV over 60 min; Maintenance: 0.25–0.75 µg/kg/min	Both inotropy and lusitropy ↓ Vascular tone in pulmonary and systemic circulation	• Main role in postcardiac surgery • Useful adjunct to iNO in presence of PPHN • More effective than dobutamine in presence of diastolic dysfunction • Cautious in presence of hypotension
Vasopressin	0.01–0.12 units/kg/hr	↑ SVR; releases cortisol in presence of ACTH	• Indicated in warm and vasopressor resistant shock • Caution in presence of myocardial dysfunction • Watch for oliguria as ↓ renal blood flow is known
Noradrenaline	0.02–1 µg/kg/min	↑ SVR	Limited evidence of efficacy
Levosimendan	0.1–0.4 µg/kg/min	Positive inotropy and lusitropy ↓ SVR	• Limited evidence of efficacy • Useful in postoperative care of congenital heart diseases

(ACTH: adrenocorticotropic hormone; HR: heart rate; iNO: inhaled nitric oxide, PPHN: persistent pulmonary hypertension of the neonate; SVR: systemic vascular resistance)

Very Low Birth Weight Neonates with Hemodynamically Significant Patent Ductus Arteriosus

The principles of management include restoring hemodynamic stability as well as pharmacological closure of PDA. To decrease left-to-right shunt through PDA, one should use maneuvers to keep slightly higher pulmonary vascular resistance, e.g., adjusting ventilator settings to avoid hyperoxia, keeping PCO_2 values on the higher side of normal range, higher positive end expiratory pressure, etc. There are no well-controlled trials comparing different vasoactive agents in the management of shock in neonates with PDA. Bouissou et al. found that dopamine (<10 µg/kg/min) increased BP and systemic blood flow in preterm hypotensive neonates with PDA.[24] Therefore dopamine in inotropic doses (5–10 µg/kg/min) or dobutamine (10–20 µg/kg/min) should be the first line of management in such cases. Epinephrine (0.1–0.5 µg/kg/min) should be used if there is no response to dopamine and dobutamine.[25]

Shock in Neonates with Severe Birth Asphyxia

In severely asphyxiated neonates, multiple derangements such as capillary leak syndrome, myocardial dysfunction, and persistent pulmonary hypertension of the neonate (PPHN) may occur together. Therefore, therapy must be individualized and constantly adjusted.[9] Fluids should be given cautiously in absence of setting of volume loss. In normotensive patients with poor peripheral circulation, dobutamine should be used. In normotensive neonates with presence of poor peripheral circulation and concomitant PPHN, milrinone can be considered. In cases of hypotension, dopamine ≥10 µg/kg/min should be started and gradually titrated. Inhaled nitric oxide should be considered for neonates with PPHN, poor cardiac indices (<3.3 L/m^2/min) or poor superior vena cava (SVC) flow (<40 mL/kg/min).[1,10]

Septic Shock

Fluid resuscitation should be given initially as there is relative hypovolemia. The initial choice of vasoactive drug is dopamine (10–20 µg/kg/min) in hypotensive neonates. Epinephrine (0.2–0.5 µg/kg/min) should be added, if neonates remain hypotensive despite dopamine infusion. Use of epinephrine as a first line vasoactive drug is upcoming, however, currently there is no conclusive evidence of its superiority over dopamine.[26] In contrast, a normotensive septic neonate, with signs of peripheral circulatory failure, should be treated with dobutamine or dopamine (5–10 µg/kg/min).[1,10]

Late-onset Glucocorticoid Responsive Circulatory Collapse

It occurs after the first week of life in VLBW infants in the absence of other common causes such as sepsis, PDA, blood loss, or other obstructive causes of shock. Relative adrenal insufficiency is implicated in its pathophysiology. It is characterized by sudden-onset hypotension which is usually resistant to fluid resuscitation and vasoactive support. Hydrocortisone is given at 1.0 mg/kg every 6–8 hourly till 48 hours followed by 1 mg/kg 12 hourly for next three days. If poor response persists vasopressin can be considered.[27,28]

Catecholamine-resistant Hypotension

Steroids are indicated at the onset of catecholamine-resistant hypotension. There is no universal definition of catecholamine resistant hypotension but most followed definition is persistence of shock despite >10 μg/kg/min dopamine and a directly acting vasoactive agent (either epinephrine > 0.3 μg/kg/min or dobutamine > 10 μg/kg/min). They increase BP and decrease vasopressor requirement in such neonates.[29] Given the lack of long-term safety data of steroids on developing brain and prolonged half-life of steroids in preterm neonates, lower doses are preferred. Hydrocortisone is given at 1.0 mg/kg every 6–8 hourly till 48 hours followed by 1 mg/kg 12 hourly for next three days.[30]

Supportive Management

Broad-spectrum antibiotics (as per the local sensitivity pattern) should be started, wherever the possibility of sepsis cannot be ruled out. First dose should be administered as early as possible within the first hour of shock. Enteral feeds should be withheld. However, trophic feeding can be continued, if abdominal examination is normal and shock is in improving trend. Parenteral nutrition may be considered. Routine sedation is not required. Avoid hyperglycemia and maintain electrolytes and calcium in their normal range. Maintain hematocrit >35%. In bleeding tendencies, vitamin K injection, platelet concentrates for platelet count <50,000/mm^3, and fresh frozen plasma (FFP) transfusions should be considered for coagulopathy. Consider urgent chest tube drainage if there is pneumothorax. Consider venoarterial extracorporeal membrane oxygenation (ECMO) for refractory shock.[1]

Other specific management like prostaglandin E1 (PGE1) can be considered to maintain systemic circulation, if duct-dependent systemic circulation is suspected.

■ OUTCOMES

Neonates with shock are likely to have longer duration of hospital stay, chronic lung disease, growth failure, retinopathy of prematurity, and adverse neurodevelopmental outcomes. Mortality rates up to 40–50% are reported in VLBW in various studies from developed nations; and studies from developing countries have shown 70–80% mortality in septic shock. A recent hospital-based study from India reported the case fatality rates of 62% in neonatal shock among 392 neonates developing shock over 2-year study period.[5]

Poor prognostic factors in such studies are refractory shock at onset, acute renal failure, disseminated intravascular coagulation (DIC), neutropenia, metabolic acidosis, and hypothermia.[10] Neurodevelopmental outcomes following septic shock at 18 months of age show higher risk of impairment especially in preterm neonates. Severe sequelae either cerebral palsy, visual impairment, severe developmental delay, or short bowel syndrome have been described up to 19% at 18 months follow-up and the combined risk of death or severe sequelae in half of them.[31,32]

■ CONCLUSION

Hypotension is a late marker of shock. Septic shock is the most common form of shock in neonatal age group especially in the developing countries. Early recognition of shock at the compensated stage and appropriate intervention can maximize survival and neurodevelopmental outcomes. Apart from the clinical signs, laboratory parameters such as base excess and lactate may be useful in identification in borderline cases. Functional echocardiography is a noninvasive tool for assessment of neonates with shock. The management of shock begins with IV fluid resuscitation unless there is clear evidence that the preload is optimum in the neonate. Conventionally, dopamine is the first-line inotrope for fluid-refractory neonatal shock. However, the choice of vasoactive agent(s) may change with the underlying pathophysiology. Hydrocortisone should be given in catecholamine resistant shock. Despite everything, the case fatality rates are astonishingly high.

■ KEY POINTS

- Shock is a clinical syndrome of acute circulatory dysfunction, resulting in insufficient delivery of oxygen and vital nutrients to the body tissues relative to their metabolic demand.
- The incidence of shock is higher in very and extremely premature neonates.
- Septic shock is the most common form of shock followed by cardiogenic shock.
- Hypotension is a late manifestation of shock.
- The clinical assessment of shock involves both measuring BP and parameters of peripheral perfusion.
- Functional echocardiography is a useful supplement for clinical assessment and management of shock.
- Management involves early stabilization of temperature, airway, breathing, and IV fluid resuscitation.
- Vasoactive agents are indicated in fluid-refractory shock.
- Dopamine is generally the first line vasoactive agent for the management of neonatal shock. However, the choice depends on the underlying pathophysiology and severity of shock. The escalation of dose of vasoactive drugs should be done every 10–15 minutes intervals during management of shock.
- Hydrocortisone is indicated in catecholamine resistant shock.
- Long-term neurodevelopmental follow-up is essential for neonates with shock.

REFERENCES

1. Brierley J, Carcillo JA, Choong K, Cornell T, Decaen A, Deymann A, et al. Clinical practice parameters for hemodynamic support of pediatric and neonatal septic shock: 2007 update from the American College of Critical Care Medicine. Crit Care Med. 2009;37(2):666-88.
2. Barrington KJ. Hypotension and shock in the preterm infant. Semin Fetal Neonatal Med. 2008;13(1):16-23.
3. Wong J, Shah P, Yoon E, Yee W, Lee S, Dow K. Inotrope use among extremely preterm infants in Canadian neonatal intensive care units: variation and outcomes. Am J Perinatol. 2015;32:9-14.
4. Chan KH, Sanatani S, Potts JE, Harris KC. The relative incidence of cardiogenic and septic shock in neonates. Paediatr Child Health. 2020;25(6):372-7.
5. Saini SS, Shrivastav AK, Kumar J, Sundaram V, Mukhopadhay K, Dutta S, et al. Predictors of mortality in neonatal shock: a retrospective cohort study. Shock. 2021.
6. Angus DC, van der Poll T. Severe sepsis and septic shock. N Engl J Med. 2013;369:840-51.
7. Vesoulis ZA, Mathur AM. Cerebral Autoregulation, Brain Injury, and the Transitioning Premature Infant. Front Pediatr. 2017;5:64.
8. Noori S, Seri I. Neonatal blood pressure support: the use of inotropes, lusitropes, and other vasopressor agents. Clin Perinatol. 2012;39:221-38.
9. Seri I, Noori S. Diagnosis and treatment of neonatal hypotension outside the transitional period. Early Hum Dev. 2005;81:405-11.
10. Wynn JL, Wong HR. Pathophysiology and treatment of septic shock in neonates. Clin Perinatol. 2010;37:439-79.
11. Saini SS, Kumar P, Kumar RM. Hemodynamic changes in preterm neonates with septic shock: a prospective observational study. Pediatr Crit Care Med. 2014;15:443-50.
12. McNamara PJ WD, Giesinger RE, Jain A. Hemodynamics. In: MacDonald MG SM (Ed). Avery's Neonatology: Pathophysiology and Management the Newborn. Philadelphia: Wolters Kluwer; 2016. pp. 457-86.
13. Dionne JM, Bremner SA, Baygani SK, Batton B, Ergenekon E, Bhatt-Mehta V, et al. Method of Blood Pressure Measurement in Neonates and Infants: A Systematic Review and Analysis. J Pediatr. 2020;221:23.
14. Batton B, Li L, Newman NS, Das A, Watterberg KL, Yoder BA, et al. Early blood pressure, antihypotensive therapy and outcomes at 18-22 months' corrected age in extremely preterm infants. Arch Dis Child Fetal Neonatal Ed. 2016;101:F201.
15. Osborn DA, Evans N, Kluckow M. Clinical detection of low upper body blood flow in very premature infants using blood pressure, capillary refill time, and central-peripheral temperature difference. Arch Dis Child Fetal Neonatal Ed. 2004;89:F168-73.
16. Giesinger RE, McNamara PJ. Hemodynamic instability in the critically ill neonate: an approach to cardiovascular support based on disease pathophysiology. Semin Perinatol. 2016;40:174-88.
17. Goldstein B, Giroir B, Randolph A. International pediatric sepsis consensus conference: definitions for sepsis and organ dysfunction in pediatrics. Pediatr Crit Care Med. 2005;6:2-8.
18. Shah BA, Padbury JF. Neonatal Sepsis: an old problem with new insights. Virulence. 2014;5:170-8.

19. Mertens L, Seri I, Marek J, Arlettaz R, Barker P, McNamara P, et al. Targeted neonatal echocardiography in the neonatal intensive care unit: practice guidelines and recommendations for training. Eur J Echocardiogr. 2011;12(10):715-36.
20. Singh Y, Katheria AC, Vora F. Advances in diagnosis and management of hemodynamic instability in neonatal shock. Front Pediatr. 2018;6:2.
21. Dempsey E, Rabe H. The use of cardiotonic drugs in neonates. Clin Perinatol. 2019;46(2):273-90.
22. Kirupakaran K, Mahoney L, Rabe H, Patel BA. Understanding the stability of dopamine and dobutamine over 24 h in simulate neonatal ward conditions. Paediatr Drugs. 2017;19(5):487-95.
23. Seri I. Management of hypotension and low systemic blood flow in the very low birth weight neonate during the first postnatal week. J Perinatol. 2006;26:S8-13.
24. Bouissou A, Rakza T, Klosowski S, Tourneux P, Vanderborght M, Storme L. Hypotension in preterm infants with significant patent ductus arteriosus: effects of dopamine. J Pediatr. 2008;153:790-4.
25. Evans N. Which inotrope for which baby? Arch Dis Child Fetal Neonatal Ed. 2006;91:F213-20.
26. Baske K, Saini SS, Dutta S, Sundaram V. Epinephrine versus dopamine in neonatal septic shock: a double-blind randomized controlled trial. Eur J Pediatr. 2018;177(9):1335-42.
27. Kawai M. Late-onset circulatory collapse of prematurity. Pediatr Int. 2017; 59(4):391-6.
28. Iijima S. Late-onset glucocorticoid-responsive circulatory collapse in premature infants. Pediatr Neonatol. 2019;60(6):603-10.
29. Higgins S, Friedlich P, Seri I. Hydrocortisone for hypotension and vasopressor dependence in preterm neonates: a meta-analysis. J Perinatol. 2010;30:373-8.
30. Watterberg K. Evidence-based neonatal pharmacotherapy: postnatal corticosteroids. Clin Perinatol. 2012;39:47-59.
31. Kermorvant-Duchemin E, Laborie S, Rabilloud M, Lapillonne A, Claris O. Outcome and prognostic factors in neonates with septic shock. Pediatr Crit Care Med. 2008;9:186-91.
32. Davis AL, Carcillo JA, Aneja RK, Deyman AJ, Lin JC, Nguyen TC, et al. American College of critical care medicine clinical practice parameters for hemodynamic support of pediatric and neonatal septic shock. Crit Care Med. 2017;45:1061-93.

Nutrition

CHAPTER 2: Junk and Ultra-processed Foods

Sumaira Khalil, Dheeraj Shah

■ INTRODUCTION

Globally, there has been an increase in the consumption of fast foods.[1] The recent National Family Health Survey-5 (NFHS-5, 2019–20) data reported a dramatic increase in the prevalence of obesity in children below the age of 5 years as 4.6% in urban areas and 3.5% in rural areas.[2] This reflects that obesity has doubled amongst under-5 children from 2015–16 to 2018–19. The main reasons attributed to this increase were the lack of physical activity and unhealthy eating habits among children. The prevalence of junk food consumption was reported as 51.3% in a multicountry study conducted on 72,900 children (6–7 years) from 17 countries and 199,135 adolescents (13–14 years) from 36 countries.[3]

India is currently facing a major challenge of dealing with a state of dietary dichotomy. Rising prevalence of malnutrition along with overweight and obesity, especially in the youth and adolescents in the last two decades is very alarming. According to the Comprehensive National Nutrition Survey (2016–18), overall prevalence of overweight and obesity in under-5 children was 1–2% which was significantly higher than expected, indicating an upsurge of overweight and obesity in the country.[4] The highest prevalence was seen in Mizoram, Tripura, and Uttarakhand. Among 5–9-year-old children, the overall prevalence of overweight reported was 4% and obesity 1%. States such as Goa and Nagaland reported the maximum prevalence of overweight in 5–9-year-old children (15%), whereas Bihar and Jharkhand reported the least (<1%). In the adolescent age group, overweight and obesity were reported as 5% and 1%, respectively. Delhi, Goa, and Tamil Nadu reported the highest prevalence (>12%) of overweight amongst the adolescents and Bihar, Jharkhand, Rajasthan, Uttar Pradesh, and Madhya Pradesh, reported the lowest prevalence (<3%) amongst the adolescents.[4]

■ DEFINITIONS

Fast Food

Cambridge Dictionary defines fast food as food already cooked and served hot, and food you can take away easily to eat, e.g., hamburgers, fried chicken.[5]

Merriam Webster Online Dictionary defines fast food as food that is available easily and can be cooked and served quickly; with little consideration given to quality and significance.[6] New Oxford American Dictionary defines fast food as food that can be prepared easily and quickly and sold in restaurants as take away meals or quick meals In India, apart from the fried chicken, pizza and burgers, foods such as *pav bhaji, bhujia, bhelpuri,* and vegetable sandwiches may also be considered as fast food.

Junk Foods

Junk food is defined as energy-dense food with low nutritional value but high content of fat, salt, and sugar. The National Institute of Nutrition has defined junk food as food that contains minimal or no protein, vitamin, or minerals but is rich in salt, fat, and energy.[7] Very often fast food and junk food are terms used interchangeably but not all fast foods are junk foods although most of the junk foods are fast foods. Junk foods are usually tasty and full of coloring agents, preservatives, and artificial flavors but have low nutritional value and high caloric content.

High Fat, Salt, and Sugar Foods

The World Health Organization (WHO) defines high fat, salt, and sugar (HFSS) foods as foods that are high in salt, sugar, and fats with minimal amounts of proteins, vitamins, phytochemicals, minerals, and dietary fiber.[8] They are known to have harmful effects on the health if consumed regularly or in large amounts, e.g., chocolates, chips, bakery products, and fried foods. Other terms used in some countries include *"Foods of Minimal Nutritional Value" (FMNV),* in the USA,[9] *"Energy-Dense Low-Nutrient Density Foods" (EDLNF)*[10] or *"Energy-Dense and Nutrient-Poor Foods for Children" (EDNPFC),*[11] in the Republic of Korea. Consumption of these foods has a negative impact on health due to an imbalance of nutrients. Excess consumption of foods with high content of fats, sugar, and salt negatively impacts the health and nutrients such as proteins, mineral, and fiber that positively enhances health are either absent or present in negligible amounts in these kinds of foods. But these terms have not got popular due to the complicated terminologies.

Junk food also contains preservatives and trans-fatty acids (TFA) commonly found in processed and packaged food which again have detrimental effects on the health. Trans-fatty acids are made of hydrogenated oils, which are used to make *vanaspati* or they contain polyhydrogenated vegetable oils. The process of hydrogenation increases their shelf-life and improves the texture of polyhydrogenated vegetable oils.[7] TFA are found commonly in snacks that are deep-fried and bakery products.

Delhi High Court in 2015 ordered a restriction on the sale of junk foods—foods high in fat, salt, and sugar—in and around schools in India thereby regulating its consumption. It also directed the Food Safety and Standards Authority of India (FSSAI) to implement guidelines on making wholesome and nutritious food available to schoolchildren in a time-bound manner. This judgement was welcomed as a significant step toward understanding the link between unhealthy food consumption and increasing incidence of obesity.[12]

■ NEW CLASSIFICATIONS

NOVA Classification

The new and evolving method of classifying foods gives emphasis to what is done to the food stuff and the nutrients present in them rather than the nutrient content only. Therefore, the emphasis is on *food processing*, i.e., the extent, nature, and purpose of processing and the effect it has on the food and our health.

The NOVA classification categorizes foods not according to the nutrient content but according to the nature, purpose, and extent of food processing.[13] NOVA identifies *food processing* as physical, biological, and chemical processes used after foods are separated from nature, and before being consumed or prepared as dishes and meals. Based on the processing, Professor Carlos Monteiro developed the NOVA classification as he noticed that increased consumption of the ultra-processed and highly processed foods led to an increased prevalence of obesity and type 2 diabetes. A small study was conducted by the National Institute of Health (NIH) where ultra-processed and unprocessed food were given to participants with same amount of carbohydrates, calories, fat, fiber, and sugar for 2 weeks. People who consumed the ultra-processed food ate 500 calories more, gained more weight, and ate faster as compared to those who consumed unprocessed food. Scientific evidence available reveals that a 10% increase in consumption of ultra-processed foods, approximately causes a 10% rise in the occurrence of obesity, cardiovascular disease, asthma, and diabetes even in the pediatric population.

According to the NOVA classification, foods are classified into four groups according to their processing.

Group 1: Unprocessed or Minimally Processed Food

These include natural and raw foods including the edible parts of animal (eggs, muscle, and milk) or plants (seed, roots, fruits, leaves, and stems) and of fungi, algae, and water after they are separated from nature. They are consumed frozen, fried, ground, crushed, roasted, boiled, pasteurized, cooled, and fermented. None of these processes add sugar, fats, oils, salt, and other preservatives to natural foods. These foods are made at home and not processed in factories and sometimes difficult to consume raw. These include fruits and vegetables such as banana, carrots, onion, and potatoes; grains such as ragi, corn, wheat, rice, oats and nuts; and raw chicken. Minimally processed foods are natural foods that are changed due to processes such as removal of inedible part, and drying, roasting, boiling, crushing, filtering, grinding, fractioning, refrigeration, pasteurization, nonalcoholic fermentation, chilling and freezing. These processes preserve the natural foods and make them edible or pleasant for consumption and more suitable for storage.

Group 2: Processed Culinary Ingredients

These ingredients are added to food to enhance its taste and flavor while cooking or for seasoning. They are extracted from group 1 foods or directly from minimally processed and unprocessed foods by milling, spray drying, grinding, refining, and pressing. Some examples include salted butter, vinegar, sugar, salt, iodized salt, and oil or butter extracted from milk. Such processes make products durable and they can be used at home or restaurants to cook or season group 1 foods. They are also used to make different and varied handmade meals such as soups, salads, stews, desserts, and breads. They are usually consumed in combination with group 1 foods while making prepared meals and not consumed by themselves.

Group 3: Processed Foods

Processed foods are also derived from combining unprocessed or minimally processed with group 2 foods and are made by adding salt, sugar, or oil and processed by baking, cooking, and nonalcoholic fermentation. These foods are unhealthy by virtue of the quantity of sugar, salt, and oil added to them. Processing increases the durability of group 1 foods or enhances their sensory qualities. Canned fruits and vegetables, pickles made from vegetables and preserved with added oil and salt water, *murabba* and jams made from fruits preserved with sugar syrup, and cheese made from milk are some examples of processed foods. They are modified versions of group 1 foods and are edible either by themselves or in combination with other foods.

Group 4: Ultra-processed Foods

This group does not contain any natural food but is processed in factories and sold as ready to eat foods or instant food. They are entirely made from substances derived from foods and additives and are not modified from group 1 food. They are the most harmful attributed by high-energy densities and low micronutrient content. They contain five to six ingredients and one additive and undergo processing by whipping, defoaming, bulking and de-bulking, and carbonating. The additives include emulsifiers, dyes, coloring agents, nonsugar sweeteners, and flavors. Ultra-processed food incorporates large amounts of salt, sugar, oil, fats, and antioxidant stabilizers and soy protein isolate, maltodextrin, hydrogenated oils, whey, gluten which are directly extracted. They also contain other sources of nutrients, which are normally not used in culinary preparations. Chocolates, cakes, processed fruit juices, protein bars, carbonated drinks, instant noodles, *upma,* and energy drinks are some examples. The overall purpose of the ultra-processed food is to create highly durable, convenient, ready-to-eat, highly palatable, branded and highly marketed food products ready to displace all other food groups. But this definition also has a few pitfalls. It mainly caters to packaged foods and seems to focus on process of making/packaging foods rather than the content. As a result, home prepared or freshly prepared (as in restaurants) nutritionally inappropriate foods may be left out if this definition is used.

Nutrient Profiling

Nutrient profiling is the science of ranking foods according to their nutritional content for prevention of disease and promoting health.[14] It is a scientific method to assess the quality of food products and beverages depending on the nutrient content such as quantity of sugar, salt, fats, dietary fiber, minerals, and vitamins. Based on this, several countries have developed their own specific models, which need to be simple to understand and apply in practice. Most models on nutrient profiling categorize foods based on "negative" food components whereas some balance the positive and negative food components. But the drawback of this type of profiling is the varied interpretations of this model can lead to confusion. Therefore, a set of guiding principles is required along with a validated approach so that national authorities can use suitable models.

Food Labeling

Food labeling as green, yellow, and red categories to those suggested for school canteens by Report of Working Group on Addressing Consumption of Foods High in Fat, Salt, and Sugar (HFSS) and Promotion of Healthy Snacks in Schools of India.[8] However, these guidelines have not been approved by the FSSAI as yet. The Food Safety and Standard Regulations were brought about in 2020 regarding safe food and balanced diet for children in schools.[15] According to these regulations, sale of food products high in saturated fat or trans fat or added sugar or sodium is not allowed in the school premises. It is mandatory to put a board displaying the same at the entrance gate. Any advertising banner or wallpaper on food products high in saturated fat or trans fat or added sugar or sodium is not allowed on the school computers. It also regulates to convert school campus into "Eat Right Campus" that focuses on serving of safe food and balanced diet, local and seasonal food without any food waste. Advertising or marketing or permission for the sale of food products high in saturated fat or trans fat or added sugar or sodium in school campus or to school children in an area within 50 meters from the school gate in any direction is banned.

The Center for Science and Environment (CSE) raised the issue of need for strengthening the nutritional information and had also recommended labeling of calories, sugar, fat, saturated fat, and salt on the front of pack (FoP) of foods.[16] However, the FSSAI decided to delink FoP labeling norms from the general labeling regulations. According to the FSSAI, FoP labeling requirement is largely related to the declaration of the threshold of salt, sugar, and fat and its depiction. However, FoP norms would help consumers to make informed decision on its consumption by better understanding of the food.

In the United Kingdom, Natasha's Law, or the UK Food Information Amendment, which comes into effect from October 2021, requires that all "Prepacked for Direct Sales (PPDS)" food clearly display the name of the food with full list of ingredients including allergenic ingredients emphasized on the packaging. This legislation is brought about to protect those who suffer from allergy and to give them confidence about the food they are buying. This law will apply to all businesses in England, Wales, Northern Island, and Scotland.[17]

IAP Nomenclature: JUNCS

With so many confusing definitions, a new term was coined by the Indian Academy of Pediatrics (IAP) Guidelines on fast and junk foods, sugar, sweetened beverages, and energy drinks, irrespective of fastness or processing techniques or place of serving which may include all nutritionally poor or harmful food for children and adolescent consumption. This was termed as JUNCS as described in **Table 2.1**. This term includes all unhealthy components such as fat, salt content, sugar content, or contents of harmful non-nutritional substances, or ultra-processed foods which are consumed

TABLE 2.1: IAP nomenclature of junk, ultra-processed, foods: The "JUNCS".*

J	Junk food (foods high in fats, especially saturated and trans fats, sugars and salts, and foods lacking in micronutrients/minerals)
U	Ultra-processed foods (as defined in the fourth category of NOVA classification)
N	Nutritionally inappropriate foods. Home-made foods can also qualify to be nutritionally inappropriate if prepared in recycled oil, or contain high amount of sugar, fat, or salt
C	Caffeinated/colored/carbonated beverages
S	Sugar-sweetened beverages

(IAP: Indian Academy of Pediatrics)
Note: *Reproduced with permission from Gupta P, Shah D, Kumar P, Bedi N, Gupta Mittal H, Mishra K, et al. Indian Academy of Pediatrics Guidelines on the Fast and Junk Foods, Sugar Sweetened Beverages, Fruit Juices, and Energy Drinks. Indian Pediatr. 2019;56:849-63.

> **BOX 2.1:** Factors contributing to increased consumption of JUNCS.
> - Urbanization
> - High percentage of working age population and young population
> - Increase in number of nuclear families
> - Digitalization and online deliveries
> - Increasing percentage of working women
> - Rising middle class population
> - Changing consumer preferences
> - Aggressive marketing and advertising of JUNCS food
> - Changing cooking practices
> - Increased intake of ready-to-use food and processed food

in high quantity.[18] Factors leading to increased consumption of JUNCS are described in **Box 2.1**.

■ HARMFUL EFFECTS OF JUNK FOODS

Metabolic Effects

Increased consumption of junk food and ultra-processed foods leads to higher body mass index (BMI) and obesity. This is attributed to high palatability of fat and high-energy density of fast food. Evidence suggests that increased frequency of fast food consumption also leads to higher BMI levels and higher chances of developing obesity later. Fast food consumption leads to higher consumption of saturated fats, calories, higher sodium consumption, and lower intake of vitamin A and C. Milk consumption is reduced. Food rich in saturated fats, salts, and sugars cause obesity, hypertension, dyslipidemia, and metabolic syndrome. Deficiency of calcium and magnesium in fast foods results in osteoporosis. High-sugar content leads to dental caries.[19-21]

Abnormal Cardiometabolic Biomarkers

Increased consumption of fast food is known to cause increased levels of adiponectin,[22] interleukin-6 (IL-6), triglycerides, low-density lipoprotein cholesterol (LDL-c) and increased concentration of glucose and is inversely related to high-density lipoprotein cholesterol (HDL-c) levels. Children having higher adherence to fast food intake patterns have a two-fold higher chances of developing insulin resistance. Fast food pattern has a positive association with LDL-c levels and blood pressure and a negative association with HDL-c levels. Increased consumption of ultra-processed food is known to cause metabolic syndrome and its consumption at preschool age is a significant predictor of increased levels of total and LDL cholesterol at school age.[23]

Hypertension

There is paucity of data from controlled studies regarding association between consumption of fast food and blood pressure. The data is variable due to lack of intervention trials. Whatever cross-sectional data is available, suggests that fast food dietary pattern is positively associated with hypertension in children and adolescents.[24,25]

Abnormal Psychological Behavior

Attention deficit hyperactive disorders (ADHD), abnormal psychological behavior, and oppositional disorders are associated with a diet associated with increased fast food pattern, meat pattern, and sugar sweetened beverage pattern. High dietary consumption of fats causes psychiatric distress, violent behavior leading to bad physical fights, and bullying behavioral pattern.[26-28]

■ HARMFUL EFFECTS OF ENERGY DRINKS

Energy drinks have increased concentration of caffeine, sugar, taurine, herbal supplements and vitamins. Caffeine acts as an adenosine receptor blocker, a neurological stimulant, and a phosphodiesterase inhibitor. It is a ventilator stimulant and has bronchoprotective properties. It causes diuresis and in toxic levels is known to cause dyselectrolytemia. Energy drinks are known not to have any nutritional benefits. Numerous additives are added to energy drinks that enhance the effect of caffeine, such as taurine, guarana, L-carnitine, ginseng, and yohimbine.

Higher Consumption of Calories, Carbohydrates, and Fats

Energy drinks are known to have increased levels of caffeine and guarana, which act as stimulants. Therefore, replacement of water with energy drinks and its frequent consumption leads to misbalance in the caloric, carbohydrate, and fat intake predisposing children to overweight and obesity. A positive association is seen with energy drinks consumption and consumption of other sweetened carbonated drinks thereby further increasing caloric intake and sugar consumption.[28]

Cardiovascular Effects

High caffeine content in energy drinks is known to have deleterious cardiovascular side effects due to its adenosine receptor blocking properties. Caffeine has cardiac chronotropic and inotropic effects and causes tachycardia and hypertension and in toxic doses can also lead to arrhythmias and hypotension. Increased intracellular concentration of calcium causes supraventricular and ventricular tachycardias, atrial fibrillation, and sudden cardiac arrest. Energy drinks contain additives such as taurine that add to the caffeine content worsening its cardiotoxic effects. Taurine has an inotropic action on cardiac muscle leading to coronary vasospasm. Other detrimental cardiac effects of energy drinks reported are acute coronary thrombosis, aortic aneurysm dissection, cardiomyopathy, heart failure, QT prolongation, ST segment elevation, and sudden cardiac death.[29,30]

Central Nervous System Manifestations

Energy drink overdose can lead to jitteriness, seizures, headaches, raised intracranial pressure, cerebral vasospasm, cerebral edema, hallucinations, stroke, rigidity, and altered sensorium. These are again attributed to high content of caffeine. Caffeine intoxication syndrome is characterized by nervousness, anxiety, insomnia, diarrhea, palpitations, tremors, tachycardia, and irritability.

Defective Bone Mineralization

Energy drinks containing high concentrations of caffeine lead to defective bone mineralization by interfering with the intestinal absorption of calcium.

Altered Sleep Pattern

Caffeine-containing energy drinks are known to alter the sleep pattern by reducing the percentage of time spent in deep sleep phase, and produces difficulty in sleeping and morning fatigue.

Psychiatric Disturbances and High-risk Behavior

Depression, suicidal tendencies, suicide attempts, and stress are some of the psychiatric manifestations associated with increased frequency of consumption of caffeinated energy drinks (CEDs). Energy drinks are known to cause instant mood elevations, therefore anyone dealing with severe stress has increased propensity for consumption of energy drinks due to its instant mood elevation effects, resulting in its toxicity and further worsening of mood. Fast food consumption with energy drinks has a synergistic effect on aggressive behavior, delinquency, and hyperactivity. This is attributed to its high sugar content, and food additives present in energy drinks along with lack of micronutrients and polyunsaturated fatty acids in fast foods.[30]

There is a positive association between frequency of energy drinks consumption and high-risk behavior, especially in the adolescent age group. Increased consumption of energy drinks is associated with alcohol addiction, marijuana, and tobacco smoking and addiction to many prescription drugs. There is a consistent association with energy drinks consumption with violent risk-taking behavior, especially in the adolescent age group, which can be extrapolated to younger population as well.[31]

Dental Erosions

Citric acid content of energy drinks and sports drinks makes its pH acidic leading to enamel demineralization causing dental erosions.[30]

Health Effects of Food Coloring Agents

Food coloring agents are dye molecules added as additives to foods to enhance its appeal, flavor, texture, and storage. They can be used as stabilizers, sweeteners, preservatives, and emulsifying agents. Some of the artificial food dyes approved by the Food and Drug Administration (FDA) are tartrazine, Allura red, erythrosine, brilliant blue, sunset yellow, and indigotine.[32] Some natural food coloring agents derived from plants and animal sources are used commonly in foods, textiles, and drugs. These include saffron, turmeric, grape skin extract, carotenoids, chlorophyll, and anthocyanin and are nontoxic in nature. In general, the artificial food dyes and coloring agents are known to have detrimental health effects. Food dyes are being used five times more than what they used to be in the past. Artificial food coloring agents are causing a public health hazard nowadays. Increased consumption is known to cause behavioral problems such as ADHD, irritability, restlessness, and sleep disorders. Other harmful effects, food coloring agents, are known to cause are allergic reactions, learning disorders, aggressive behavior, disturbed sleep patterns, memory loss, and depression. Chromosomal damage, lymphomas, brain tumor, and bladder tumors also have been reported.[33]

The harmful effects of JUNCS food, energy drinks, and dyes and food coloring agents are summarized in **Table 2.2**.

■ STRATEGIES TO REDUCE CONSUMPTION OF JUNK FOODS
Regulation on Consumption of Fast Food in Schools

Brazil has one of the oldest and largest foods and nutrition programs promoting good eating habits and improving students' nutritional status in all the public schools. To facilitate eating healthy habits, a law was passed (Lei no. 11.947) regarding funding at least 30% of federal school meals to purchase food directly from family farms, in addition to meeting students' nutritional needs during school hours.[33] This complements other programs that integrate health promotion into school activities and ensures access to healthy foods. In partnership with the Education Department, the "School Health Program"[34] has been implemented in public schools of around 50% of the Brazilian municipalities. A survey to study the impact of school meals on food consumption in 86,600 ninth-grade students in public and private schools of Brazil reported that 22.8% children consumed school meals regularly out of the 86,600 children enrolled; and concluded that regular consumption of school meals positively influenced the eating habits of ninth-grade students, promoting a healthy diet.[35]

The Government of Australia has developed policies in schools regulating healthy food options in school canteens. But extensive data is available reporting that a large number of school menus are not compliant with the policy and banned foods continue to be served in school canteens.[36] A study from Western Australia concluded that a majority of school canteens were not complying with the state or territory guidelines, especially the ones which were not regularly monitored.[37]

TABLE 2.2: Harmful effects of JUNCS foods, energy drinks, and food coloring agents.

JUNCS food	Energy drinks	Dyes/coloring agents

• *Metabolic*:
   – Obesity
   – Hypertension
   – Osteoporosis
   – Dyslipidemia
 • *Cardiometabolic biomarkers*:
   – Increased IL-6
   – Increased LDL-c
   – Increased adiponectin
   – Decreased HDL-c
   – Insulin resistance
 • *Psychological disorders*
   – ADHD
   – Violent behavior
   – Bullying
   – Physical fights
   – Oppositional disorders
 • *Hypertension*
	• Obesity/overweight
	 • *Cardiac*:
	   – Aortic aneurysm dissection
	   – Arrhythmias
	   – Tachycardia
	   – Hypertension
	   – Coronary vasospasm
	   – Acute coronary thrombosis
	   – Hypotension
	   – Cardiomyopathy
	   – Sudden cardiac death
	   – ST elevation
	   – QT prolongation
	 • *CNS*:
	   – Cerebral vasospasm
	   – Seizures
	   – Stroke
	   – Altered sensorium
	   – Headache
	   – Raised ICT
	   – Cerebral edema
	   – Tremors
	   – Irritability
	 • *Altered sleep pattern*
	 • *Dental erosions*
	 • *Psychiatric*:
	   – Depression
	   – Hallucinations
	   – High-risk behavior
	   – Suicidal tendencies
	   – Aggressive behavior
	   – Delinquency
	   – Hyperactivity
	 • *Defective bone mineralization*
		• Hypersensitivity
		 • Anaphylactic reactions
		 • Urticaria
		 • *Disturbed sleep pattern*
		 • *ADHD*
		 • *Malignancy*
		   – Lymphoma
		   – Brain tumors
		   – Bladder tumor
		 • *Aggressive behavior*
		 • *Learning disorders*
		 • *Hearing loss*
		 • *Genotoxicity*
		   – Frameshift mutation
		   – Chromosomal breakage
		   – DNA damage
		   – Base substitution
		   – Base pair mutation

(ADHD: attention deficit hyperactivity disorder; ICT: intracranial tension; IL-6: interleukin-6; LDL-c: low-density lipoprotein cholesterol; HDL-c: high-density lipoprotein cholesterol)

School salad bars are another initiative that promotes healthier eating options amongst school children. Michelle Obama in the United States in 2010 launched the "Let's Move Salad Bars to School" as a part of the "Let's move" movement.[38] This helps to raise awareness of having salad bars in school canteens to improve child nutrition.

A survey conducted in 18 Municipal Corporation of Delhi [MCD] schools,[39] private schools and government schools revealed that junk food was readily available around public schools as compared to others; half the students carry junk food in their lunch boxes every day and while majority (84.4%) of the students stated that their schools were taking measures to make them aware. Only 23% of the students said that healthy food was easily available in their school canteens. This led to the Delhi High Court setting a ban on the sale of junk food including sugar-sweetened, carbonated and noncarbonated beverages within the school or within 50 meters of its premises in 2015.[39]

Food Labeling

There is enough evidence to prove that nutrition labeling of food items helps consumers to make healthier choices at point of purchase. A systematic review on labeling regulations to examine the current scenario of food labeling in the country reported that food labeling regulations in India are at par to the developed countries, but consumers while making food choices rarely read the food labels. Perhaps, there is a need to evolve and experiment symbol-based labeling of foods in India.[40] A survey based on Delhi schoolchildren revealed that only 24.6% of children always looked at the content label, 46.5% children checked it sometime, and 28.8% never checked the label.[39] Numerous countries have different labeling systems such as the 'keyhole' symbol in Nordic countries, a "traffic light" labeling system in UK, "Health of Star Rating System" in Australia.[41-43]

Regulation of Advertisements

Unhealthy food choices are promoted by advertising JUNCS foods leading to obesity. 85% students at Delhi school reported that television (TV) was a major source of advertising junk food, followed by magazines (78.5%), internet (29.5%), and billboards in and around their schools (22%). Eighty-nine percent students also said that junk food advertising also creates a desire to consume them.[39] Systematic review and meta-analysis reported that food advertising on TV resulted in their increased intake amongst children.[44] Apart from TV, print media, and online portals (such as YouTube) significantly impacted its consumption and adversely affected the BMI. Evidence is available to prove that children perceive food item with licensed characters to taste better than those presented in plain packages.[45,46]

Taxes and Subsidies

To encourage healthy eating habits, the WHO has recommended a fiscal policy on levy taxation on unhealthy food. Pricing strategies can act as a promising intervention to effect dietary habits. Taxes on sugar-sweetened beverages (SSB) are associated with reductions in their purchases.[47,48]

Marketing

Marketing strategies directed to children, promotion using popular personalities, and premiums such as free toys all influence children's decision regarding purchase of advertised products. A possible role of licensed cartoon characters positively influencing the intake of traditionally healthy fruits and vegetables has been demonstrated in numerous studies. Therefore, it is suggested that food-branding cues can be used to promote healthy food intake because food branding does influence the eating behavior of children.[49,50]

■ STRATEGIES TO REDUCE CONSUMPTION OF ENERGY DRINKS

Marketing, Advertising, and Sales

Evidence supports precautionary approach of advertisement and marketing of CEDs in Canada and discourages use of alcohol mixed with energy drinks, especially among the adolescents. An online survey done on children and adults (12–24 years) to evaluate the exposure to energy drink marketing and educational messages that warn about the potential health risks of energy drinks reported that 80% of respondents saw energy drink marketing through at least one channel, most commonly TV (58.8%), posters or signs in a convenience or grocery store (48.5%), and online ads (45.7%). Overall, 32% of respondents reported ever seeing an educational message about energy drinks; and the most frequently reported sources of exposure were at school (16.2%), online (15.0%), and on TV (12.6%). Therefore, they concluded that despite regulations in Canada prohibiting the marketing of CEDs to children, CED advertisements are still perceived as targeting young people.[51]

Labeling

All CEDs sold in Canada must contain labels noting that they are "not recommended for children, pregnant/breastfeeding women." The American Beverage Association in 2014 published the "Guidance for the Responsible Labeling and Marketing of Energy Drinks," which allowed energy drinks companies to voluntarily commit to report total quantities of caffeine from all sources, to restrict marketing of energy drinks to children, and voluntarily report adverse events after consumption of energy drinks to the FDA. Studies have reported that energy drink consumers are sensitive to price and that adolescent energy drink consumers are sensitive to caffeine content and warning labels. This evidence could be used for formulation of potential regulations that may discourage energy drink purchasing, especially among adolescents.[52,53]

Restriction on Sales and Banning of Energy Drinks

Currently, there are no laws that restrict the sale of energy drinks in retail stores in Canada. Sales might indirectly be affected by policies promoting healthy lifestyles. For example, the Ontario Ministry of Education, as part of a comprehensive health policy for schools has restricted the sale of energy drinks. Liquor Control Board of Ontario does not sell energy drinks and has sponsored health-promoting literature for parents and guardians regarding health hazards of energy drinks and its harmful effects on mixing with alcohol. The Toronto City Council in 2011 adopted the policy of prohibiting the sales of energy drinks in vending machines at parks and recreational places. Many municipalities in Ontario, as a part of their municipal alcohol policy have specifically restricted the sale of energy drinks along with alcohol in events hosted on the municipal property. There is evidence to support consumption of inappropriate quantity of energy drinks in children and adolescents, but due to lack of scientific evidence, a statutory ban on sale of energy drinks is not justified. It also said that a voluntary approach is the quickest and most effective way of implementing change, rather than resorting to legislation.[51,54,55]

In India, the FSSAI had released draft regulations called Food Safety and Standards (safe food and healthy diets for school children) Regulation, 2019 which ensures a ban on selling junk food or food high in sugar, salt, or fats within and 50 meters around school premises with an aim to modify school campuses into "Eat right school campuses" promoting provision of safe and nutritious food and healthy eating. According to these guidelines, all vendors involved with manufacturing or selling of food products in and around 50 meters of school premises must be registered under the FSS Act and regular periodic inspection in schools would be conducted to check the quality and safety of food served in schools.[15]

The IAP Guidelines and Recommendation on Fast Food, Fruit Juice, and Energy Drinks in Children and Adolescents

Based on the review of evidence, the IAP came up with a consensus guidelines of fast food, fruit juice, and energy drinks in children and adolescents.[18] These are detailed in below (reproduced with permission from Indian Pediatrics. Originally published as IAP Guidelines on the Fast and Junk Foods, Sugar Sweetened Beverages, Fruit Juices, and Energy Drinks in Indian Pediatr.[18]

Guidelines for Children and Families

General recommendations:
- Avoid consumption of the JUNCS foods and beverages by all children and adolescents, as far as possible.

Junk and Ultra-processed Foods

- Alternatively, limit consumption of the JUNCS foods at home/outside and suggest having not more than one serving per week; serving not exceeding 50% of total daily energy intake for that age.
- Do not consume foods while watching TV screen.
- The Group endorses the WHO guidelines to eliminate trans fat and reduce free sugars to 5% of total energy intake.
- Traditional and acceptable home-made snacks with long shelf-line can be offered to children as alternative to the JUNCS foods.
- Freshly cooked home foods with minimal addition of sugar and no trans fats should be preferred over restaurant/packaged foods.
- Lunch boxes packed only with healthy food should be carried to school if school does not have provision of providing healthy mid-day meal.
- The JUNCS food should not be offered as reward/gift to any child as this gives undue promotion to unhealthy foods.

Fruit juices:
- Encourage intake of regional and seasonal whole fruits over fruit juices in children and adolescents.
- Fruit juices/fruit drinks/sugar, sweetened beverages (SSBs) should not be offered to infants and young children aged below 2 years.
- For children and adolescents (2–18 years) fruit juices, fruit drinks, and SSBs should be avoided as far as possible. Water should be encouraged as the best drink and should be promoted over fruit juices/drinks at home and school.
- Fruit juices/drinks, if given, should be limited to 125 mL per day for children aged between 2 and 5 years, and 250 mL per day for age >5 years; and these should preferably be given as fresh juices.

Caffeinated drinks:
- Caffeinated energy drinks should not be consumed by children and adolescents. Intake of carbonated drinks tea and coffee is to be completely avoided by children <5 years.
- In school-going children and adolescents, tea/coffee intake should be limited to maximum of half cup/day (100 mL) in 5–9 years, and one cup/day (200 mL) in adolescents (10–18 years), provided no other caffeinated products (cola, chocolates) are being consumed.

Policy Recommendations for Schools, Labeling, Advertising, and Marketing

Guidelines for schools:
- The Group supports Ministry of Women and Child Development recommendations of ban on sale of HFSS foods in school canteens and in near vicinity of 200 meters. We also suggest expanding these recommendations to all the JUNCS foods.

- Efforts to regulate availability of the JUNCS foods in schools must be coupled with ensuring availability and affordability of a variety of healthy snacks and foods in mid-day meals or school canteens.
- School authorities should ensure availability of safe and potable drinking water in schools to reduce consumption of SSBs.
- Ensuring ongoing support, provision of resources, monitoring, feedback, and recognition will help to increase the compliance of schools to provide healthy food to children.

Guidelines for labeling:
- We support and advocate traffic light coding of all packaged food as suggested by FSSAI. Labeling of nutritional content of packaged foods should be further strengthened.
- The Group also supports labeling "not suitable for children" and advocates addition of "adolescents" for unsuitability of CEDs.
- The Group supports traffic light coding of food available in school canteens (LOE 5), for their nutritional value, and advocates its extension to all packaged/ultra-processed foods in future.

Guidelines for Advertisements

- The Group agrees that advertising has strong impact on dietary intake. Advertisement of the JUNCS foods may lead to unhealthy food choices and is likely to be associated with increasing obesity.
- The Group recommends legal ban of screen/print/digital advertisements of all JUNCS foods for channels/magazines/websites/social media catering to children and adolescents through legislative measures.
- The Group recommends ban of branding and use of licensed characters for promoting fast foods/SSBs.
- Advertisements ridiculing healthy foods need to be legally banned.
- The Group also recommends screen/print/digital advertisements promoting healthy foods for channels catering to children and adolescents and use of licensed characters for branding and promoting healthy foods. Modalities for funding of same need to be explored.

Guidelines for marketing:
- The Group suggests providing tax discounts on healthy foods and beverages and regulation of discounts on large portions and multiple purchases of the JUNCS foods.
- Differential taxation on the JUNCS and healthy foods/beverages should be considered to promote healthy eating.
- Ensuring availability of variety of healthy food menu at markets/restaurants will give better options for public, thereby promoting healthy lifestyle.

- Steps should be taken to curb round the clock availability of the JUNCS food on order through mobile Apps.

Behavioral Change and Communication

- School-based interventions are more effective than home-based strategies. All schools should promote balanced diets and highlight adverse impacts of unhealthy foods in a structured curriculum.
- Nutrition education initiatives should be taken to increase awareness among school children. Schools should be motivated to organize poster-easy competitions, debates, etc., on adverse effects of the JUNCS foods, besides teaching about healthy and balanced diet.
- Parents should themselves follow healthy eating habits and serve as role models for children thereby providing them a nutrition-sensitive and enabling environment

■ KEY POINTS

- Junk food includes foods high in fat, sugars, and salts, lacking micronutrients and minerals. They also include carbonated, caffeinated drinks, and sugar-sweetened beverages.
- "JUNCS" foods cause hypertension, osteoporosis, dyslipidemia, and insulin resistance.
- Energy and carbonated drinks lead to cardiac arrhythmias, coronary vasospasm, acute coronary thrombosis, and sudden cardiac death. They are a risk factor for causing stroke, seizures, raised ICT and cerebral vasospasms. Altered sleep patterns, psychiatric disorders, and dental erosions are some harmful effects caused by them.
- The IAP recommends avoidance of consumption of JUNCS foods and beverages by all children and adolescents, as far as possible.
- The IAP also recommends limiting consumption of JUNCS foods to not more than one serving per week, serving not exceeding 50% of total daily energy intake for that age.
- Eating while watching screen/television is not recommended.
- The IAP also recommends that fruit juices/fruit drinks/SSBs should not be offered to infants and young children aged below 2 years, and intake of regional and seasonal fruits must be encouraged over fruit juice.
- The IAP also recommends against intake of carbonated drinks, tea, and coffee in children <5 years.
- A healthy eating home atmosphere promotes a nutrition-sensitive and enabling environment for children.

■ REFERENCES

1. Fast Food FACTS. (2021). Fast food advertising: Billions in spending, continued high exposure by youth. [online] Available from: https://www.fastfoodmarketing.org › media. [Last accessed December, 2021].
2. National Family Health Survey. (2020). National Family Health Survey-5. [online] Available from: rchiips.org/nfhs/NFHS-5_FCTS/FactSheet_DD.pdf. [Last accessed December, 2021].

3. Dubois L, Farmer A, Girard M, Peterson K. Regular sugar-sweetened beverage consumption between meals increases risk of overweight among preschool-aged children. J Am Diet Assoc. 2007;107:924-34.
4. National Health Mission. (2018). Comprehensive Nation Nutrition Survey (2016-2018). [online] Available from: https://nhm.gov.in/WriteReadData/l892s/1405796031571201348.pdf. [Last accessed December, 2021].
5. Definition of FAST FOOD in the Cambridge English Dictionary. [online] Available from: https://dictionary.cambridge.org/us/dictionary/english/fast-food. [Last accessed December, 2021].
6. Definition of fast food. [online] Available from: https://www.merriam-webster.com/dictionary/fast-food. [Last accessed December, 2021].
7. Khurana A, Dhangar I. In: Banerjee S (ed). Junk food targeted at children. New Delhi: Centre for Science and Environment; 2014.
8. Ministry of Women & Child Development. (2015). The Report of Working Group on Addressing Consumption of Foods High in Fat, Salt and Sugar (HFSS) and Promotion of Healthy Snacks in Schools of India. [online] Available from: https://wcd.nic.in/acts/report-working-group-addressing-consumption-foods-high-fat-salt-and-sugar-hfss-and-promotion. [Last accessed December, 2021].
9. Furbish LK. (2003). Nutritious and non-nutritious food definitions. [online] Available from: https://www.cga.ct.gov/2003/rpt/2003-R-0224.htm. [Last accessed December, 2021].
10. Dahl WJ, Foster L. Energy and nutrient density. [online] Available from: https://edis.ifas.ufl.edu/publication/FS176. [Last accessed December, 2021].
11. Nicklas TA, O'Neil CE, Mendoza J, Liu Y, Zakeri IF, Berenson GS. Are energy dense diets also nutrient dense? J Am Coll Nutr. 2008;27:553-60.
12. Cerefoodlabs. (2021). What is the new "Junk" Food Law in India? [online] Available from: https://ceresfoodlabs.com/what-is-the-new-junk-food-law-in-india/. [Last accessed December, 2021].
13. Monteiro CA, Cannon G, Moubarac J-C, Levy RB, Louzada MLC, Jaime PC. The UN Decade of Nutrition, the NOVA food classification and the trouble with ultra-processing. Public Health Nutr. 2018;21:5-17.
14. Kowsalya T, Parimalavalli R. Categorisation of junk foods based on nutrient profiling model of UK and cut-off criteria of India. PSGCAS Search: A Journal of Science and Technology. 2016;4(2):2349-5456.
15. Food Safety and Standards Authority of India. (2020). FSSAI Regulation 2020. [online] Available from: https://fssai.gov.in/cms/food-safety-and-standards-regulations.php. [Last accessed December, 2021].
16. Maindola A. (2019). FSSAI decides to delink front-of-pack labelling norms from general ones. . [online] Available from: http://www.fnbnews.com/Top-News/fssai-decides-to-delink-frontofpack-labelling-regns-from-general-ones-53549. [Last accessed December, 2021].
17. UK Food labelling resource. [online] Available from: https://natashas-law.com/. [Last accessed December, 2021].
18. Gupta P, Shah D, Kumar P, Bedi N, Mittal HG, Mishra K, et al. Pediatric And Adolescent Nutrition Society (Nutrition Chapter) of Indian Academy of Pediatrics. Indian Academy of Pediatrics Guidelines on the fast and junk foods, sugar sweetened beverages, fruit juices, and energy drinks. Indian Pediatr. 2019;56:849-63.

19. Goon S, Bipasha MS, Islam MS. Fast food consumption and obesity risk among university students of Bangladesh. Eur J Prev Med. 2014;2:99-104.
20. Asgary S, Nazari B, Sarrafzadegan N, Parkhideh S, Saberi S, et al. Evaluation of fatty acid content of some Iranian fast foods with emphasis on trans fatty acids. Asia Pac J Clin Nutr. 2009;18:187-92.
21. Kaushik JS, Narang M, Parakh A. Fast food consumption in children. Indian Pediatr. 2011;48:95-101.
22. Kennedy A, Spiers JP, Crowley V, Williams E, Lithander FE. Postprandial adiponectin and gelatinase response to a high-fat versus an isoenergetic low-fat meal in lean, healthy men. Nutrition. 2015;31:863-70.
23. Isganaitis E, Lustig RH. Fast Food, central nervous system insulin resistance, and obesity. Arterioscler Thromb Vasc Biol. 2005;25:2451-62.
24. Shang X, Li Y, Liu A, Zhang Q, Hu X, Du S, *et al.* Dietary pattern and its association with the prevalence of obesity and related cardiometabolic risk factors among Chinese children. PLoS One. 2012;7(8):e43183.
25. Payab M, Kelishadi R, Qorbani M, Motlagh ME, Ranjbar SH, Ardalan G, *et al.* Association of junk food consumption with high blood pressure and obesity in Iranian children and adolescents: the CASPIAN-IV Study. J Pediatr (Rio J). 2015;91:196-205.
26. Xu H, Sun Y, Wan Y, Zhang S, Xu H, Yang R, et al. Eating pattern and psychological symptoms: A cross-sectional study based on a national large sample of Chinese adolescents. J Affect Disord. 2019;244:155-63.
27. Jacka FN, Mykletun A, Berk M, Bjelland I, Tell GS. The association between habitual diet quality and the common mental disorders in community-dwelling adults: the Hordaland Health study. Psychosom Med. 2011;73:483-90.
28. Field AE, Sonneville KR, Falbe J, Flint A, Haines J, Rosner B, et al. Association of sports drinks with weight gain among adolescents and young adults. Obesity (Silver Spring). 2014;22:2238-43.
29. Mangi MA, Rehman H, Rafique M, Illovsky M. Energy drinks and the risk of cardiovascular disease: A review of current literature. Cureus. 2017;9:e1322.
30. Seifert SM, Schaechter JL, Hershorin ER, Lipshultz SE. Health effects of energy drinks on children, adolescents, and young adults. Pediatrics. 2011;127:511-28.
31. Arria AM, Caldeira KM, Kasperski SJ, O'Grady KE, Vincent KB, Griffiths RR, et al. Increased alcohol consumption, nonmedical prescription drug use, and illicit drug use are associated with energy drink consumption among college students. J Addict Med. 2010;4:74-80.
32. Kobylewski S, Jacobson MF. Toxicology of food dyes. Int J Occup Environ Health. 2012;18:220-46.
33. DiasIsis PC, de Oliveira Barbosa R, Barbosa RMS, Ferreira DM, Kamilla Carla Bertu Soares KCB, da Silva Bastos Soares D, Henriques P, et al. Purchases from family agriculture for school feeding in Brazilian capitals. REVISTA DE SAÚDE PÚBLICA. 2020;54.
34. Jaime PC, da Silva ACF, Gentil PC, Claro RM, Monteiro CA. Brazilian obesity prevention and control initiatives. Obes Rev. 2013;14:88-95.
35. Locatelli NT, Canella DS, Bandoni DH. Positive influence of school meals on food consumption in Brazil. Nutrition. 2018;53:140-4.
36. Chandrika UG, Prasad Kumarab PA. Gotu Kola (Centella asiatica): Nutritional properties and plausible health benefits. Adv Food Nutr Res. 2015;76:125-57.

37. Woods J, Bressan A, Langelaan C, Mallon A, Palermo C. Australian school canteens: menu guideline adherence or avoidance? Health Promot J Austr. 2014;25:110-5.
38. Harris DM, Seymour J, Grummer-Strawn L, Cooper A, Collins B, DiSogra L, et al. Let's move salad bars to schools: A public–private partnership to increase student fruit and vegetable consumption. Child Obes. 2012;8:294-7.
39. Delhi High court orders curb on junk food sale in school all over India. [online] Available from: https://www.downtoearth.org.in/news/delhi-high-court-orders-curb-on-junk-food-sale-in-schools-across-india-49038. [Last accessed December, 2021].
40. Indian Council of Medical Research. (2009). Assessment of current scenario of food labelling in India: NIN Annual Report (2009-2010). [online] available from: https://www.nin.res.in/annualreports/AnnualReport_2009-10.pdf. [Last accessed 2021]. .
41. Nordic Council of Ministers. The keyhole: Healthy Choices Made Easy. [online] Available from: http://norden.diva-portal.org/smash/get/diva2:700822/FULLTEXT01.pdf. [Last accessed December, 2021].
42. Food Standards Agency. (2013). Front-of-pack nutrition labelling. [online] Available from: https://www.foodstandards.gov.scot/downloads/Front_of_pack_nutrition_labelling_joint_responses.pdf. [Last accessed December, 2021].
43. Australia Food News. (2013). Australian ministers approve front-of-pack labeling system but dairy products approach still to be finalized. [online] Available from: www.ausfoodnews.com.au/2013/06/17/australian-ministers-approve-front-of-pack-labellingsystem-but-dairy-products-approach-still-to-be-finalised.html. [Last accessed December, 2021].
44. Russell SJ, Croker H, Viner RM. The effect of screen advertising on children's dietary intake: A systematic review and meta-analysis. Obes Rev. 2019;20:554-68.
45. Manganello JA, Smith KC Sudakow K, Summers AC. A content analysis of food advertisements appearing in parenting magazines. Public Health Nutr. 2013;16:2188-96.
46. Swinburn B, Kraak V, Rutter H, Vandevijvere S, Lobstein T, Sacks G, et al. Strengthening of accountability systems to create healthy food environments and reduce global obesity. Lancet. 2015;385:2534-45.
47. World Health Organization. (2008). 2008–2013 action plan for the global strategy for the prevention and control of noncommunicable diseases. [online] Available from: https://www.who.int/bulletin/volumes/88/8/09-070987/en/. [Last accessed December, 2021].
48. Thow AM, Jan S, Leeder S, Swinburn B. The effect of fiscal policy on diet, obesity and chronic disease: a systematic review. Bull World Health Organ. 2010;88:609-14.
49. Brand JE. Television advertising to children: a review of contemporary research on the influence of television advertising directed to children. Canberra: Australian Communications and Media Authority, Commonwealth of Australia; 2007.
50. Keller KL, Kuilema LG, Lee N, Yoon J, Mascaro B, Combes A-L, et al. The impact of food branding on children's eating behavior and obesity. Physiol Behav. 2012;106:379-86.

51. Toronto Public Health. (2017). Caffeinated Energy Drinks. Technical Report on Public Health Concerns and Regulation in Canada. [online] Available from: https://www.toronto.ca/legdocs/mmis/2017/hl/bgrd/backgroundfile-101646.pdf. [Last accessed December, 2021].
52. Heckman MA, Sherry K, De Mejia EG. Energy drinks: an assessment of their market size, consumer demographics, ingredient profile, functionality, and regulations in the United States. Compr Rev Food Sci Food Saf. 2010; 9:303-17.
53. Temple JL, Ziegler AM, Epstein LH. Influence of Price and Labeling on Energy Drink Purchasing in an Experimental Convenience Store. J Nutr Educ Behav. 2015;48:54-9.
54. City of Toronto (Government Management Committee). GM2.16 Healthy Vending Criteria - Cold Drink Vending Request for Proposal (Ward: All). [online] Available from: http://app.toronto.ca/tmmis/viewAgendaItemDetails.do?function=getMinutesItemPreview&agendaItemId=28764. [Last accessed December, 2021].
55. UK Parliament. (2018). Energy Drinks inquiry launched.[online] Available from: https://committees.parliament.uk/committee/135/science-and-technology-committee/news/100907/energy-drinks-inquiry-launched/. [Last accessed December, 2021].

Infectious Diseases

CHAPTER 3: SARS-CoV-2 Infection

Dhiren Gupta, Ashish Kumar Simalti

■ INTRODUCTION

Coronavirus has been drawing global attention since 2019 and is not a new species of virus. Even before the coronavirus disease-2019 (COVID-19) pandemic, almost 15–30% of the cases of common cold could be attributed to four different strains of coronaviruses.[1] This virus was first described in 1931 and it was labeled as *infectious bronchitis virus* (IBV). Besides being a common infectious agent causing common cold, it was not considered to be an important pathogen, but since 2003 new strains of coronavirus have been detected which were responsible for severe acute respiratory distress syndrome (SARS) and Middle East respiratory syndrome (MERS)[2] **(Fig. 3.1)**. The current ongoing pandemic of COVID-19 is caused by a novel strain of coronavirus, which has been labeled by World Health Organization (WHO) as SARS-CoV-2.

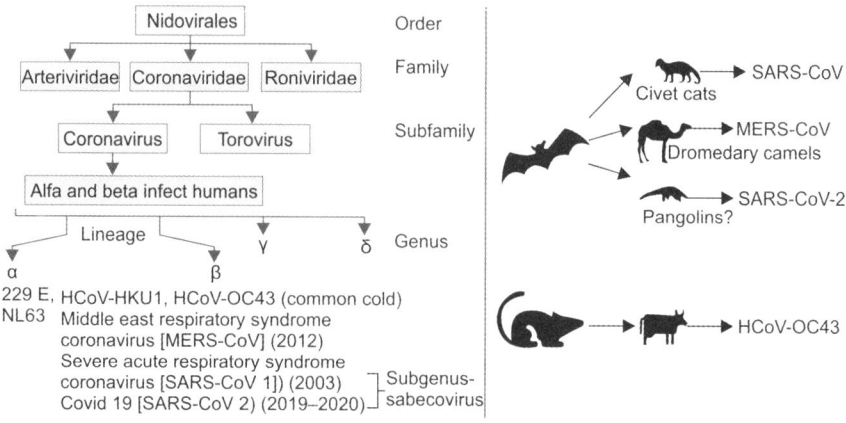

Fig. 3.1: Types of coronavirus and their modes of spread.

■ EPIDEMIOLOGY

The Global Burden

Coronavirus was first considered as a threat to public health in 2003 when it was found to be responsible for SARS; this strain was designated as SARS-CoV-1. The coronavirus responsible for MERS in 2012 was designated as MERS-CoV. The first case of virus (pneumonia), which later evolved into COVID-19 pandemic originated from Wuhan, China in December 2019. Although the origin of this strain is not clear, epidemiological investigations have linked the primary source of infection to a seafood and animal wholesale market. Because of the interconnected nature of world, this disease spread rapidly all over the continents. At the time of writing this article there were more than 233 million confirmed cases with almost 5 million deaths.

The Indian Scenario

India reported its first case on January 30, 2020 in a returnee from Wuhan, China.[3] Over the next few months many more travelers from affected countries returned to India and introduced this virus to all the states. Cases started increasing in March 2020; surge in cases has been periodic in India with the peak of first wave continuing till November 2020. After a significant dip during the first few months of 2021, cases rose again from April 2021. This was designated as second wave of COVID-19 and this time a mutant of the original virus, the delta variant was the predominant strain. Around 33 million cases were confirmed in India and 5 lakh deaths were reported till 30 September 2021.

■ ETIOLOGY

Coronavirus belongs to the *Coronaviridae* family of the order *Nidovirales*. *Corona* means "crown" or "wreath" in Latin. On electron microscopy there are large, bulbous surface projections on the surface of this virus, giving the appearance of a "crown", because of which the name "coronavirus" was given. There are around 45 species of these viruses identified so far, which are grouped into four genera, *alphacoronavirus, betacoronavirus, gammacoronavirus* and *deltacoronavirus*.

Coronaviruses are enveloped viruses with round and sometimes pleomorphic virions of approximately 80–120 nm in diameter. **Figure 3.2** depicts the structure of coronavirus. Coronaviruses contain one of the largest known RNA genomes with size between 27 and 32 kb. This genome encodes four or five structural proteins—the spike (S), envelop (E), membrane (M), hemagglutinin-esterase (HE) and nucleocapsid (N). The characteristic spikes of coronavirus are formed by S protein, which binds with membrane of the host cell and allows entry into the cell. SARS-CoV-2 differs from other coronaviruses in having cleavage site in its spike, which may have a role in the increased infectivity of

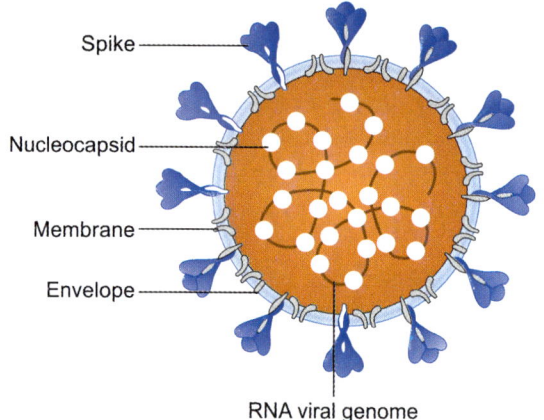

Fig. 3.2: Structure of coronavirus. (SARS-CoV-2 structure)

this virus. The spike protein changes its configuration after fusion leading to membrane fusion. The type of spike determines which host coronavirus can infect and the type of tissue it can get access to. Same spikes are also relevant for immunity, as they contain major antigens used by host cells as targets for cytotoxic lymphocytes and also stimulate neutralizing antibody.

■ VIRAL TRANSMISSION

Coronaviruses are widespread among mammals and birds. In fact, this virus was first reported as a causative agent behind respiratory infection among chickens. Bats are hosts to many different genotypes. One of them is the bat-origin SARS-like coronavirus, which may have mutated into SARS-CoV-2, the strain responsible for COVID-19. How the strain first got transmitted to humans is not clear but as of now the only proven mode of transmission is from human to human.

The principal *mode of transmission* is through respiratory droplets. Exposure occurs through inhalation, deposition of infected droplets on mucous membranes (eyes, mouth and nose) by direct splashes and sprays, or through contaminated hands touching mucous membranes. Droplet transmission is usually limited to a closer range up to 6 feet but in enclosed spaces with inadequate ventilation people at distances beyond 6 feet have also been affected leading to suspicion that the virus may also be airborne. Therefore, airborne precautions should be practiced whenever there is risk of transmission through aerosol generation.[4]

Experiments have shown that virus can be viable up to 28 days at 20°C on glass, stainless steel, and paper.[5] Infectivity reduces as temperature increases from 20 to 40°C. These studies are based on experimental models; therefore applicability in actual condition is doubtful and the main mode of transmission seems to be through air only.

■ PATHOGENESIS

Before COVID-19, human coronaviruses were associated with common cold. Two prototype variants were OC43 and 229E. Although they have not been known to cause any serious illness, their role in some illnesses such as multiple sclerosis and hepatitis was speculated.[6] They have also been documented to cause neonatal enteritis.[7]

As mentioned earlier, the spikes of virus get attached to specific cellular receptors and undergo conformational change resulting in fusion between the viral and host cell membranes. The entry receptors in host cells are angiotensin converting enzyme-2 (ACE2) and cluster of differentiation 147 transmembrane spike protein (CD147-SP, also known as basigin or EMMPRIN) and the tissue tropism toward alveolar cells is because of abundant expression of ACE2 receptors in alveolar cells. Dendritic-cell specific intercellular adhesion molecule-3-grabbing nonintegrin (DC-SIGN) is another target of attachment for SARS-CoV-2 virus, which is highly expressed in immune cells of lungs. Nucleocapsid of virus gains entry into the cell, which leads to production of multiple viral specific enzymatic activities essential for metabolism of coronavirus RNA as well as in interfering with the host cell activities.[8]

The pathogenesis of COVID-19 can be divided in two phases—viral replication and hyperactivity of immune system leading to pulmonary destruction characterized by proliferation of epithelial cells and macrophages and alveolar damage. This concept of two phases of pathogenesis has implication on the treatment and is shown in **Figure 3.3**.

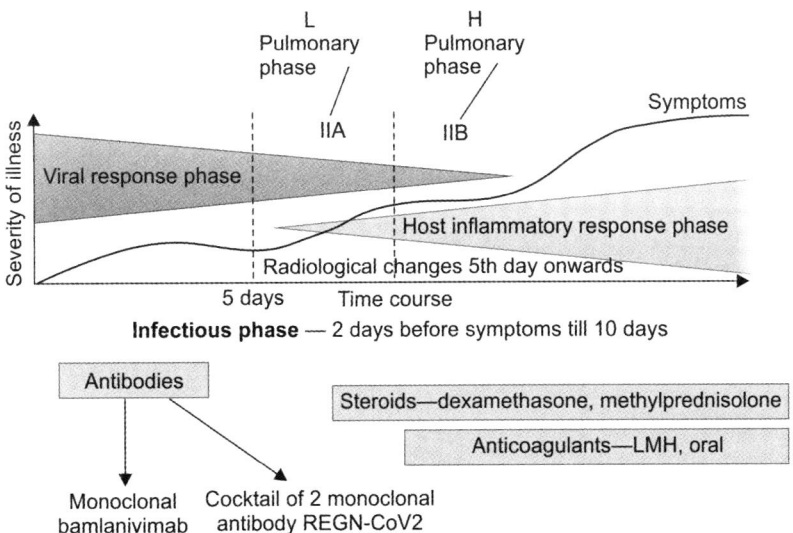

Fig. 3.3: Two phases of coronavirus infection and their implication on treatment. (H: high elastase type; L: low elastase type; LMH: low molecular weight heparin; REGN-CoV2: a combination of two monoclonal antibodies)

Coronavirus infection is associated with multinucleate giant cell infiltrates of macrophage or epithelial origin producing syncytium-like formation. Stimulated alveolar macrophages release many proinflammatory cytokines. The presence of lymphopenia and hemophagocytosis suggests cytokine dysregulation. Interestingly SARS-CoV also replicates in enterocytes but does not disrupt intestinal architecture. The mechanism of this lack of destruction could be antiapoptotic host cellular response and upregulation of transforming growth factor-β.[9] COVID-19 is associated with extrapulmonary dissemination, which causes viral shedding in urine, stool and sweat besides respiratory secretions.

Among unexposed hosts, the response is that of an innate immunity response, rather than a specific immune activity against coronavirus. Innate immune cells in lungs are dendritic cells (DCs) and macrophages, which travel to lymph node and act as antigen presenting cell (APC) to lymphocytes. Stimulation of lymphocytes leads to release of proinflammatory cytokines such as interleukin (IL)-6 and IL-10. Endothelial cells, which make one-third of lung cells, get damaged leading to increased permeability, thrombosis, and pulmonary embolism. Clinical consequence of this is pneumonia or acute respiratory distress syndrome (ARDS).[10] Increased gene expressions of fibrinogen gamma chain, fibroblast growth factor, and serin proteases induced by this virus, lead to upregulation of coagulation cascade factors generating a procoagulable state. Widespread pulmonary thrombosis and near normal lung compliance are unusual features of this disease as compared to classic ARDS.[11] Most of the symptoms after first week can be attributed to immune dysregulation fueled by viral debris.

■ CLINICAL FEATURES

Incubation Period

Incubation period ranges from 2 to 11 days depending on the viral load, host factors such as age and comorbidities.[12] Mean incubation period was found to be 5.1 days, at Wuhan with almost 97.5% of individuals developing symptoms within 11.5 days of acquiring infection.

General Features

COVID-19 infection in most cases presents either as an asymptomatic infection or mild flu-like illness. Fever, cough, malaise, headache and myalgia are the common symptoms at this stage. At this stage, it is not possible to clinically distinguish COVID-19 from other viral illness although some features such as loss of smell and taste are more common with COVID-19. According to initial surveys approximately 10–15% of infected cases may have severe illness.[13]

Some of the *predisposing factors* identified for severe illness include male sex, old age and comorbidities such as diabetes mellitus, hypertension and obesity. Blood group A has also been associated with increased risk of respiratory failure.[14] The second wave occurred due to the delta strain, which had the capability of more airborne spread as well as predilection toward younger age group.

Pulmonary Involvement

SARS-CoV-2 virus shows tissue tropism toward the alveoli and pneumonia is the most common presentation in severe COVID-19. Pneumonia can rapidly progress to ARDS as defined by hypoxia and chest X-ray findings. ARDS associated with COVID-19 can be classified into two categories—high elastase type (H) or classical ARDS and low elastase type (L) type in which compliance is not very low but hypoxia is present due to increased alveolar arterial oxygen gradient. In L type of ARDS, anti-inflammatory and antithrombotic therapy is more important than invasive ventilation.[15]

Extrapulmonary Symptoms

Coagulopathy

Marked inflammation and endothelial damage constitute a prothrombotic stage presenting as deep vein thrombosis, pulmonary embolism and catheter-related thrombosis. Besides these macrothrombotic events, alveolar capillary microthrombi are very common and contribute to refractory hypoxia.

Cardiac Involvement

SARS-CoV-2 infection can affect heart directly or indirectly due to hypoxia or thrombotic complications. The cardiovascular manifestations include acute coronary syndromes, myocardial damage, cardiomyopathy, cor pulmonale and cardiogenic shock. Cardiac arrhythmias such as new-onset atrial fibrillation, ventricular arrhythmias or heart block can present at any stage of illness and require vigilance.[16]

Neurological Involvement

COVID-19 can present with nonspecific symptoms related to neurological system such as headache, dizziness, myalgia, fatigue, anorexia, anosmia (loss of smell) and ageusia (loss of taste). The most serious neurological involvement can be in the form of stroke or coma. Other reported neurological sequelae include hemorrhagic posterior reversible encephalopathy, Guillain-Barré syndrome, meningoencephalitis, and acute necrotizing encephalopathy. Neurological involvement can either be because of neuroinvasion by the virus or could be secondary to systemic disorders such as hypoxia, coagulopathy, etc., as shown in **Flowchart 3.1**.

Other Systems

Other extrapulmonary manifestations include acute kidney injury, gastrointestinal (GI) symptoms such as anorexia, nausea, vomiting, diarrhea

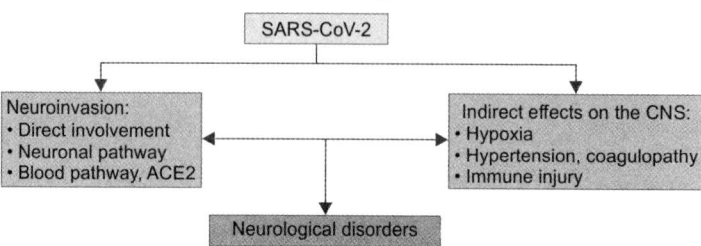

Flowchart 3.1: Mechanism of neurological involvement in coronavirus.

and abdominal pain, dermatological manifestations such as erythematous rash, urticaria and vesicles resembling varicella infection.[17]

Multisystem Inflammatory Syndrome in Children

In case of a child presenting with fever, pain abdomen and rash one must consider multisystem inflammatory syndrome in children (MIS-C), or pediatric multisystem inflammatory syndrome temporally associated with SARS-CoV-2 (PIMS-TS). MIS-C is an aberrant immune response, which is associated with cardiac dysfunction.[18] Clinical features of MIS-C include fever, erythema of tongue and oral mucosa, conjunctival congestion and rash, which are similar to Kawasaki disease (KD) and toxic shock syndrome (TSS). Unlike KD, the coronary aneurysm is not a common complication of MIS-C, but these children may develop shock because of reduced ejection fraction.

■ DIFFERENTIAL DIAGNOSIS

Initial phase of fever, cough and myalgia is indistinguishable from other viral fevers and COVID-19 can be diagnosed only by investigations based on local epidemiology. Loss of taste or smell and development of dyspnea after the onset of initial symptoms are suggestive of COVID-19. Pulmonary involvement resembles other causes of infectious pneumonia and ARDS. Differentiating features are refractory hypoxia despite relatively preserved lung compliance. Another issue is the incidental presence of antibodies post-epidemic because of high seroprevalence in a patient presenting with another illness. Clinicians need to exercise their judgment before labeling a child as MIS-C in such situations.

Differential Diagnosis for MIS-C

In children MIS-C needs to be differentiated from KD and TSS. The differentiating features of various symptoms and signs of COVID-19 include the following:
- *Fever with rash*: Scarlet fever, toxic shock syndrome, dengue fever, KD
- *Fever with early multiple organ dysfunction syndrome (MODS)*: Scrub typhus, dengue, leptospirosis

- *Fever with shock*: Septic shock (staphylococcal), gram-negative sepsis, enteric fever
- *Fever with eye congestion*: Adenovirus, KD, leptospirosis
- *Fever with abdominal catastrophe*: Diabetic ketoacidosis (DKA), appendicitis, pancreatitis
- *Viral myocarditis*: Infection due to Epstein-Barr virus, cytomegalovirus, adenovirus, enteroviruses
- *Cutaneous manifestations with systemic illness*: Systemic lupus erythematosus (SLE), other vasculitis.

INVESTIGATIONS

Investigations to Confirm Diagnosis

Reverse Transcription Polymerase Chain Reaction

Nucleic acid amplification testing (NAAT) with reverse transcription polymerase chain reaction (RT-PCR) targeting coronavirus RNA in respiratory secretions is currently the gold standard test for diagnosis. In this test two genes are targeted. One is a generic coronavirus gene while the other gene is specific for SARS-CoV-2 virus. The turnaround time is usually less than 24 hours.

Cycle threshold (Ct) value is reported along with positive report, which gives estimation for the viral load. This value suggests number of cycles required to detect virus RNA. Higher the viral load, lesser the number of cycles required thus, low Ct value indicates high infectivity, which is usually present during the early stage of infection. Ct values should not be used to make treatment decisions, as these are not standardized and vary depending on the platform used for RT-PCR test and its use has not been validated in any management protocol.

Sensitivity of the test also depends on the sample. Bronchoalveolar lavage (BAL) sample has the highest sensitivity (95%) as compared to samples from nasopharyngeal swab (50%) and oropharyngeal swab (30%). Nasal swabs should not be used as they have very low sensitivity (20%).

Point-of-care testing for NAATs has become available but its sensitivity is lower than the conventional test.[19]

Rapid Antigen Tests

RT-PCR test is the gold standard but because of delay in results, it cannot be used for screening in an emergency. For rapid diagnosis of COVID-19 a rapid antigen test (RAT) has been available since May 2020. It is performed as a point-of-care test with results being available within 15 minutes. Positive report can be taken as SARS-CoV-2 infection, but, as RAT is not a very sensitive test and negative antigen tests should be confirmed by

RT-PCR. In case of nonavailability of RT-PCR, Center for Disease Control and Prevention (CDC), USA suggests repeating RAT every 3–7 days for 14 days to label it negative.

Antibody Test

Serologic tests to detect antibodies against SARS-CoV-2 have been validated in identification of previous SARS-CoV-2 infection or current infection, if symptomatic for more than 3–4 weeks but antibody tests are not recommended for diagnosis in a symptomatic patient.[10] Enzyme-linked immunosorbent assay (ELISA), lateral flow assay and chemiluminescence enzyme immunoassays (CLIA) are the techniques used to detect antibodies. The main use of antibody testing is to diagnose MIS-C in pediatric population and for seroprevalence studies among asymptomatic population. According to Infectious Diseases Society of America (IDSA), IgG or total antibody tests are preferred over IgM antibody, because of their better accuracy.[20]

Computed Tomography Scan of Chest

Computed tomography (CT) scans of chest for evaluation of a breathless patient may be performed when RT-PCR report is awaited. Subpleural ground glass opacities in a patient with pneumonia are considered specific to COVID pneumonia. Ground glass opacities, consolidation, crazy-paving pattern, and fibrosis are commonly seen. A CT score based on the extent of lobar involvement has been validated to correlate with laboratory findings and disease severity. However, because of the cost and radiation, CT scan is not recommended to be used as screening tool.

Investigations Related to Management

In a confirmed case of COVID-19 pneumonia investigations are required to monitor the stage of the disease and make decisions related to management. These tests include:

- *Complete blood count (CBC) with differential lymphocyte count.* Neutrophil and lymphocyte ratio (NLR) more than 4 is associated with severe disease. In MIS-C, children may show neutrophilia with platelet counts ranging from normal or low unlike KD where platelet counts tend to be high.
- Elevated *D-Dimer* levels suggest ongoing coagulopathy.
- *Prothrombin time (PT), partial thromboplastin time (PTT) and fibrinogen* should also be monitored for assessing coagulation function.
- Monitoring levels of *C-reactive protein (CRP), erythrocyte sedimentation rate (ESR), IL-6 and ferritin* can quantify ongoing inflammation.
- Assessment of cardiac status:
  - *Troponin-I* levels may be elevated in case of cardiac involvement.

- *Electrocardiograph (ECG)* for arrhythmia and *echocardiography* for assessing ejection fraction should be performed as indicated.
- *Echocardiography* would also be needed to look for early signs of coronary artery dilatation while managing a patient with MIS-C.

■ MANAGEMENT
General Aspects

Most of the patients with COVID-19 infection do not require more than supportive care consisting of antipyretics and hydration like any other viral fever. Patients are advised isolation either at home or a quarantine center. Patient or caregiver should monitor temperature and oxygen saturation with a pulse oximeter daily. Patient should be able to contact medical facility in case of warning signs such as dyspnea or drop in oxygen saturation.

Oxygen

Hypoxia is the main cause of death in COVID-19 pneumonia and oxygen forms the mainstay of therapy. Oxygen delivery devices include nasal prongs, facemask and nonrebreathing facemasks in ascending order of oxygen requirement. Awake-proning or lying-in prone position helps in improving oxygenation.[11] High-flow nasal oxygen (HFNO) and noninvasive ventilation (NIV) with mask are the next steps in escalation. Widespread use of HFNO is limited by its availability and the high volume of oxygen required. These modes of oxygen delivery are associated with a risk of airborne transmission hence suitable precautions related to airborne transmission should be in place.

Mechanical Ventilation

Patients suffering from respiratory failure and refractory hypoxemia may need invasive ventilation. Overall experience with invasive ventilation in severe COVID-19 pneumonia has not been very encouraging.[21] Lung-protective strategies should be followed during invasive ventilation. Prone positioning helps in improving oxygenation. Extracorporeal membrane oxygenation (ECMO) where available can be tried as next step in refractory cases of hypoxia.

Steroids

Steroids could impact ARDS by modifying systemic immune responses. Downregulation of the inflammation leads to an improvement in alveolar-capillary membrane permeability and also improves tissue repair. The RECOVERY trial showed survival benefit with dexamethasone. Dose of dexamethasone used in the RECOVERY trial was 6 mg once daily for 10 days.[22]

These observations suggest that all patients with hypoxia should be given steroids as they may benefit. Theoretically, methylprednisolone has quicker onset and a shorter duration of action compared to the dexamethasone. However care should be taken, as steroids are associated with many complications including predisposition to secondary bacterial infection.

Anticoagulation

Besides steroids the only other pharmacological intervention with significant benefit from mortality is therapeutic anticoagulation in high-risk individuals.[23] All patients with dyspnea, tachypnea, oxygen saturation below 90%, and laboratory findings of elevated CRP, D-dimer and fibrinogen levels are at high risk for thrombosis. Anticoagulation strategies should be considered only when indicated. European Society of Cardiology recommends parenteral heparin in intensive care units (ICU) with the goal of keeping active prothromboplastin time (APPT) between 60 to 85 seconds. The more commonly used intervention is subcutaneous low molecular weight heparin in a dose of 1 mg/kg twice a day. Point-of-care ultrasound should be used to monitor deep venous thrombosis.[24]

Antiviral Agents

At the beginning of pandemic, many available antiviral agents including antiretroviral drugs such as lopinavir and ritonavir were tried in COVID-19 pneumonia, but without any benefit. Similarly, many antiparasitic agents and antibiotics such as hydroxychloroquine, ivermectin and azithromycin were also evaluated, but no benefit either in prophylaxis or management could be proven. Remdesivir has shown some statistically insignificant benefit in a randomized control trial (RCT) in hypoxic patients but not in those requiring invasive ventilation.[25] It should ideally be given to hypoxic patients before they require ventilation. Pediatric dose of remdesivir is 5 mg/kg on first day followed by 2.5 mg/kg daily for 5 days.

Immunomodulation

Very high levels of IL-6 in some of the patients led to the introduction of anti-IL-6 agents such as tocilizumab. It is a monoclonal antibody against the IL-6 receptor. As tocilizumab leads to significant immunosuppression, preexisting bacterial or fungal infection should be ruled out. Pediatric dose of tocilizumab is 4–8 mg/kg. A single dose is sufficient, but it can also be repeated after 12–24 hours if considered appropriate by the treating physician. However, a recent RCT failed to show any benefit in an interim analysis. Itolizumab, anakinra and sarilumab are other immunomodulators available but none of these is recommended as of now.[16]

Convalescent plasma has not shown any benefit either on duration of disease or survival rates, so it is no longer being recommended.[26] For the management of MIS-C, immunomodulation is the mainstay of management. Intravenous immunoglobulin (IVIG) and methylprednisolone are the most used agents but the subset, which benefits with immunomodulation, has not been defined clearly.

Monoclonal Antibodies

Monoclonal antibodies against spike protein have shown a role in preventing coronavirus infection in households. Food and Drug Administration (FDA) of USA has authorized three combinations of monoclonal antibodies for emergency use. These combinations are bamlanivimab and etesevimab combination, casirivimab and imdevimab combination and sotrovimab alone. Theoretically these antibodies have a role before the host has developed antibodies against the virus; hence treatment should be started within the first 10 days of reporting positive. It would be useful for patients with risk factors associated with severe disease such as obesity, hypertension, chronic renal disease and chronic lung disease. At present monoclonal antibody treatment is very expensive and not easily available in India.[27]

The treatment algorithm for adults and children is summarized in **Flowcharts 3.2 and 3.3**, respectively.

■ EMERGENCE OF OMICRON VARIANT

The **Omicron variant**, the new SARS-CoV-2 variant (B.1.1.529) is another coronavirus that causes COVID-19 infection. It was first reported to the WHO from South Africa on 24 November 2021 and has rapidly spread to the rest of the world. Compared to the previous variants of concern (VOC), Omicron is believed to be far more contagious (spreading much quicker)[8] and spreads around 70 times faster than any previous variants in the airways including bronchi and lungs. But it is less able to penetrate the deep lung tissue, and perhaps for this reason there is a considerable reduction in the risk of severe disease requiring hospitalization. However, the extremely high rate of spread combined with its ability to evade both double vaccination and the body's immune system, means that the total number of patients requiring hospital care at any given time is still of great concern. CDC has recommended the following treatment modalities for Omicron infection:

1. *Nirmatrelvir* 300 mg with *ritonavir* 100 mg (Paxlovid™) orally twice daily for 5 days, initiated as soon as possible and within 5 days of symptom onset in those aged ≥12 years and weighing ≥40 kg (it is not available in India). Caution should be taken, as there are a lot of drug interactions due to ritonavir. Hence review all drugs being used in the management.
2. *Sotrovimab*, an investigational monoclonal antibody, retains in vitro activity against the full known spike protein of the SARS-CoV-2 variant Omicron. Sotrovimab 500 mg as a single IV infusion is administered as soon as possible and within 10 days of symptom onset in those aged ≥12 years and weighing ≥40 kg living in areas with a high prevalence of the

SARS-CoV-2 Infection

Flowchart 3.2: Treatment plan for an adult having suspected symptoms of COVID 19.

```
Treatment plan for adult having suspected
         symptoms of COVID-19
                    │
                    ▼
         RT-PCR, rapid antigen test
          │                    │
       Positive              Negative
          │                    │
          ▼                    ▼
   Classify into:       Repeat test negative,
   Low risk/high risk   other differentials ruled
                        out, symptoms persisting
```

Upper respiratory tract infection/ fever less than 5 days	High-risk comorbidity—Obesity, poorly controlled hypertension, poorly controlled diabetics (HbA1C >7.5), immunocompromised unvaccinated or last dose 6 months back or more	High-grade fever persisting after 5–7 days, hypoxemia	HRCT scan with CORAD scoring (after 5 days of symptoms; 97% sensitive)
Monitor signs and symptoms till day 10 (second phase when patient can develop pneumonia –8 to 10th day)	Check for anti-RBD antibodies Consider monoclonal antibodies	Consider use of steroids/ anticoagulant/ monoclonal antibody	HRCT scan severity score > 12/25– evaluate for inflammatory markers like CRP— consider steroids/ anticoagulants (Note-Treatment should not be initiated based on the HRCT images alone)

Duration of steroids/anticoagulant depends on disease progression/resolution clinically/inflammatory markers such as CRP
Poor response to steroids—use IL-6 inhibitors, JAK inhibitors

(Anti-RBD antibodies: anti-spike protein receptor-binding domain antibodies; CORAD: COVID-19 Reporting and Data System; CRP: C-reactive protein; HbA1C: glycosylated hemoglobin; HRCT: high resolution computed tomography; IL-6: interleukin-6; JAK: Janus kinase; RT-PCR: reverse transcription polymerase chain reaction)

Flowchart 3.3: Treatment plan for child having suspected symptoms of COVID-19.

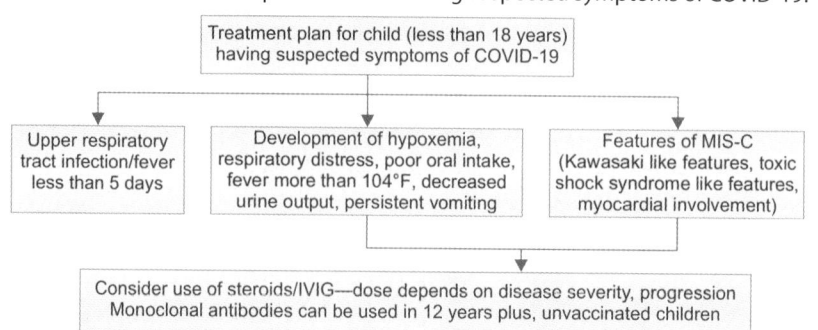

(MIS-C: multisystem inflammatory syndrome in children; IVIG: intravenous immunoglobulin)

Omicron. Neutralizing antibodies against Omicron are three times less but still can be effective. (Present REGN-antibodies available in India are not effective against Omicron and should not be used).
3. *Remdesivir*: 3-day course is approved by CDC. Remdesivir 200 mg IV on day 1, followed by remdesivir 100 mg IV daily on days 2 and 3, initiated as soon as possible and within 7 days of symptom onset in those aged ≥12 years and weighing ≥40 kg.
4. *Molnupiravir* 800 mg orally twice daily for 5 days, initiated as soon as possible and within 5 days of symptom onset in those aged ≥18 years, *only when none of the above options can be used.*

Above drugs are not indicated as a routine treatment unless patient has uncontrolled comorbidity and is unvaccinated or the last dose of vaccine was taken more than 6 months back.

CONCLUSION

Despite being around for a long-time, coronavirus has drawn global attention only since 2019. The pandemic has brought significant changes in every aspect of human interaction. The COVID-19 epidemic is still unfolding at the time of writing this article. However, with better insight into epidemiology and vaccination one hopes to see recession of this unprecedented pandemic.

KEY POINTS

- The ongoing pandemic of COVID-19 is caused by a novel strain of coronavirus, SARS-CoV-2.
- COVID-19 spreads mainly through droplets— by inhalation, deposition of infected droplets on mucous membranes (eyes, mouth and nose) by direct splashes and sprays, or through touch of contaminated hands.
- COVID-19 infection is mostly asymptomatic or presents as a mild flu-like illness. Anosmia and ageusia are characteristic features.
- Pneumonia is the most common presentation in severe COVID-19, which may rapidly progress to ARDS characterized by hypoxia and typical radiological findings.
- Extrapulmonary involvement occurs as coagulopathy, cardiac involvement (acute coronary syndromes, myocardial damage, and cardiomyopathy) and nonspecific neurologic illness.
- Multisystem inflammatory syndrome in children (MIS-C) should be suspected in a child presenting with fever, pain abdomen and rash.
- Nucleic acid amplification testing (NAAT) with reverse transcription polymerase chain reaction (RT-PCR) targeting coronavirus RNA in respiratory secretions is currently the gold standard for diagnosis.
- For rapid diagnosis of COVID-19, a rapid antigen test (RAT) is available as a point-of-care test with results available within 15 minutes.
- Subpleural ground glass opacities in a patient with pneumonia are considered specific to COVID-19 pneumonia. CT chest helps to grade the disease.

- Hypoxia is the main cause of mortality in COVID-19 pneumonia and oxygen forms the mainstay of therapy. Oxygen can be delivered through nasal prongs, facemask and nonrebreathing facemasks; those suffering from respiratory failure and refractory hypoxemia may need invasive ventilation. All patients with hypoxia should be given steroids as trials showed survival benefit with dexamethasone. The recommended dose of dexamethasone is 6 mg once daily for 10 days.
- European Society of Cardiology recommends parenteral heparin in patients admitted to intensive care units (ICU) with the goal of keeping APPT between 60 and 85 seconds.
- Antiviral agents including remdesivir, antiparasitic agents, antibiotics, convalescent plasma and IVIG have been tried but not shown any significant benefit so far.
- FDA has authorized combinations of monoclonal antibodies for emergency use in patients at high risk and severe forms of disease.

■ REFERENCES

1. Paules CI, Marston HD, Fauci AS. Coronavirus infections—more than just the common cold. JAMA. 2020;323(8):707-8.
2. de Wit E, van Doremalen N, Falzarano D, Munster VJ. SARS and MERS: recent insights into emerging coronaviruses. Nat Rev Microbiol. 2016;14(8):523-34.
3. Andrews MA, Areekal B, Rajesh KR, Krishnan J, Suryakala R, Krishnan B, et al. First confirmed case of COVID-19 infection in India: A case report. Indian J Med Res. 2020;151(5):490.
4. Lendacki FR, Teran RA, Gretsch S, Fricchione MJ, Kerins JL. COVID-19 Outbreak among attendees of an exercise facility — Chicago, Illinois, August–September 2020. MMWR Morb Mortal Wkly Rep. 2021;70(9):321-5.
5. Fiorillo L, Cervino G, Matarese M, D'amico C, Surace G, Paduano V, et al. COVID-19 surface persistence: a recent data summary and its importance for medical and dental settings. Int J Environ Res Pub Health. 2020;17(9):3132.
6. Lopez M, Bell K, Annaswamy T, Juengst S, Ifejika N. COVID-19 Guide for the rehabilitation clinician: A review of non-pulmonary manifestations and complications. Am J Phys Med Rehab. 2020;99(8):669-73.
7. Davis E, Rush BR, Cox J, DeBey B, Kapil S. Neonatal enterocolitis associated with coronavirus infection in a foal: a case report. J Vet Diagn Invest. 2000;12(2):153-6.
8. Rothan HA, Acharya A, Reid SP, Kumar M, Byrareddy SN. Molecular aspects of COVID-19 differential pathogenesis. Pathogens. 2020;9(7):538.
9. Filippi CM, Juedes AE, Oldham JE, Ling E, Togher L, Peng Y, et al. Transforming growth factor-β suppresses the activation of CD8+ T-cells when naive but promotes their survival and function once antigen experienced: a two-faced impact on autoimmunity. Diabetes. 2008;57(10):2684-92.
10. Perrotta F, Matera MG, Cazzola M, Bianco A. Severe respiratory SARS-CoV2 infection: Does ACE2 receptor matter? Resp Med. 2020;168:105996.
11. Giannis D, Ziogas IA, Gianni P. Coagulation disorders in coronavirus infected patients: COVID-19, SARS-CoV-1. MERS-CoV and lessons from the past. J Clin Virol. 2020;127:104362.
12. Lauer SA, Grantz KH, Bi Q, Jones FK, Zheng Q, Meredith HR, et al. The Incubation period of coronavirus disease 2019 (COVID-19) from publicly reported confirmed cases: Estimation and application. Ann Intern Med. 2020: M20-0504.

13. Wu Z, McGoogan JM. Characteristics of and important lessons from the coronavirus disease 2019 (COVID-19) outbreak in China: summary of a report of 72 314 cases from the Chinese Center for Disease Control and Prevention. JAMA. 2020;323(13):1239-42.
14. Ellinghaus D, Degenhardt F, Bujanda L, Buti M, Albilios A, Invernizzi P, et al. The ABO blood group locus and a chromosome 3 gene cluster associate with SARS-CoV-2 respiratory failure in an Italian-Spanish genome-wide association analysis. medRxiv. 2020.
15. Gupta D, Simalti A, Gupta N, Bhardwaj P, Bansal A, Sachdev A. Management principles of COVID 19 in adolescents and children. Indian J Adolesc Med. 2020;2(1):48-58.
16. Clerkin KJ, Fried JA, Raikhelkar J, Sayer G, Griffin JM, Masoumi A, et al. COVID-19 and cardiovascular disease. Circulation. 2020;141(20):1648-55.
17. Gupta A, Madhavan MV, Sehgal K, Nair N, Mahajan S, Sehrawat TS, et al. Extrapulmonary manifestations of COVID-19. Nat Med. 2020;26(7):1017-32.
18. Carlotti AP, de Carvalho WB, Johnston C, Rodriguez IS, Delgado AF. COVID-19 Diagnostic and Management Protocol for Pediatric Patients. Clinics (Sao Paulo). 2020;75:e1894.
19. Mlcochova P, Collier D, Ritchie A, Assennato SM, Hosmillo M, Goel N, et al. Combined point-of-care nucleic acid and antibody testing for SARS-CoV-2 following emergence of D614G spike variant. Cell Rep Med. 2020;1(6):100099.
20. Hanson KE, Caliendo AM, Arias CA, Englund JA, Hayden MK, Lee MK, et al. Infectious Diseases Society of America Guidelines on the Diagnosis of COVID-19: Serologic Testing. Clin Infect Dis. 2020;ciaa1343.
21. King CS, Sahjwani D, Brown AW, Feroz S, Cameron P, Osborn E, et al. Outcomes of mechanically ventilated patients with COVID-19 associated respiratory failure. PLoS One. 2020;15(11):e0242651.
22. RECOVERY Collaborative Group; Horby P, Lim WS, Emberson JR, Mafham M, Bell JL, Linsell L, et al. Dexamethasone in hospitalized patients with Covid-19. N Engl J Med. 2021;384(8):693-704.
23. Rico-Mesa JS, Rosas D, Ahmadian-Tehrani A, White A, Anderson AS, Chilton R. The role of anticoagulation in COVID-19-induced hypercoagulability. Curr Cardiol Rep. 2020;22(7):53.
24. Atallah B, Mallah SI, AlMahmeed W. Anticoagulation in COVID-19. Eur Heart J Cardiovasc Pharmacother. 2020;6(4):260-1.
25. Singhal T. A review of coronavirus disease-2019 (COVID-19). Indian J Pediatr. 2020;87(4):281-6.
26. Gharbharan A, Jordans C, Geurtsvan Kessel C, den Hollander JG, Karim F, Mollema FPN, et al. Convalescent plasma for COVID-19. A randomized clinical trial. MedRxiv. 2020.
27. Jiang S, Hillyer C, Du L. Neutralizing antibodies against SARS-CoV-2 and other human coronaviruses. Trends Immunol. 2020;41(5):355-9.

Infectious Diseases

CHAPTER 4: Systemic Antifungal Therapy

Vidya Krishna

■ INTRODUCTION

Invasive fungal infections (IFIs) are on the rise globally especially, in the critical care settings in view of invasive lines and broad-spectrum antibiotic therapy especially in patients on immunosuppressive therapy for malignancies or autoimmune disorders and in post-transplant settings, both solid organ and hematopoietic stem cell transplants. They are often associated with significant morbidity, mortality, treatment costs and delays in diagnosis and treatment due to various factors including lack of clinical suspicion, improper or inadequate sampling and culture techniques, and lack of cheap and easily available biomarkers.

Early and appropriate systemic antifungal therapy is known to reduce morbidity and mortality in IFIs. Thus, there is a great need to balance risk of empirical over-usage of these agents leading to antifungal resistance. Globally, antifungal resistance is increasingly being recognized as much as, if not as a greater threat than antibacterial resistance and hence, antifungal stewardship is being strongly advocated.

The current repertoire of systemic antifungal agents is small and most of these drugs have significant side effects, drug interactions and are expensive. Hence, a thorough working knowledge of the pharmacology and clinical indications is necessary for all clinicians dealing with patients with risk factors for IFIs. This chapter, however, only focuses on systemic antifungal drugs and the treatment of some specific infections, e.g., *Pneumocystis jirovecii* is not included.

■ HISTORY OF ANTIFUNGAL THERAPY

Some of the landmarks in the development of antifungal therapy are listed here:
- Amphotericin B deoxycholate was the first systemic antifungal drug to be introduced in 1958. Despite potent, broad-spectrum antifungal activity, it has been associated with significant renal toxicity and infusion-related reactions.

Systemic Antifungal Therapy

- Flucytosine was introduced in 1973 and it has activity against *Candida* and *Cryptococcus*. This drug can rapidly develop resistance when used alone.
- The first-generation azoles, fluconazole and itraconazole were introduced in 1990s. They have good activity against yeasts and are orally bioavailable. They show significant CYP450-mediated drug-drug interactions.
- Lipid-based formulations of amphotericin B were introduced in the mid-1990s. They retained the potency and broad spectrum of action, with less toxicity when compared to the deoxycholate preparation.
- The echinocandins have been available since 2000s and have good activity against *Candida*, including a few azole-resistant species. This class of drugs has very few drug-drug interactions and a favorable toxicity profile.
- The second-generation azoles including voriconazole, posaconazole and isavuconazole have been available since 2000s. They have good activity against filamentous fungi.[1]

■ BACKGROUND

Clinically important fungi can be classified into three major groups **(Fig. 4.1)**. *Candida*, *Cryptococcus*, and the filamentous fungi act as opportunistic pathogens while the dimorphic fungi are usually found in the soil in endemic areas and cause disease in normal hosts.

Dermatophytes (e.g., *Microsporum*) cause superficial infections of skin, hair and nails but rarely, systemic mycoses.

■ DIAGNOSIS OF SYSTEMIC FUNGAL INFECTIONS

Systemic fungal infections should be suspected in the appropriate clinical context and usually require a combination of imaging, appropriate tissue sampling with histopathology (to demonstrate tissue invasion) and fungal cultures to make a conclusive diagnosis **(Table 4.1)**. Biomarkers such as beta-D-glucan and galactomannan have gained interest but are not yet fully validated in the pediatric population. There is increasing interest in specific or generic fungal polymerase chain reactions (PCRs) but well-validated commercial PCRs are not readily available.

Beta-D-Glucan

Beta-D-glucan (BDG) is present in the cell wall of *Aspergillus*, *Candida* and *Pneumocystis jirovecii* (PCP). It is typically negative in patients with

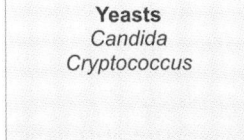

Fig. 4.1: Classification of fungi causing systemic mycoses.

TABLE 4.1: Diagnosis of systemic fungal infections.

Suspected infection	Clinical syndromes	Diagnostics
Candidiasis	Invasive candidiasis	• Send blood cultures (at least one peripheral) prior to starting antifungal agent • Send a blood culture from all the lines if present • Send serum BDG • In neonates, send urine culture and image kidneys if culture is positive. Do CSF analysis and dilated retinal examination if blood/urine culture is positive for candida species • Consider abdominal-pelvic imaging if neutropenic or if hepatosplenic infection is suspected, e.g., in neonate with persistently positive blood cultures
Aspergillosis	Pulmonary/disseminated aspergillosis in a neutropenic host/post-HSCT/solid organ transplant/T cell immunosuppression	• Send good quality lower respiratory tract samples; ideally BAL or tissue for fungal stain and culture. Send *Aspergillus* PCR if available • Send BAL for GM • Send serum GM in neutropenic host • HRCT of chest and sinuses or other site-specific imaging
Mucormycosis	Rhino-orbito-cerebral, pulmonary, gastric, disseminated mucormycosis in a diabetic/immunosuppressed host as per EOSRTC-MSG criteria[2]	• Send BAL/tissue for fungal stain and culture • Site-specific imaging • Fungal biomarkers such as BDG and GM are negative in mucormycosis
Cryptococcosis	–	• Send blood culture and serum cryptococcal antigen • Perform CSF analysis with opening pressure and send for CSF cryptococcal antigen, India ink stain and fungal cultures
Endemic fungi- like histoplasma	–	Histopathology and fungal cultures, specific serology/antigen tests

(BAL: bronchoalveolar lavage; BDG: beta-D-glucan; CSF: cerebrospinal fluid; EOSRTC-MSG: European Confederation of Medical Mycology in cooperation with the Mycoses Study Group; GM: galactomannan; HRCT: high resolution computed tomography; HSCT: hematopoietic and stem cell transplant; PCR: polymerase chain reaction) cryptococcosis or mucormycosis. BDG is generally measured in a serum sample. Limitations of this test include false positives in a number of scenarios [previous administration of intravenous immunoglobulin (IVIG) and other blood products, hemofiltration, mucositis and use of some beta-lactam antibiotics due to cultivation process]. Interpreting the results of serial testing should be done with caution, as changes in levels of BDG are not always associated with treatment failure or success.

Galactomannan

Galactomannan (GM) is found in the cell wall released from the growing tips of *Aspergillus*. A serum or bronchoalveolar lavage (BAL) biomarker assay positive for the presence of GM is not specific for the presence of invasive *Aspergillus* disease, as a number of other molds release GM (e.g., *Fusarium* species, *Penicillium* species). GM assay sensitivity is reduced with concurrent antimold therapy, e.g., azole or liposomal amphotericin. False positivity may occur with concurrent beta-lactam use such as piperacillin-tazobactam and co-amoxiclav. Decreases in GM are associated with favorable treatment outcomes.

■ SYSTEMIC ANTIFUNGAL AGENTS

There are four main classes of antifungal agents **(Table 4.2)** and the antifungal susceptibility of different group of fungi is discussed in **Table 4.3**.

■ SITE OF ACTION

The systemic antifungal agents act on the fungal cell wall, cell membrane or by inhibiting protein synthesis.

The fungal cell wall is essential for structural integrity and viability of the cell. They take part in other functions such as metabolism and ion exchange;

TABLE 4.2: Classification of systemic antifungal agents.

Azoles	Echinocandins	Polyenes	Pyrimidine analogs/ Antimetabolite
• Fluconazole • Itraconazole • Voriconazole • Posaconazole • Isavuconazole	• Micafungin • Caspofungin • Anidulafungin	• Amphotericin B deoxycholate (AmBd) • Liposomal Amphotericin (L-AmB) • Lipid complex Amphotericin B (ABLC) • Amphotericin B colloidal dispersion (ABCD)	Flucytosine

TABLE 4.3: Antifungal susceptibility of different fungi.

Fungus	Flu	Itr	Vori	Posa	AmB	Ech	5-FC	DOC
Candida species								
C. albicans	+	+	+	+	+	+	+	Echinocandin for primary therapy, fluconazole for step-down[6]
C. tropicalis	+	+	+	+	+	+	+	Echinocandin for primary therapy, fluconazole for step-down[6]
C. glabrata	±	±	+	+	+	+	+	Echinocandin for primary therapy, high dose fluconazole/voriconazole for step-down if sensitive[6]
C. krusei	-	±	+	+	+	+	±	Echinocandin for primary therapy, voriconazole for step-down if sensitive[6]
C. parapsilosis	+	+	+	+	±	+	+	Fluconazole is the drug of choice[6]
C. lusitaniae	+	+	+	+	-	+	+	Echinocandin for primary therapy, fluconazole for step-down[6]
Cryptococcus spp.	+	+	+	+	+	-	+	• Severe cases/meningitis—Amphotericin B plus flucytosine for induction therapy followed by fluconazole for consolidation and maintenance • Mild-moderate pulmonary disease—Fluconazole[7]
Aspergillus species								
A. niger	-	±	+	+	+	+	-	• Voriconazole is the preferred first line therapy • Amphotericin B is less preferred alternate agent • Combination therapy with echinocandin (especially, Anidulafungin) has been shown to reduce mortality in patients with positive radiographic findings and serum galactomannan positivity[8,9]
A. terreus	-	+	+	+	-	+	-	
A. flavus	-	+	+	+	±	+	-	
A. fumigatus	-	+	+	+	+	+	-	

Contd...

Contd...

Fungus	Flu	Itr	Vori	Posa	AmB	Ech	5-FC	DOC
Mucorales	-	-	-	+	+	-	-	• Amphotericin B is the drug of choice • Posaconazole can be used as salvage therapy in refractory cases/amphotericin B toxicity[10]
Blastomyces dermatitidis	+	+	+	+	+	±	-	• Mild-moderate disease—Itraconazole • Severe disease—Amphotericin B followed by itraconazole[5]
Histoplasma capsulatum	+	+	+	+	+	±	-	• Amphotericin B is recommended first line in severe cases/disseminated disease • Itraconazole is preferred first line for mild-moderate disease[5]
Coccidioides immitis	+	+	+	+	+	±	-	• Fluconazole is the preferred first line agent • Itraconazole is alternate agent in mild-moderate disease • Amphotericin B is recommended as initial therapy for severe osseous disease and disseminated disease[11]
Paracoccidioides spp.	-	+	+	-	+	-	-	• Mild-moderate disease—Itraconazole • Severe disease—Amphotericin B. Voriconazole is used as alternate therapy[5]
Fusarium spp.	-	-	+	+	±	-	-	Voriconazole or amphotericin B depending on the sensitivity pattern[5]
Scedosporium spp.	-	±	±	±	±	-	-	Voriconazole is the preferred agent. *Scedosporium apiospermum* is resistant to Amphotericin B[5]

(Flu: Fluconazole; Itr: Itraconazole; Vori: Voriconazole; Posa: Posaconazole; Ech: Echinocandin; 5-FC: Flucytosine; DOC: drug of choice) and some parts of the cell wall are immunogenic. The cell wall is made of glucans, chitin and various glycoproteins. The β-1,3-D-glucan is the most important structural component of the cell wall and is synthesized by a group of enzymes called as glucan synthases in the plasma membrane. The genes encoding β-1,3-D-glucans are the FKS1 and FKS2.[3] The *echinocandins* act by inhibiting the glucan synthase and thereby the cell wall synthesis. FKS mutations can lead to echinocandin resistance. They are fungicidal.

The fungal cell membrane is made up of predominantly lipids including glycerophospholipids, sphingolipids and sterols. Unlike animal cell membranes, where cholesterol is the major component, ergosterol is the main sterol present in fungal cell membranes.[4] The *azole* antifungals act by inhibiting the fungal cell membrane synthesis. They inhibit C-14α-demethylase [a cytochrome P450 (CYP450) enzyme], thereby blocking the demethylation of lanosterol to ergosterol. They are fungistatic agents.

The *polyenes* have a detergent like action on the cell membrane. They integrate into the fungal cell membrane by binding to sterols, especially ergosterol, forming micropores and increasing membrane permeability. Loss of intracellular potassium and other molecules contributes to the fungicidal effect.[5]

The pyrimidine analog, *flucytosine,* is taken up by the fungal cell and converted to 5-fluorodeoxyuridine 5'-monophosphate. This metabolite inhibits thymidylate synthase, thereby depriving the organism of thymidylic acid, an essential component of DNA. 5-fluorodeoxyuridine 5'-monophosphate is further metabolized to a trinucleotide, which incorporates into fungal RNA and inhibits nucleic acid and protein synthesis.[5] It is fungistatic.

■ AZOLES

The azole group of antifungals includes imidazoles (clotrimazole, ketoconazole and miconazole) and triazoles (fluconazole, itraconazole, voriconazole, posaconazole, and isavuconazole). The imidazoles have a significant toxicity when administered systemically and have been relegated to topical use for vaginal candidiasis and superficial mycoses. The triazoles have a better safety profile when administered systemically. **Tables 4.4 and 4.5** discuss the properties and dosing of azoles.

■ SPECTRUM OF ACTION

Fluconazole

Fluconazole has excellent activity against most of the *Candida* species including the common species such as *C. albicans, C. tropicalis, C. lusitaniae, C. dubliensis,* etc. It is not active against *C. krusei*. It is not a good drug for *C. glabrata, C. guilliermondii* and *C. rugosa* as minimum inhibitory concentrations (MIC) are higher. Fluconazole has very good activity against *Cryptococcus neoformans*.

Among the dimorphic fungi, it is used in the treatment of Coccidioidomycosis. It has no activity against any of the filamentous fungi.

Itraconazole
Itraconazole is predominantly used in the treatment of dimorphic fungi such as B. *dermatitidis, H. capsulatum, coccidioides species, paracoccidioides species,* and *Sporothrix schenckii*. It has activity against most *Candida* species with higher MICs for *C. glabrata* and *C. krusei*. Itraconazole is also active against many *Aspergillus* species, including *A. fumigatus, A. flavus, A. nidulans,* and *A. terreus*. Itraconazole exhibits minimal activity against *Fusarium* species and the mucorales.

Voriconazole
Voriconazole is primarily used for its activity against *Aspergillus* species. It acts on *A. terreus* which is amphotericin B-resistant. It has activity against yeasts, *Cryptococcus* species and *Candida* species including fluconazole-resistant *C. glabrata* strains. Voriconazole has activity against dimorphic fungi *B. dermatitidis, Coccidioides immitis,* and *H. capsulatum* and on filamentous fungi, *Fusarium* and *Scedosporium* but does not act on *Mucorales*.

Posaconazole
Posaconazole has a spectrum of action similar to voriconazole but exhibits activity against most *Mucorales* species.

Isavuconazole
Isavuconazole has a spectrum of action similar to voriconazole but exhibits activity against some of the *Mucorales* and *Scedosporium* species.

■ CLINICAL INDICATIONS
Fluconazole
It is mainly used in the treatment of candidiasis and cryptococcosis. Fluconazole can be used as empirical and targeted therapy for candidemia in non-neutropenic patients who are not critically ill, with no recent azole exposure or at risk of harboring an azole-resistant species. In stable neutropenic hosts with no azole exposure, it is a less preferred alternative agent to echinocandin for empiric therapy.

In critically ill patients and in neutropenic hosts with suspected candidemia, echinocandins are the preferred agents both for empirical and early-targeted therapy. Once the patient is clinically stable, has documented blood culture clearance and isolate is confirmed to be sensitive, step-down therapy to fluconazole to complete duration of treatment is recommended.

TABLE 4.4: Properties of azole drugs.[1,12]

Drug	Route of administration	Oral bioavailability	Metabolism/Excretion	Tissue concentrations
Fluconazole	Oral, parenteral	90%, not affected by food or gastric pH	Renal—primarily excreted unchanged in urine and hence, attains high urinary concentrations	Good including CSF, ocular tissues
Itraconazole	Oral (capsule and solution)	• Capsule—55%, taken with acidic beverage and food • Avoid concomitant PPIs/ H₂ blockers • Solution—80% not affected by gastric pH or food • Achieves 30% higher serum concentration than capsule preparation	• Hepatic—by CYP450 isoenzyme 3A4 • Excreted in urine and feces but urinary metabolites are inactive • Cannot be used to treat lower urinary tract infections	• Highly protein bound and hence, poor CSF and ocular concentrations • Good concentrations in skin and nails and hence, excellent agent for cutaneous and nail mycoses
Voriconazole	Oral (tablet and suspension), parenteral formulation complexed with β-cyclodextrin	• Oral formulations have bioavailability > 90% • Absorption best in fasted state and not affected by gastric acidity	• Hepatic—CYP450 enzyme mediated • CYP2C19 polymorphisms lead to slow or rapid metabolizers leading to toxicity or therapeutic failure • Urinary concentrations are low and hence, not used to treat urinary tract infections	Good penetration including CSF, ocular tissues

Contd...

Contd...

Drug	Route of administration	Oral bioavailability	Metabolism/Excretion	Tissue concentrations
Posaconazole	Oral (suspension, delayed release tablet), parenteral formulation complexed with β-cyclodextrin	• Solution best absorbed when taken with high-fat food • Avoid concomitant PPIs/ H₂ blockers • Tablet has more reliable absorption and serum concentrations as absorption not affected by acidity or food	Metabolized by hepatic uridine diphosphate (UDP)— glucuronidation and is excreted via the bile and feces	Poor CSF and ocular penetration
Isavuconazole	Both oral capsule and parenteral formulation contain Isavuconazonium, the water-soluble prodrug of isavuconazole	Oral capsule is highly bioavailable, and absorption is not affected by acidity or food	Metabolized by hepatic CYP450 enzymes and metabolites are excreted in the feces	Highly protein bound (>99%) and hence, poor CSF and ocular concentrations

(CSF: cerebrospinal fluid; PPI: proton pump inhibitors)

TABLE 4.5: Dosing of azole drugs.[13,14]

Drug	Plasma half-life (t₁/₂)	Dosing	Comments	Adverse effects
Fluconazole	20–50 hours	*Prophylaxis:* Infants, children and adolescents: 6 mg/kg (maximum 400 mg) oral/IV once daily Term neonates: Week 1 of life: 3 mg/kg/dose to 6 mg/kg/dose oral/IV twice weekly Week 2–4 of life: 6 mg/kg/dose oral/IV every 72 hourly *Treatment:* Infants, children, adolescents: Loading dose: 12 mg/kg (maximum 800 mg) IV/oral as single dose Maintenance dose: 6 mg/kg (maximum 400 mg) IV/oral once daily Use 12 mg/kg once daily if immunocompromised child/severe infection Term Neonates: Loading dose: 25 mg/kg IV as a single dose. *Maintenance dose:* Week 1 of life: 12 mg/kg IV/oral every 48 hourly Week 2–4 of life: 12 mg/kg IV/oral once daily	Dose reduction is needed in renal failure and not in hepatic failure Oral formulation can be taken with or without food	GI symptoms, headache, rash, raised AST, rarely, severe hepatotoxicity and QT prolongation

Contd...

Systemic Antifungal Therapy

Drug	Plasma half-life ($t_{1/2}$)	Dosing	Comments	Adverse effects
Itraconazole	35–40 hours	*Oral solution:* (not readily available in India) 1 month to <12 years: 5 mg/kg oral twice daily (maximum dose 600 mg/day) *Neonates:* Limited data *Oral capsules:* 12–18 years: 2.5 mg/kg oral twice daily (maximum 200 mg/dose)	Dose adjustment needed in renal failure *Liquid:* Administer on an empty stomach at least 1 hour before food with an acidic beverage (e.g., cola, orange juice) *Capsules:* Administer with or after food. For patients on gastric acid suppressant medications, separate administration by at least 2 hours and administer with an acidic beverage (e.g., cola, orange juice)	Same as fluconazole
Voriconazole	6 hours	*Infants and children up to 2 years:* 9 mg/kg IV/oral twice daily *2–12 years (up to 50 kg):* Loading dose: 9 mg/kg IV/oral twice daily for 2 doses Maintenance dose: Intravenous: 8 mg/kg IV twice daily and titrate according to TDM results Oral: 9 mg/kg oral twice daily [maximum 350 mg/dose, titrate according to therapeutic drug monitoring (TDM) results]	Cyclodextrin component of parenteral preparation can accumulate in renal insufficiency and hence, dose reduction is required for CrCl <50 mL/min In mild to moderate hepatic impairment (Child-Pugh score of 7–9; class B—significant functional compromise, after loading dose, reduce maintenance dose by 50% and perform therapeutic drug monitoring	Same as fluconazole Visual disturbances as in photopsia, visual hallucinations are dose related, self-limiting and rarely require cessation of therapy Long-term use (> 6 months) can lead to increased risk of skin cancers

Contd...

Drug	Plasma half-life ($t_{1/2}$)	Dosing	Comments	Adverse effects
		12–15 years (less than 50 kg): Use dose for children 2–12 years 12–15 years (more than 50 kg): Use dose for adolescents 15–18 years (below) 15–18 years (more than 50 kg): Loading dose: 6 mg/kg IV/oral twice daily for 2 doses Maintenance dose—Intravenous: 4 mg/kg IV twice daily and titrate according to TDM results Maintenance dose—Oral: 4 mg/kg oral twice daily (maximum initial dose of 200 mg/dose then titrate according to TDM results) Neonates: Limited data Treatment and prophylaxis dose are same in children due to lack of good data	Therapeutic drug monitoring: Prophylaxis—timing: Trough level on day 5 Target: Trough level 1–2 mg/L Treatment: Timing: Take trough level (30 minutes predose) before 4th dose as a safety check If level > 4 mg/L, needs dose adjustment Repeat trough level on day 5 (steady state) after starting drug or changing dose Target: Trough level 1–5 mg/L A higher target (e.g., >2 mg/L) should be used if there is disease with a poor prognosis (e.g., CNS infection, bulky disease, multifocal infection) Note: A trough level of more than 5 or 6 mg/L is associated with an increased probability of neurological and ocular toxicity Administer 1 hour before or after food (absorption reduced with high fat meals) Council on avoidance sun exposure. Reports of skin cancer with prolonged (more than 6 months) use Concurrent omeprazole may increase IV voriconazole levels (boosting via CyP 2C19 interaction)	

Drug	Plasma half-life ($t_{1/2}$)	Dosing	Comments	Adverse effects
Posaconazole	>24 hours	*Treatment:* Oral modified release tablets (preferred over suspension if able to swallow tablets): Weight 10–20 kg: 200 mg 12 hourly on day one, followed by 200 mg 24 hourly thereafter Weight 20–30 kg: 300 mg 12 hourly on day one, followed by an alternating daily dose of 300 mg and 200 mg once daily Weight >30 kg: 300 mg 12 hourly on day one, followed by 300 mg 24 hourly thereafter *Oral suspension (use only if tablets not suitable):* 1–6 years: 200 mg 6 hourly 7–12 years: 300 mg 6 hourly ≥13 years: 200 mg 6 hourly *IV Infusion:* Weight <30 kg: 10 mg/kg 12 hourly on day one, followed by 10 mg/kg 24 hourly thereafter Weight ≥30 kg: 300 mg 12 hourly on day 1, followed by 300 mg 24 hourly thereafter	*Oral suspension:* Absorption is very variable and is affected by the presence of food It is important to ensure that posaconazole is administered during or after a high-fat meal for best absorption If this is not possible, administration with any meal or food supplement or an acidic, carbonated drink will improve absorption No dosage adjustments are required in renal or hepatic impairment *All formulations: Therapeutic drug monitoring:* Trough level (30 minutes predose) on day 5–7 after starting drug or changing dose *Prophylaxis:* Trough > 0.5–0.7 mg/L *Treatment:* Trough 1 to 3 mg/L Avoid antacids, H2 receptor antagonists, and proton pump inhibitors	Same as fluconazole

Contd...

Contd...

Drug	Plasma half-life ($t_{1/2}$)	Dosing	Comments	Adverse effects
		Prophylaxis: Oral modified release tablets (preferred over suspension if able to swallow tablets): *7–12 years old and able to swallow whole tablets:* 5–7 mg/kg/dose (to a maximum of 300 mg) 12 hourly on day one, followed by 5–7 mg/kg (to a maximum of 300 mg) 24 hourly thereafter *Children ≥13 years old:* 300 mg 12 hourly on day 1, followed by 300 mg 24 hourly thereafter *Oral suspension (use only if tablets not suitable):* *Children ≥8 months to 12 years old:* 4 mg/kg/dose (to a maximum of 200 mg) 8 hourly *Children ≥13 years old:* 200mg 8 hourly		
Isavuconazole	>75 hours	Safety and efficacy not established in children < 18 years	–	Same as fluconazole except it causes QT shortening

(AST: aspartate aminotransferase; CrCl: creatinine clearance; CNS: central nervous system; TDM: therapeutic drug monitoring)

Systemic Antifungal Therapy

For neonatal candidiasis, while amphotericin B deoxycholate (AmBd) is the preferred agent, fluconazole is a reasonable alternative if the baby has not been on fluconazole prophylaxis.

Fluconazole is a good agent for *Candida* endophthalmitis and can be used as step-down to liposomal AmB (LAmB) for central nervous system (CNS) candidiasis.

Fluconazole is also recommended as a single dose agent for vulvovaginal candidiasis. It is used in moderate-severe oropharyngeal and esophageal candidiasis.

Fluconazole is the preferred agent of treatment of mild to moderate pulmonary cryptococcosis. In CNS/disseminated disease, it is less preferred to amphotericin B, which is preferred agent for induction, and is used only in the consolidation and maintenance phase of therapy.

Fluconazole is recommended for prophylaxis of candidemia in newborns with a weight < 1,000 g admitted to neonatal units with high rates of invasive candidiasis (>10%). Fluconazole can be used as prophylaxis in low-risk neutropenic patients who are not at risk for mold infections.

Itraconazole

It is primarily recommended for treatment of mild to moderate disease in endemic mycoses such as histoplasmosis, blastomycosis, sporotrichosis, coccidioidomycosis and paracoccidioidomycosis. It has no CNS penetration and hence, should not be used upfront in severe or disseminated disease. It can be used as step-down therapy to amphotericin B if CNS disease has been excluded.

It is recommended for treating chronic pulmonary aspergillosis and allergic bronchopulmonary aspergillosis.

It is no longer recommended therapy for mucosal candidiasis, prophylaxis in oncology patients and in invasive aspergillosis.

Voriconazole

It is the preferred first-line therapy for invasive aspergillosis. It has good CNS and tissue penetration and is recommended for severe and deep-seated infections as well. In invasive candidiasis, it can be used as a step-down therapy for fluconazole-resistant *C. krusei*, and *C. glabrata*.

It can be used to treat mucosal candidiasis if proven to be due to fluconazole-resistant organisms. It is used in the treatment of fusariosis and scedosporiosis. It is used as prophylaxis in neutropenic settings where mold-coverage is recommended. It has no action against mucormycosis.

Posaconazole

It is primarily used as a prophylaxis agent in high-risk neutropenic patients, e.g., post-stem cell transplant recipients with graft versus host disease as it has activity against *Candida, Aspergillus* and *Mucor*. It can be used for salvage therapy as it also has activity against *Fusarium, Scedosporium* and in refractory endemic mycosis.

Isavuconazole

It is recommended in the treatment of invasive aspergillosis and invasive mucormycosis.

■ DRUG INTERACTIONS

Azole drugs act as substrates and inhibitors of the CYP450 enzymes (CYP3A4, CYP2C19, and CYP 2C9) and the affinities for each enzyme vary significantly by individual drug.[15] The common drug classes, that they can interact with, include antiarrhythmics, antipsychotics, immunosuppressants, migraine medications, antibiotics, anticoagulants, antidepressants, antiepileptics, antiretrovirals, chemotherapeutics, antihypertensives, lipid lowering agents, narcotics, sedatives, hormonal therapies, and antidiabetic drugs. Hence, a careful review of drug chart for potential drug interactions should be undertaken when azoles are prescribed.

■ ECHINOCANDINS
Spectrum of Action and Clinical Indications

The echinocandins have excellent activity against most candida species except *C. parapsilosis* and *C. guilliermondii*. They also are used as salvage therapy in invasive aspergillosis in adults with refractory disease and intolerance to other agents. They are fungicidal against *Candida* and fungistatic against *Aspergillus*. Echinocandins have no activity against dimorphic fungi, *Mucorales, Cryptococcus, Fusarium* and *Scedosporium*.

Caspofungin and micafungin are approved for usage in children while anidulafungin is not well studied in the pediatric population. Based on clinical trial data demonstrating safety and efficacy, caspofungin is FDA approved for pediatric patients aged 3 months of age with esophageal candidiasis (that is severe/refractory/resistant to azoles), empiric therapy for presumed fungal infections in febrile neutropenic patients and in invasive candidiasis. Anecdotal experience in neonatal infections also is reported.

Micafungin is approved by the FDA for intravenous treatment of pediatric patients aged 4 months and older with invasive candidiasis, esophageal candidiasis and prophylaxis of invasive *Candida* infections in patients undergoing hematopoietic stem cell transplantation.[16]

Pharmacology

These drugs are only available as intravenous preparations and are not absorbed orally. They are primarily eliminated through nonenzymatic degradation to inactive products and excreted via the fecal route. As they are

Systemic Antifungal Therapy

excreted poorly in the urine, they should not be used for treatment of urinary tract infections. Also, they do not penetrate CNS and ocular tissues.

They do not have significant drug-drug interactions, as they are not significantly metabolized by the CYP450 enzymes.

Both caspofungin and micafungin undergo hepatic metabolism and dose reduction is recommended in patients with hepatic dysfunction. Echinocandins are very well tolerated and adverse effects are rarely reported. Gastrointestinal (GI) upset, headache, elevation of transaminases and infusion-related reactions may occur.

Dosing

Caspofungin

Treatment:

- *Infants (>3 months), children and adolescents*: Loading dose: 70 mg/m^2 IV on day 1 (maximum 70 mg/day). Maintenance dose: 50 mg/m^2 IV on day 2 onward (maximum 50 mg/day). In critically ill patients, maintenance dose can be increased to 70 mg/m^2/day (maximum 70 mg/day).
- *1–3 months of age*: 25 mg/m^2 IV daily (maximum 25 mg/day)
- *Neonates*: Limited data.

Prophylaxis: Infants (>3 months), children and adolescents: 50 mg/m^2 IV daily (maximum 50 mg/day). 1–3 months of age: 25 mg/m^2 IV daily (maximum 25 mg/day).

Micafungin

Treatment:

- *1 month – 2 years*: 5 mg/kg IV once daily (maximum 100 mg/day).
- *2–16 years (up to 40 kg)*: 3 mg/kg IV once daily (maximum 100 mg/day*).
- *16–18 years (more than 40 kg)*: 3 mg/kg IV once daily (maximum 150 mg/day) (*Increase to maximum 200 mg once daily if response is inadequate).
- *Term neonates*: General: 4 mg/kg IV once daily; CNS infection: 10 mg/kg IV once daily.

Prophylaxis: Infants, children, and adolescents: 1 mg/kg IV daily (maximum 50 mg/day).

■ POLYENES

Amphotericin B is the only agent in this class and is available as amphotericin B deoxycholate (AmBd) and three lipid-based preparations—liposomal amphotericin B (LAMB), lipid complex amphotericin B (ABLC) and amphotericin B colloidal dispersion (ABCD). Amphotericin B, the active component in all preparations, is a lipophilic molecule, derived from *Streptomyces nodosus*, a soil actinomycete.

Spectrum of Action

Amphotericin B is a broad-spectrum, potent, systemic antifungal agent with activity against most of the invasive fungi. Among the yeasts, it works against *Candida* species (except *C. lusitaniae*) and *Cryptococcus* species. It has good activity against *Aspergillus* (except *A. terreus*) and *Mucorales* but poor activity against *Fusarium* and *Scedosporium*. It is potent against all the dimorphic fungi including *B. dermatitidis, H. capsulatum,* coccidioides species, paracoccidioides species, and *Sporothrix schenckii*.

Pharmacology

All available preparations of amphotericin B are suitable only for intravenous administration. Ratio of the peak serum concentration to the MIC is the pharmacodynamics parameter driving in vivo response. Good tissue concentrations are attained in liver, spleen, bone marrow, kidney, and lungs. The lipid formulations attain better CNS and ocular concentration.

Amphotericin B Deoxycholate

This must be dissolved in 5% dextrose solution as the colloidal nature causes clouding when mixed with sodium chloride or bicarbonate. It is given as slow infusion over at least 10–12 hours to avoid infusion related infusions. Rapid infusions, especially in patients with renal dysfunction can lead to hyperkalemia and ventricular fibrillation. Preloading with saline helps to reduce nephrotoxicity.

Lipid Formulations of Amphotericin B

They need higher doses when compared to the deoxycholate preparation and attain good tissue levels except in the kidneys. They can be infused over shorter durations of 2–4 hours. Lipid complex formulation consists of amphotericin B complexed with two lipid bilayer ribbons, while the liposomal formulation consists of a vesicular bilayer liposome with amphotericin B intercalated within the membrane. LAMB is the only preparation that can be used with an in-line filter.

Table 4.6 lists the dosing of amphotericin B preparations.

Clinical Indications

Amphotericin B is approved as first-line agent for treatment of the following infections:
- Mucormycosis
- Neonatal candidiasis, hepatosplenic candidiasis, *Candida* meningitis and endophthalmitis.
- Severe forms of endemic mycoses—histoplasmosis, blastomycosis, sporotrichosis, coccidioidomycosis and paracoccidioidomycosis.

TABLE 4.6: Dosing of Amphotericin B.

Amphotericin B deoxycholate	• 0.3–1.5 mg/kg/day as single infusion depending on clinical indication • Higher doses (1–1.5 mg/kg) are recommended in invasive aspergillosis and mucormycosis
Liposomal Amphotericin B	• 5 mg/kg/day as single infusion • 5–10 mg/kg/day may be required in mucormycosis
Amphotericin B lipid complex	3–5 mg/kg/day as single infusion

- Cryptococcal meningitis/disseminated disease.
- Visceral and mucosal leishmaniasis.

It is a second-line agent for treatment of aspergillosis.

Toxicity

The common adverse reactions encountered with amphotericin B preparation are infusion-related reactions, nephrotoxicity, and electrolyte disturbances.

Infusion-related reactions including fever, chills and tachypnea are common with the deoxycholate preparation, especially in adults. They start about 30–45 minutes after initiating the infusion and can last for 2–4 hours. It is due to the activation of toll-like receptor 2 resulting in proinflammatory cytokine storm. Premedication with paracetamol, steroids and antihistamines may be helpful. True allergic reaction is rare, though desensitization may be done if required.

Nephrotoxicity is also more common with the deoxycholate preparation in adults. It is due to the vasoconstrictive effect of the drug on real arterioles and causes a dose-dependent decrease in glomerular filtration rate (GFR). Preloading with saline is associated with reduced nephrotoxicity. Long-term and permanent renal damage can occur due to damage to the renal tubules and is attributed to the cumulative dose.

It also causes potassium, bicarbonate and magnesium wasting and decreased erythropoietin production. Strict monitoring of serum potassium and magnesium should be done with replacement as required.

It is advisable to avoid concomitant nephrotoxic medications and hypovolemia in patients receiving amphotericin B deoxycholate. Also, the lipid-based preparations are the preferred agents in patients with preexisting renal failure and postrenal transplant patients.

Other less common toxicities, especially on prolonged use include bone marrow suppression and neurological side effects including tinnitus, dysesthesias of soles and encephalopathy. Phlebitis is common if peripheral venous catheters are used for infusion.

Comparison of the Different Preparations

Lipid formulations of amphotericin B have not consistently demonstrated superior efficacy to the deoxycholate preparation though they have fewer rates of nephrotoxicity and infusion related reactions.[17]

Liposomal amphotericin-B (LAMB) is the preferred preparation as per most guidelines, as it has been shown to have equal efficacy to the deoxycholate preparation with much better tolerability profile. It has been shown to have superior efficacy to the deoxycholate preparation in histoplasmosis.[18] They have good CNS and ocular penetration but have poor urinary concentrations. The limiting factor for usage of LAMB in India is the cost.

Amphotericin B colloidal dispersion is not recommended due to the infusion-related reactions.

Amphotericin B lipid complex (ABLC) is better tolerated than AmBd, is less studied than LAMB and is almost as expensive as LAMB.

Children generally tolerate the deoxycholate preparation much better than adults.

■ FLUCYTOSINE

It is a pyrimidine analog and acts by inhibiting protein synthesis. It has activity against both *Candida* and *Cryptococcus* species, but is only clinically used in the treatment of cryptococcosis. It can rapidly develop resistance when used as monotherapy.

Pharmacology

It is available as an oral formulation (capsule) with an excellent bioavailability of 80–90%. It has a short half-life (t1/2) and is hence, dosed frequently (6 hourly). It is excreted unchanged in urine and dose adjustment is hence, recommended in patients with creatinine clearance (CrCl) < 50 mL/min. It has excellent CNS and ocular penetration. It has no significant drug-drug interactions.

Clinical Indications

The clinical indications for administration of flucytosine include the following:
1. Cryptococcal meningitis—it is used along with amphotericin B preparation in the induction phase.
2. *Candida* cystitis—it can be used as a treatment option in view of high urinary concentrations and short duration of therapy.[19]

Toxicity

These include GI upset, rash, bone marrow suppression (dose-dependent) and hepatic toxicity. Cell counts should be monitored regularly while on therapy, especially in patients with renal insufficiency, as adverse effects are more common in them.

■ KEY POINTS

- Early and appropriate systemic antifungal therapy is known to reduce morbidity and mortality in invasive fungal infections. However, antifungal resistance is increasingly being documented.
- Systemic fungal infections should be suspected in the appropriate clinical context and usually require a combination of imaging, tissue sampling with histopathology to demonstrate tissue invasion and fungal cultures to make a conclusive diagnosis.
- Serum beta-D-glucan (BDG) is a good marker of infections due to invasive *Aspergillus, Candida* and *Pneumocystis jirovecii*.
- Estimation of galactomannan (GM) in bronchoalveolar lavage is an evidence of invasive Aspergillus disease but not specific.
- The common antifungal agents used in clinical practice are azoles, echinocandins, polyenes and pyrimidine analogs.
- Itraconazole is predominantly used in the treatment of dimorphic fungi.
- Fluconazole is mainly used in the treatment of candidiasis and cryptococcosis, while amphotericin B deoxycholate (AmBd) is the preferred agent for neonatal candidiasis.
- Voriconazole is the preferred first-line therapy for invasive aspergillosis.
- Amphotericin B is a broad spectrum, potent, systemic antifungal agent with activity against most of the invasive fungi. It is the first-line agent in the treatment of mucormycosis, neonatal candidiasis, cryptococcal disease and severe forms of endemic mycoses.
- The common adverse reactions encountered with amphotericin B preparation are infusion-related reactions, nephrotoxicity, and electrolyte disturbances.
- Flucytosine is clinically used only in the treatment of cryptococcal meningitis and candida cystitis.
- The current repertoire of systemic antifungal agents is small and most of these drugs have significant side effects, drug interactions and are expensive.

■ REFERENCES

1. Nett JE, Andes DR. Antifungal agents: spectrum of activity, pharmacology, and clinical indications. Infect Dis Clin North Am. 2016;30(1):51-83.
2. Donnelly JP, Chen SC, Kauffman CA, Steinbach WJ, Baddley JW, Verweij PE, et al. Revision and Update of the Consensus Definitions of Invasive Fungal Disease From the European Organization for Research and Treatment of Cancer and the Mycoses Study Group Education and Research Consortium. Clin Infect Dis. 2020;71(6):1367-76.
3. Garcia-Rubio R, de Oliveira HC, Rivera J, Trevijano-Contador N. The Fungal Cell Wall: Candida, Cryptococcus, and Aspergillus Species. Front Microbiol. 2020;10:2993.
4. Sant DG, Tupe SG, Ramana CV, Deshpande MV. Fungal cell membrane-promising drug target for antifungal therapy. J Appl Microbiol. 2016;121(6):1498-510.
5. Rex JR, Stevens DA. Drugs active against Fungi, Pneumocystis, and Microsporidia. In: Bennett JE, Dolin R, Blasser MJ (Eds). Mandell, Doulas, and Bennett's Principles and Practice of Infectious Diseases, 8th edition. Philadelphia: Elsevier Saunders; 2015.
6. Pappas PG, Kauffman CA, Andes DR, Clancy CJ, Marr KA, Ostrosky-Zeichner L, et al. Clinical Practice Guideline for the Management of Candidiasis: 2016 Update by the Infectious Diseases Society of America. Clin Infect Dis. 2016;62(4):e1-50.

7. Perfect JR, Dismukes WE, Dromer F, Goldman DL, Graybill JR, Hamill RJ, et al. Clinical practice guidelines for the management of cryptococcal disease: 2010 update by the Infectious Diseases Society of America. Clin Infect Dis. 2010;50(3):291-322.
8. Patterson TF, Thompson GR 3rd, Denning DW, Fishman JA, Hadley S, Herbrecht R, et al. Practice Guidelines for the Diagnosis and Management of Aspergillosis: 2016 Update by the Infectious Diseases Society of America. Clin Infect Dis. 2016;63(4):e1-e60.
9. Marr KA, Schlamm HT, Herbrecht R, Rottinghaus ST, Bow EJ, Cornely OA, et al. Combination antifungal therapy for invasive aspergillosis: a randomized trial. Ann Intern Med. 2015;162(2):81-9. Erratum in: Ann Intern Med. 2019;170(3):220.
10. Cornely OA, Alastruey-Izquierdo A, Arenz D, Chen SCA, Dannaoui E, Hochhegger B, et al; Mucormycosis ECMM MSG Global Guideline Writing Group. Global guideline for the diagnosis and management of mucormycosis: an initiative of the European Confederation of Medical Mycology in cooperation with the Mycoses Study Group Education and Research Consortium. Lancet Infect Dis. 2019;19(12):e405-e421.
11. Galgiani JN, Ampel NM, Blair JE, Catanzaro A, Geertsma F, Hoover SE, et al. 2016 Infectious Diseases Society of America (IDSA) Clinical Practice Guideline for the Treatment of Coccidioidomycosis. Clin Infect Dis. 2016;63(6):e112-46.
12. Ashley ESD, Lewis R, Lewis JS, Martin C, Andes D. Pharmacology of systemic antifungal therapy. Clin Infect Dis. 2006;43(Suppl 1):S28-39.
13. Children's Health Queensland Health and Hospital Service. Antifungal Prophylaxis and Treatment in Paediatric Oncology Patients and other Immunocompromised Children. [online] Available from: https://www.childrens.health.qld.gov.au/wp-content/uploads/PDF/ams/DUG-Antifungal.pdf. [Last Aaccessed January, 2022].
14. Government of Western Australia Child and Adolescent Health Service. Posaconazole Monograph—Paediatric. Perth Children's Hospital. [online] Available from: https://pch.health.wa.gov.au/-/media/Files/Hospitals/PCH/General-documents/Health-professionals/ChAMP-Monographs/Posaconazole.pdf. [Last Aaccessed January, 2022].
15. Brüggemann RJ, Alffenaar JW, Blijlevens NM, Billaud EM, Kosterink JG, Verweij PE, et al. Clinical relevance of the pharmacokinetic interactions of azole antifungal drugs with other coadministered agents. Clin Infect Dis. 2009;48(10):1441-58.
16. Red Book. (2018). Antimicrobial Agents and Related Therapy. Antifungal Drugs for Systemic Fungal Infections. [online] Available online: https://redbook.solutions.aap.org/book.aspx?bookid=2205. [Last Aaccessed January, 2022].
17. Hamill RJ. Amphotericin B formulations: a comparative review of efficacy and toxicity. Drugs. 2013;73(9):919-34.
18. Johnson PC, Wheat LJ, Cloud GA, Goldman M, Lancaster D, Bamberger DM, et al; U.S. National Institute of Allergy and Infectious Diseases Mycoses Study Group. Safety and efficacy of liposomal amphotericin B compared with conventional amphotericin B for induction therapy of histoplasmosis in patients with AIDS. Ann Intern Med. 2002;137(2):105-9.
19. Fisher JF, Sobel JD, Kauffman CA, Newman CA. Candida urinary tract infections-treatment. Clin Infect Dis. 2011;52(Suppl 6):S457-66.

Infectious Diseases

CHAPTER 5

Meningococcal Disease

Rashna Dass Hazarika

■ INTRODUCTION

Meningococcal disease, also known as "invasive meningococcal disease (IMD)" poses a major public health threat because of its rapidly progressive nature with high mortality and morbidity. It has a potential to lead to major epidemics, especially affecting young children below 5 years of age, adolescents, and young adults. Vieusseux in 1805 first described the disease in an outbreak with 33 deaths that occurred in the vicinity of Geneva, Switzerland.[1] Marchiafava and Celli from Italy in 1884 first described the intracellular structure of *Neisseria meningitidis* from cerebrospinal fluid (CSF).[2] Based on the structural differences in the polysaccharide capsule, *N. meningitidis* has been divided in to 12 serotypes designated as A, B, C, H, I, K, L, M, X, Y, Z, 29E, and W-135. Serotypes A, B, C, Y, and W-135 are responsible for most infections.[3] The emergence of sulfonamide-resistant strains in the 1963 epidemic in two military bases in California served as the trigger for the development of the meningococcal vaccine. Currently, several effective vaccines are available against IMD and are the best way to protect from this dreadful infection.

■ EPIDEMIOLOGY

Global Perspective

Neisseria meningitidis is now recognized as the main etiological agent of bacterial meningitis beyond infancy and in young adults.[4] It is endemic across the world with some areas being hyperendemic, epidemic, or pandemic. About 80 countries around the world are affected by the disease, with an annual caseload of 1.2 million and 135,000 deaths.[5] Ninety percent of the cases are caused by serogroups A, B, C, Y, and W-135. Serogroup A and C predominate in Asia.[6] In developed countries serogroup B is responsible for most cases. Nearly 30–40% of the cases in the Unites States and 90% in Europe and Australia are caused by the serogroup B.[6,7] Serogroup W-135 is also becoming increasingly important especially related to the Hajj pilgrimage.[8] Epidemic rates of meningococcal disease however vary from <1–3/100,000 in many developed countries to as high as 10–25/100,000 in some developing countries.[5] The different pathogenic properties of *N. meningitidis* strains and different socioeconomic, environmental, and climatological conditions are responsible for the varying attack rates across the globe.

Meningococcal disease is often seasonal in nature with serogroup A and C mostly increasing during the dry season in Africa whereas serogroup B and C peaking during the winter months in the developed countries. The largest and most frequently recurring outbreaks have been in the semi-arid area of sub-Saharan Africa for the last 100 years, otherwise known as the "meningitis belt."[9] The last 30 years have seen many epidemics in Asia with the largest reported from China in 1980.[10]

Indian Scenario

One of the first attempts to look at the burden of meningococcal disease in India was done by Sinclair et al. in 2010.[11] In this report, tertiary care centers had about 3.3% cases of bacterial meningitis out of the total admissions during the non-epidemic periods. *N. meningitidis* accounted for about 1.9% of the total admissions, with serotype A being the most common followed by serotype C. Epidemic cases were first reported in 1878. The first documented reports of cerebrospinal fever were by Patel describing 170 cases from Bombay (now Mumbai) from 1921 to 1924, occurring in overcrowded areas and mostly in winter and spring, and affecting adults > 20 years of age. The first major epidemics were reported in the 1930's from Delhi, Kolkata, and Ahmedabad. Subsequently there have been many epidemics of meningococcal disease in India nearly every 20 years with small outbreaks in between. The largest epidemic was reported from New Delhi in 1984 with 6,133 cases and 799 deaths reported at the peak of the epidemic. Subsequent epidemics were again reported in 2004–2005 from New Delhi, 2008–2009 from Meghalaya, and 2009 from Tripura. The epidemics mostly occur in the dry months of the end of winter and beginning of spring.[11] In the interepidemic period, the disease remains endemic. The disease mostly occurs in young children and infants but has an age shift to adolescents and young adults during epidemics.

About 10 years later in 2020, Dutta et al. reviewed the meningococcal data and found that there is no routine surveillance of meningococcal disease in India.[12] Therefore, data on endemic disease is lacking due to insufficient surveillance and lack of diagnostic facilities. A total of 262 publications were screened and finally 32 original studies were used for reviewing the epidemiology of meningococcal disease in India. Data from 9 papers from 2002 onward showed that the incidence of meningococcal disease in an epidemic setting varied from 4.5 to 23.4% with a mortality ranging from 0–21.8%. The most common serogroup was A, and one study reported 20% of the cases to be due to serogroup A and 30% due to A,C, W, and Y. Data from twelve papers showed the incidence of disease in nonendemic period to be about 0.1–7.6% with the disease occurring mostly in adolescents and young adults. Serogroup A was the most common followed by few cases reports of serogroups B, C, and Y. However, the authors felt that the disease is severely underreported and underrecognized.

ETIOPATHOGENESIS

The four conditions that must be fulfilled for the etiopathogenesis of IMD include exposure to a pathogenic strain, colonization of the nasopharyngeal mucosa, survival and passage through the nasopharyngeal mucosa, and finally survival of the bacteria in the bloodstream.[10] Transmission happens following direct contact to a patient or exposure to droplets of a susceptible individual for a distance up to 1 meter. The spread usually occurs from a nasopharyngeal carrier. The carriage rate of *N. meningitidis* has been described to range from 10-35%.[13] However, the carriage rate can reach up to 100% in close contacts such as students, military recruits, and pilgrims.[14]

The nasopharyngeal colonization is influenced by temperature, humidity, host defense, and bacterial factors.[13] It is, however, unclear why some humans become carriers and others do not. Nasopharyngeal colonization is facilitated by damage to the ciliated epithelium by either passive or active smoking. The colonization and occurrence of the invasive forms of the disease can also be facilitated by stressful events such as a preceding viral infection.[15] The serogroups A, B, and C are more invasive in nature.

Pathogenesis of meningococcal disease involves three steps, i.e., interaction of the host and pathogen, activation of the host immune response followed by effect on various organ systems.

Interaction of Host and Pathogen

This interaction involves nasopharyngeal colonization by the bacteria followed by invasion of the vascular compartments and meninges, and lastly by continued survival in the bloodstream. Adhesion factors such pili and opacity proteins (Opa and Opc) facilitate nasopharyngeal colonization. Two other proteins widely expressed in virulent *N. meningitidis* strains known as *Neisseria* hia homologue A (NhhA), and adhesion and penetration protein (app) help in adhesion and penetration of the meningococci into the nasopharyngeal epithelial cells.[16] After internalization in the nasopharynx, the meningococci enter the endothelial cells lying next to the nasopharyngeal epithelium. Crossing of the bacteria through the choroid plexus in the ventricles and the capillary endothelia which make up the blood-brain barrier (BBB) helps the meningococci to enter the brain. This is influenced to a great extent by the flow rate and shear stresses in the BBB. Areas with low blood flow and low shear stress allow more adhesion and transport of meningococci to the brain.[17] Further the pili and Opa and Opc enhance the entry and survival of the bacteria in the meninges. Once the BBB is breached, the meningococci interact with the leptomeningeal epithelial cells and release proinflammatory cytokines and result in meningitis.[16]

In the bloodstream, the meningococci are exposed to a lot of inhibitory factors such as antibody/complement complexes and opsonophagocytic mechanisms. This is overcome by the presence of the lipo-oligosaccharide (LOS) in the capsule of meningococci. They also bypass the complement system by various mechanisms and survive in the bloodstream.

Activation of the Host Immune Response

Once the viable meningococci survive in the bloodstream, the subsequent behavior of the bacteria in the human body depends on the degree of bacteremia, and the status of the host immune system. In patients with low bacteremia, the organism is cleared spontaneously following a mild and transient flu-like infection.[18] In others where the host immune factors do not clear the infection, the meningococci survive and lead to overt clinical manifestations. The severity of the clinical manifestations is dependent on the capacity of the bacteria to survive in the blood and its ability to multiply rapidly in the blood.[19] Immunoprotection in the human host depends on the production of specific antibodies.[19] The degree of host immune response is determined by the release of endotoxins from the outer membrane blebs.[20] The factor responsible for the striking difference in the acute and severe presentation seen in patients with meningococcal septicemia compared to the more benign course of patients with chronic meningococcemia is the secretion of more toxic endotoxin from the meningococcal strains in the septicemic patients.[21] The host response to these endotoxins differs from person to person. Complement and macrophage activation and neutrophil killing, all determine the clinical manifestation.[22,23]

Effect on Various Organ Systems

By utilizing the various mechanisms of immune escape, the viable meningococci cause diverse effects on various organ systems as described below.

Microvascular Injury

Four processes are affected. The first is increased vascular permeability, which causes volume loss by capillary leak in all vascular beds resulting in hypovolemia and shock. Subsequently, loss of cardiac compensatory mechanisms leads to impaired cardiac output. Loss of albumin in the urine compounds the physiologic instability by increasing the loss of both fluids and electrolytes. The accumulation of protein-rich fluid in the lungs and abdominal cavities also leads to pulmonary edema and respiratory failure.[24,25]

The second effect of microvascular injury is the intense initial vasoconstriction in patients with meningococcal sepsis leading to cold and blue peripheries followed by thrombosis in the peripheral vasculature leading to gangrene. On the other hand, some patients have intense vasodilatation manifesting as warm shock.

The third effect is loss of thromboresistance and intravascular coagulation due to activation of procoagulant pathways. There is a decrease in the levels of prostacyclin and antithrombin production, decreased secretion of protein C and S, increased plasminogen activator inhibitor-1 (PAI-1) and tissue factor expression.[26] The levels of PAI-1 increase to a great extent in meningococcal sepsis and have a direct correlation with the severity of the disease and death.[27]

The fourth effect is myocardial dysfunction secondary to negative inotropic effects induced by nitric oxide, tumor necrosis factor-α, and interleukin-1β.[28] This myocardial dysfunction is further compounded by existing hypoxia, acidosis, hypoglycemia, hypokalemia, hypocalcemia, and hyperphosphatemia. The above four processes result in impairment of microvascular blood flow to the tissues and organs of the body leading to shock and multiorgan failure.

Renal Impairment

Some degree of renal impairment always exists in patients with meningococcal septicemia secondary to the vascular leak and hypovolemia. Oliguria and rise in serum creatinine may be seen. This is transient and responds well to appropriate fluid therapy.[19]

Pulmonary Effects

Capillary leak leads to early respiratory involvement in the form of tachypnea and progression to respiratory failure. Aggressive fluid management can compound the problem by causing pulmonary edema.

Gastrointestinal Effects

Majority of patients will have some gastrointestinal manifestations secondary to shock and hypoxia leading to ileus and occasional perforation.[28]

Central Nervous System Effects

The central nervous system (CNS) effects can be because of both direct invasion of meninges and effect of shock and hypoxia. A significant proportion of patients have raised intracranial tension (ICT) and decreased consciousness and risk of cerebral hypoperfusion and infarcts.

■ CLINICAL FEATURES

Based on the pathophysiology, patients with meningococcal infection can be broadly classified into four categories:[29]
1. Septicemia without shock

2. Shock but no meningitis
3. Septicemia and meningitis both
4. Meningitis.

An easier way of clinical classification is presentation as meningitis, meningococcemia (septicemia), or a combination of both. This sort of a clinical classification helps in the management of these patients aggressively and appropriately.

Meningococcal Meningitis

Patients with meningitis present with fever, headache, vomiting, photophobia, drowsiness, and confusion and have neck stiffness with positive meningeal signs on clinical examination. Many would expect that such cases would also have the classical rash at presentation. This, however, is not true. Our own experience from Meghalaya showed that rash was seen in approximately 24% of the cases.[30] Forty percent of the cases present with seizures. Symptoms in the young infants are usually nonspecific such as fever, decreased activity, poor feeding, drowsiness, and seizures mimicking any other viral illness in contrast to older children and adolescents. Rash is rarely seen in infants.[31]

Meningococcemia and Septicemia

Meningococcemia has a more abrupt presentation with fever, chills, nausea, vomiting, muscle pains, and the classical purpura or petechial rash with or without bullae formation. One should be cautious if there is no meningitis as it indicates a poor prognosis. Some studies have shown that children under 16 years frequently have leg pains, cold extremities, and abnormal skin color in the first 12 hours of IMD (median onset 7–12 hours) suggestive of a septicemic process, particularly in severe meningococcemia. The classic features of hemorrhagic rash, meningism, and impaired consciousness are late signs (median onset 13–22 hours).[32] Some may present with chronic meningococcemia. These patients present with intermittent fever, rashes, arthritis, headaches, splenomegaly, endocarditis, and immune reactions.

Meningococcal septicemia is primarily characterized by a classic purpura in a patient who has fever and tachycardia. The clinical pearl is to always consider meningococcemia in an unwell child with a purpura unless proven otherwise.[31,32] The purpura may vary widely in patients with faint rashes in some and more prominent ones known as purpura fulminans in others **(Figs. 5.1A to D)**. Capillary leak can manifest as periorbital puffiness and generalized anasarca **(Fig. 5.2)**.

The Center for Disease Control (CDC), USA has provided the updated case definitions for meningococcal meningitis and septicemia in 2015 as follows:[33]

Meningococcal Disease

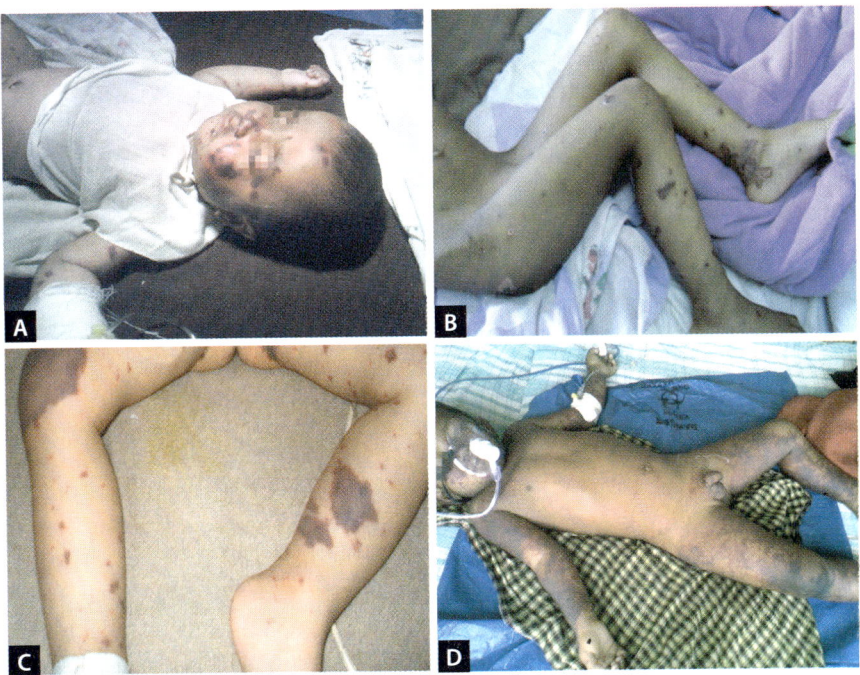

Figs. 5.1A to D: Various forms of the rash in IMD. Figure D shows purpura fulminans.
(IMD: invasive meningococcal disease)

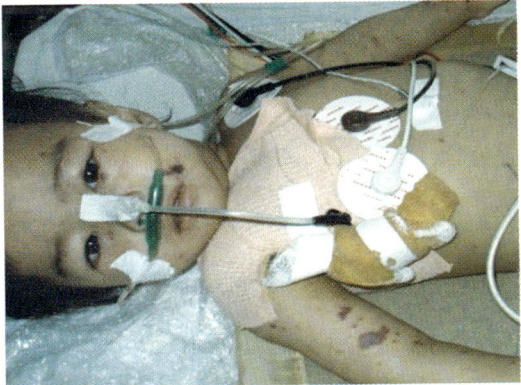

Fig. 5.2: Periorbital swelling in a patient with meningococcemia (secondary to capillary leak).

Suspect:
- Clinical purpura fulminans in the absence of a positive blood culture, OR
- Gram-negative diplococci, not yet identified, isolated from a normally sterile site (e.g., blood or CSF)

Probable:
- Detection of *N. meningitidis* antigen:
  - In formalin-fixed tissue by immunohistochemistry (IHC) OR
  - In CSF by latex agglutination

Confirmed:
- Detection of *N. meningitidis*-specific nucleic acid in a specimen from a normally sterile body site (e.g., blood or CSF) using a validated polymerase chain reaction (PCR) assay OR
- Isolation of *N. meningitidis*:
  - From a normally sterile body site (e.g., blood or CSF, or less commonly, synovial, pleural, or pericardial fluid), OR
  - From purpuric lesions

Meningococcal septicemia progresses rapidly to shock, multiorgan failure, and death in less than a day. In our own experience from Meghalaya some of the very sick patients died within hours of admission to the hospital and while on treatment.[30] The first 4–6-hour period is characterized by nonspecific symptoms such as fever, drowsiness, nausea, and poor feeding. By the next 12 hours, nonspecific signs of sepsis such as leg pains, cold hands and feet, and abnormal color appear. After 12 hours, the classic rapidly evolving purpuric rash, neck pain, and stiffness usually develop.[34] Unfortunately, most of the cases of meningococcal septicemia get diagnosed only after the appearance of the late signs. Initial misdiagnosis is common in admitted children.

Literature promotes the *"tumbler test"* to parents (i.e., compression of the rash by a transparent tumbler or glass for a few seconds and looking for nonblanching nature of the rash).[35] Presence of a nonblanching purpuric rash (>2 mm in diameter) in an ill febrile child in all probability points to meningococcal disease unless proved otherwise. About 11% of children with the petechial rash will eventually be diagnosed with meningococcal disease.[36] Many others will have viral infections. Up to 30% of children with meningococcal disease may present with a nonspecific maculopapular rash.[37]

Various complications such as shock, respiratory failure, azotemia, metabolic acidosis, hypo and hyperglycemia, coagulopathy, electrolyte imbalance, and neuropsychiatric manifestations can occur.

■ DIFFERENTIAL DIAGNOSIS

Meningococcal meningitis presents like any other bacterial or viral meningitis, and in the initial period it may be missed for a flu-like illness. The other differentials are those of illnesses with fever with rash such as invasive pneumococcal disease, dengue, leptospirosis, Lyme disease, rickettsiosis, human immunodeficiency virus (HIV) with CNS infections, tubercular meningitis, infective endocarditis, or conditions such as acute disseminated encephalomyelitis, and hematological malignancy. Septicemia with shock may mimic an adrenal failure.

Meningococcal Disease

■ DIAGNOSIS

Once a clinical suspicion of IMD is made, all attempts must be made to isolate the organism. Here one must remember that *N. meningitidis* is a fastidious organism highly susceptible to cold, heat, and drying. It grows best in a carbon dioxide-rich humid environment at 89.6–98.6°F and a pH of 7–7.5.[38] So, it can die even before or during plating in a culture medium and result in negative cultures. It is also highly susceptible to antibiotics and even a single dose of antibiotic may yield a negative culture.[39] Other barriers to the diagnosis of IMD are unaffordability, lack of after-hours diagnostic facilities, lack of laboratory expertise in detecting *N. meningitidis* and lack of other techniques such as latex agglutination test (LTA) and PCR for establishing a diagnosis.[38] PCR and LTA are specially useful in those who have already received prior antibiotics.

The investigations to be sent are for:
1. Confirmation of diagnosis
2. To detect complications.

Tests for Confirmation of Diagnosis

Blood cultures should be sent in all patients as far as possible prior to antibiotic therapy, and positive blood cultures are seen in about 40% of cases.[40] Once the patient is stable and there is no evidence of raised ICT, a lumbar puncture (LP) is done and the CSF is divided into three parts—first part is sent for physical examination routine microscopy, biochemical analysis and Gram stain, second part is for latex agglutination test (LAT) and/or PCR if available, and the third part is incubated for culture on blood or chocolate agar **(Fig. 5.3)**. The yield is better if the CSF can be plated directly on to a blood or chocolate agar plate during the LP and the plates are then sent to the laboratory at room temperature. The typical CSF findings in bacterial meningitis are shown in **Table 5.1**.

Latex agglutination tests (LAT) use the principle of detecting the specific polysaccharide antigen on the surface of the bacteria. In India, the available

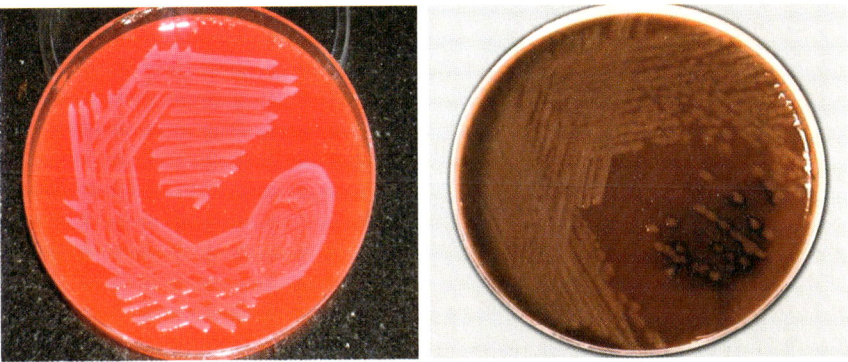

Fig. 5.3: Colonies of *Neisseria meningitidis* on blood and chocolate agar culture plates.

Meningococcal Disease

TABLE 5.1: Typical CSF findings in bacterial meningitis.

CSF parameter	Typical finding
Cell count	1000–5000/mm^3 (range 10–10000)
Neutrophils	80%
Glucose	<40 mg/dL
Protein	100–500 mg/dL
CSF to serum glucose levels	<0.4
Gram stain	Positive in 60–90% of cases
Culture	Positive in 70–85% of cases
Latex agglutination test (LAT) and Polymerase chain reaction (PCR)	Yield increases many folds

(CSF: cerebrospinal fluid)

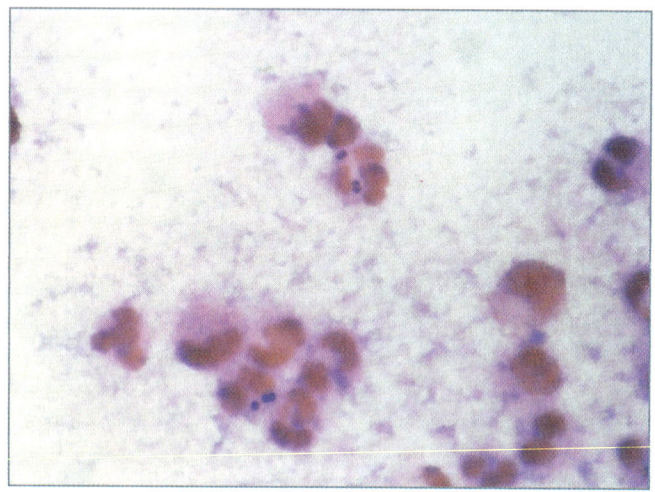

Fig. 5.4: Diplococci in pairs in a Gram stain of CSF. (CSF: cerebrospinal fluid)

LAT can test for *Haemophilus influenzae B, Streptococcus pneumoniae, Escherichia coli K1, N. meningitidis A, B, C,* and *Y, Group B streptococcus, and Streptococcus agalactiae.* LAT is more sensitive than culture for detection of *N. meningitidis* in the CSF, the positivity ranging from 22–93.5%. LAT is useful because of its high negative predictive value which helps to rule out acute bacterial meningitis.[40] The other advantage of LAT is that the results are available in about 10–15 minutes.

Gram stain of the CSF should always be done and is positive for the typical gram-negative diplococci **(Fig. 5.4)** in 75% of the cases. Other samples such as blister fluid, skin scrapings from site of the purpura fulminans lesions, other body fluids such as abscesses, and joint fluids are to be sent for both culture and Gram staining. Nasopharyngeal swabs are useful to detect the carriers of the organism. A molecular test like real-time PCR (RTPCR) is extremely sensitive (87–100%) and specific (98–100%) for detection of meningococcal infection, as it remains positive even after institution of antibiotic therapy and nonviability of the organism.[41] RTPCR is considered as a confirmatory test for meningococcal infection.

Tests to Detect Complications

All patients should have a complete blood count, C-reactive protein, serum procalcitonin (if available and affording), serum electrolytes, random blood glucose, serum creatinine, blood urea and coagulation parameters. This helps to look at the baseline parameters and to follow-up the patients during the hospital stay, as many of them are likely to have a stormy course and develop various complications such as electrolyte imbalances, coagulopathy, and multisystem failure. Chest X-rays are ordered if there is a suspicion of a respiratory involvement or in those cases requiring intubation and respiratory support. Neuroimaging studies are done if there is suspicion of complications such as a subdural abscess, intracerebral abscess, or raised ICT. A contrast-enhanced CT scan or MRI of the brain may be done. In an extremely sick child, a CT scan would be preferred because the procedure takes less time, but an MRI brain is always better for good image quality and zero radiation exposure.

■ MANAGEMENT

Aggressive and appropriate management greatly impact the outcome of the disease. The prognosis is greatly affected by the *"door-to-needle time"* (i.e., the time between the first arrival at a health facility and the first dose of antibiotic), as it greatly improves the outcomes and reduces mortality significantly.[42] Therefore, treatment receives priority over investigations. The cases can rapidly progress to shock and other complications even after admission and institution of antibiotics.[43] So during the initial treatment, no differentiation should be made between meningitis and meningococcemia, and one must manage these cases in a pediatric intensive care unit (PICU). The management begins with a quick assessment of the airway, breathing and circulation, and management of the airway, institution of oxygen therapy and securing an intravenous (IV) access. Some good early interventions, especially in the septicemic child, are insertion of nasogastric tube, early intubation, and start of mechanical ventilation with 100% oxygen even if there is no evidence of respiratory failure.

Important Issues in Management

Shock

Shock occurs due to widespread capillary leak, loss of vasomotor tone, and maldistribution of intravascular volume, impaired myocardial function, and impaired cellular function. Early recognition of shock is crucial as it leads to early intervention and improved outcome.[42] A simple sign like tachycardia may be the only early sign present to indicate fluid requirement and should be enough to start fluid resuscitation. Repeated fluid boluses comprising of 20 mL/kg of isotonic saline are given initially till shock resolves. Fluids >60 mL/kg increase the risk of pulmonary edema and such patients need transfer to a tertiary unit or PICU for elective intubation, mechanical ventilation, and insertion of a central venous pressure (CVP) line.

Fluid resuscitation is then continued followed by addition of epinephrine or norepinephrine based on volume status assessments by using the blood pressure, pulse volume, capillary refill time, and CVP measurements.[44] Many children with meningococcal disease may require as high as 100–200 mL/kg of fluid resuscitation but such patients also require mechanical ventilation. In our own experience, we had to use normal saline ranging from 20–200 mL/kg, and dopamine and dobutamine with good response.[30] Pollard et al. have shown that 4.5% albumin is more useful as a resuscitating fluid.[43] Children with meningococcal disease are known to present with lower serum albumin levels and may therefore benefit from 5% albumin. Many British pediatric intensivists routinely use albumin in the septicemic patients and demonstrated a significant reduction in the mortality (decrease up to 2%) in patients with meningococcal disease.[42] The National Institute for Health and Clinical Excellence (NICE), UK guidelines recommend using 20 mL/kg of isotonic saline or 4.5% albumin solution for the subsequent boluses.[45] However, in our experience, we have used only normal saline or Ringer's lactate as a resuscitating fluid and not albumin.

Persistent shock adversely impacts the survival in a time-dependent manner with at least a two-fold increase in mortality for every hour of delay in treatment.[35] Reversal of shock within 75 minutes of presentation leads to a 94% rate of survival.[42] Shock with hepatomegaly or rales may indicate coexistent myocardial dysfunction, and fluid resuscitation must be done with extreme care and caution in this group of patients. Maintenance fluids are continued by concurrent and continued careful assessment of the intravascular status. There is no role of fluid restriction unless there is evidence of raised ICT or syndrome of inappropriate antidiuretic hormone secretion (SIADH).[45]

Airway and Breathing

It is mandatory to ventilate patients with shock not only to avoid risk of pulmonary edema but also to reduce the work of breathing and oxygen consumption. The NICE guidelines recommend elective intubation and mechanical ventilation with vasoactive drugs when 60 mL/kg of fluids are required for volume resuscitation.[45] A low Glasgow coma scale (GCS < 8), hypoxia, respiratory failure, pulmonary edema, and raised ICT are also other indications for elective intubation. Rapid sequence intubation is the preferred method. However, shock should be corrected before intubation as induction of anesthesia may exacerbate the shock. If there is no evidence of raised ICT, ketamine may be used because of its ability to have a positive effect on the hemodynamic status along with atropine to circumvent reflex bradycardia which may worsen shock. Intubation must be performed by a professional with good experience in pediatric airway management.

Antibiotic Choices

The cornerstone of therapy in meningococcal disease is institution of the right antibiotic at the right time. The factors, which influence the success of antibiotic therapy, are the timing of the antibiotic (door to needle time), the ability of the antibiotic to penetrate the tissues, and the presence of antibiotic resistance. Broad-spectrum antibiotics should be used.

The most widely used antibiotics the world over are penicillin G, ceftriaxone, and cefotaxime. Increasing reports of reduced susceptibility of *N. meningitidis* to penicillin has come from various parts of the world[46,47] and therefore the recommended first-line therapy in the present scenario is ceftriaxone. There are recent reports on emergence of meningococcal strains resistant to penicillin, ceftriaxone, and ciprofloxacin.[48] Ciprofloxacin and ceftriaxone resistance has also been reported from India.[49,50] We had a similar experience while managing the meningococcal epidemic in Meghalaya in 2008-09, where patients had an excellent response to ceftriaxone in the beginning of the epidemic but after about 6 months of the epidemic, there was poor clinical response to ceftriaxone and antibiotic policy in our unit was revised to IV chloramphenicol for 7 days with good response.[30]

The second-line therapy consists of vancomycin and azithromycin. Though there are no studies to demonstrate the adequate duration of antibiotic therapy for *N. meningitidis*, classically a 7-day course of antibiotic is followed.[51]

Correction of Metabolic Abnormalities

Metabolic acidosis, hypokalemia, hypocalcemia, hypomagnesemia, hypophosphatemia, hyponatremia, and hypernatremia are common and require management accordingly. Hyponatremia is usually caused by SIADH, cerebral salt wasting, or adrenal insufficiency due to Waterhouse-Friderichsen syndrome. Magnesium replacement is required in cases of persistent hypokalemia. Bicarbonate infusion is indicated if the pH is <7.2.

In our experience, there are a significant number of patients who progress rapidly to develop diabetes insipidus (DI) which required aggressive management with hypotonic fluids and vasopressin. All our patients with DI had 100% mortality.[30] Hyperglycemia is quite common. In children with meningococcal disease, a small cohort of patients showed an association between hyperglycemia and severity of disease. In these patients, hyperglycemia was associated with low levels of insulin in contrast to findings in adults.[52] Severe hyperglycemia (blood glucose > 200 mg/dL) should be treated with insulin.

Raised Intracranial Tension

The standard management of raised ICT is with mannitol, 3% saline, and controlled mechanical ventilation aiming at a pCO_2 of 30–35 mm Hg and sedation if required. If patients have shock with raised ICT, the management of shock must be done first. Control of raised ICT is best achieved by adequate control of blood pressure. So, the general guidelines that are to be followed in managing raised ICT are avoidance of cannulation of the internal jugular vein, deferring lumbar puncture, especially in patients with reduced or fluctuating level of consciousness, i.e., GCS < 9 or a drop of 3 or more, relative bradycardia and hypertension, in those with focal neurological signs, abnormal posture or posturing, unequal, dilated, or poorly responsive pupils, papilledema, abnormal "doll's eye" movements, shock, extensive or spreading purpura, recent convulsions and a child yet to be stabilized, coagulation abnormalities, local infection at the LP site and cardiorespiratory insufficiency. All children with a GCS of ≤9 mandatorily require management in a PICU.

Seizures

The seizures are treated with benzodiazepines, phenytoin, or phenobarbitone. These patients also require monitoring for respiratory depression and a low threshold for elective intubation and mechanical ventilation, especially in those with status epilepticus.

Steroids

The NICE guidelines on steroid use in meningococcal meningitis state that children <3 months should not be given steroids. In older children, dexamethasone at 0.15 mg/kg per dose to a maximum of 10 mg, four times a day for 4 days for suspected or confirmed bacterial meningitis is recommended as soon as possible if lumbar puncture shows any of the following:
- Frankly purulent CSF
- CSF with white blood cell (WBC) count >1000/mm^3
- Increased CSF WBC count with protein concentration >1 g/L
- Bacteria on Gram stain.

Dexamethasone reduces neuronal damage if given prior to the first dose of antibiotic. In meningococcal shock (with a suspicion of adrenal insufficiency), hydrocortisone is given in a dose of 1 mg/kg every 6 hours.

Coagulation Disorders

Coagulopathy occurs secondary to endothelial damage, vasculitis, and disseminated intravascular coagulation (DIC). The best treatment of coagulopathy is the optimal management of shock. Mild clotting abnormalities are well tolerated and need no treatment. Fresh frozen plasma (FFP) is recommended in severe coagulopathy. In our own experience, IV vitamin K and if required FFP work with good results.[30]

Limb Ischemia and Gangrene

Necrotic areas must be monitored carefully as they become areas of bacterial colonization and multiplication. Surgical debridement is preferred in extensive wounds. Hyperbaric oxygen can also be tried in such necrotic tissues.[53]

Arthritis

Arthritis can be a result of direct bacterial seeding of the joints in the early phase of the illness or can be secondary to an immune-complex-mediated phenomenon in the subacute or convalescent phase of the illness. Treatment of the bacterial arthritis consists of antibiotics and drainage of joint fluid if needed. Immune complex reactions are usually treated with nonsteroidal anti-inflammatory drugs or steroids. A patient with immune-complex-mediated arthritis had a dramatic response to intravenous immunoglobulin (IVIG) used as a last resort.[54]

■ PROGNOSIS OF INVASIVE MENINGOCOCCAL DISEASE

The overall case fatality in invasive meningococcal disease is about 10% and rises to approximately 50–60% in those with fulminant disease and most deaths are due to respiratory or cardiac failure.[55] There are various scoring systems devised for prognostication in IMD. The most popular scoring systems are the Stiehm and Damrosch **(Box 5.1)** and the Glasgow Meningococcal Septicemia Prognostic Score (GMSPS) **(Box 5.2)**.[56,57] Among the survivors, about 30% have significant morbidity in the form of skin loss or scarring,

---

BOX 5.1: Stiehm and Damrosch criteria.

- Petechiae present for <12 hours before admission
- Hypotension (systolic blood pressure < 70 mm Hg)
- Absence of meningitis (<20 WBCs in CSF)
- Peripheral white cell count < 10,000 /mm^3
- ESR < 10 mm/hour

When three or more factors were present, mortality was 90%, and when two or less factors were present, mortality was 9%.

(CSF: cerebrospinal fluid; ESR: erythrocyte sedimentation rate; WBC: white blood cell)

> **BOX 5.2:** Glasgow meningococcal septicaemia prognostic score (GMSPS).
>
> | Criteria | Score |
> |---|---|
> | Hypotension* | 3 |
> | Skin/rectal temperature difference > 3°C | 3 |
> | Base deficit (capillary sample) < 8 mmol/L | 1 |
> | Modified pediatric coma score < 8 anytime or deterioration of ≥ 3 in an hour | 3 |
> | Lack of meningitis | 2 |
> | Parental opinion that the child's condition has become worse over the past hour | 2 |
> | Widespread ecchymoses or extending lesions on review | 1 |
>
> *Systolic BP < 75 mm Hg if below 4 years of age, < 85 mm Hg if older.
> Note: Any score >8 out of 15 in the GMSPS and presence of three or more factors in the Stiehm and Damrosch systems have a fatal outcome.

limb loss or amputation, hearing deficits, hemiplegia, neurodevelopmental delay, epilepsy, and neuropsychological effects such as post-traumatic stress disorder, depression, psychosis, anxiety, and learning difficulties.[58]

■ PREVENTION OF INVASIVE MENINGOCOCCAL DISEASE

This consists of two aspects—immediate chemoprophylaxis of close contacts and definitive prevention by immunization.

Chemoprophylaxis

The household contacts have a 100-fold more chance of contracting the disease. Household members, child-care center contacts and anyone directly exposed to the patient's oral secretions in the 7 days preceding symptoms qualify for being labeled as close contacts. Secondary disease occurs mostly after onset of disease in the index patient. Therefore, there is a need for immediate preventive chemoprophylaxis, as vaccination will require a minimum of 14 days for production of effective antibodies. Several drugs are available for chemoprophylaxis **(Table 5.2)**.[59] However, one must keep in mind that chemoprophylaxis is a temporary measure and cannot be used for long periods because of the issue of emergence of antimicrobial resistance.

Vaccination

Vaccines remain the best solution for control of IMD. Several good conjugate vaccines are available for use containing various strains. The conjugate vaccines currently used across the world are the monovalent vaccines such as Men A-TT (Men Afri A®, Serum Institute of India), monovalent Men B vaccine (available as Trumenda®, Pfizer, and Bexsero®, GlaxoSmithKline), and

TABLE 5.2: Drugs for chemoprophylaxis against meningococcal disease.[59]

Ciprofloxacin				
Adults and children over 12 years	500 mg	Single dose	PO	
Children aged 5–12 years	250 mg	Single dose	PO	
Children aged 1 month to 4 years	125 mg	Single dose	PO	
Alternative regimens *Rifampicin*				
Adults and children over 12 years	600 mg	BD	PO	2 days
Children aged 1–12 years	10 mg/kg (max 600 mg)	BD	PO	2 days
Neonates and infants under 1 year	5 mg/kg	BD	PO	2 days
Prophylaxis of meningococcal meningitis in pregnant contact:				
Ceftriaxone*	250 mg	Single dose	IM	
Ofloxacin	400 mg	Single dose	Oral	

*Not licensed for this indication, therefore counselling should be given.

the HibMen C (conjugated with TT, GlaxoSmithKline), and the conjugate tetravalent Men ACYW-135-DT (Menactra®, Sanofi Pasteur), Men ACYW-135-CRM 197 (Menveo®, GlaxoSmithKline), Men ACYW-135-TT (Nimenrix®, GlaxoSmithKline). The Men Afri A vaccine has been successful in reducing the incidence of IMD in sub-Saharan Africa to a remarkable extent. Currently, work is on for development of a pentavalent thermostable meningococcal vaccine (ACYW135X) by Serum Institute of India.

The schedules and strain recommendations vary from country to country based on local epidemiology. The Advisory Committee on Immunization Practices of the Centers for Disease Control and Prevention (CDC) recommends that the quadrivalent meningococcal conjugate vaccine (ACYW-135) to all children between 11 and 18 years of age with a booster at 16 years, and to those between 2 and 55 years of age who are at increased risk for meningococcal disease (C3, properdin, factor D and late complement deficiencies), persons with anatomic or functional asplenia, those who have prolonged exposure (e.g., microbiologists routinely working with *N. meningitidis*, or travelers to, or residents of countries where meningococcal disease is hyperendemic or epidemic), persons with HIV and first year college students in resident halls. It also recommends the meningococcal B vaccine to those children above 10 years at increased risk for meningococcal disease.[60]

The vaccines currently available in India are the conjugate ACYW-135 vaccines Menveo® and Menactra®. Menveo is recommended as a single dose from 2 to 70 years of age and Menactra is recommended in a two-dose schedule from 9 to 24 months given 3 months apart, and a single dose above 2 years of age up to 55 years. Currently, the Advisory Committee on Vaccines and Immunization Practices (ACVIP) of the Indian Academy of Pediatrics (IAP) recommends the use of the conjugate ACYW-135 meningococcal vaccines only in special groups.[61] The National Centre for Disease Control (NCDC) recommends the ACYW-135 conjugate meningococcal vaccines in India for those going to Hajj as pilgrims, and other travelers visiting countries where meningococcal disease is a major problem, or where frequent outbreaks occur, in high-risk groups such as children in orphanages, jail inmates and soldiers in barracks, and in mass vaccination during epidemics.[62]

■ KEY POINTS

- Invasive meningococcal disease has a high mortality and morbidity.
- An emerging infectious disease, IMD occurs as frequent epidemics at regular intervals with an endemic presence in many parts of the world including India.
- Serogroups A, C, Y and W-135 are seen in developing countries mostly, and serogroup B is more common in developed countries and in infants.
- Clinical effects are sudden and potentially fatal.
- Cases may present as septicemia, meningitis, or both with multiorgan involvement.
- Survival is dramatically affected by early and aggressive therapy.
- Prognosis is greatly affected by a reduced "house-to-hospital" and reduced "door-to-needle" time.
- Early suspicion and recognition of the disease by the practicing pediatrician and simple early interventions and early referral contribute to significant reduction of mortality.
- Pediatric ICU management improves survival and all patients (even if not sick at admission) must be kept under intensive monitoring.
- Chemoprophylaxis of close contacts and vaccination of high-risk groups are the best preventive measures.
- The current available conjugate vaccines are highly immunogenic.
- Vaccination is the only way to prevent IMD.

■ REFERENCES

1. Vieusseux M. Mémoire sur la maladie qui a regné a Genêve au printemps de 1805. J Med Chir Pharmacol. 1805;11:163.
2. Weichselbaum A. Ueber die aetiologie der akuten meningitis cerebospinalis. Fortschr Med. 1887;57:573-83.
3. Frash CE, Zollinger WD, Poolman JT. Serotype antigens of *Neisseria meningitidis* and a proposed scheme for designation of serotypes. Rev Infect Dis. 1985; 7:504-10.
4. Brouwer MC, Tunkel AR, van de Beek D. Epidemiology, diagnosis and antimicrobial treatment of acute bacterial meningitis. Clin Microbiol Review. 2010;23:467-92.
5. Jafri RZ, Ali A, Messonnier NE, Tevi-Benissan C, Durrheum D, Eskola J, et al. Global epidemiology of invasive meningococcal disease. Popul Health Metr. 2013;11(1): 17.

6. Steinhoff MC. Global epidemiology of meningococcal infections. In: Nelson KE, Williams CM (Eds). Text Book of Infectious Disease Epidemiology-Theory and Practice, 2nd edition. Sudbury, Massachusetts: Jones and Bartlett; 2007. pp. 637-51.
7. Australian meningococcal surveillance programannual report 2010. Commun Dis Intell Q Rep. 2011;35:217-28.
8. Lingappa JR, Al-Rabeah AM, Hajjeh R, Mustafa T, Fatani A, Al-Bassam T, et al. Serogroup W-135 meningococcal disease during the Hajj, 2000. Emerg Infect Dis 2003;9:665-71.
9. Greenwood B. 100 years of epidemic meningitis in West Africa-Has anything changed? Trop Med Int Health. 2006;11:773-80.
10. Schwartz B, Moore PS, Broome CV. Global epidemiology of meningococcal disease. Clin Microbiol Rev. 1989;2:S118-24.
11. Sinclair D, Preziosi MP, John TJ, Greenwood B. The epidemiology of meningococcal disease in India. Trop Med Int Health. 2010;15:1421-35.
12. Dutta AK, Swaminathan S, Abitbol V, Kolhapure S, Sathyanarayanan S. A comprehensive review of meningococcal disease burden in India, Infect Dis Ther. 2020;9 537–59.
13. Nelson JD. Jails, microbes, and the three-foot barrier. NEJM. 1996;335:885-6.
14. Caugant DA, Hoiby EA, Rosenqvist E, Froholm LO, Selander RK. Transmission of Neisseria meningitidis among asymptomatic military recruits and antibody analysis. Epidemiol Infect. 1992;109:241-53.
15. van Deuren M, Brandtzaeg P, van der Meer JWM. Update on meningococcal disease with emphasis on pathogenesis and clinical management. Clin Microbiol Rev. 2000;13:144-66.
16. Stephens DS, Farley MM. Pathogenic events during infection of the human nasopharynx with Neisseria meningitis and Haemophilus influenzae. Rev Infect Dis. 1991;13:22-3.
17. Leimkugel J, Hodgson A, Forgor AA, Fluger V, Dangy JP, Smith T, et al. Clonal waves of Neisseria colonisation and disease in the African meningitis belt: eight-year longitudinal study in northern Ghana. PLoS Med. 2007;4:e101.
18. Massari P, Ho Y, Wetzler LM. *Neisseria meningitidis* porin Por b interacts with mitochondria and protects cells from apoptosis. Proc Natl Acad Sci USA. 2000;97:9070-5.
19. Sullivan TD, LJ LaScolea Jr. *Neisseria meningitidis* bacteremia in children: Quantification of bacteremia and spontaneous clinical recovery without antibiotic therapy. Pediatrics. 1987;80:63-7.
20. Brandtzaeg P, Kierulf P, Gaustad P, SkulbergA, Bruun JN, Halvorsen S, et al. Plasma endotoxin as a predictor of multiple organ failure and death in systemic meningococcal disease. J Infect Dis. 1989;159:195-204.
21. Anderson BM. Endotoxin release from *Neisseria meningitidis*. Relationship between key bacterial characteristics and meningococcal disease. Scand J Infect Dis. 1989;64:1-43.
22. Prins JM, Lauw FN, Derkx BHF, Speelman P, Kuijper EJ, Dankert J, et al. Endotoxin release and cytokine production in acute and chronic meningococcemia. Clin Exp Immunol. 1998;114:215-9.
23. Lewis LA, Ram S. Meningococcal disease and the complement system. Virulence. 2014;5:98-126.

24. Klein NJ, Shennan GI, Heydermann RS, Levin M. Alteration in glycosaminoglycan metabolism and surface change on human umbilical vein endothelial cells induced b cytokines, endotoxin, and neutrophils. J Cell Sci. 1992;102 (Pt. 4):821-32.
25. Oragui EE, Nadel S, Kyd P, Levin M. Increased excretion of urinary glycosaminoglycans in meningococcal septicaemia and their relationship to proteinuria. Crit Care Med. 2000;28:3002-8.
26. Kornelisse RF, Hazelzet JA, Salvelkoul HF, Hop WCJ, Suur MH, Borsboom ANJ, et al. The relationship between plasminogen activator inhibitor-1 and proinflammatory and counter-inflammatory mediators in children with meningococcal septic shock. J Infect Dis. 1996;173;1148-56.
27. Hermans PW, Hibberd ML, Booy R, Daramola O, Hazeljet JA, de Groot R, et al. 4G/5G promoter polymorphism in the plasminogen activator inhibitor-1 gene and outcome of meningococcal disease. Meningococcal Research Group. Lancet. 1999;354:556-60.
28. Britto J, Nadel S, Habibi P, Levin M. Gastrointestinal perforation complicating meningococcal disease. Pediatr Infect Dis J. 1995;14:393-4.
29. Gedde-Dahl TW, Hoiby EA, Schillinger A, Lystad A, Bovre K. An epidemiological, clinical, and microbiological follow-up study of incident meningococcal disease cases in Norway, winter 181-1982. Material and epidemiology in the menOPP project. NIPP Ann. 1990;6:155-68.
30. Hazarika RD, Deka NM, Khyriem AB, Lyngdoh WV, Barman H, Duwarah SG, et al., Invasive meningococcal disease: An analysis of 110 cases from a tertiary care centre in Northeast India. Indian JPediatr. 2013;80:359-64.
31. Huang HR, Chen HL, Chu SM. Clinical spectrum of meningococcal infection in infants younger than six months of age. Chang Gung Med J. 2006;29:107-13.
32. Strelow VL, Vidal JE. Invasive meningococcal disease. Arq. Neuropsiquiatr 2013;71(9-B):653-8.
33. Centers for Disease Control and Prevention. Meningococcal Disease (*Neisseria meningitidis*): 2015 Case Definition. [online] Available from https://ndc.services.cdc.gov/case-definitions/meningococcal-disease-2015/. [Last accessed December, 2021].
34. Hart CA, Thomson APJ. Meningococcal disease and its management in children. BMJ. 2006;333:685-90.
35. Branco RG, Amoretti CF, Tasker RC. Meningococcal disease and meningitis. J Pediatr (Rio J). 2007;83:S46-53.
36. Wells LC, Smith JC, Weston VC, Collier J, Rutter N. The child with a non-blanching rash: How likely is meningococcal disease? Arch Dis Child. 2001;85:218-22.
37. Marzouk O, Thomson APJ, Sills J, Hart CA, Harris F. Features, and outcome in meningococcal disease presenting with maculopapular rash. Arch Dis Child. 1991;66:485-7.
38. Vyse A, Wolter JM, Chen J, T Ng, Soriano-Gabarro M. Meningococcal disease in Asia: An under recognized public health burden. Epidemiol Infect. 2011;139:967-85.
39. Yang YH, Fu SG, Peng H, Shen AD, Yue SJ, Go YF, et al. Abuse of antibiotics in China and its potential interference in determining the etiology of pediatric bacterial diseases. Pediatr Infect Dis. 1993;12:986-8.

40. Chanteau S, Dartevelle S, Mahmane AE, Djibo S, Boisier P, Nato F. New rapid diagnostic assays for Neisseria meningitidis serogroup A, W135, C and Y. PLoS Medicine. 2006;3:1579-86.
41. Richardson DC, Louie L, Louie M, Simor AE. Evaluation of a rapid PCR assay for diagnosis of meningococcal meningitis. J Clin Microbiol. 2003;41:3851-53.
42. Riordan FAI, Thompson APJ, Sills JA, Hart CA. Prospective study of door to needle time in meningococcal disease. J Accid Emerg Med. 1998;15:249-51.
43. Pollard AJ, Britto J, Nadel S, Munter C de, Habibi P,Levin M. Emergency management of meningococcal disease. Arch Dis Child 1999;80:290-6.
44. Sahoo T, Aradhya AS, Gulla KM. International guidelines 2020 for the management of septic shock in children. Indian Pediatr. 2020;57:671-5.
45. Visintin C, Mugglestone MA, Fields EJ, Jacklin P, Murphy SM, Pollard AJ. Management of bacterial meningitis and meningococcal septicaemia in children and young people: summary of NICE guidance. BMJ. 2010;341:c3209
46. Mortensen J E, Gerrety M J, Gray LD. Surveillance of antimicrobial resistance in *Neisseria meningitidis* from patients in the Cincinnati tristate region (Ohio, Kentucky, and Indiana). J Clin Microbiol. 2006;44:1592-3.
47. Vázquez, J A., Enriquez, R. Abad R, Alcalá B, Salcedo C, Arreaza L. Antibiotic resistant meningococci in Europe: Any need to act? FEMS Microbiology Rev. 2007;31:64-70.
48. Zouheir Y, Atany T, Boudebouch N. Emergence and spread of resistant *N. meningitidis* implicated in invasive meningococcal diseases during the past decade (2008-2017). J Antibiot (Tokyo). 2019;72:185-8.
49. Manchanda V, Bhalla P. Emergence of non-ceftriaxone-susceptible *Neisseria meningitidis* in India. J Clin Microbiol. 2006;44:4290-1.
50. Singhal S, Purnapatre KP, Kalia V, Dube S, Nair D, Deb M, et al. Ciprofloxacin-resistant *Neisseria meningitidis*, Delhi, India. Emerg Infect Dis. 2007;13:1614-6.
51. Tunkel AR, van de Beek D, Scheld WM. Acute meningitis. In: Mandell, Douglas, and Bennett's Principles and Practice of Infectious Diseases, 7th edition. London: Churchill Livingstone, Elsevier; 2010. pp. 1189-229.
52. DeKleijn ED, Joosten KF, Van Rijn B, Westerterp M, De Groot R, Hokken-Koelega ACS, et al. Low serum cortisol in combination with high adrenocorticotrophic hormone concentrations are associated with poor outcome in children with severe meningococcal disease. Pediatr Infect Dis J. 2002;21:330-6.
53. Takac I, Kvolik S, Divkovic D, Kalajdzic-Candrlic J, Puseljic S, Izakovic S. Conservative surgical management of necrotic tissues following meningococcal sepsis: case report of a child treated with hyperbaric oxygen. Undersea Hyperb Med. 2010;37:95-9.
54. Dass R, Barman H, Duwarah SG, Deka NM, Jain P, Choudhury V. Immune complex reaction after successful treatment of meningococcal disease: an excellent response to IVIG. Rheumatol Int. 2013;33:231-3
55. Naeini AE. Importance of scoring systems in prognosticating meningococcaemia. J Res Med Sciences. 2005;1:34-7.
56. Stiehm RE, Damrosch DS. Factors in the prognosis of meningococcal infection. Medical Progress. 1966;68:457-67.
57. Thomson AP, Sills JA, Hart CA. Validation of Glasgow meningococcal septicaemia prognostic score: a 10 year retrospective study. Crit Care Med. 1991;19:26-30.

58. Nadel S, Ninis N. Invasive meningococcal disease in the vaccine era. Front Pediatr. 2018;6:321.
59. Antimicrobial prophylaxis: Meningococcal meningitis. Meningitis: prevention of secondary cases of meningococcal meningitis/septicaemia. East Kent Hospital University,NHS Foundation Trust. [online] Available from http://www.ekhuft.nhs.uk/staff/clinical/antimicrobial-guidelines/antibiotic-prophylaxis/meningitis-prophylaxis/meningococcal-meningitis/. [Last accessed December, 2021].
60. Meningococcal vaccination: Recommendations of the Advisory Committee on Immunization Practices, 2020. MMWR. 2020;69: No 9.
61. Kasi SG, Shivananda S, Marathe S, Chatterjee K, Agarwalla SK, Dhir SK, et al. Indian Academy of Pediatrics (IAP) Advisory Committee on Vaccines and Immunization Practices (ACVIP): Recommended Immunization Schedule (2020-21) and Update on Immunization for Children Aged 0 Through 18 Years. Indian Pediatr. 2021;58:44-53.
62. National Centre for Disease Control. (2009). Meningococcal disease: Need to remain alert. CD Alert. [online] Available from https://ncdc.gov.in/WriteReadData/linkimages/OCT-NOV_098132922884.pdf. [Last accessed December, 2021].

Immunizations

SARS-CoV-2 Vaccines

Srinivas G Kasi

■ INTRODUCTION

On December 31, 2019, the Country Office of the World Health Organization (WHO) in the People's Republic of China picked up a media statement by the Wuhan Municipal Health Commission from their website on cases of "viral pneumonia" in Wuhan, People's Republic of China. Following a rapid spread across the globe, on March 11, 2020, the WHO declared it as a pandemic.[1] Globally, as on December 23, 2021, there have been 276, 436, 619 confirmed cases of Coronavirus-19 (COVID-19), including 5, 374, 744 deaths, reported to WHO. Corresponding figures for India are 34, 765, 976 confirmed cases and 478,759 deaths.[2]

The observations that the novel strain of COVID-19, labeled as SARS-CoV-2 by WHO is transmitted from asymptomatic infected individuals and it has spread rapidly across the globe, imply that control of this viral infection by inducing herd immunity will be challenging without the prospect of a vaccine.

■ IMMUNOLOGY AS RELATED TO VACCINATION

The mechanisms of the human immune response to natural severe acute respiratory syndrome–related coronavirus (SARS-CoV-2) infection are incompletely understood. Entry into humans occurs through the respiratory tract. At initial contact, the receptor-binding domain (RBD) of the spike protein (S-protein) interacts with the angiotensin-converting enzyme-2 (ACE2) receptor. Interaction with a specific cellular serine protease, the transmembrane protease serine-2 (TMPRSS2), helps the virus to enter the human alveolar and bronchial mucosal cells.

Evidence to date suggests that the SARS-CoV-2 suppresses activation of the innate immune system. Immunoglobulin-M (IgM) and immunoglobulin-G (IgG) antibodies to SARS-CoV-2 are detectable within 1–2 weeks after the onset of symptoms in most infected individuals, with the magnitude of the antibody titers correlating with the severity of the illness. Subjects with asymptomatic or mild illness have faster waning of antibody titers. Neutralizing antibodies target the RBD of the S-protein and include IgG, IgM and IgA antibodies. Antibody responses to other proteins are also elicited, but their role in protection is uncertain.[3]

Emerging evidence suggests an important and crucial role of the T cell-mediated immunity for protection against SARS-CoV-2. Convalescent subjects have high titers of both neutralizing antibodies and T cells, with the highest titers in those with severe disease. Milder disease elicits a predominantly T helper type 1 (Th1) response while subjects with severe lung involvement are seen to have a type 2 (Th2) response.[3]

In a study examining the immunological memory to SARS-CoV-2 assessed for up to 8 months after infection, IgG to the S-protein was relatively stable over 6+ months. Spike-specific memory B cells were more abundant at 6 months than at 1 month post-symptom onset. SARS-CoV-2-specific CD4+ T cells and CD8+ T cells declined with a half-life of 3–5 months.[4] The duration of the immune response may have implications regarding the need for boosters.

■ PANDEMIC SPEED VACCINES

Developing COVID-19 vaccines in record time is a challenging process and involves different stages of vaccine development running in parallel versus the traditional sequential process that needs several years. Parallel developmental processes compress the vaccine development process from the usual decade to a year or two. This process involves massive investments and significant financial risks.

Rapid development of COVID-19 vaccines has been enabled by various factors including knowledge derived from trials of previous coronavirus vaccines that pinpointed the role of the spike protein in the pathogenesis of infection and the observation that neutralizing antibodies against the spike protein are protective. Exploring multiple platforms simultaneously will increase the chances of overall success in the development of a COVID-19 vaccine. Multiple platforms are also essential, as different types of vaccines may be needed for different population groups. Some vaccines may elicit a better immune response in older individuals, while some may not be safe in the immunocompromised. Development of novel vaccine platforms (e.g., the nucleic acid platforms) has made possible the rapid development and scaling up of production of COVID-19 vaccines. Knowledge about the genetic sequence of the pathogen enables creation, modification, and rapid scale-up of COVID-19 vaccines.[5]

The speed of the pandemic and vaccine development is illustrated by the sequence of development of the Moderna/NIH mRNA vaccine. On January 11, 2020, two Chinese authorities shared the genetic sequence of the novel coronavirus. On January 13, 2020, the National Institute of Health (NIH) and the infectious disease research team of Moderna finalized the sequence for mRNA-1273. Moderna mobilized toward clinical manufacture. On February 7, 2020, the first clinical batch of mRNA-1273 was completed, a total of 25 days from sequence selection to vaccine manufacture. The batch then proceeded to analytical testing for release.[6]

■ VACCINE PLATFORMS

Various platforms, conventional and new, are being explored for COVID-19 vaccines. These are listed here.

Inactivated Vaccines

Undesired immunopotentiation in the form of eosinophilic infiltration or increased infectivity, which was noted with the earlier SARS and MERS vaccines, has not been noted with the inactivated COVID-19 vaccines. Adjuvants play an important role in skewing the immune response to a Th1 type. The inactivated COVID-19 vaccines, presently, in clinical trials, have not demonstrated any disease enhancement. There are six inactivated vaccines in phase 3 trials and four in phase 4 trials.[7]

Live Attenuated Vaccines

For COVID-19 vaccines, attenuation is achieved by deleting or modifying the genes responsible for virulence. A novel method in use for COVID-19 vaccines is the codon-deoptimizing technology. In this technology, viral genomes are recoded synthetically, producing suboptimal codon pairs. This results in instability of mRNA and reduced efficiency of translation of the codon pair-deoptimized genes, resulting in virus attenuation. There is only one such live attenuated vaccine, being jointly developed by Codagenix and Serum Institute of India, which is in phase 3 trial.[7]

Viral Vectored Vaccines

In viral vectored vaccines, one or more genes that encode an antigen of interest, is inserted into the genome of an unrelated virus (viral vector) by genetic engineering. The viral vector can be replication competent (live attenuated) or replication deficient. Commonly used viral vectors include adenovirus (Ad), measles virus (MV), vesicular stomatitis virus (VSV), alphaviruses, poxviruses and herpes viruses. Viral vectors induce potent CD4+ and CD8+ responses even in the absence of an adjuvant, which makes them a suitable vaccine vector for vaccines against viral infections. The disadvantages include a longer production timeframe, the need for biosafety level 2 laboratories and the observation that preexisting immunity in vaccine recipients to viral vectors may decrease the vaccine effectiveness. The latter can be minimized by using low human prevalence adenoviral serotypes (Ad26 or Ad35). The first vectored vaccine to enter human usage is the (rVSV-ZEBOV) Ebola vaccine, the recombinant vesicular stomatitis virus-Zaire Ebola virus (rVSV-ZEBOV).[8] Several vectored vaccines against COVID, are in various stages of clinical development. As of

December 21, 2021, there are 20 non-replicating vectored viral vaccines (two in phase 3 and three in phase 4) and two replication-competent vectored viral vaccines (one in phase 3) in various stages of clinical development.[7]

Subunit Vaccines

Subunit vaccines consist of parts of the pathogen, which have the capability to trigger a strong immune response. Subunit vaccines may contain protein or polysaccharide components of the pathogen. Subunit vaccines are considered very safe. While these vaccines are relatively cheap and easy to produce, they may lack the pathogen-associated molecular patterns (PAMPS) necessary for an efficient immune response. To overcome this problem, subunit vaccines are usually combined with potent adjuvants and booster doses may be required. Only protein subunit vaccines are being developed against the virus that causes COVID-19. As on December 21, 2021, there are 47 subunit vaccines in clinical development of which 13 are in phase 3 and 1 is in phase 4.[7]

Nucleic Acid Vaccines

These are of two types—(1) RNA vaccines and (2) DNA vaccines.

RNA vaccines

RNA vaccines, which encode the genes for the protective antigen, utilize the cell's machinery for synthesizing protein of interest, which is recognized as a foreign protein and results in a protective immune response by the recipient's immune mechanism. In the protein synthesis pathway by cells, mRNA is the intermediate step between the translation of the DNA encoding the antigen and the production of the protein by the ribosomes in the cytoplasm.[8,9]

The major advantages of the mRNA platform include safety (as there is no potential risk of infection or insertional mutagenesis), efficacy, rapid uptake, and expression in the cytoplasm and finally robust adaptive humoral and cellular immune responses. The versatility and rapidity of production enables rapid production within days of obtaining gene sequence information.[10,11]

The disadvantages include instability and rapid degradation in the cytosol by RNAase enzymes, aberrant immune reactions and the need for strict storage conditions.

Since the entire process occurs in the cytoplasm and reversion of RNA into DNA is a property found only in retroviruses, which contain reverse transcriptase enzymes, there is no risk of insertional mutagenesis by RNA vaccines. As of December 21, 2021, 23 RNA vaccines are in clinical development, 3 are in phase 4 and 3 in phase 3.[7]

DNA vaccines

A DNA vaccine is composed of the gene/s encoding the antigenic determinant from the pathogen, which when administered, enters the nucleus of the host, wherein it is translated to messenger RNA (mRNA), which exits the nucleus into the cytoplasm, combines with the ribosomes, in which it is transcribed to the corresponding protective peptide sequence. Since this peptide sequence is foreign to the host, it induces a protective immune response against the antigen of interest. DNA vaccines elicit robust cellular and humoral immunity. Since the foreign protein is processed intracellularly and presented to the immune system in the context of the MHC class I system, it induces potent cell-mediated immune responses (CMI), which is crucial for vaccines against viruses and parasites.

The advantages of DNA vaccines include the stimulation of both potent CMI and humoral immunity, temperature stability, improved vaccine stability, lack of any infectious agent and the relative ease of large-scale manufacture. Rapid designing and optimization of pathogen sequences and synthesis, facilitates speed in preclinical testing with rapid transition to clinical scale up.[12]

Potential issues with DNA vaccines include the risk of insertional mutagenesis, anti-DNA antibody formation and the possibility of autoimmune diseases.

As on December 21, 2021, there are 15 DNA vaccines against COVID-19, in clinical development, 6 in phase 1 and 2 in phase 3 trials. The only DNA vaccine, which has completed phase 3 trial, is ZyCov-D, developed by Zydus Healthcare in India.[7]

Other Platforms

Other platforms being investigated include, virus like particles (VLP)—6 in clinical development, non-replicating viral vector with antigen presenting cells (APC)—2 in clinical development and replicating viral vector with antigen presenting cells (APC)—1 in clinical development.

■ WHO TARGET PRODUCT PROFILES FOR COVID-19 VACCINES

On April 29, 2020, the WHO published the preferred target product profile (TPP) for COVID-19 vaccines.[13] The preferred TPP stated that the vaccine should be suitable for active immunization of persons for prevention of COVID-19 in the area of an on-going outbreak. The vaccine should be suitable for all ages, including the elderly; mild and transient adverse effects are acceptable; and the benefit-risk ratio should be favorable. For outbreak control the vaccine should have at least 50% efficacy against variable endpoints, disease, severe disease, and/or shedding/transmission. For long-term usage, the vaccine should demonstrate at least 70% efficacy (on population basis), with consistent results in the elderly.

While single dose regimens are preferred, the schedule should not have more than two doses, with some need for boosters. While any route of administration is acceptable during an outbreak, non-parental routes are preferred for long-term usage.

The product should have a shelf life of at least 6–12 months, at temperatures of +2°C to +8°C. The product should be presented as unit dose or multi-dose vials, conforming to the WHO multi-dose vial policy and the maximum parenteral volume should be <1 mL. Rapid scale-up of production should be possible and the cost/dose should permit broad usage in low-income countries (LIC) and low-middle income countries (LMIC). Emergency use authorization (EUA) or emergency use listing (EUL) procedures should be granted by the national regulatory agencies (NRA).

■ EMERGENCY USE AUTHORIZATION

Approval for use of vaccines and medicines is granted after a detailed assessment of safety and effectiveness, based on data from trials. This is a long process and approval from the regulator is required at every stage of these trials. This process assures that a medicine or vaccine is absolutely safe and effective.[14]

In an emergency, such as the present pandemic, mechanism to facilitate the accelerated availability and use of medical countermeasures, including vaccines, is known as "emergency use authorization (EUA)". EUA is granted provided there is evidence of reasonable efficacy and safety. The National Regulatory Authority (NRA) must determine that the known and potential benefits outweigh the known and potential risks of the vaccine. This is an interim approval. Final approval is granted only after completion of the trials and analysis of full data.

As on December 20, 2021, the following vaccines have received EUL by the WHO:
- Pfizer/BioNTech: BNT162b2
- Moderna: mRNA-1273
- COVID-19 vaccine (ChAdOx1-S): Covishield
- Janssen (Johnson and Johnson): Ad26.COV2.S
- Covaxin
- COVID-19 vaccine (SARS-CoV-2 rS protein nanoparticle): Covovax
- CoronaVac COVID-19 vaccine (Vero Cell)
- Inactivated COVID-19 vaccine (Vero Cell): BIBP.

Assessment is ongoing for Sputnik V, Inactivated SARS-CoV-2 vaccine (Vero cell): WIBP, Ad5-nCoV of CanSinoBio, CoV2 preS dTM-AS03 vaccine of Sanofi and SCB-2019 of Clover Biopharmaceuticals.[15]

The only COVID-19 vaccine to receive full approval by the Food and Drug Administration of USA (US-FDA) is the Pfizer-BioNTech COVID-19 vaccine.[16] It will now be marketed as 'Comirnaty' (the name represents a combination of the terms COVID-19, mRNA, community and immunity, to highlight the first authorization of a messenger RNA 9mRNA) vaccine, as well as the joint global efforts that made this achievement possible) for the prevention of COVID-19 disease in individuals 16 years of age and older. The vaccine also continues to be available under EUA, including for individuals 12 through 15 years of age and for the administration of a third dose in certain immunocompromised individuals.

Draft Landscape of COVID-19 Vaccine Candidates

As of December 21, 2021, there are 194 vaccines in preclinical development, 137 in clinical development, of which 41 are in phase 1, 32 in phase 1–2, 11 in phase 2, 11 in phase 2–3, 29 in phase 3 and 10 in phase 4.[7]

■ VACCINES THAT ARE IN CLINICAL USAGE: (COMPLETED PHASE 3 TRIALS)

Oxford/AstraZeneca Vaccine (UK/US)

The AZD1222 (ChAdOx1 nCOV-19) vaccine by the University of Oxford in the UK and AstraZeneca in Cambridge is based on a replication-deficient chimpanzee adenovirus. The use of chimpanzee adenoviruses may to some extent reduce the negative effects of preexisting immunity in the population.[17] AZD1222, previously known as ChAdOx1, carries certain gene deletions that inhibit replication. It expresses the full-length structural surface glycoprotein (spike protein) of SARS-CoV-2, with a tissue plasminogen activator leader sequence.

In the *phase 1 of the phase 1–2 study*, 1,077 healthy adults aged 18–55 years who did not have any history of a positive laboratory confirmed SARS-CoV-2 infection or of COVID-19-like symptoms, were randomized (1:1) to receive ChAdOx1 nCoV-19 at a dose of 5×10^{10} viral particles or MenACWY as a single intramuscular injection.[18] The vaccine-induced adverse effects, were generally of mild to moderate intensity. Spike-specific T-cell responses peaked on day 14. The IgG antibody response peaked at day 28 (median 157 EU) and remained elevated till day 56 (median 119 EU). At day 56, 28 days after a booster dose, the median titers were 639 EU. After the first dose, 91% of the participants demonstrated a neutralizing response, while the same rose to 100% after the booster dose.

In the *phase 2 component of the phase 2–3 trial,* most of the reported local and systemic adverse events were mild to moderate in severity. Fewer adverse events were reported after the booster vaccination than after the prime vaccination and reactogenicity reduced with increasing age. The lower dose of vaccine was less reactogenic than the standard dose of vaccine across all age groups.[19] By day 28, total IgG (RBD + S-Protein) were elevated and were similar in the low dose (LD) and standard dose (SD) groups. Titers decreased with increasing age. By day 28 after the booster dose, similar antibody titers were seen regardless of age and dose of vaccine. Higher titers were found in the boosted group. Neutralizing antibody (Nab) titers peaked by day 42 in the 2-dose group. The titers were similar in all age groups and LD/SD groups. Almost >99% achieved neutralizing antibodies by day 14 after the booster dose. A good correlation was observed between the IgG titers and the neutralizing antibody titers. T-cell responses peaked by day 14 after the priming dose and no significant increase was observed after the booster dose.

The interim primary efficacy analysis of the *phase 3 studies* was done on 11,636 participants (7,548 in the UK, 4,088 in Brazil).[20] The interim analysis is based on data generated from four ongoing blinded, randomized, controlled trials studies done in three countries—COV001 (phase 1/2; UK), COV002 (phase 2/3; UK), COV003 (phase 3; Brazil), and COV005 (phase 1/2; South Africa). The primary end point of the study was symptomatic COVID-19, with a positive RT-PCR for COVID-19, in seronegative participants, more than 14 days after a second dose of vaccine. About 12.2% of the total cohort in the current analysis, were above 56 years of age.

Due to some quantification error, some subjects in the 18–55 years cohort received a lower dose of vaccine as the first dose. This constituted the low dose (LD) cohort in the study. This cohort received their second dose after a substantial gap. The vaccine efficacy (VE) (%) values in this study are given in **Table 6.1**.

As the interval between doses varied due to various factors, the VE also varied to some extent, as shown in **Table 6.2**.

TABLE 6.1: Oxford/AstraZeneca Vaccine: The vaccine efficacy values of phase 3 studies.[20]

Parameter	Vaccine efficacy (%)
All LD/SD and SD/SD recipients	70.4% (54.8–80.6)
COV002 (UK)	73.5% (55.5–84.2)
LD/SD recipients	90.0% (67.4–97.0)
SD/SD recipients	60.3% (28.0–78.2)
COV003 (Brazil; all SD/SD)	64.2% (30.7–81.5)
All SD/SD recipients	62.1% (41.0–75.7)
Any symptomatic COVID-19 disease	67.1% (52.3–77.3)
Asymptomatic or symptoms unknown (COV002)	27.3% (−17.2 to 54.9)
LD/SD recipients	58.9% (1.0–82.9)
SD/SD recipients	3.8% (−72.4 to 46.3)
Any NAAT-positive swab	55.7% (41.1–66.7)
(LD: low dose; SD: standard dose; NAAT: nuclei acid amplification test)	

TABLE 6.2: Oxford/AstraZeneca Vaccine: The vaccine efficacy values of phase 3 studies based on age and dosage interval.[20]

Parameter	Vaccine efficacy (%)
COV002 (UK), age 18–55 years	
LD/SD recipients	90.0% (67.3–97.0)
SD/SD recipients	59.3% (25.1–77.9)
COV002 (UK), age 18–55 years with >8 weeks' interval between vaccine doses	
LD/SD recipients	90.0% (67.3–97.0)
SD/SD recipients	65.6% (24.5–84.4)
All SD/SD (UK and Brazil)	
<6 weeks' interval between vaccine doses	53.4% (−2.5 to 78.8)
>6 weeks' interval between vaccine doses	65.4% (41.1–79.6)
(LD: low dose; SD: standard dose)	

Vaccine efficacy (VE) in older age groups could not be assessed because of insufficient data.

Serious adverse events (SAEs) and adverse events of special interest were balanced across the study arms, indicating a good safety profile of the vaccine. Around 79 in the vaccine group and 89 in the control group had SAEs. A case of *transverse myelitis* occurring 14 days after the booster dose was suspected to be due to the vaccination. There were four deaths, not due to COVID, in the study. None were considered related to the vaccine.

The overall VE and effect of interval between doses, evaluated in a pooled analysis of four randomized trials—one phase 1/2 study in the UK (COV001), one phase 2/3 study in the UK (COV002), and a phase 3 study in Brazil (COV003 and one double-blind phase 1/2 study in South Africa (COV005)—is shown in **Table 6.3**.[21] The VE after a single standard dose of vaccine from day 22 to day 90 after vaccination was 76.0% (59.3–85.9).[22] There was a minimal waning of antibodies over 90 days after 2 doses and modeling analysis indicated that protection did not wane during this initial 90-day period.

Vaccine Induced Thrombotic Thrombocytopenia

Post-authorization surveillance of adenovectored COVID-19 vaccines has identified unusual cases of thrombocytopenia with thrombosis, some manifesting as a very serious condition termed vaccine-induced immune thrombotic thrombocytopenia (VITT).[22] This condition is characterized by presentation with a combination of symptoms including thrombosis, particularly at unusual sites, mild to severe thrombocytopenia, high levels of antibodies to platelet factor-4 (PF4)–polyanion complexes identified by enzyme-linked immunosorbent assay (ELISA), as well by assays based on platelet activation, which, when tested, was enhanced by addition of PF4.

TABLE 6.3: Oxford/AstraZeneca Vaccine: The overall vaccine efficacy and effect of interval between doses, evaluated in a pooled analysis of four randomized trials.[21]

Parameter	Vaccine efficacy (%)
Prespecified analyses: Cases more than 14 days after second dose	
Primary symptomatic COVID-19	66.7% (57.4–74.0)
SD/SD	63.1% (51.8–71.7)
LD/SD	80.7% (62.1–90.2)
Asymptomatic or unknown infection (COV002 UK only) SD/SD	22.2% (–9.9 to 45.0)
SD/SD	2.0% (–50.7 to 36.2)
LD/SD	49.3% (7.4–72.2)
Primary symptomatic COVID-19: Cases more than 14 days after second dose- according to interval between doses (SD/SD)	
<6 weeks	55.1% (33.0–69.9)
6–8 weeks	59.9% (32.0–76.4)
9–11 weeks	63.7% (28.0–81.7)
>12 weeks	81.3% (60.3–91.2)
(LD: low dose; SD: standard dose)	

Cerebral venous sinus thrombosis (CVST) is the most dreaded manifestation of this condition. This condition has been associated with the ChAdOx1 CoV-19 vaccine and the Ad26.COV2.S vaccine (Janssen; Johnson and Johnson), but not with the other adenovectored vaccines.

The incidence of VITT is around 1 per 100,000 to 250,000 vaccine recipients. CVST is estimated to occur at a rate of 1 per 100,000 vaccine recipients with the Ch-AdOx1 vaccine and 1 per 1,000,000 with the Ad26.COV2.S vaccine. More than 90% of patients with CVST have been younger than 60 years, with more women being affected than men (2.5:1 ratio). There was neither any history of receipt of heparin nor any risk factors for thrombosis. Most patients presented late and up to one-third of the initial reported patients died. The median (range) onset of symptoms was 10 (5–24) days after the ChAdOx1 vaccine and 8 (6–15) days after the Ad26.COV2.S vaccine.[10,11,23]

On April 13, 2021, the US-FDA, paused the use of this vaccine, pending further investigations.[24] On April 23, 2021, the CDC Advisory Committee on Immunization Practices voted to recommend that the JJ vaccine again be available for persons aged 18 years and older under the EUA of US-FDA.[25]

In the UK, the Medicines and Healthcare products Regulatory Agency (MHRA) issued a guidance that people of any age who are at higher risk of blood clots because of their medical condition should be considered only if benefits from the protection from COVID-19 infection outweigh potential risks. Similar guidance has been issued for administration in pregnancy.[26]

The WHO has also commented that the benefits of vaccination far outweigh the risk associated with the AstraZeneca vaccine.[27] Several countries, including Austria, Norway, Denmark, Iceland, Romania, Bulgaria, Ireland, Netherlands, have temporarily halted the use of the AstraZeneca vaccine.[28]

Pfizer BNT162b2 mRNA COVID-19 Vaccine

This is a lipid nanoparticle-formulated, 5 nucleoside-modified RNA (modRNA) encoding the SARS-CoV-2 full-length spike. Two proline mutations lock the SARS-CoV-2 full-length spike, in the prefusion conformation.

In the phase 1 study, two formulations were assessed, BNT162b1, which encodes a secreted trimerized SARS-CoV-2 receptor–binding domain (RBD) and BNT162b2, which encodes a membrane-anchored SARS-CoV-2 full length spike, stabilized in the prefusion conformation.[29]

BNT162b2 was chosen as the candidate for further clinical studies. *The phase 2/3 part of the global phase 1/2/3 trial* was conducted in 43,548 participants, > 16 years of age, who underwent randomization. About 43,448 received injections—21,720 with BNT162b2 and 21,728 with placebo.[23]

The primary safety end points of this trial were solicited—*specific local or systemic adverse events* and use of antipyretic or pain medication within 7 days after the receipt of each dose of vaccine or placebo. The first efficacy primary end point was the efficacy of BNT162b2 against confirmed COVID-19 with onset at least 7 days after the second dose, in participants who had been without serologic or virologic evidence of SARS-CoV-2 infection up to 7 days after the second dose; the second primary end point was efficacy in participants with and participants without evidence of prior infection.

In general, more local reactions were reported by BNT162b2 recipients than placebo recipients. The most commonly reported local side effect was mild-moderate pain at the site of the vaccination. Less than 1% reported severe pain. Pain was more frequent in the younger participants, <55 years than the older participants, >55 years. Injection-site redness or swelling was less frequently reported and the local reactogenicity did not increase after the second dose. Systemic reactogenicity was more common in the younger participants and after the second dose. Fatigue and headache were the most commonly reported systemic side effects. Nearly 16% of younger subjects and 11% of older subjects reported fever, generally after the second dose. Lymphadenopathy was reported by 0.3% of vaccine recipients and <1% of placebo recipients. No deaths in the study were causally linked to the vaccine or placebo.

The efficacy of the vaccine in preventing COVID-19 occurrence at least 7 days after the second dose, in participants without evidence of infection, was 95.0% (90.3–97.6) with 8 cases in the vaccine group and 162 cases in the placebo group. In participants with and those without evidence of infection, the VE was 94.6% (89.9–97.3), 9 cases in the vaccine group and 169 cases in the placebo group.

Vaccine efficacy was fairly uniform across age groups, 95.6% (89.4–98.6%) in the 16–55 year group, 93.7% (80.6–98.8%) in those > 55 years, 94.7% (66.7–99.9%) in those > 65 years and 100.0% (–13.1 to 100.0%) in those > 75 years. Approximately 39 cases occurred in the BNT162b2 group and 82 cases in the placebo group, between doses 1 and 2, resulting in a VE of 52% (95% CI, 29.5–68.4). Protection was observed as early as 12 days after the first dose.

Moderna mRNA-1273 SARS-CoV-2 Vaccine

This vaccine is a lipid-nanoparticle (LNP)-encapsulated mRNA vaccine expressing the prefusion-stabilized S-2 spike glycoprotein, consisting of the SARS-CoV-2 glycoprotein with a transmembrane anchor and an intact S1-S2 cleavage site. Two consecutive proline substitutions at amino acid positions 986 and 987 confer stability to the prefusion conformation.

In the phase 1 study, with three formulations, 25 µg, 100 µg, and 250 µg, the highest titers were elicited in the 250 µg subjects, with a significant boost after the second dose.[30] Following the second dose, serum neutralizing antibody titers were similar to those in the upper half of the distribution of a panel of control convalescent serum specimens. Strong CD4 T-cell responses were elicited in the 25 µg and 100 µg doses, with a predominantly Th1 response. Pain at the injection site was the most common solicited local adverse event and was mild or moderate in intensity.

The dose of 100 µg was used in the *phase 3 trials*. The phase 3 randomized, observer-blinded, placebo-controlled trial, of the mRNA-1273 (100 µg), was conducted in a cohort of 30,420, in 99 centers across USA.[31] Solicited injection site adverse effects and systemic adverse effects occurred more frequently in the vaccine group as compared to the placebo (84.2% vs. 19.8%) and more after the second dose (88.6% vs. 18.8%) as compared to after the first dose.

Solicited systemic adverse effects occurred more frequently in the vaccine group as compared to the placebo and more after the second dose (88.6% vs. 18.8%) as compared to after the first dose. Both, the vaccine group and the placebo group had a similar frequency of unsolicited adverse events, unsolicited severe adverse events, and serious adverse events during the 28 days after injection.

The overall VE was 94.1% (89.3–96.8%) with 11 cases in the vaccine group and 185 cases in the placebo group. The VE in those between 18 and 65 years was 95.6% (90.6–97.9%) and in those > 65 years was 86.4% (61.4–95.2%).

Thirty participants in the trial had severe COVID-19 and all were in the placebo group.

In a press release on November 16, 2020, Moderna stated that further tests revealed that revealed their vaccine was found to remain stable at 2–8°C for 30 days, at –20°C for up to 6 months and at room temperature for up to 12 hours.[32]

Myopericarditis and mRNA Vaccines

Myocarditis has been reported as a rare complication of COVID-19 mRNA vaccinations.[33] According to the Vaccine Adverse Effects Reporting System (VAERS) data, out of the ~300 million COVID-19 mRNA vaccine doses administered through June 11, 2021, there were 1,226 reports of probable myocarditis/pericarditis cases in VAERS, 67% of which followed the second dose.[34] Of these, 79% were in males, with the majority in individuals <30 years of age with a median age of 24 years. Symptom onset occurred at a median of 3 days, with the highest rate at day 2 after vaccination among patients 16–18 years of age. Almost all presented with chest pain, about two-thirds of patients had ST-T changes and/or abnormal cardiac enzymes. Hospitalization was necessary in 96%.

Centers for Disease Control and Prevention (CDC) of USA Vaccine Safety Datalink with data from 9 participating integrated health care organizations, showed that the risk of myo/pericarditis was higher in the age group 12–39 years, with an estimated rate of 12.6 cases per million doses with second-dose mRNA vaccine.[35]

Gam-COVID-Vac (Sputnik V)

Gam-COVID-Vac is a recombinant vector vaccine, in which the priming is done with recombinant adenovector type 26 (rAd26) and boosting is done with the recombinant adenovector type 5 (rAd5)—both of which carry the gene for SARS-CoV-2 full-length glycoprotein S (rAd26-S and rAd5-S). The two doses are administered at an interval of 21 days. This vaccine has been developed by the NF Gamaleya National Research Center for Epidemiology and Microbiology, Moscow, Russia.

Each dose contains 10^{11} viral particles per dose for both recombinant adenoviruses. Frozen (Gam-COVID-Vac) and lyophilized (Gam-COVID-Vac-Lyo) formulations were prepared with the frozen vaccine having a volume of 0.5 mL (per dose) and the lyophilized vaccine, which needs to be reconstituted in 1.0 mL of sterile water for injection (per dose).

The phase 1–2 study was conducted in 76 participants aged 18–60 years.[36] The solicited local and systemic adverse effects were mild and included pain at injection site [44 (58%)], hyperthermia [38 (50%)], headache [32 (42%)], asthenia [21 (28%)], and muscle and joint pain [18 (24%)]. No serious adverse effects were noted. At day 42, robust receptor binding domain-specific IgG titers (14,703 with the frozen formulation and 11,143 with the lyophilized formulation) and neutralizing antibodies (49.25 with the frozen formulation and 45.95 with the lyophilized formulation) were elicited. The seroconversion rate was 100%. Cell-mediated responses were detected in all participants at day 28, with a predominantly Th1 response.

The phase 3 study was done in 21,977 adults, aged at > 18 years, who had a negative SARS-CoV-2 PCR and IgG and IgM tests, no infectious diseases in the 14 days before enrolment, and no other vaccinations in the 30 days before enrolment.[37] The interim analysis of the phase 3 study was done when 78 COVID-19 cases in participants was confirmed, after receiving the second dose. Most reported adverse events (94%) were grade 1. The distribution of serious adverse events was similar in the vaccine and placebo groups. None were considered associated with vaccination. Of the four deaths reported during the study, none were considered related to the vaccine.

The vaccine was found to be highly immunogenic with detection of RBD-specific IgG in 98% of subjects, geometric mean titer (GMT) of 8,996 (95% CI 7,610–10,635), and a seroconversion rate of 98.25%. Those in 18–30 years age group had a significantly higher GMT than the other age groups. The GMTs of neutralizing antibodies on day 42 after first vaccination was 44.5 (95% CI 31.8–62.2) and the seroconversion rate was 95.83% in the vaccine group, which was much higher than in the placebo group. Robust cellular immune responses were elicited in the form of significantly higher levels of interferon-gamma (IFN-γ) secretion upon antigen restimulation [median 32.77 pg/mL (interquartile range, IQR 13.94–50.76)] compared with the day of administration of the first dose.

The VE was measured as the first COVID-19 occurrence from 21 days after dose 1 (day of dose 2). Overall VE was 91.6% (85.6–95.2%). It was similar across the age bands, with VE of 91.8% (67.1–98.3%) in those > 60 years. The VE against moderate-severe COVID-19 was 100%, with all cases reported in the placebo group. From 15 to 21 days after the first dose, efficacy was 73.6% (p = 0.048).

Sputnik Light

Sputnik Light is the first component [recombinant human adenovirus serotype number 26 (rAd26)] of the 2-dose Sputnik V vaccine.

In a phase 1/2 study, by day 10, RBD specific IgG increased to a level of 26,899 from a baseline value on 594.4.[38] In those who were seronegative, the titers increased to 29.09 on day 10. Seroconversion and GMT in seropositive and seronegative subjects were 92.9% and 100% and 19,986 and 1648 on day 42. The seroconversion and GMT of neutralizing antibodies in seropositive and seronegative subjects, on day 42, were

92.9% and 81.7% and 579.9 and 15.18 respectively. T cell responses against the S-protein were demonstrated in 100% of seropositives and 96% of seronegatives.

After dose 1 of Sputnik V, among seronegatives, the seroconversion rate was 94% with GMT of 244 (180–328) and after two doses corresponding values were 100% and 2148 (1742–2649). In seropositives, after dose 1, the titers rose to 9850 (8460–11,480) from a baseline of 531 (380–742). After dose 2, the titers rose to 9590 (7410–12,408). Thus, in seropositives, the increase in titers following dose 2, were statistically non-significant as compared to the titers after dose 1.

Nearly 21 days after dose 1, neutralizing antibodies (Nab) were found in 90% of subjects who were seronegative at baseline with GMT of 12 (10–14). 21 days after dose 2, the Nab GMT was 42 (33–53). A robust increase in Nab activity was observed after a single vaccine dose in participants with prior infection.

The overall VE against the delta variant in the 18–29-year-old group was 88.61% and 75.28% in the 18–59 group.

Sputnik Light has received approval in 22 countries.

BBV152 (Covaxin™ Manufactured by Bharat Biotech)

This is a whole-virion inactivated vaccine, inactivated with β-propiolactone. The COVID-19 strain, NIV-2020-770, contains the Asp614Gly mutation. The vaccine is formulated with Algel-IMDG, an imidazoquinoline class molecule (TLR7 and TLR8 agonist) adsorbed onto Algel. This adjuvant skews the immune response to a Th1 type and greatly reduces the risk of vaccine associated enhanced disease (VAED).

The phase 1 study was conducted in 11 hospitals across nine states of India in 375 subjects aged 18–55 years, in 2-dose schedule 28 days apart, with 3 μg and 6 μg groups in combination with Algel-IMDG, or only Algel.[39] The most common *solicited adverse events* were injection site pain, headache, fever and nausea or vomiting. All solicited adverse events were mild to moderate in severity and were more frequent after the first dose. IgG Ab titers (GMT) to spike protein, RBD, and nucleocapsid protein (N-protein) were elevated after the administration of both doses. The titers were similar with the 3 μg and 6 μg with Algel-IMDG groups. The ratios of IgG1/IgG4 was greater than 1 for all vaccinated groups, indicating a predominantly Th1 response.

High seroconversion rates were observed after the second dose, with the highest titers in the 6 μg with Algel-IMDG group. The vaccine-induced responses were similar to those observed in the convalescent sera. Estimations in a small number of samples showed a CD3+, CD4+, and CD8+ T-cell responses that were reflected in the IFN-γ production, in the Algel-IMDG groups.

The phase 2 trial showed comparable levels of anti-S1 protein, anti-RBD, and anti-N protein GMT elicited by both formulations, with a high IgG1/IgG2 ratio, indicating a predominant Th1 response.[40] After 4 weeks of the second dose, the 6 µg with Algel-IMDG group elicited significantly higher neutralizing antibody GMT than that in the 3 µg with Algel-IMDG group and were comparable to those observed in convalescent serum collected from COVID-19 recovered patients.

The phase 3 study was a randomized, double-blind, placebo-controlled, multicentre, clinical trial in 25 Indian hospitals or medical clinics to evaluate the efficacy, safety, and immunological lot consistency of BBV152 in adults (age ≥18 years) who were healthy or had stable chronic medical conditions. About 25,798 participants were recruited.[41] The interim results regarding immunogenicity and safety outcomes were assessed on days 0 to 56 and the efficacy results at a median of 99 days. The reactogenicity profile of the vaccine was favorable with the rate solicited, unsolicited, and serious adverse events and adverse events of special interest, similar in the placebo and vaccine groups. The incidence of serious adverse events was similar in the placebo and vaccine groups, 0.3% in the vaccine group and 0.5% in the placebo group.

The efficacy analysis was done after the occurrence of 130 symptomatic COVID-19 cases during follow-up beginning 2 weeks after the second vaccination. There were no statistically significant differences in the Nab titers according to age and gender. The GMT was significantly higher in those who were positive for SARS-CoV-IgG as compared to those who were negative. The efficacy results are provided in **Tables 6.4 and 6.5**.

NVX-CoV2373 (Covovax)

This is a recombinant SARS-CoV-2 (rSARS-CoV-2) nanoparticle vaccine, constructed from the full-length wild-type SARS-CoV-2 spike glycoprotein, adjuvanted with Novavax's patented saponin-based Matrix-M.

TABLE 6.4: BBV152 vaccine efficacy against SARS-CoV-2 after at least 14 days after the second dose in the per-protocol population (N = 16,973).[41]

Clinical condition	Vaccine efficacy, % (95% CI)
Symptomatic COVID-19	77.8% (65·2–86·4)
Severe symptomatic COVID-19	93.4 (57.1–99.8)
Symptomatic COVID-19 in participants aged 18–59 years	79.4% (66·0–88·2)
Symptomatic COVID-19 in participants aged >60 years	67.8 (8.0–90.0)
Symptomatic COVID-19 in participants with a pre-existing chronic medical condition	66.2% (33·8–84·0)
Asymptomatic COVID-19	63.6 (29.0–82.5)

TABLE: 6.5: BBV152 efficacy against COVID-19 variants.[41]

Variant	Vaccine efficacy, % (95% CI)
All variants	70.8 (50.0–83.8)
B.1.1.7 (Alpha)	NS
B.1.617.1 (Kappa)	90.1 (30.4–99.8)
B.1.617.2 (Delta)	65.2 (33.1–83.0)

TABLE: 6.6: Vaccine efficacy data of NVX-CoV2373 of UK Phase 3 trials.[43]

Analysis group	Vaccine efficacy % (95% CI)
Per-protocol population	89.7 (80.2–94.6)
18 to <65 year	89.8 (79.7–95.5)
≥65 to 84 year	88.9 (20.2–99.7)
Non-B.1.1.7	96.4 (73.8–99.5)
B.1.1.7	86.3 (71.3–93.5)
With coexisting illness	90.9 (70.4–97.2)
Without coexisting illness	89.1 (76.2–95.0)

In the *phase 1–2 study,* adverse effects seen were generally mild in nature, more in the group receiving the adjuvanted vaccine and of short duration (<2 days).[42] The geometric mean fold rises (GMFR) achieved were 10 times more than that seen in the unadjuvanted subjects, on day 7 and 100 times higher by day 35 and were similar to those in convalescent serum from patients hospitalized with COVID-19.

The UK Phase 3 study enrolled 15,000 participants between 18 and 84 years of age, including 27% over the age of 65.[43] During the study period, over 50% of the PCR-confirmed symptomatic cases were variant strains. The safety assessment demonstrated a low level, balanced occurrence of severe, serious, and medically attended adverse events between vaccine and placebo groups. The efficacy data is given in **Table 6.6**.

In *the Phase 2b clinical trial,* conducted in South Africa, in human immunodeficiency virus (HIV) negative subjects, a VE of 60% (95% CI: 19.9–80.1) was observed.[44] This was when 92.6% (25 out of 27 cases) were the South Africa escape variant. The overall VE in HIV positive and negative subjects was 49.4% (95% CI: 6.1–72.8).

A phase 3, randomized, observer-blinded, placebo-controlled trial was conducted in 29,949 adults >18 years of age, in the United States and Mexico to evaluate the efficacy and safety of NVX-CoV2373 in adults (≥18 years of age) who were seronegative for SARS-CoV-2 infection.[45] The results are presented in **Table 6.7**.

TABLE: 6.7: Vaccine efficacy data of NVX-CoV2373 phase 3 trials.[45]

Analysis group	Vaccine efficacy (95% CI)
Per protocol efficacy population	90.4 (82.9–94.6)
Age of 18–64 year	91.5 (84.2–95.4)
With coexisting conditions	90.8 (79.2–95.9)
Without coexisting conditions	89.9 (77.1–95.6)
At high risk for COVID-19[#]	91.0 (83.6–95.0)

[#]Included those 65 years of age or older and those of any age with chronic health conditions or an increased risk for COVID-19 because of work or living conditions.

TABLE 6.8: The primary vaccine efficacy data of Janssen COVID-19 vaccine.[46]

	Vaccine efficacy (%)	
	Moderate to severe/Critical	Severe/Critical
14 days post-vaccination		
All subjects	66.9 (59.0; 73.4)	76.7 (54.6; 89.1)
18 to 59 years of age	63.7 (53.9; 71.6)	
>60 years	76.3 (61.6; 86.0)	
28 days post-vaccination		
All subjects	66.1 (55.0; 74.8)	85.4 (54.2; 96.9)
18–59 years of age	66.1 (53.3; 75.8)	
>60 years	66.2 (36.7; 83.0)	

Covovax, which is the trade name for the NVX-CoV2373, being developed by Serum Institute India, was granted EUA by the WHO on December 17, 2021.

Janssen COVID-19 (Ad.26.COV2.S)

This vaccine is a recombinant, replication-incompetent adenovirus serotype 26 (Ad26) vector vaccine, encoding the stabilized prefusion spike glycoprotein of SARS-CoV-2, which is administered intramuscularly, in a single dose containing 5×10^{10} virus particles per 0.5 mL dose.

The primary efficacy analysis was done in 39,321 individuals (19,630 in the Janssen COVID-19 vaccine group and 19,691 in the placebo group). About 34.6% of the study population was >60 years of age.[46] The median length of follow up for efficacy for individuals in the study was 8 weeks post-vaccination. **Table 6.8** lists the primary VE data of Janssen COVID-19.

In USA, during the trial period, 96.4% of the circulating strains in the study carried the Wuhan D614G mutation. In South Africa 94.5% was the B 1.351 mutant strain and in Brazil, 69.4% was of the P.2 lineage. The VE in these settings are given in **Table 6.9**.

TABLE 6.9: Vaccine efficacy of Janssen COVID-19 vaccine against various strains of SARS-CoV-2.

Variable	Vaccine efficacy (95% CI) >14 days after dosing	Vaccine efficacy (95% CI) >28 days after dosing
Worldwide		
Moderate to severe–critical COVID-19	66.3 (59.9–71.8)	65.5 (57.2–72.4)
Severe–critical COVID-19	76.3 (57.9–87.5)	83.5 (54.2–96.9)
United States		
Moderate to severe–critical COVID-19	74.4 (65.0–81.6)	72.0 (58.2–81.7)
Severe–critical COVID-19	78.0 (33.1–94.6)	85.9 (–9.4 to 99.7)
Brazil		
Moderate to severe–critical COVID-19	66.2 (51.0–77.1)	68.1 (48.8–80.7)
Severe–critical COVID-19	81.9 (17.0–98.1)	87.6 (7.8–99.7)
South Africa		
Moderate to severe–critical COVID-19	52.0 (30.3–67.4)	64.0 (41.2–78.7)
Severe–critical COVID-19	73.1 (40.0–89.4)	81.7 (46.2–95.4)

The common solicited local adverse reactions reported in the 7 days following vaccination in individuals 18–59 years of age were injection site pain, injection site erythema and injection site swelling, which were generally mild and more in the 18–59 years group. Similar results were noted with the solicited systemic adverse reactions reported in the 7 days following vaccination.

CoronaVac (Sinovac Research and Development Co.)

This is a purified, β-propiolactone inactivated virus alum-adjuvanted candidate vaccine of the CN2 strain of SARS-CoV-2.

In the phase 2 studies, comparing a 3 µg or 6 µg dose, both dosages elicited a seroconversion rate (SCR) of >90% with a good tolerability profile.[47] The *Phase 3 clinical trials* are being conducted in a two-dose injection regimen with a 14-days interval, in Brazil (NCT04456595), Indonesia (INA-WXFM0YX), and Turkey. The phase 3 trial of CoronaVac was conducted in Brazil among healthy healthcare professionals in 16 centers, with participants receiving two doses of vaccine (3 µg in 0.5 mL) vaccine or placebo at day 0 and 14.[48] The primary efficacy against symptomatic COVID-19 was 50.7% (95% CI 36.0–62.0). All adverse effects were not causally related to the vaccine. In a subset of participants, neutralizing antibody assays showed similar seroconversion and geometric mean titers against B.1.128, P.1, and P.2 variants. The WHO granted EUA for CoronaVac.

Other Inactivated Vaccines in Clinical Trials

Other inactivated vaccines in clinical trials include Wuhan Institute of Biological Products/China National Biotech Group-Sinopharm inactivated vaccine and the inactivated vaccine by BBIBP-CorV (Beijing Institute of Biotechnology/China National Biotech Group-Sinopharm.[7] ZF2001 (Anhui Zhifei Longcom Biopharmaceutical/Chinese Academy of Medical Sciences), an adjuvanted RBD-dimeric antigen subunit vaccine candidate, has entered phase 3 clinical trials in China and Uzbekistan. Indonesia, Pakistan and Ecuador are the study sites outside China. The trial will involve 22,000 subjects.[7]

ZyCov-D

ZyCoV-D is a DNA plasmid based COVID-19 vaccine developed by Cadila Healthcare. *The phase 1–2 study,* which was conducted in a cohort of 1,048 subjects between 18 and 60 years, demonstrated the safety and immunogenicity of two 0.1 mL doses administered intradermally, on the upper arm, on day 0–28–56 (CTRI/2020/07/026352).[49] *The phase 3 trial,* involving a cohort of 28,216 between 12 and 99 years, who received two 0.1 mL doses, intradermally, on the upper arm, on day 0–28–56, showed an efficacy of 66.6% against symptomatic RTPCR positive COVID-19. (CTRI/2020/07/026352).[50] An additional phase 1–2 trial is evaluating a 2-dose schedule, on day 0 and 28, in 18–60 years-old subjects (CTRI/2021/03/032051). Results of the trials have not been published.

EUA was granted by the Government of India on August 20, 2021, in a 3-dose schedule in the age group >12 years. This is the world's first DNA vaccine that has entered clinical usage.

■ EQUITABLE DISTRIBUTION OF COVID-19 VACCINES

COVID-19 attacks everyone, rich and the poor. As long as COVID-19 exists anywhere, no one is safe. There is a threat of COVID-19 vaccines being monopolized by the affluent countries. This occurred during the 2009 influenza A (H1N1) pandemic, when the wealthy nations monopolized all supplies of vaccines and left LIC and LMIC countries with very limited supplies, which were delivered too late.[51] To prevent the occurrence of similar situations during the present COVID-19 pandemic, the Global Alliance for Vaccines and Immunizations (GAVI,) the Coalition for Epidemic Preparedness Innovations (CEPI), and WHO, have created COVAX, which is the vaccines pillar of the "Access to COVID-19 Tools (ACT) Accelerator, which is a global public-private-philanthropic collaboration to accelerate the development, production, and equitable rollout of COVID-19 tests, treatments, and vaccines.[52] This is being facilitated by the COVAX facility, with an aim of securing and enabling equitable allocation of 2 billion doses of COVID-19 vaccines by the end of 2021, to the WHO-defined priority populations, including frontline healthcare workers and other groups at high risk. Almost 191 countries, including the 92 countries that are eligible for donor-funded doses through the COVAX Advance Market Commitment (AMC), have joined COVAX.

Equitable vaccine distribution is not just ethical—it is essential for controlling the spread.

As of December 30, 2021, the COVAX Facility has delivered >907 million doses of COVID-19 vaccines to over 144 countries and territories.[53]

■ PRIORITIZATION OF COVID VACCINES

In the initial phase of the COVID-19 vaccine rollout, shortage of vaccines necessitated the prioritization of available vaccines, to ensure maximization of benefits of vaccination to both individual recipients and the population overall. In the WHO-SAGE publication on *"Roadmap for prioritizing uses of COVID-19 vaccines in the context of limited supply"*, published in November 2020, frontline healthcare workers (HCWs) have received priority, as positive COVID-19 test reporting was 11 times higher than in the general population.[54,55] Vaccination of HCWs will also ensure uninterrupted functioning of the healthcare system.

The next highest priority group is older adults defined by age-based risk specific to country/region.

Once vaccine availability improves, sufficient to cover 11–20% of the country's population, the next priority groups are groups with comorbidities or health states determined to be at significantly higher risk of severe disease or death. This will include younger age groups with comorbidities including diabetes, severe asthma and various other medical conditions, including hypertension, which are risk factors for a COVID-19 related death. Frontline essential workers such as fire fighters, police officers, food and agricultural workers, postal workers, manufacturing workers, grocery store workers, public transit workers, and those who work in the educational sector (teachers, support staff, and daycare workers), are also prioritized in this phase. Sociodemographic groups at significantly higher risk of severe disease or death are also included in this phase.

As vaccine availability increases, vaccination recommendations will expand to include more groups.

■ COVID VACCINES IN CHILDREN

Children of all age groups are susceptible to COVID-19 infection. Asymptomatic children constitute a significant proportion of all cases.

When symptomatic, the illness is of milder nature. The incidence of critical illness, hospitalization, intensive care unit (ICU) admission, and mechanical ventilation is much lower than that seen in adults. Death is extremely rare in pediatric COVID-19. In the pediatric age group, the incidence of critical illness is highest in those <1 year of age.[56] However, the association between recent or past COVID and the recently described novel Kawasaki disease-like multisystem inflammatory syndrome in children (MIS-C), emphasizes the need for continued surveillance in children.[57]

Unlike influenza, children may not be major drivers of transmission of COVID-19. In family outbreaks, children are rarely the index case.[58] Following school reopening, outbreaks in schools have been rarely reported and when reported, the transmission has usually occurred from staff to the students. Outbreaks of COVID-19 have been reported in schools and school camps.[59] Recent data suggests that school-age children and adolescents can efficiently transmit SARS-CoV-2 to household members, which may lead to hospitalization of high-risk adults in the household.[60] Adolescents contribute significantly to household transmission, and rates of transmission by this age group (11–18 years) may be higher than that in adults.[61]

It needs to be noted that children under the age of 15 account for 26% of the global population. Unless this population is immunized, the goal of herd immunity against COVID-19 will remain unattained.

The *phase 3 trial*, of the *Pfizer BNT162b2 vaccine*, in adolescents 12–15 years of age, enrolled 2,260 adolescents in the United States.[62] In the trial, 18 cases of COVID-19 were observed in the placebo group (n = 1,129) versus none in the vaccinated group (n = 1,131) with a VE of 100%.[62] The GMT in this group was noninferior to GMT elicited by participants aged 16 to 25 years in an earlier analysis. Further, BNT162b2 administration was well tolerated, with side effects generally consistent with those observed in participants 16–25 years of age.

On May 10, 2021, the US-FDA expanded the EUA for the Pfizer-BioNTech COVID-19 vaccine to include adolescents 12 through 15 years of age. Children aged 5 to 11 years received two-doses of 10 µg each.[63] The SARS-CoV-2-neutralizing antibody GMT in the 5–11 years was 1197.6 (95% CI, 1106.1, 1296.6), as compared to the 16–25 years cohort [1146.5 (95% CI: 1045.5, 1257.2)], proving non-inferiority in the 5–11 years cohort. The reactogenicity and adverse effects profile was similar to that observed in the 16–25 years age group. On October 29, 2021, EUA was granted by the US-FDA for use in children 5–11 years.

Moderna is conducting two trials of its *mRNA-1273 SARS-CoV-2 vaccine*, in two age groups, 12–17 years and 6 months to 11 years. In the *phase 2-3 placebo-controlled trial*, adolescents aged 12–17 year received two doses of 100 µg/dose of Moderna vaccines, at 0–28 days.[64] The GMT of neutralizing antibodies was 1401.7 (1276.3–1539.4) compared to levels of 1301.3

(1177.0–1438.8) in young adults, establishing non-inferiority. The VE against COVID-19 in per protocol cohort 14 days after the second dose was 100% (28.9 to NE: not estimated). On September 4, 2021, this vaccine was granted EUA by the US-FDA, for adolescents 12–17 years.

The *KidCOVE Study,* which is a phase 2/3 study, will assess the safety and effectiveness of the mRNA-1273, in children between the ages of 6 months and 11 years, in a cohort of 6,750 participants (NCT04796896). In part 1 of the study, participants will receive two intramuscular (IM) injections of mRNA-1273 at up to 3 doses prespecified for this study, 28 days apart, on day 1 and day 29. In part 2, participants will receive two IM injections of mRNA-1273 at the dose selected from part 1, 28 days apart, on day 1 and day 29. The comparator is a placebo.

The estimated primary completion date is June 10, 2023.

The University of Oxford had launched the first study of *ChAdOx1 nCoV-19 COVID-19 vaccine* in 300 children and young adults in three age groups, 12–18 years (group 1), 6–12 years (group 2) and 2–6 years (group 3).[65] Following the association of the vaccine with VITT, this trial is kept on hold.

Bharat Biotech (the makers of *Covaxin*™), has completed a phase 2/3 trial in three age groups, 12–18 years (group 1), 6–12 years (group 2) and 2–6 years (group 3) with 175 subjects in each group. Each participant was administered two doses of Covaxin (6 µg/0.5 mL) on 0–28 days.[66] The immune responses as measured by microneutralization (MNT) antibody titers and plaque reduction neutralization test (PRNT) titers, were similar in all three age groups. Robust antibody responses were elicited against the S-protein, RBD and N-protein. The results are displayed in **Tables 6.10** and **6.11**. On December 25, 2021, Covaxin received approval from the Drug Controller General of India (DGCI) for use in children 12–18 years.

TABLE 6.10: Covaxin™ phase 2/3 trial in children: The immune responses as measured by microneutralization (MNT) antibody titers and plaque reduction neutralization test (PRNT) titers.[66]

	MNT_{50}		$PRNT_{50}$	
	GMT	SCR (%)	GMT	SCR (%)
Group 1 12–18 years	138.8 (111.0–173.6)	90.3 (84.9–94.2)	317.4 (224.4–449.2)	94.9 (90.5–97.6)
Group 2 6–12 years	137.4 (99.1–167.5)	89.8 (84.0–94.1)	366.9 (297.0–453.3)	98.2 (94.9–99.6)
Group 3 2–6 years	197.6 (176.4–221.4)	96.6 (92.8–98.7)	358.6 (287.2–447.8)	98.3 (95.0–99.6)
GMT ratio All children/adults	0.98 (0.80–1.19)		1.76 (1.32–2.33)	

(GMT: geometrical mean titer; MNT: microneutralization test; PRNT: plaque reduction neutralization test; SCR: seroconversion rate)

TABLE 6.11: Covaxin™ phase 2/3 trials in children: The immune responses as measured by the S-protein, RBD and N-protein IgG levels.[66]

	ELISA S-protein IgG		ELISA RBD IgG		ELISA N-protein IgG	
	GMT	SCR (%)	GMT	SCR (%)	GMT	SCR (%)
Group 1 12–18 years	8,985 (7,735–10,437)	97.1 (84.9–93.9)	5,513 (4,487–6,773)	87.4 (81.6–91.6)	10,308 (8,521–12,470)	95.4 (91.1–97.8)
Group 2 6–12 years	8,198 (7,015–9,580)	95.3 (84.0–94.7)	5,278 (4,529–6,151)	92.4 (87.3–95.6)	11,040 (9,356–13,027)	92.9 (88.0–96.8)
Group 3 2–6 years	7,066 (5,653–8,832)	82.1 (75.5–87.5)	5,149 (4,220–6,281)	82.1 (75.5–82.1)	6,548 (5,404–7,933)	84.9 (78.8–89.9)

(GMT: geometrical mean titer; SCR: seroconversion rate; S-protein: spike protein, RBD: receptor-binding domain; N-protein: nucleocapsid protein)

Other vaccines, which have received approval for studies in children in India, include ZyCov-D, Covovax (a subunit vaccine developed by Novavax and being developed by Serum Institute India), Corbevax (an adjuvanted subunit vaccine by Biological E Limited) and the Janssen vaccine.

■ VARIANTS AND VACCINES

Genetic variants of SARS-CoV-2 have been emerging and circulating around the world throughout the COVID-19 pandemic. The *D614G mutation* was the first major mutation detected and by May 2020, had become the predominant strain, world over. Subsequently, mutations have been detected in different countries with varied consequences on the transmissibility and severity of the resultant infections, with, over a period of time, the more transmissible variants displacing the previous ones, as occurred in the case of the *delta variant*.

Currently, as per the WHO, there are 5 variants of concerns (VOC)—Alpha (B.1.1.7), Beta (1.351), Gamma (P1), Delta (1.617.2) and Omicron (B.1.1.529), 2 variants of interest (VOI)—lambda (C.37) and Mu (B.1.64) and 3 variants under monitoring (VUM)—AZ 5, C.12 and B.1640.[67] **Figures 6.1** and **6.2** show the rapidity of spread of the Omicron variant in UK and India.

Current COVID-19 vaccines are based on the SARS-CoV-2 spike protein of the original Wuhan-hu-1 strain. The variants of concern generally have mutations in the spike protein, raising concerns of VE against these variants. Both, the D614G and the B.1.1.7 mutations, were fairly susceptible to neutralization by infection and vaccine-induced antibodies. On the other hand, the B.1.351 and P.1 lineages that emerged in South Africa and Brazil respectively have sequence changes in key positions, which may adversely affect neutralization by antibodies induced by past infection or vaccines.[68]

SARS-CoV-2 Vaccines

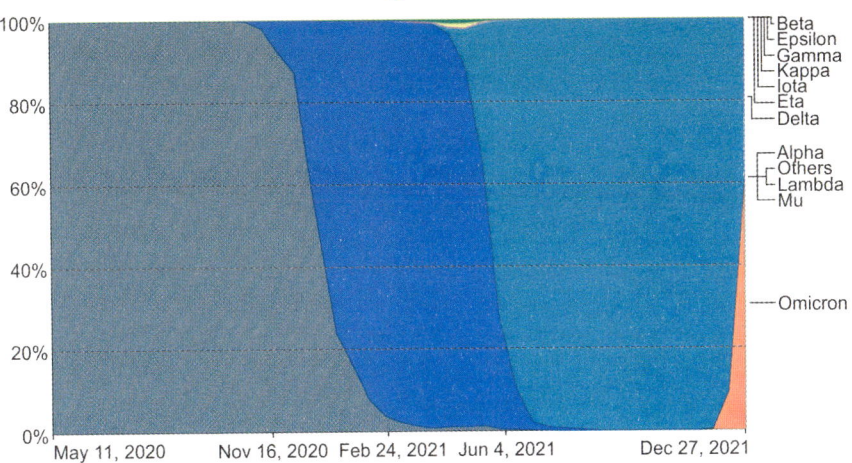

Fig. 6.1: SARS-CoV-2 variants in analyzed sequences, UK.
Source: CoVariants.org and GISAID – Last updated December 31, 2021, 20:00 (London time). OurWorldInData.org/coronavirus • CC BY
Note: Recently-discovered or actively-monitored variants may be overrepresented, as suspected cases of these variants are likely to be sequenced preferentially or faster than other cases.

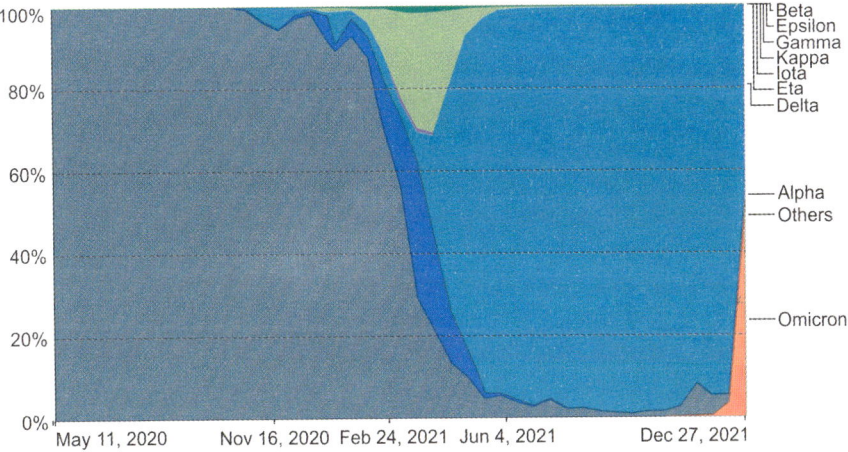

Fig. 6.2: SARS-CoV-2 variants in analyzed sequences, India.
Source: CoVariants.org and GISAID – Last updated December 31, 2021, 20:00 (London time). OurWorldInData.org/coronavirus • CC BY
Note: Recently-discovered or actively-monitored variants may be overrepresented, as suspected cases of these variants are likely to be sequenced preferentially or faster than other cases.

This has been demonstrated with the Pfizer and Moderna mRNA vaccines, AstraZeneca, Novavax and the Janssen vaccines.[69,70]

Worldwide the *delta variant* has become the most prevalent variant in circulation. Studies have demonstrated the significantly reduced efficacy against symptomatic COVID infection, while the efficacy against severe infection and hospitalization remains relatively unaffected. In the UK, the vaccine effectiveness, after one dose of vaccine (BNT162b2 or ChAdOx1 nCoV-19) was 30.7%; (95% CI, 25.2–35.7) against the delta variant as 48.7% (95% CI, 45.5–51.7) against the alpha variant, with similar results for both vaccines.[71] Two doses of the BNT162b2 vaccine resulted in vaccine effectiveness of 93.7% (95% CI, 91.6–95.3) against the alpha variant as against 88.0% (95% CI, 85.3–90.1) among those with the delta variant. Two doses of the ChAdOx1 nCoV-19 vaccine conferred a vaccine effectiveness of 74.5% (95% CI, 68.4–79.4) against the alpha variant and 67.0% (95% CI, 61.3–71.8) against the delta variant.[71]

The neutralization capability of Covaxin was assessed by plaque reduction neutralization test (PRNT50) using sera collected from the vaccine recipients against hCoV-19/India/20203522 (UK-variant) and hCoV27 19/India/2020Q111 (heterologous strain). Similar neutralization efficacy was shown against the UK-variant and the heterologous strain.[72] 12 isolates of the variant, B.1.617, were propagated in Vero cells and characterized. Convalescent sera and sera from BBV152 vaccinees, had similar neutralizing capacity against the variant B.1.617.[72] In the phase 3 study of Covaxin, a VE of 65.2% (33.1–83) was observed against the delta variant.[41]

The *Omicron variant* was first detected in specimens collected on November 11, 2021 and on November 26, 2021. WHO designated the variant B.1.1.529 (Omicron) as a variant of concern. This variant with increased transmissibility now (as of December 27, 2021) accounts for 42.6% of isolates in USA, 61.2% in UK and 47.3% in India.[73] While it is believed that the omicron variant is more transmissible, its effect on severity and susceptibility to vaccine-induced protection is uncertain.

A test-negative design, case control study, was conducted to estimate the vaccine effectiveness against the Omicron and delta variants, in England, between November 27, and December 6, 2021.[74] Two doses of the AstraZeneca vaccine did not confer any protection against symptomatic Omicron infection from 15 weeks after the second dose. In subjects who received two doses of the Pfizer vaccine the efficacy fell from 88% (65.9 to 95.8) 2–9 weeks after dose 2 to 34.2% (−5 to 58.7) at 25+ weeks. During the same period, vaccine effectiveness of the A-Z vaccine against the delta variant fell from 76.2% (63.7–84.5) at 2–9 weeks to 41.8% (39.4–44.1) at 25+ weeks. Figures for the Pfizer vaccine were 88.2% (86.7–89.5) and 63.5% (61.4–65.5).

■ DURABILITY OF RESPONSES AFTER SARS-CoV-2 VACCINATION

No correlate of protection has been established for the COVID-19 vaccines. The duration of humoral immunity following natural COVID-19 infection is variable and robust memory B-cell responses have been demonstrated despite falling levels of plasma neutralizing antibodies. Vaccines, which have been granted EUA, have follow up data till 2 months following vaccination. Follow up at 90 days following the second dose of the mRNA-1273, has demonstrated robust binding antibody levels and neutralizing antibody levels, which were higher than those found in convalescent plasma.[75]

At 180 days after the second dose of the mRNA-1273, binding antibodies as measured by ELISA, against SARS-CoV-2 spike receptor–binding domain remained elevated. Detectable activity was present in all participants by the pseudovirus neutralization assay and the live-virus focus-reduction neutralization. The lowest levels of GMT were found in the subjects 71 years of age or older, the highest levels in those 56–70 years of age and intermediate levels in those 18 to 55 years of age. The immune responses beyond 6 months are being evaluated in ongoing studies.[76]

■ EFFECTIVENESS OF COVID VACCINES

With the vaccine rollout in December 2020, studying the real-world effects of these vaccines is an urgent requirement.

In Scotland, about 1,331,993 people were vaccinated over the study period between December 8, 2020 and February 22, 2021 with the BNT162b2 mRNA vaccine or the ChAdOx1 vaccine.[77] The VE against COVID-19 hospital admission at 28–34 days post-vaccination was 91% (95% CI 85–94) for the BNT162b2 mRNA vaccine and 88% (95% CI 75–94) for the ChAdOx1 vaccine. Overall combined VE against hospital admission due to COVID-19 was 83% (95% CI 72–89) in those aged 80 years and older, at 28–34 days post-vaccination.

In an analysis of the early effectiveness of COVID-19 vaccination with BNT162b2 mRNA vaccine and ChAdOx1 adenovirus vector vaccine on symptomatic disease, hospitalizations and mortality in older adults in England, the following observations were made.[78] In individuals >80 years, VE for BNT162b2, was 70% (95% CI 59–78%) from day 28 to 34 and then plateauing. The VE, 14 days after dose 2 was 89% (95% CI 85–93%). In individuals > 70 years, VE for BNT162b2, was 61% (95% CI 51–69%) from day 28–34 and then plateauing. For the ChAdOx1 vaccine the VE was 73% (95% CI 27–90%) from day 35 onward. The BNT162b2 vaccine conferred an additional protection of 43% (95% CI 33–52%) against emergency hospitalization and an additional protection of 51% (95% CI 37–62%) against death due to COVID. One dose of the ChAdOx1 vaccine conferred an additional protection of 37% (95% CI 3–59%) against emergency hospitalization. The combined VE against symptomatic COVID and emergency hospitalizations was 80%.

Robust data has emerged from Israel, one of the first countries to achieve over 95% coverage with the BNT162b2 mRNA vaccine.[79] All persons who received their first dose between December 20, 2020 and February 1, 2021, were matched to unvaccinated controls in a 1:1 ratio. VE against documented

TABLE 6.12: BNT162b2 mRNA vaccine trials in Israel.[79]

End point	Day 14–20 after dose 1	> 7 days after dose 2
Documented infection	46 (95% CI, 40–51)	72 (95% CI, 88–95)
Symptomatic infection	57 (95% CI, 50–63)	94 (95% CI, 87–98)
Hospitalization	74 (95% CI, 56–86)	87 (95% CI, 55–100)
Severe disease	62 (95% CI, 39–80)	92 (95% CI, 75–100)
Death	72 (95% CI, 19–100)	

infection with COVID-19, symptomatic COVID-19, COVID-19–related hospitalization, severe illness, and death, was estimated. The results are mentioned in **Table 6.12**.

A study estimating the interim VE of the BNT162b2 and mRNA-1273 COVID-19 vaccines in preventing SARS-CoV-2 infection among health care personnel, first responders, and other essential and frontline workers in eight US locations, between December 2020 and March 2021, demonstrated an adjusted VE of 80% (59–90) ≥14 days after receiving first dose and 90% (68–97) ≥14 days after the second dose.[80]

■ BOOSTER DOSES

The successive waves of COVID-19 caused by the highly contagious and virulent delta variant of SARS-CoV-2 and now the highly transmissible Omicron variant, combined with emerging data that vaccine and infection induced immunity tends to fade over time, have led to strong considerations for boosting those who have been fully vaccinated. A growing number of countries have already initiated booster doses for their populations.

Neutralizing antibody responses show biphasic decay over the first few months after infection. The first phase of rapid decay in the first 1–2 months after infection, is due to the decay of IgA responses and IgM responses, whereas the second phase of slower decay is due to the slow decay of IgG responses. T cell responses decay at a slightly slower rate than IgG over the first few months after infection, whereas memory B cell responses are seen to increase during that period. A similar response has been observed after vaccination.[81] While it is well known that efficacy of vaccines against symptomatic RTPCR positive infections tend to wane over time, protection against severe disease remains high.

A study was done in Israel, estimating the breakthrough infection rates in those >16 years, who received the second dose of the Pfizer vaccine between January to April. A statistically significant 51% (95% CI 40–68%) increased risk for breakthrough infection was found in early vaccinees (Jan–Feb) versus the late vaccinees (Mar–Apr).[82]

In a systematic review and meta-regression analysis of the duration of effectiveness of vaccines against SARS-CoV-2 infection and COVID-19 disease, it was seen that following full vaccination, up to 6 months after the final dose, the VE (VE) against SARS-CoV-2 infection fell by 18.5% (95% CI 8.4–33.4) overall and 19.9% (95% CI 9.2–36.7), in those >65 years.[83] Similar data for symptomatic COVID-19 disease was 25.4% (95% CI 13.7–42.5) and 32.0% (95% CI 11.0–69.0), respectively; and for severe COVID-19 disease, 8.0% (95% CI 3.6–15.2) and 9.7% (95% CI 5.9–14.7), respectively. The majority of VE estimates against severe disease remained over 70% for all time points. This analysis was done with four widely used vaccines—Pfizer-BioNTech-Comirnaty, Moderna-mRNA-1273, Janssen-Ad26.COV2.S, and AstraZeneca-Vaxzevria.

A booster dose results in significantly elevated levels of neutralizing antibodies against the pathogen. The memory B-cell pool is expanded leading to a faster, stronger response to subsequent exposures. Boosters also promote enhanced affinity maturation and T-cell responses, which result in the production of more broadly neutralizing antibodies, which may be more effective against emerging variants. However, there is insufficient data and too little follow-up to assess the kinetics and duration of the response.[84]

The first priority of a COVID-19 vaccination program is to reduce mortality and severe disease and to protect health systems. Hence maximization of coverage among the high-risk groups is of primary importance. Ongoing global vaccine supply constraints and inequities are facts to be considered when planning any booster programs.

Heterologous boosting schedules are being studied for added program flexibility in situations of uncertain vaccine supplies, reducing reactogenicity, increasing immunogenicity, and enhancing vaccine effectiveness.[85] A study done in Chile investigated the effects of heterologous boosting with either ChAdOx1-S BNT162b2 in Sinovac-CoronaVac primed individuals.[85] The results are given in **Table 6.13**.

■ SECOND-GENERATION COVID-19 VACCINES

The main disadvantages of the first-generation COVID-19 vaccines include a variant specific efficacy, short duration of protection against symptomatic disease, and the stringent refrigeration requirements for some of the first-generation vaccines and poorer immunogenicity in the elderly and immunocompromised. Thus, there is a potential requirement for different technologies, which might be able to provide a more robust and widespread immune response.

Thus, the second-generation vaccines aim to have a broad efficacy against variants, elicit high neutralizing antibodies, reduce transmission, and

TABLE 6.13: The effects of heterologous boosting with either ChAdOx1-S BNT162b2 in Sinovac-CoronaVac primed individuals.[85]

	Vaccine efficacy (%) of booster with		
	ChAdOx1-S	BNT162b2	CoronaVac
Infection	90	93	68
Symptomatic disease	93	95	71
Hospitalization	96	98	75
ICU admission	98	90	79

(VE: vaccine efficacy; ICU: intensive care units)

be cheap and convenient to produce and administer en masse. There are four oral and eight intranasal vaccines in clinical development.

Other platforms being investigated are the self-amplifying RNA platform (saRNA) and non-modified mRNA platforms.[86] Vaccines based on the RBD with adjuvants are in preclinical studies.[87,88] NVX-CoV2373, a second-generation subunit COVID-19 vaccine adjuvanted with Matrix-M, has demonstrated 90% overall efficacy as well as a high level of efficacy against circulating variants in phase 3 clinical trials, although there is no data about its efficacy against the delta and omicron variants.

Subunit vaccines are relatively easy to manufacture and have less stringent refrigeration requirements, which make it easier to distribute in countries lacking advanced health systems.

A universal COVID vaccine should preferably prevent infection by all sarbecoviruses and merbecoviruses and infections by viral drift and recombination variants. One such vaccine being investigated is the Spike Ferritin Nanoparticle COVID-19 vaccine (SPFN_1B-06-PL). This vaccine is a combination of a polymerized version of ferritin, attached to a modified spike protein sequence and adjuvanted with a unique adjuvant ALF-Q. The preclinical study results showed that the SpFN COVID-19 vaccine elicits a potent immune response with a broad protection against the SARS-CoV-2 beta-coronavirus variants of concern as well as other coronaviruses. Enrolment for a phase 1 study has begun.[89]

■ KEY POINTS

- The platforms being explored for COVID vaccines include inactivated, live attenuated, viral vectored, subunit, nucleic acid (RNA and DNA) and virus-like particle based.
- As on December 20, 2021, the following vaccines have received EUL by the WHO: Pfizer/BioNTech: BNT162b2; Moderna: mRNA-1273; COVID-19 vaccine (ChAdOx1-S): Covishield; Janssen (Johnson and Johnson): Ad26.COV2.S; Covaxin; COVID-19 vaccine (SARS-CoV-2 rS protein nanoparticle: Covovax); CoronaVac COVID-19 vaccine (vero cell); and Inactivated COVID-19 Vaccine (vero cell): BIBP.

- The only COVID vaccine to receive full approval by the US-FDA is the Pfizer-BioNTech COVID-19 vaccine.
- Astra Zeneca AZD1222 vaccine is based on a replication-deficient chimpanzee adenovirus; the vaccine efficacy after a single standard dose of vaccine from day 22 to day 90 after vaccination was 76.0%.
- Post-authorization surveillance of adenovectored COVID-19 vaccines has identified vaccine-induced immune thrombotic thrombocytopenia (VITT) manifesting as cerebral venous sinus thrombosis (CVST).
- Pfizer BNT162b2 mRNA COVID-19 Vaccine is a lipid nanoparticle–formulated, 5 nucleoside-modified RNA (modRNA) with VE of 95.0%.
- Myopericarditis has been reported as a rare complication of COVID-19 mRNA vaccinations.
- Covaxin™ is manufactured by Bharat Biotech is a whole-virion inactivated vaccine, received approval from the Drug Controller General of India (DGCI) for use in children 12–18 years.
- Covaxin, a vaccine efficacy of 65.2% (33.1–83) was observed against the delta variant.
- The omicron variant (B.1.1.529) is more transmissible, its effect on severity and susceptibility to vaccine-induced protection is uncertain.
- The main disadvantages of the first-generation COVID-19 vaccines include a variant specific efficacy, short duration of protection against symptomatic disease and the stringent refrigeration requirements for some of the first-generation vaccines and poorer immunogenicity in the elderly and immunocompromised.

■ REFERENCES

1. World Health Organization. WHO Director General's opening remarks at the media briefing on COVID-19 – 11 March 2020. [online] Available from: https://www.who.int/director-general/speeches/detail/who-director-general-s-opening-remarks-at-the-media-briefing-on-covid-19. [Last Accessed January, 2022].
2. World Health Organization. Coronavirus (COVID-19) Dashboard. [online] Available from: https://covid19.who.int/. [Last Accessed January, 2022].
3. Moderbacher R, Ramirez SI, Dan JM, Grifoni A, Hastie KM, Weiskof D, et al. Antigen-specific adaptive immunity to SARS-Cov-2 in acute COVID-19 and associations with age and disease severity. Cell. 2020;183(4):996-1012.e19.
4. Dan JM, Mateus J, Kato Y, Hastie KM, Yu ED, Faliti CE, et al. Immunological memory to SARS-Cov-2 assessed up to 8 months after infection. Science. 2021;371(6529):eabf4063.
5. Lurie N, Saville M, Hatchett R, Halton J. Developing Covid-19 Vaccines at Pandemic Speed. N Engl J Med. 2020;382(21):1969-73.
6. Moderna's Work on Our COVID-19 Vaccine. [online] Available from: https://www.modernatx.com/modernas-work-potential-vaccine-against-covid-19. [Last Accessed January, 2022].
7. World Health Organization. COVID-19 vaccine tracker and landscape. [online] Available from: https://www.who.int/publications/m/item/draft-landscape-of-covid-19-candidate-vaccines. [Last Accessed January, 2022].
8. Juan-Giner A, Tchaton M, Jemmy JP, Soumah A, Boum Y, Fag EM, et al. Safety of the rVSV ZEBOV vaccine against Ebola Zaire among frontline workers in Guinea. Vaccine. 2019;37(48):7171-7.

9. Pardi N, Hogan MJ, Porter FW, Weissman D. mRNA vaccines — a new era in vaccinology. Nat Rev Drug Discov. 2018;17(4):261-79.
10. Ulmer JB, Geall AJ. Recent innovations in mRNA vaccines. Curr Opin Immunol. 2016;41:18-22.
11. Corbett KS, Edwards DK, Leist SR, Abiona OM, Boyoglu-Barnum S, Gillespie RA, et al. SARS-CoV-2 mRNA vaccine design enabled by prototype pathogen preparedness. Nature. 2021;586(7830):567-71.
12. Hobernik D, Bros M. DNA Vaccines–How Far From Clinical Use? Int J Mol Sci. 2018;19(11):3605.
13. World Health Organization. WHO Target Product Profiles for COVID-19 Vaccines. [online] Available from: https://www.who.int/docs/default-source/blue-print/who-target-product-profiles-for-covid-19-vaccines.pdf. [Last Accessed January, 2022].
14. US Food and Drug Administration. Emergency Use Authorization. [online] Available from: https://www.fda.gov/emergency-preparedness-and-response/mcm-legal-regulatory-and-policy-framework/emergency-use-authorization. [Last Accessed January, 2022].
15. World Health Organization. Status of COVID-19 Vaccines within WHO EUL/PQ evaluation process. [online] Available from: https://extranet.who.int/pqweb/sites/default/files/documents/Status_COVID_VAX_23Dec2021.pdf. [Last Accessed January, 2022].
16. US Food and Drug Administration. FDA News Release. FDA Approves First COVID-19 Vaccine. [online] Available from: https://www.fda.gov/news-events/press-announcements/fda-approves-first-covid-19-vaccine. [Last Accessed January, 2022].
17. Tan WG, Jin HT, West EE, Penaloza-MacMaster P, Wieland A. Comparative analysis of simian immunodeficiency virus gag-specific effector and memory CD8+ T cells induced by different adenovirus vectors. J Virol. 2013,87(3):1359-72.
18. Folegatti PM, Ewer KJ, Aley PK, Angus B, Becker S, Belij-Rammerstorfer S, et al. Safety and immunogenicity of the ChAdOx1 nCoV-19 vaccine against SARS-CoV-2: a preliminary report of a phase 1/2, single-blind, randomised controlled trial. Lancet. 2020;396(10249):467-78.
19. Ramasamy MN, Minassian AM, Ewer KJ, Flaxman AL, Folegatti PM, Owens DR, et al. Safety and immunogenicity of ChAdOx1 nCoV-19 vaccine administered in a prime-boost regimen in young and old adults (COV002): a single-blind, randomised, controlled, phase 2/3 trial. Lancet. 2020;396(10267):1979-93.
20. Voysey M, Costa Clemens SA, Madhi SA, Weckx LY, Folegatti PM, Aley PK, et al. Safety and efficacy of the ChAdOx1 nCoV-19 vaccine (AZD1222) against SARS-CoV-2: an interim analysis of four randomised controlled trials in Brazil, South Africa, and the UK. Lancet. 2021;397(10269):99-111.
21. Voysey M, Costa Clemens SA, Madhi SA, Weckx LY, Folegatti PM, Aley PK, et al. Single-dose administration and the influence of the timing of the booster dose on immunogenicity and efficacy of ChAdOx1 nCoV-19 (AZD1222) vaccine: a pooled analysis of four randomized trials. Lancet. 2021;397(10277):881-91.
22. GOV.UK. Coronavirus (COVID-19) Latest updates and guidance. [online] Available from: https://www.gov.uk/government/publications/coronavirus-covid-19-vaccine-adverse-reactions/coronavirus-vaccine-summary-of-yellow-card-reporting. [Last Accessed January, 2022].

23. Walsh EE, Frenck Jr. RW, Falsey AR, Kitchin N, Absalon J, Gurtman A, et al. Safety and Immunogenicity of Two RNA-Based Covid-19 Vaccine Candidates. N Engl J Med. 2020;383(25):2439-50.
24. CDC Newsroom. Joint CDC and FDA Statement on Johnson & Johnson Covid-19 Vaccine. [online] Available from: https://www.cdc.gov/media/releases/2021/s0413-JJ-vaccine.html. [Last Accessed January, 2022].
25. Centers for Disease Control and Prevention. COVID-19. Selected Adverse Events Reported After COVID-19 Vaccination. [online] Available from: https://www.cdc.gov/coronavirus/2019-ncov/vaccines/safety/JJUpdate.html. [Last Accessed January, 2022].
26. GOV.UK. Coronavirus (COVID-19) Latest updates and guidance. [online] Available from: https://www.gov.uk/government/news/mhra-issues-new-advice-conclu...ce=3fbfe68a-be2d-4b92-9097-23e76232941f&utm_content=immediately. [Last Accessed January, 2022].
27. World Health Organization. Regional Office for Europe. [online] Available from: https://www.who.int/news/item/07-04-2021-interim-statement-of-the-c...ubcommittee-of-the-who-global-advisory-committee-on-vaccine-safety. [Last Accessed January, 2022].
28. AlJazeera. News. Coronavirus pandemic. [online] Available from: https://www.aljazeera.com/news/2021/3/15/which-countries-have-halted-use-of-astrazenecas-covid-vaccine assessed on21/4/21. [Last Accessed January, 2022].
29. Polack FP, Thomas SJ, Kitchin N, Absalon J, Gurtman A, Lockhart S, et al. Safety and Efficacy of the BNT162b2 mRNA Covid-19 Vaccine. N Engl J Med. 2020;383(27):2603-15.
30. Jackson LA, Anderson EJ, Rouphael NG, Roberts PC, Makhene M, Coler RN, et al. An mRNA Vaccine against SARS-CoV-2 — Preliminary Report. N Engl J Med. 2020;383(20):1920-31.
31. Baden LR, El Sahly HM, Essink B, Kotloff K, Frey S, Novak R, et al. Efficacy and Safety of the mRNA-1273 SARS-CoV-2 Vaccine. N Engl J Med. 2021; 384(5):403-16.
32. Moderna. News. [online] Available from: https://investors.modernatx.com/news-releases/news-release-details/moderna-announces-longer-shelf-life-its-covid-19-vaccine". [Last Accessed January, 2022].
33. Centers for Disease Control and Prevention (CDC). Advisory Committee on Immunization Practices (ACIP). Coronavirus disease 2019 (COVID-19) vaccines. [online] Available from: https://www.cdc.gov/vaccines/acip/ meetings/slides-2021-06.html. [Last Accessed January, 2022].
34. Hause AM, Gee J, Baggs J, Abara WE, Marquez P, Thompson D, et al. COVID-19 Vaccine Safety in Adolescents Aged 12–17 Years — United States, December 14, 2020–July 16, 2021. MMWR Morb Mortal Wkl Rep. 2021;70(31):1053-8.
35. Klein NP, Lewis N, Goddard K, Fireman B, Zerbo O, Hanson KE, et al. Surveillance for adverse events after COVID-19 mRNA vaccination. JAMA. 2021:326(14):1390-9.
36. Logunov DY, Dolzhikova IV, Zubkova OV, Tukhvatulin AI, Shcheblyakov DV, Dzharullaeva AS, et al. Safety and immunogenicity of an rAd26 and rAd5 vector-based heterologous prime-boost COVID-19 vaccine in two formulations: two open, non-randomised phase 1/2 studies from Russia. Lancet. 2020; 396(10255):887-97.

37. Logunov DY, Dolzhikova IV, Shcheblyakov DV, Tukhvatulin AI, Zubkova OV, Dzharullaaeva AS, et al. Safety and efficacy of an rAd26 and rAd5 vector-based heterologous prime-boost COVID-19 vaccine: an interim analysis of a randomised controlled phase 3 trial in Russia. Lancet. 2021;397(10275):671-81.
38. Tukhvatulin AI, Dolzhikova IV, Shcheblyakov DV, Zubkova OV, Dzharullaeva A, Kovyrshina AV, et al. An open, non-randomised, phase 1/2 trial on the safety, tolerability, and immunogenicity of single-dose vaccine "Sputnik Light" for prevention of coronavirus infection in healthy adults. Lancet. 2021:11.100241.
39. Ella R, Vadrevu KM, Jogdand H, Prasad S, Reddy S, Sarangi V, et al. Safety and immunogenicity of an inactivated SARS-CoV-2 vaccine, BBV152: a double-blind, randomised, phase 1 trial. Lancet Infect Dis. 2021;21(5):637-46.
40. Ella R, Reddy S, Jogdand H, Sarangi V, Ganneru B, Prasad S, et al. Safety and immunogenicity of an inactivated SARS-CoV-2 vaccine, BBV152: interim results from a double-blind, randomised, multicentre, phase 2 trial, and 3-month follow-up of a double-blind, randomised phase 1 trial. Lancet Infect Dis. 2021;21(70):950-61.
41. Ella R, Reddy S, Blackwelder W, Poddar V, Yadav P, Sarangi V, et al. Efficacy, safety, and lot-to-lot immunogenicity of an inactivated SARS-CoV-2 vaccine (BBV152): interim results of a randomised, double-blind, controlled, phase 3 trial. Lancet. 2021;398(10317):2173-84.
42. Keech C, Albert G, Cho I, Robertson A, Reed P, Neal S, et al. Phase 1-2 Trial of a SARS-CoV-2 Recombinant Spike Protein Nanoparticle Vaccine. N Engl J Med, 2020;383(24):2320-32.
43. Heath PT, Galiza EP, Baxter DN, Boffito M, Browne D, Burns F, et al. Safety and Efficacy of NVX-CoV2373 Covid-19 Vaccine. N Engl J Med. 2021;385(13):1172-83.
44. Novavax. Novavax COVID-19 vaccine demonstrates 89.3% efficacy in UK phase 3 trial. [online] Available from: https://ir.novavax.com/node/15506/pdf". [Last Accessed January, 2022].
45. Dunkle LM, Kotloff KL, Gay CL, Áñez G, Adelglass JM, Hernández AQB, et al. Efficacy and Safety of NVX-CoV2373 in Adults in the United States and Mexico. N Eng J Med. 2021.
46. Sadoff J, Gray G, Vandebosch A, Cárdenaz V, Shukarev G, Grinsztejn B, et al. Safety and Efficacy of Single-Dose Ad26.COV2.S Vaccine against Covid-19. N Engl J Med. 2021;384(23):2187-2201.
47. Xia S, Zhang Y, Wang Y, Wang H, Yang Y, Gao GF, et al. Safety and Immunogenicity of an inactivated SARS-CoV-2 vaccine, BBIBP-CorV: a randomized, double-blind, and placebo-controlled phase 1/2 trial. Lancet Infect Dis. 2021;21(1):39-51.
48. Palacios R, Batista AP, Albuquerque CSN, Patiño EG, Santos JP, Conde MTRP, et al. Efficacy and safety of a COVID-19 inactivated vaccine in healthcare professionals in Brazil: The PROFISCOV Study. SSRN Elec J. 2020.
49. Momin T, Kansagra K, Patel H, Sharma S, Sharma B, Patel J, et al. Safety and Immunogenicity of a DNA SARS-CoV-2 vaccine (ZyCoV-D): Results of an open-label, non-randomized phase I part of phase I/II clinical study by intradermal route in healthy subjects in India. EClin Med. 2021;38:101020.
50. Zydus dedicated to life. Zydus Cadila receives approvals from DCGI to start Phase III Clinical Trial of ZyCoV-D – fully indigenously developed vaccine.

[online] Available from: https://zyduscadila.com/public/pdf/pressrelease/Zydus_Cadila_receives_approvals_from_the_DCGI_to_start_Phase_III_Clinical_Trial_of_ZyCoV_D_fully_indigenously_developed_vaccine_-3_1_2021.pdf. [Last Accessed January, 2022].

51. Fidler DP. Negotiating equitable access to influenza vaccines: global health diplomacy and the controversies surrounding avian influenza H5N1 and pandemic influenza H1N1. PLoS Med. 2010;7(5):e1000247.
52. World Health Organization. The Access to COVID-19 Tools (ACT) Accelerator. [online] Available from: https://www.who.int/initiatives/act-accelerator/covax". [Last Accessed January, 2022].
53. GAVI. COVAX. [online] Available from: http://gavi.org/covax-facility". [Last Accessed January, 2022].
54. Nguyen LH, Drew DA, Graham MS, Joshi AD, Guo CG, Ma W, et al. Risk of COVID-19 among front-line health-care workers and the general community: A prospective cohort study. Lancet Public Health. 2020;5(9):e475-e483.
55. World Health Organization. WHO SAGE Roadmap for prioritizing uses of COVID-19 vaccines in the Context of Limited Supply. [online] Available from: https://www.who.int/publications/m/item/who-sage-roadmap-for-prioritizing-uses-of-covid-19-vaccines-in-the-context-of-limited-supply. [Last Accessed January, 2022].
56. Dong Y, Mo X, Hu Y, Qi X, Jiang Z, Tong S, et al. Epidemiology of COVID-19 Among Children in China. Pediatrics. 2020;145(6):e20200702.
57. Jiang L, Tang K, Levin M, Irfan O, Morris SK, Wilson K, et al. COVID-19 and multisystem inflammatory syndrome in children and adolescents. Lancet Infect Dis. 2020;20(11):e276-e288.
58. Lee B, Raszka Jr WV. COVID-19 Transmission and Children: The Child Is Not to Blame. Pediatrics. 2020;146(2):e2020004879.
59. Szablewski CM, Chang KT, Brown MM, Chu VT, Yousaf AR, Anyalechi N, et al. SARS-CoV-2 Transmission and Infection Among Attendees of an Overnight Camp — Georgia, June 2020. MMWR Morb Mortal Wkly Rep. 2020;69(31):1023-5.
60. Goldstein E, Lipsitch M, Cevik M. On the effect of age on the transmission of SARS-CoV-2 in households, schools, and the community. J Infect Dis. 2021;223(3):362-9.
61. Park YJ, Choe YJ, Park O, Park SY, Kim YM, Kim J, et al. Contact tracing during Coronavirus Disease Outbreak, South Korea, 2020. Emerg Infect Dis. 2020;26(10):2465-8.
62. Frenck, Jr RW, Klein NP, Kitchin N, Gurtman A, Absalon J, Lockhart S, et al. Safety, Immunogenicity, and Efficacy of the BNT162b2 Covid-19 Vaccine in Adolescents. N Engl J Med. 2021;385(3):239-50.
63. Walter EB, Talaat KR, Sabharwal C, Gurtman A, Lockhart S, Paulsen GC, et al. Evaluation of the BNT162b2 Covid-19 Vaccine in Children 5 to 11 Years of Age. N Engl J Med. 2022;386(1):35-46.
64. Ali K, Berman G, Zhou H, Deng W, Faughnan V, Cornado-Voges M, et al. Evaluation of mRNA-1273 SARS-CoV-2 vaccine in adolescents. N Eng J Med. 2021;385(24):2241-51.
65. Pharmaceutical Technology. Oxford University launches COVID-19 vaccine study in children. [online] Available from: https://www.pharmaceutical-technology.com/news/oxford-university-study-children/. [Last Accessed January, 2022].

66. Vadrevu KM, Reddy S, Jogdand H, Ganneru B, Mirza N, Tripathy VN, et al. Immunogenicity and safety of an inactivated SARS-CoV-2 vaccine (BBV152) in children from 2 to 18 years of age: an open-label, age-de-escalation phase 2/3 study. medRxiv. 2021.
67. World Health Organization. Tracking SARS-CoV-2 variants. [online] Available from: https://www.who.int/en/activities/tracking-SARS-CoV-2-variants/". [Last Accessed January, 2022].
68. GISAID. Tracking of variants. [online] Available from:https://www.gisaid.org/hcov19-variants/. [Last Accessed January, 2022].
69. Liu Y, Liu J, Xia H, Zhang X, Fontes-Garfias CR, Swanson KA, et al. Neutralizing Activity of BNT162b2-Elicited Serum. N Engl J Med. 2021;384(15):1466-8.
70. Wu K, Werner AP, Koch M, Choi A, Narayanan E, Stewart-Jones GBE, et al. Serum Neutralizing Activity Elicited by mRNA-1273 Vaccine. N Engl J Med. 2021;384(15):1468-70.
71. Bernal JL, Andrews N, Gower C, Gallagher E, Simmons R, Thelwall S, et al. Effectiveness of Covid-19 Vaccines against the B.1.617.2 (Delta) Variant. N Engl J Med. 2021;385(7):585-94.
72. Sapkal GN, Yadav PD, Ella R, Deshpande GR, Sahay RR, Gupta N, et al. Neutralization of UK-variant VUI-202012/01 with COVAXIN vaccinated human serum. bioRxiv. 2021.
73. Our World in Data. Coronavirus Pandemic (COVID-19). [online] Available from: https://ourworldindata.org/coronavirus#coronavirus-country-profiles. [Last Accessed January, 2022].
74. Andrews N, Stowe J, Kirsebom F, Toffa S, Rickeard T, Gallagher E, et al. Effectiveness of COVID-19 vaccines against the Omicron (B.1.1.529) variant of concern. medRxiv. 2021.
75. Widge AT, Rouphael NG, Jackson LA, Jackson AJ, Roberts PC, Makhene M, et al. Durability of Responses after SARS-CoV-2 mRNA-1273 Vaccination. N Engl J Med. 2021;384(1):80-2.
76. Doria-Rose N, Suthar MS, Makowski M, O'Connell S, McDermott AB, Flach B, et al. Antibody Persistence through 6 Months after the Second Dose of mRNA-1273 Vaccine for Covid-19. N Eng J Med. 2021;384(23):2259-61.
77. Vasileiou E, Simpson CR, Shi T, Kerr S, Agarwal U, Akbari A, et al. Interim findings from first-dose mass COVID-19 vaccination roll-out and COVID-19 hospital admissions in Scotland: a national prospective cohort study. Lancet. 2021;397(10285):1646-57.
78. Bernal JL, Andrews N, Gower C, Stowe J, Robertson C, Tessier E, et al. Early effectiveness of COVID-19 vaccination with BNT162b2 mRNA vaccine and ChAdOx1 adenovirus vector vaccine on symptomatic disease, hospitalisations and mortality in older adults in England. medRxiv. 2021.
79. Dagan N, Barda N, Kepten E, Miron O, Perchik S, Katz MA, et al. BNT162b2 mRNA Covid-19 Vaccine in a Nationwide Mass Vaccination Setting. N Engl J Med. 2021;384(15):1412-23.
80. Thompson MG, Burgess JL, Naleway AL, Tyner HL, Yoon SK, Meece J, et al. Interim Estimates of Vaccine Effectiveness of BNT162b2 and mRNA-1273 COVID-19 Vaccines in Preventing SARS-CoV-2 Infection Among Health Care Personnel, First Responders, and Other Essential and Frontline Workers - Eight U.S. Locations, December 2020-March 2021. MMWR Morb Mortal Wkly Rep. 2021;70(13):495-500.

81. Mortaz E, Tabarsi P, Varahram M, Folkerts G, Adcock IA. The Immune Response and Immunopathology of COVID-19. Front Immunol. 2020;11:2037.
82. Mizrahi B, Lotan R, Kalkstein N, Peretz A, Perez G, Ben-Tov A, et al. Correlation of SARS-CoV-2-breakthrough infections to time-from-vaccine. Nat Comm. 2021;12:6379.
83. Feikin DR, Higdon MM, Abu-Raddad LJ, Andrews N, Araos R, Goldberg Y, et al. Duration of effectiveness of vaccines against SARS-CoV-2 infection and COVID-19 disease: results of a systematic review and meta-regression. Lancet. 2021;18:42.
84. Nature. COVID vaccine boosters: the most important questions. [online] Available from: https://www.nature.com/articles/d41586-021-02158-6. [Last Accessed January, 2022].
85. World Health Organization. Interim recommendations for heterologous COVID-19 vaccine schedules. [online] Available from: https://www.who.int/publications/i/item/WHO-2019-nCoV-vaccines-SAGE-recommendation-heterologous-schedules. [Last Accessed January, 2022].
86. Gebre MS, Rauch S, Roth N, Yu J, Chandrashekar A, Mercado NB, et al. Optimization of Non-Coding Regions for a Non-Modified mRNA COVID-19 Vaccine. Nature. 2021.
87. Pino M, Abid T, Ribeiro SP, Edara VV, Floyd K, Smith JC, et al. A yeast-expressed RBD-based SARS-CoV-2 vaccine formulated with 3M-052 –alum adjuvant promotes protective efficacy in non-human primates. Sci Immunol. 2021;6(61):eabh3634.
88. Malladi SK, Patel UR, Rajmani RS, Singh R, Pandey S, Kumar S, et al. Immunogenicity and Protective Efficacy of a Highly Thermotolerant, Trimeric SARS-CoV-2 Receptor Binding Domain Derivative. ACS Infect Dis. 2021;7(8):2546-64.
89. Carmen JM, Shrivastava S, Lu Z, Anderson A, Morrison EB, Sankhala RS, et al. SARS-CoV-2 ferritin nanoparticle vaccine induces robust innate immune activity driving polyfunctional spike-specific T cell responses. NPJ Vaccines. 2021;6(1):151.

Neurology

CHAPTER 7: Autoimmune Encephalitis

Naveen Sankhyan, Renu Suthar

■ INTRODUCTION

The causes of encephalitis in children are numerous, and despite extensive workup, the cause in most children remains uncertain. In the past decade and a half, the discovery of autoantibodies implicated in several clinical syndromes has changed the approach to the diagnosis and treatment of encephalitis. The first significant advance in this field was the identification of antibodies against the N-methyl-D-aspartate receptor (NMDAR) and its associated clinical syndrome.[1] Autoantibodies may be directed against the synaptic receptors, cell surface proteins or ion channels, or intracellular neuronal antigens or proteins on glial cells. While, a host of antibody-associated encephalitis are described, only a few are commonly seen in children. The most common autoantibodies associated with autoimmune encephalitis (AE) in children are directed against NMDAR, myelin oligodendrocyte glycoprotein (MOG), and glutamic acid decarboxylase 65 (GAD65) antigens.[2,3] Most of the other AE are seen in the context of tumors in adults and are very uncommon in children.

From a clinical perspective, it is essential to remember that autoimmune encephalitides are an important and treatable cause of acute encephalitis. However, given the myriad of ways it can present, overlap in clinical presentations with other diseases, and the complexity of normal behavior changes in children make it challenging to diagnose. It is also known that children with a clinical phenotype of AE may not have a known autoantibody. They are often termed as "seronegative AE" in the presence of highly suggestive clinical features and other supportive investigations, and in the absence of known AE antibodies.

The subsequent sections in this chapter describe the current understanding of autoimmune encephalitides in children. The focus is clinical and on common syndromes found in children. Though anti-MOG and anti-aquaporin-4 (AQp4) antibodies are also within the ambit of AE, they have a different clinical phenotype. Consequently, most of the discussion will focus on the more prototypical AE and the anti-NMDAR encephalitis.

EPIDEMIOLOGY

The recent discovery of the AE group of disorders means that epidemiological trends are difficult to ascertain. However, specific important facts are emerging from studies on the subject. AE is reported to be either more common or at least as common as viral encephalitis in many parts of the world.[3,4] In some prospective cohorts, including adults and children, AE was the single most common cause of encephalitis, more than any single viral etiology.[5] This fact may not be accurate in areas with a high incidence of viral encephalitis, particularly in epidemic settings. It is likely that with the increase in testing facilities and more awareness, an increasing number of AE is being diagnosed in children as well as adults. Consequently, the potential contribution of immune-mediated encephalitis in the overall incidence of encephalitis globally may well surpass infectious encephalitis.

Anti-NMDAR encephalitis is the leading cause of AE in children, responsible for about 4% of cases of pediatric encephalitis and is more frequent than *Herpes simplex virus* type 1 (HSV1) and enteroviruses.[3] This fact has emerged from large countrywide cohorts as well as the California encephalitis project.[3,6] Within the individuals with anti-NMDAR encephalitis, it has been reported that 65% occurred in patients aged ≤18 years and females have a predilection for this disorder.[3] More recent studies from developed countries have reported an increased frequency of the diagnosis of anti-NMDAR encephalitis, responsible for as many as 26% of cases of acute encephalitis in children.[7]

In many studies, anti-MOG antibodies have not formed a subgroup of AE, but, anti-MOG antibody-associated demyelination and encephalitis are widespread in children and are possibly the most common antibody-mediated clinical neurological syndrome in children.[8,9] The presentation of the anti-MOG syndrome is, however, distinct and usually defined by radiological findings.[9] This contrasts with AE, where the clinical picture and radiological findings may differ based on the antibodies involved.

ETIOPATHOGENESIS

Autoimmune encephalitis is characterized by an immune response triggered by infection, tumor, or unknown genetic or environmental factors leading to antibodies or cellular response against the neuronal epitopes. The antibodies in AE are directed toward extracellular surface antigens or intracellular antigens. The pathogenic antibodies targeting the neuronal surface antigens alter the cellular function without causing cell death, hence are responsive to immunotherapy. Anti-NMDAR antibodies were the first identified antibodies against cell surface synaptic receptor in 2007 in women with ovarian teratoma.[1] Subsequently, antibodies were identified against the glycine receptor (GlyR), the α-amino-3-hydroxy-5-methyl-4-isoxazolepropionic acid receptor (AMPAR), the leucine-rich glioma-inactivated protein-1 (LGI1), the contactin-associated protein-2 (Caspr2), the γ-aminobutyric acid-A receptor (GABA$_A$R) and γ-aminobutyric acid-B receptor (GABA$_B$R), the metabotropic glutamate receptor 5 (mGluR5), the dopamine-2 receptor (D2R), the dipeptidyl peptidase-like protein-6 (DPPX), and the immunoglobulin-like cell adhesion molecule-5 (IgLON5).[3-10] Autoantibodies may be directed against the synaptic receptors (NMDA, AMPA, GABA$_A$R, GABA$_B$R, and D2R receptors), cell surface proteins or ion channels (LGI1, CASPR2 and DPPX) or intracellular neuronal antigens (glutamic acid-decarboxylase [GAD], Hu, and Ma2), or proteins on glial cells (e.g., MOG). Intracellular antigens are usually associated with paraneoplastic syndromes and have a poor prognosis.[10] Currently, the most common autoantibodies associated with pediatric AE target NMDAR, MOG, and GAD65 antigens.[2] It is also known that children with a clinical phenotype of AE may not have a known autoantibody.

■ CLINICAL FEATURES

Children with AE typically present with a variable combination of acute or subacute onset neuropsychiatric symptoms, seizures, and/or movement disorder.[11,12] Typically, onset is abrupt with an acute or subacute course of <3 months duration and relapsing and remitting symptoms. Immune reaction in AE is diffuse, often leading to multifocal presentation. While the prototypical anti-NMDAR encephalitis is by and large the most common AE, other AE syndromes may rarely also be encountered in practice. Though there are some common features, the symptomatology of AE depends partly on the age and the inciting autoantibody **(Box 7.1** and **Table 7.1)**.

Cognitive impairment and memory disturbances are other cardinal features of AE. The presence of cognitive impairment differentiates AE

BOX 7.1: Proposed diagnostic criteria for autoimmune encephalitis (AE).*

A diagnosis of AE can be made when all three of the following criteria have been met:
1. Subacute onset (rapid progression of <3 months) of working memory deficits (short-term memory loss), altered mental status, or psychiatric symptoms
2. At least one of the following:
   - New focal neurological findings
   - Seizures not explained by a previously known seizure disorder
   - Cerebrospinal fluid (CSF) pleocytosis (white blood cell count of >5 cells per mm^3)
   - Magnetic resonance imaging (MRI) features suggestive of encephalitis
3. Reasonable exclusion of alternative causes

Source: Graus F, Titulaer MJ, Balu R, Benseler S, Bien CG, Cellucci T, et al. A clinical approach to diagnosis of autoimmune encephalitis. *Lancet Neurol.* 2016;15(4):391–404

from pediatric neuropsychiatric autoimmune syndromes (PNAS), where cognition is preserved and movement disorder is self-limiting. Assessment of cognitive regression or impairment can be difficult in children; however certain degree of developmental regression, language regression, mutism, and speech impairment is always present. Chronic presentation is reported

TABLE 7.1: Selected phenotypes and associated autoantibodies in children with autoimmune encephalitis.

Feature/s	Antibody targets typically involved
Polysymptomatic encephalopathy and movement disorder	NMDAR, $GABA_BR$, mGluR5
Epilepsy and neuropsychiatric symptoms	LGI1, CASPR2, NMDAR, $GABA_BR$, GAD65, Hu, DNER
Status epilepticus or very high seizure burden	NMDAR, LGI1, $GABA_A$, $GABA_B$, GAD65
Brainstem encephalitis (Bickerstaff encephalitis)	GQ1b
Limbic encephalitis	LGI1, CASPR2, $GABA_BR$, GAD65, Hu, DNER
Cerebellitis or autoimmune cerebellar syndrome	DNER, NMDAR, mGluR1a
Opsoclonus myoclonus syndrome	Hu, GAD65
Progressive encephalomyelitis with rigidity and myoclonus (PERM)	GAD65, GlyR, LGI1
Demyelinating diseases	MOG, AQp4
Female preponderance	GAD65, NMDAR – Adolescents Other autoimmune disorders with overlap - e.g., SLE
Pre-existing autoimmune disorder	GAD65
After viral encephalitis (e.g., HSE)	NMDAR
Viral prodrome	MOG
Neoplasm	NMDAR (teratoma), anti-Hu (neuroblastoma), mGluR5 (Hodgkin disease)

Source: Adapted from Bien CG, Bien CI. Autoimmune encephalitis in children and adolescents. Neurol Res Pract. 2020;2:4.

(AQp4: aquaporin-4; CASPR: contactin-associated protein receptor; DNER: delta/notch-like EGF-related receptor; GABABR: γ-aminobutyric acid-B receptor; $GABA_BR$:- γ-aminobutyric acid-B receptor; GAD65: glutamic acid decarboxylase 65 kDa; GQ1B: antibodies to ganglioside Q1B; GlyR: glycine receptor; HSE: herpes simplex encephalitis NMDAR: N-methyl-D-aspartate receptor; mGluR5: metabotropic glutamate receptor 5; LGI1: leucine-rich glioma inactivatedprotein1; mGluR1a: metabotropic glutamate receptor 1a; MOG: myelin oligodendrocytic glycoprotein; SLE: systemic lupus erythematosus)

TABLE 7.2: Clinical features and phenotypes of autoimmune encephalitis in relation to specific autoantibodies in children.

Antibody type	Selected features or phenotypes
Anti-NMDAR*	Psychosis, movement disorder, sleep disturbances, seizures, psychiatric problems, language problems, and autonomic dysfunction
Anti-MOG*	Acute disseminated encephalomyelitis, optic neuritis, transverse myelitis, neuromyelitis optica spectrum disorders, encephalitis, and relapsing demyelination
Anti-AQp4 *	Neuromyelitis optica spectrum disorders
Anti-GAD65	Subacute headache, memory disturbances, psychiatric symptoms, and seizures
Anti-GlyR	Progressive encephalomyelitis with rigidity and myoclonus (PERM), stiff-person syndrome, epilepsy, limbic encephalitis, cerebellar ataxia, transverse myelitis, optic neuritis, neuromyelitis optica, and multiple sclerosis
Anti-LGI1	Limbic encephalitis, faciobrachial dystonic seizures (FBDS) hyponatremia, Morvan syndrome, neuromyotonia, progressive encephalomyelitis with rigidity and myoclonus, chorea, hemianesthesia, and neurocardiac problems
Anti-CASPR2	Encephalopathy, seizures, limbic encephalitis, cerebellar ataxia, Morvan syndrome, peripheral nerve hyperexcitability, neuromyotonia, neuropathic pain, insomnia, and dysautonomia
Anti-GABA$_A$R	Limbic encephalitis, ataxia, and opsoclonus-myoclonus ataxia syndrome
Anti-GABA$_B$R	Encephalitis, refractory seizures, and stiff-person syndrome opsoclonus-myoclonus-ataxia syndrome
Anti-D2R	Movement disorders (dystonia, parkinsonism, chorea, and oculogyric crises), psychiatric disturbances (agitation, emotional lability, anxiety, and psychotic symptoms), sleep disturbances, lethargy, drowsiness, brainstem dysfunction, seizure, and ataxia

Note: *The most common among the group.

with certain rare forms of AE, especially LGI1, CASPR2, DPPX-6, and anti-GAD65 antibody-mediated AE. The specific clinical features in various types of AE in children are summarized in **Tables 7.1** and **7.2**.

Clinical Features of Specific AE Subtypes

Anti-NMDAR Encephalitis

Anti-NMDAR encephalitis evolves in stages, the initial stage is often a viral prodrome or nonspecific fever, followed by an explosive onset of psychiatric and behavior disturbances and a subsequent progression to profound neurological impairment with seizures, movement disorders, insomnia, and breathing or autonomic instability.[8,12] >90% of patients with anti-NMDAR encephalitis develop a combination of these features within 1 month of onset of illness. Distinctively, the presence of seizures, sleep/wake rhythm alteration, language impairment, and catatonia as the initial symptoms were predictive of anti-NMDAR encephalitis in comparison to psychotic disorder and other noninfectious encephalitides.[13] In a pediatric series from India, behavioral changes, psychosis, seizures, orolingual dyskinesia, insomnia, irritability, and language dysfunction were prominent in children with anti-NMDAR encephalitis.[14-16] Occasionally, presentation among young children can be nonspecific.

Temper tantrums, agitation, hyperactivity, irritability, aggression, sleep-wake cycle disturbances, and progressive speech deterioration are seen frequently in children.[11,12,16] In comparison, neuropsychiatric features such as psychosis, hallucinations, aggression, catatonia, bizarre fear, insomnia, memory loss, decreased consciousness, lethargy, and mania are often seen in adolescents or adults.[8,12,15]

A combination of tremors, dyskinesia, stereotypy, dystonia, asterixis, myoclonus, and parkinsonism may be observed in children with anti-NMDAR encephalitis.[17] The most typical *movement disorder* associated with ant-NMDAR encephalitis is orofacial–lingual dyskinesia. Additionally, stereotypies, both simple and complex, are also highly suggestive of anti-NMDAR encephalitis. The movement disorder may be mild or can be complex and violent.[18] It may not be possible to classify the movement disorder into any of the known types given the bizarre nature and complexity. Often the movement disorder is accompanied by extreme agitation. The agitation may be severe, life-threatening, and enough to mandate continuous intravenous sedation. In some children catatonia may be prominent. It is also noteworthy that some clinical symptoms of anti-NMDAR encephalitis may have a fluctuant course with the child showing some period of apparent normalcy alternating with periods of symptoms.

Sleep disturbances are the next common and a distinctive clue to the diagnosis of AE and, more specifically, anti-NMDAR encephalitis in children. While most viral encephalitis will present with somnolence, anti-NMDAR encephalitis has typically varying degrees of insomnia. Most children will have a fragmented sleep, reduced sleep time, and alteration in the sleep-wake cycle. Complete lack of sleep may be seen in severely affected children.

Language dysfunction is also not uncommon in children with anti-NMDAR encephalitis and manifests as receptive and expressive language impairment.

Seizures are one of the common features of anti-NMDAR encephalitis and may be the predominant manifestation. Seizures can be focal, generalized, or multifocal in onset. Anti-NMDAR encephalitis is also known to cause the new-onset refractory status epilepticus (NORSE).

Autonomic dysfunction, although less common in children, includes central hypoventilation, urinary incontinence, and episodes of tachycardia, hypertension, or hyperthermia.

In children with viral encephalitis, the recurrence of symptoms, new onset disturbed sleep-wake cycle, language regression, stereotypies, and new-onset movement disorder should make one suspicious of AE.[19,20]

An underlying tumor is more frequently seen in adults and adolescent females and is very uncommon in younger children. In a study the frequency of ovarian teratoma was 56% in women >18 years of age, 31% in girls <18 years of age, and 9% in girls <14 years of age.[17]

Based on the typical features, diagnostic criteria have been proposed for anti-NMDAR encephalitis. The diagnostic criteria by Graus et al. (2016) have been reported to have high sensitivity and specificity in children as well **(Box 7.2)**.[10]

Autoimmune Limbic Encephalitis

This entity refers to immune-mediated inflammatory disorder of the limbic system, including the medial temporal lobes, amygdala, and cingulate

---

BOX 7.2: Diagnostic criteria for anti-NMDAR encephalitis proposed by Graus et al. (2016).

Probable anti-NMDAR encephalitis: Diagnosis can be made when all three of the following criteria have been met:
1. Rapid onset (<3 months) of *at least four of the six* following major groups of symptoms (4/6)
    - Abnormal (psychiatric) behavior or cognitive dysfunction
    - Speech dysfunction (pressured speech, verbal reduction, and mutism)
    - Seizures
    - Movement disorder, dyskinesia, or rigidity/abnormal postures
    - Decreased level of consciousness
    - Autonomic dysfunction or central hypoventilation
2. At least *one* of the following laboratory study results:
    - Abnormal EEG (focal or diffuse slow or disorganized activity, epileptic activity, or extreme delta brush)
    - CSF with pleocytosis or oligoclonal bands
3. Reasonable exclusion of other disorders

Diagnosis can also be made in the presence of *three of the above groups* of symptoms accompanied by a *systemic teratoma*.

Definite anti-NMDAR encephalitis
- Diagnosis can be made in the presence of *one or more of the six major groups* of symptoms and IgG anti-GluN1 antibodies after reasonable exclusion of other disorders.

(CSF: cerebrospinal fluid; EEG: electroencephalogram; NMDAR: N-methyl-D-aspartate receptor)

Source: Graus F, Titulaer MJ, Balu R, Benseler S, Bien CG, Cellucci T, et al. A clinical approach to diagnosis of autoimmune encephalitis. Lancet Neurol. 2016;15(4):391-404.

gyrus. Autoimmune limbic encephalitis in children is rare and is clinically characterized by memory loss, temporal lobe seizures, and behavioral changes. Two prerequisites are described for the diagnosis of limbic encephalitis; (1) signs and symptoms predominantly suggestive of limbic origin for no longer than 5 years and (2) hyperintense mediotemporal T2/FLAIR signal with no better explanation than inflammatory in origin.

Limbic encephalitis is the only AE with a distinct magnetic resonance imaging (MRI) pattern. However, the hallmark bilateral mediotemporal T2/FLAIR signal is also seen in other conditions that need exclusion before the diagnosis of limbic encephalitis can be concluded. The differentials include glioma, cortical dysplasia, poststatus epilepticus changes, and viral encephalitis (HHV6, HSV, and varicella zoster virus). This clinic-radiological phenotype has been described with LGI1, CASPR2, GABABR, GAD65, Hu, and DNER antibodies (*see* **Table 7.2**).

■ DIFFERENTIAL DIAGNOSIS

The clinical diagnosis of AE is supported by the presence of autoantibodies in the cerebrospinal fluid (CSF) and/or serum. Children with highly suggestive clinical features of AE but no detectable CSF/serum antibodies are labeled as seronegative AE. However, several disorders can mimic AE in children. Acute viral encephalitis, bacterial meningitis, toxic encephalopathy, CNS vasculitis, and an inborn error of metabolism can have a similar presentation. **Table 7.3** describes the disorders which can closely resemble AE. As children with AE require extensive immunosuppression for a long time, carefully planned investigations are essential to exclude these conditions.

■ DIAGNOSIS

Once AE is suspected clinically, a systematic workup is needed to confirm the diagnosis and exclude differential diagnoses (**Fig. 7.1**). In most cases, the evaluation begins with brain imaging and CSF analysis.

Magnetic Resonance Imaging of Brain

An MRI of the brain is important and often one of the first investigations to be done in children with the clinical phenotype of AE. Its role is not only for supporting the diagnosis of AE but, more importantly, to rule out other differential diagnoses. After the exclusion of viral encephalitis, the typical and only specific finding for AE is the presence of bilateral limbic encephalitis.[10] This pattern is uncommon in children. So effectively, there is no specific pattern that is seen in AE in children. In the most common type of AE, the anti-NMDAR encephalitis, up to half the children have normal MRI, while the other half have variable findings (**Figs. 7.2A to C**). Findings may include cortical, subcortical, striatal, or brainstem signal changes. Findings

TABLE 7.3: Differential diagnosis of pediatric autoimmune encephalitis.

Broad group of disorders	Causes or subtypes/conditions/agents
Viral infections	Japanese encephalitis, enteroviruses, HSV1, HSV2, HHV6, HHV7, CMV, EBV, Parvovirus, dengue, adenovirus, influenza, subacute sclerosing panencephalitis, HIV encephalopathy, rabies, varicella
Bacterial or fungal infections	Bacterial meningitis, tubercular meningitis, *Mycoplasma pneumoniae*, cryptococcal meningoencephalitis
Post-infectious encephalopathy	• Post-mycoplasma basal ganglia encephalitis • Poststreptococcal neuropsychiatric disorders (including Sydenham chorea) • Encephalitis lethargica
Immune-mediated disorders	• FIRES • ANE • ALERD • PANDAS/PANS • Rasmussen's encephalitis
Inflammatory disorders	• Primary CNS vasculitis • Demyelinating disorders • Hemophagocytic lymphohistiocytosis • Interferonopathies
Systemic autoimmune disorders	SLE, Sjögren syndrome, Behcet's disease, celiac disease, sarcoidosis
Toxic encephalopathies	Recreation drugs: alcohol, cocaine, marijuana, organophosphorus poisoning, ethylene glycol, methyl glycol
Genetic metabolic encephalopathies	Wilson disease, glutaric aciduria, leukodystrophy, mitochondrial disorders, urea cycle disorders
Neoplastic disorders	Primary brain tumors
Psychiatric disorders	Childhood psychosis, schizophrenia, bipolar disorder, conversion disorder, childhood disintegrative disorder, psychogenic seizures, autistic regression
Others	Abuse and neglect disorders

(ANE: acute necrotizing encephalopathy; ALERD: acute leukoencephalopathy with restricted diffusion; CNS: central nervous system; CMV: cytomegalovirus; EBV: Epstein-Barr virus; FIRES: febrile infection-related status epilepticus; HHV: human herpes virus; HIV: human immunodeficiency virus; HLH: hemophagocytic histiocytosis; HSV: herpes simplex virus; PANDAS: pediatric autoimmune neuropsychiatric disorders associated with streptococcal infections; PANS: pediatric acute-onset neuropsychiatric syndrome; SLE: systemic lupus erythematosus)

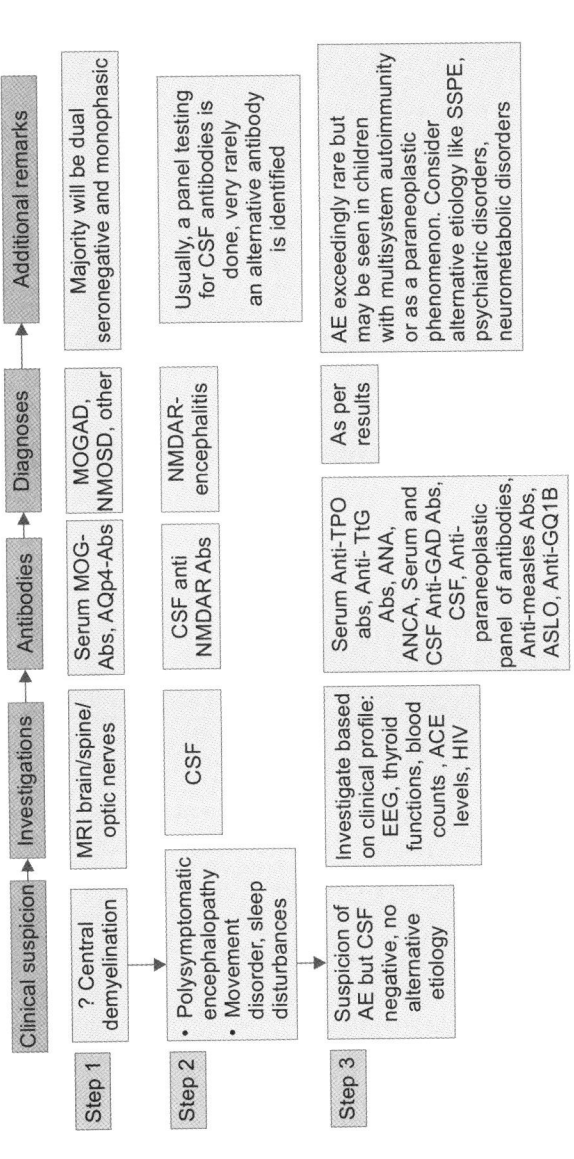

Fig. 7.1: A simplified flowchart for approaching a child with suspected autoimmune encephalitis.

(AE: autoimmune encephalitis; AQp4: aquaporin 4 antibodies; ACE: angiotensin-converting enzyme; ANA: antinuclear antibodies; ANCA: antineutrophil cytoplasmic antibodies; ASLO: antistreptolysin-O; CSF: cerebrospinal fluid; EEG: electroencephalogram; GAD: glutamic acid decarboxylase antibodies; MOGAD: myelin oligodendrocyte glycoprotein antibody-associated disease; MOG: myelin oligodendrocyte glycoprotein; NMDAR Abs: N-methyl-D-aspartate receptor antibodies; NMOSD: Neuromyelitis optica spectrum disorders; TPO: thyroid peroxidase antibodies; TTG: tissue transglutaminase antibodies)

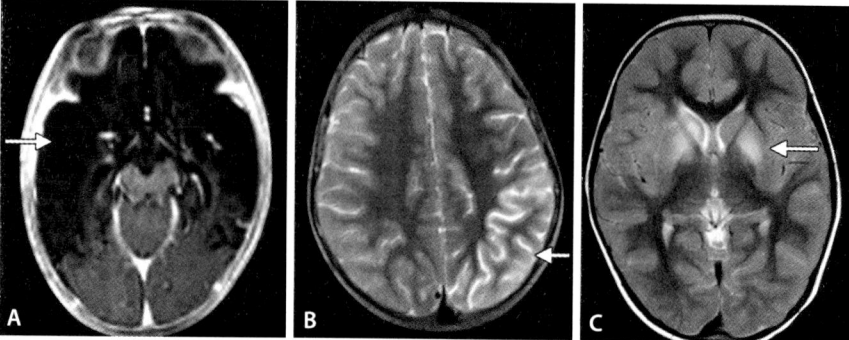

Figs. 7.2A to C: MRI brain findings in proven cases of anti-NMDAR encephalitis. (A) Axial T1 postcontrast images show extensive gliosis and encephalomalacia in temporal lobes (right > left) and basi-frontal regions in a child with anti-NMDAR encephalitis following HSV encephalitis; (B) Axial T2 image in a 6-year-old child with focal encephalitis involving left-sided high parietal lobe and subsequent anti-NMDAR encephalitis; (C) Axial T2 weighted images showing bilateral basal ganglia hyperintensities in a girl with anti-NMDAR encephalitis.

of MRI need to be supported by a positive CSF panel for the anti-NMDAR antibodies. Additionally, it is not infrequent to find nonspecific changes in MRI due to seizures. Anti-MOG syndrome, now called the MOGAD (MOG antibody-associated disorders), is usually not described in the AE rubric but has several distinctive patterns identifiable on the MRI.[21,22] Brain MRI helps exclude alternative diagnoses such as infections, stroke, neoplasm, leukodystrophies, and metabolic disorders.

Cerebrospinal Fluid Analysis

This is the most important test in the evaluation of a child with suspected AE. As discussed earlier, the MRI is usually nonspecific in AE, and CSF examination is required in all patients to exclude AE. The routine CSF analysis should be performed including sugar, protein, cytology, and additionally, oligoclonal bands, viral studies, and panel for AE is performed.

Panel testing for AE is now available in many centers in India. All methods used to detect antibodies are based on the same principle. The serum or CSF sample is incubated with matrices containing the antigens and epitopes of interest. After various steps, any bound antibodies are stained with a dye and visualized by a microscope.[23] While various testing methods have been tried such as brain tissue staining, radioimmunoassay, flowcytometry, and enzyme-linked immunosorbent assay (ELISA), the method of choice globally is the cell-based assay.[24] In most laboratories, the cell-based assay is run as a diagnostic panel test using biochip slides containing a group of antigens. These slides contain several fields with differently transfected human embryonic kidney (HEK) cells permitting testing for a broad range of surface antibody reactivities in one run. The typical biochip

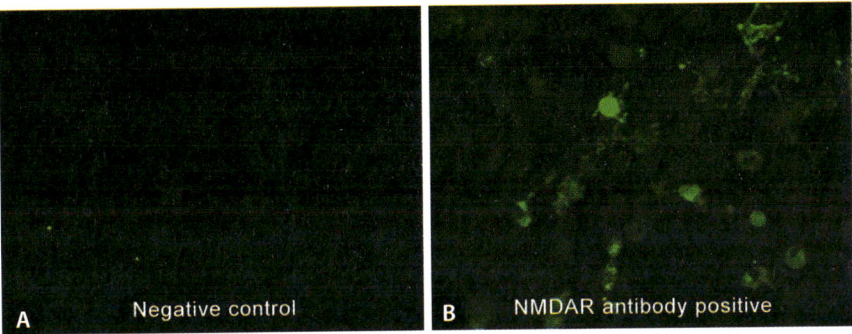

Figs. 7.3A and B: Immunofluorescence microscopic findings in a sample tested with cell-based assay from child with anti-NMDAR encephalitis. A negative control is also shown for comparison.
(*Courtesy*: Ravinder Garg, Pediatric Immunology Laboratory, PGIMER, Chandigarh)

has HEK cells transfected with the following antigens—NMDAR, AMPA1, AMPA2, LGI1, and CASPR2. The combinations of antigens available may vary depending on the kit used by the laboratory. The results are inferred by fluorescent microscopy visualization of dye-labeled antihuman immunoglobulins **(Figs. 7.3A and B)**. By serial dilutions, an estimate of titer can also be determined.

In children with negative results but continued suspicion, immunoblots containing onconeural antigens are suggested, as rarely children may have onconeural antibodies, e.g., anti-Hu antibodies in the presence of neuroblastoma.[25]

Test Serum or CSF

A frequent issue that a clinician faces is if a serum, a CSF or serum-CSF-pair testing is to be done. Experts worldwide suggest testing a CSF-serum pair for the highest sensitivity and specificity of the antibody diagnosis in AE.[26] However, this is not always feasible or financially viable. Hence knowledge of which antibody is detected well in which sample is essential. Certain antibodies are better detected in serum, and hence they are primarily tested in serum. These include anti-MOG, anti-AQp4, and anti-GAD. At the same time, some other conditions require CSF antibody testing. These include anti-NMDAR and antiglial fibrillary acidic protein (GFAP) antibodies. For some like LGI1 antibodies, the results can be inconsistent in either CSF or serum. For testing, the samples are transported uncooled as antibodies are very stable and can withstand transport for at least 3 or 4 days.[24]

Nonspecific findings of inflammation may be the only abnormality found on initial testing of CSF, and often after negative results for infections, empiric immunotherapy has to be started. The common CSF findings in AE include mild-to-moderate lymphocytic pleocytosis, raised CSF proteins and positive intrathecal oligoclonal bands. It is important to remember that routine CSF studies may be normal in some AE patients, and this does not exclude the diagnosis when clinical indicators are consistent with AE.

Blood Tests

In addition to CSF and serum testing for antibodies, several blood tests are often needed to exclude other differential diagnoses. MRI findings and the clinical presentation can guide part of the testing. Some tests that are usually suggested in this context are antithyroid antibodies, toxicology screen, ammonia, HIV, inflammatory markers, antinuclear antibodies, screen for celiac disease, antimeasles antibodies, and lupus anticoagulant antibodies, and metabolic testing (*see* Fig. 7.1). Most of these tests are often individualized based on the age and presentation of the patient.

Importantly, blood samples should be collected prior to treatment with intravenous immunoglobulins (IVIG) or plasmapheresis to avoid false-positive or false-negative results.[27]

Electroencephalogram

Electroencephalogram is commonly performed in patients with acute encephalopathy and suspected AE. The purpose is to exclude nonconvulsive status epilepticus, to monitor treatment response in patients with seizures, band to detect diagnostic patterns e.g., in subacute sclerosing panencephalitis (SSPE). AE is also a major cause of NORSE, which can be convulsive or nonconvulsive.[27] Findings suggestive of AE include focal slowing, epileptiform discharges, periodic discharges, or extreme delta brush, occasionally seen in anti-NMDAR encephalitis.[17,28] Reports in adults suggest that periodic or rhythmic patterns, seizures, and NORSE conferred an increased risk of poor outcome.[29]

Brain Positron Emission Tomography

In adults, it is suggested that obtaining a brain fluorodeoxyglucose positron emission tomography (FDG-PET) can confirm focal or multifocal brain abnormality and support a clinical suspicion of AE. It can also substitute for MRI when MRI is contraindicated.[27] Its role in children with AE is, however, less clear. There are early reports on the use of PET in children with AE, suggesting it to be a useful diagnostic modality.[30,31] However, more studies are needed before its role in children is clearly defined. Importantly, further studies are also needed to better differentiate AE patterns from those of common differentials like neuroinfections.

Tumor Screening

Ovarian teratoma is the most frequent tumor associated with anti-NMDAR encephalitis especially in adult females. Teratoma located elsewhere or other tumors are uncommon. Girls >12 years of age should be screened for tumor with MRI abdomen and pelvis every 6 monthly. However, among girls <12 years of age and boys presence of an underlying tumor is uncommon, hence regular screening is not required.[12]

■ MANAGEMENT

Several retrospective studies have reported favorable outcomes with the use of early and aggressive immunotherapy.[32] Once the diagnosis of AE is clinically suspected and infectious etiologies have been ruled out with CSF analysis (cytology, gram stain, and viral PCR), *immunotherapy* should be initiated. It is impractical and potentially hazardous to wait for the CSF antibody results to initiate immunotherapy. Delayed therapy along with persistent and ongoing brain inflammation may predispose to worse neurological outcomes.

In a large cohort of anti-NMDAR encephalitis, early initiation of immunotherapy was associated with a modified Rankin scale (mRS) score of ≤2 in 501 cases.[12] A mRS score of 2 indicates slight disability, where the patient is unable to carry out all previous activities, but able to look after his/her own affairs without assistance.

Treatment recommendations given for anti-NMDAR encephalitis are extrapolated for other AE subtypes also.[12] Most of the treatment recommendations for pediatric AE are based on the large retrospective cohorts, small case series, and expert reviews, as there are no prospectively conducted randomized controlled trials available for the treatment of AE.[11,27,33]

The general framework of immunotherapy in children with AE is divided into first-line, second-line, and third-line agents **(Fig. 7.4)**. The first-line immunotherapeutic agents include steroids, IVIG, and plasmapheresis. All three therapeutic agents have a rapid onset of action and are relatively safe. The second-line agents include rituximab and cyclophosphamide, with stronger and long-lasting immunosuppressive effect, even though they have serious adverse effects. The third-line agents are bortezomib and tocilizumab, have been used in a small number of patients with refractory disease.[33,34] The timeline for escalation of immunotherapy is not established; however, minimal or no improvement in clinical features within 10–14 days of initiation of a therapeutic agent is an indication for next-line agents.[2]

Children with refractory AE might benefit from novel therapeutic agents, and expert opinion might be useful in such situations. Maintenance therapy with slow tapering of steroids, azathioprine, and mycophenolate mofetil has been used in pediatric patients; however, there is no robust evidence for the use of maintenance therapy in pediatric AE.[27] In addition to immunotherapy, children with AE should receive symptomatic therapy for neurological complications. Tumor screening is recommended in adolescent females due to its association with ovarian teratoma.[10]

152 Autoimmune Encephalitis

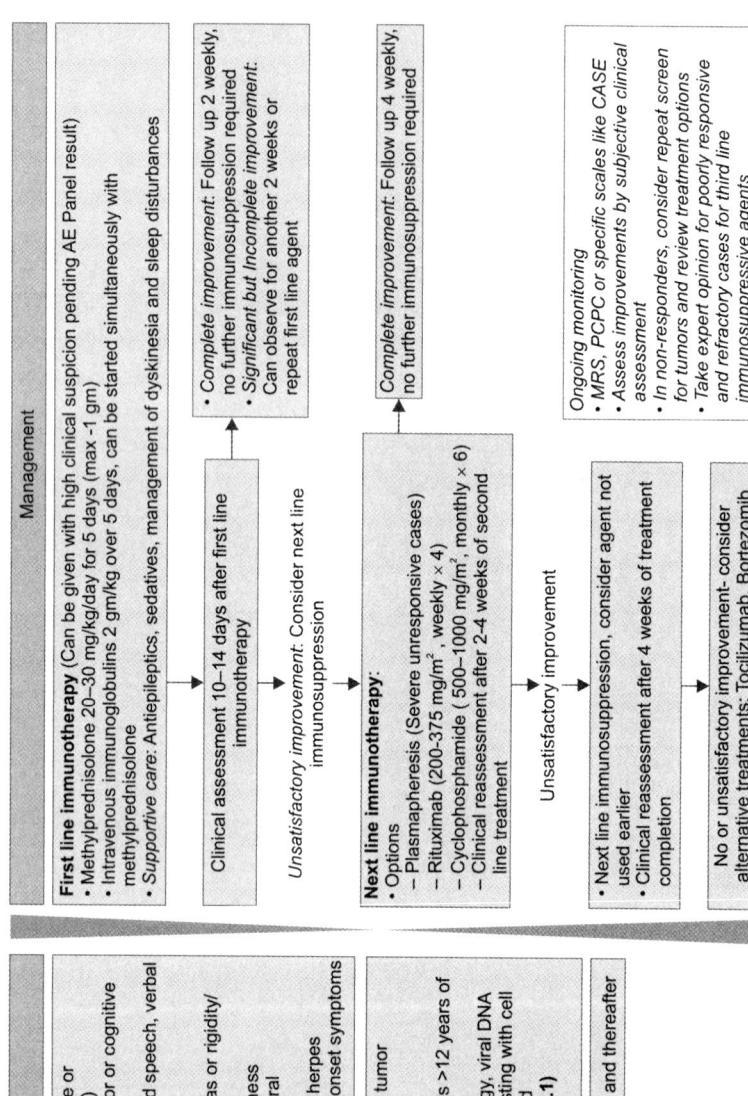

Fig. 7.4: PGIMER protocol for diagnosis, treatment, and monitoring of children with autoimmune encephalitis.

First-line Therapy
Steroids
Initiation of empirical therapy with methylprednisolone in a child with suspected AE is a reasonable approach to achieve immunosuppression rapidly. Intravenous methylprednisolone is used In a dose of 30 mg/kg/day for 3-7 days (maximum 1 g/day).[11,32,33] Intravenous methylprednisolone dosage can be repeated depending upon the response and evaluation of initial investigations. Some centers use repeated pulses of methylprednisolone once every 4 weeks or early if clinical symptoms are severe. Pulse therapy is followed by slow tapering of oral prednisolone over 4-6 weeks is also used in some centers. However, it is associated with more severe adverse events in comparison to intermittent pulses of methylprednisolone.

Intravenous Immunoglobulins
Intravenous Immunoglobulin is used along with steroids in children with AE and is occasionally used as a single agent also. The use of IVIG in children with AE is based on retrospective case series or cohort studies. The mechanism of action of IVIG is broad, with an effect on both innate and adaptive immunity. IVIG is used at the dose of 2 g/kg as an intravenous infusion over 5 days; however, more rapid administration over 48 hours is tolerated well by children. Like steroids, doses may be repeated if the response to the first dose is definite but partial.

Plasma Exchange and Plasmapheresis
Therapeutic plasma exchange (TPE) is used as adjunctive therapy for children with AE.[35,36] Rarely used as monotherapy, it is used in hospitalized patients who have no response/or partial response to steroids and IVIG. In a retrospective series, Zhan et al. studied 51 individuals with refractory AE who received steroids and IVIG with or without TPE.[36] The clinical improvement in the TPE group was significantly better than the non-TPE group at one and on 2 months follow-up. TPE is more effective for cell surface antigen-associated AE. TPE is given as 5-7 sessions every other day over 2 weeks.

Plasma exchange should not be done immediately after IVIG or rituximab therapy, as it will effectively remove all the antibodies from the circulation. TPE is invasive, requires a central venous catheter, and the most common complications include infection, hypotension, and electrolyte imbalances due to rapid fluid shift.

Combination Therapy
A combined first-line therapy is a more preferred approach by clinicians if the initial presentation is AE is very severe. However, there is a lack of high-quality

evidence for combination therapy. In a study, aggressive therapy with tumor removal, steroids, IVIG, rituximab, and tocilizumab within 1 month of diagnosis resulted in a better 1-year clinical assessment scale for autoimmune encephalitis (CASE) score and modified Rankin score in comparison to other regimens of > 1-month duration or delayed tumor removal.[37]

Second-line Therapy

In children with no or partial response in 1–2 weeks after first-line therapy, addition of a second-line agents improves the outcome. Rituximab and cyclophosphamide are the two most used second-line immunotherapeutic agents.

Rituximab

Rituximab is a monoclonal, chimeric anti-CD20 antibody that acts on CD20 expressing B-cells, and plasmablasts through both cell-meditated and complement-mediated cytotoxicity. Rituximab depletes B-cells, prevents their development into antibody-producing plasma cells, and directly depletes plasmablasts.[38] Though rituximab is classically considered a B-cell treatment, ongoing studies have demonstrated more broad anti-inflammatory effects. In addition, rituximab reduces cytokine production and proinflammatory CD4 and CD8 T cell responses.[39] Rituximab is the most common second-line agent used for AE either alone or in combination with cyclophosphamide.[32]

The typical protocol for rituximab is weekly dosage at 375 mg/m^2 for 4 weeks, or 750 mg/m^2 (maximum dose 1,000 mg) two dosages 2 weeks apart.[39] The ideal dose of rituximab in children is not known, and the immunomodulatory effect takes several weeks to months. A lower dose of 100 mg/m^2 has been used in a small pediatric series for anti-NMDAR encephalitis.[40] The reinfusion of rituximab is given when CD19+ B-cell counts of total lymphocytes in peripheral blood >1%.[40] The lower dose can deplete peripheral B-cells; however, bioavailability in CNS may also be reduced.[41]

Rituximab is well tolerated by children; only 12% of patients described infusion reaction, responding to steroids and antihistaminics.[8,42] Other adverse events include serious infection and progressive multifocal leukoencephalopathy. Monitoring of blood counts, lymphocyte subsets, and immunoglobulins is necessary as children may develop cytopenia, persistent B-cell depletion, and prolonged hypogammaglobulinemia. B-cell measurement should be done 2–4 weeks after rituximab dose to check for B-cell depletion and 3–6 monthly to look for B-cell repopulation, which may assist in redosing if clinical symptoms persist or relapse is suspected.

Cyclophosphamide

Cyclophosphamide is an alkylating agent with antimitotic and antireplicative properties through inhibition of DNA synthesis. Cyclophosphamide has a broad effect on the immune system and has good CNS bioavailability. Cyclophosphamide is used in a dose of 500–1,000 mg/m^2 as monthly doses for 6 months as second-line agent in pediatric AE.[43,44] The risk of secondary malignancy and infertility is high with cyclophosphamide, but doses used for treatment in AE are much lower than those used for cancer treatment. These serious adverse effects are generally associated with a cumulative dose of >7.5 g/m^2.[45]

Prophylaxis with cotrimoxazole is suggested along with rituximab or cyclophosphamide to prevent *Pneumocystis jirovecii* infection.[43,44]

Third-Line Agents

Third-line agents are needed when both first- and second-line agents fail. Literature regarding their use is limited to case reports. Tocilizumab, bortezomib, intrathecal steroids and methotrexate, and low-dose IL-2 have been used as third-line agents in refractory AE. Daratumumab, an anti-CD38 monoclonal antibody has also been used in refractory bortezomib cases.[46] A trial is ongoing evaluating ocrelizumab (a humanized anti-CD20 monoclonal antibody with a similar mechanism of action to rituximab) in AE.

Maintenance Therapy

The role of maintenance therapy is unclear in AE in children. Maintenance therapy is expected to maximize the therapeutic gains, provide continued improvement to the highest functional status, and complete remission without relapse. Oral prednisolone immediately after acute immunosuppression in a dose of 1–2 mg/kg/day with gradual weaning over weeks and months overlapping with a second-line or third-line agent is a common practice.[32,33] However, this approach may not be useful in children with behavioral issues and excessive steroid-induced side effects. Azathioprine and mycophenolate mofetil have been used as maintenance immunotherapy. Periodic IVIG and methylprednisolone have been used as an alternative approach. Given the low rate and mild manifestations of releases in children, long-term immunosuppression should be initiated after careful risk benefit analysis.

Acute Symptomatic Management

Autoimmune encephalitis is a polysymptomatic disorder, and often requires supportive therapy in addition to immunotherapy. Status epilepticus, respiratory depression, and severe autonomic dysfunction are indications for intensive care unit admission.[33,41] Seizures should be treated with appropriate antiseizure medications and status epilepticus as per protocol.

Sodium channel blocking agents such as carbamazepine and lacosamide are preferred in anti-LG1 encephalitis.[47] Benzodiazepines such as clobazam, clonazepam, and diazepam can be used for managing movement disorders, reduce tone, and to improve sleep.

Anticholinergics such as trihexyphenidyl, benztropine, or baclofen can be used for dystonia, and tizanidine can be used for spasticity and dystonia.[48] Dopamine blockers such as risperidone or dopamine depleters such as tetrabenazine can be used for managing chorea, athetosis, tics, and ballism. For psychosis and agitation, diazepam, clobazam, or an antipsychotic such as quetiapine can be used. For dysautonomia, intensive monitoring is required, and beta-blockers such as propranolol, and clonidine can be used. For sleep disorder, the therapeutic modalities include sleep hygiene, uninterrupted night-time sleep, melatonin, and sedating benzodiazepines such as diazepam or zolpidem.[33] Hyponatremia can occur due to syndrome of inappropriate antidiuretic hormone secretion (SIADH) and requires fluid restriction. Many manifestations like insomnia and movement disorders may not be responsive to drugs and caution should be exercised to avoid overuse of drugs, and their side effects while also maintaining their effect on functional parameters and avoiding injuries to the child.

Relapses

While acute AE is polyphasic and polysymptomatic, relapses are usually milder and monosymptomatic. Relapses are rare in children with anti-NMDAR encephalitis compared with adults and are seen in 5% or less of the children. Breakthrough seizures, sleep disturbances, fall in cognition, and memory may occur as symptoms of relapse in patients with AE. Establishing a relapse during follow-up is a difficult task—the presence of clinical symptoms, EEG, MRI, and CSF findings may support the diagnosis. Generally, reinitiation of previously effective treatment is useful in achieving remission. Within the AE spectrum, anti-AQp4 has the highest risk of relapse, mandating long-term immunosuppression. Although the majority of children with the anti-MOG antibody-associated disease have a monophasic disease, approximately 30% of children will relapse typically with acute disseminated encephalomyelitis (ADEM), optic neuritis, or myelitis. Newer consensus guidelines recommend some form of immunomodulation in relapsing anti-MOG-associated disorders.[49]

■ OUTCOME

Not much is known about long-term outcomes in AE in children. In general, antibodies against intracellular antigens are usually associated with paraneoplastic syndromes and have a poor prognosis. In a Dutch cohort of children with anti-NMDAR encephalitis, nearly two-thirds of children returned to school and were said to achieve a good outcome. However, many children had cognitive problems and fatigue, even up to adolescence, resulting in problems in academic achievement and lower quality of life.[50] In the authors' center, in a group of 35 children with anti-NMDAR encephalitis, a good functional and cognitive outcome was seen in about 70% of the children. Anti-NMDAR encephalitis following *Herpes simplex* encephalitis, abnormal MRI, and CSF pleocytosis were associated with poor long-term cognitive outcomes *(unpublished findings)*.

■ CONCLUSION

Autoimmune encephalitis in children is an under-recognized treatable condition. The diagnosis of AE should be suspected in any child with any combination of acute to subacute encephalopathy with neuropsychiatric symptoms, sleep disturbances, seizures, aphasia and movement disorder, and among children with infectious encephalitis and secondary deterioration with new onset seizures and movement disorder. The diagnosis can be easily confirmed with available cell-based assays. Early identification and diagnosis will aid in early initiation of definitive therapy. With the use of early and aggressive immunotherapy a good long-term outcome can be expected in majority of the children.

■ KEY POINTS

- Remember that autoimmune encephalitides are an important and treatable cause of acute encephalitis.
- Children with AE typically present with a variable combination of acute or subacute onset neuropsychiatric symptoms, seizures, and/or movement disorder.
- A combination of tremors, dyskinesia, stereotypy, dystonia, catatonia, asterixis, myoclonus, and parkinsonism can be observed in children with anti-NMDAR encephalitis.
- The clinical diagnosis of AE is supported by the presence of autoantibodies in the CSF and serum.
- The first-line immunotherapeutic agents include steroids, IVIG, and plasmapheresis.
- The second-line agents include rituximab and cyclophosphamide, with stronger and long-lasting immunosuppressive effect, though they have serious adverse effects.
- Autoimmune encephalitis is a polysymptomatic disorder, and often requires supportive therapy in addition to immunotherapy.
- With proper management most children can be expected to have a good long-term outcome.

■ REFERENCES

1. Dalmau J, Tüzün E, Wu H, Masjuan J, Rossi JE, Voloschin A, et al. Paraneoplastic anti-N-methyl-D-aspartate receptor encephalitis associated with ovarian teratoma. Ann Neurol. 2007;61(1):25-36.
2. Cellucci T, Van Mater H, Graus F, Muscal E, Gallentine W, Klein-Gitelman MS, et al. Clinical approach to the diagnosis of autoimmune encephalitis in the pediatric patient. Neurol Neuroimmunol Neuroinflamm. 2020;7(2):e663.

3. Gable MS, Sheriff H, Dalmau J, Tilley DH, Glaser CA. The frequency of autoimmune N-methyl-D-aspartate receptor encephalitis surpasses that of individual viral etiologies in young individuals enrolled in the California Encephalitis Project. Clin Infect Dis. 2012;54(7):899-904.
4. Dubey D, Pittock SJ, Kelly CR, McKeon A, Lopez-Chiriboga AS, Lennon VA, et al. Autoimmune encephalitis epidemiology and a comparison to infectious encephalitis. Ann Neurol. 2018;83(1):166-77.
5. Granerod J, Ambrose HE, Davies NW, Clewley JP, Walsh AL, Morgan D, et al; UK Health Protection Agency (HPA) Aetiology of Encephalitis Study Group. Causes of encephalitis and differences in their clinical presentations in England: a multicentre, population-based prospective study. Lancet Infect Dis. 2010;10(12):835-44.
6. Boesen MS, Born AP, Lydolph MC, Blaabjerg M, Børresen ML. Pediatric autoimmune encephalitis in Denmark during 2011-17: A nationwide multicenter population-based cohort study. Eur J Paediatr Neurol. 2019;23(4):639-52.
7. Erickson TA, Muscal E, Munoz FM, Lotze T, Hasbun R, Brown E, et al. Infectious and autoimmune causes of encephalitis in children. Pediatrics. 2020;145(6):e20192543.
8. Armangue T, Olivé-Cirera G, Martínez-Hernandez E, Sepulveda M, Ruiz-Garcia R, Muñoz-Batista M, et al. Associations of paediatric demyelinating and encephalitic syndromes with myelin oligodendrocyte glycoprotein antibodies: A multicentre observational study. Lancet Neurol. 2020;19(3):234-46.
9. Bruijstens AL, Lechner C, Flet-Berliac L, Deiva K, Neuteboom RF, Hemingway C, et al. EU paediatric MOG consortium consensus: Part 1 - Classification of clinical phenotypes of paediatric myelin oligodendrocyte glycoprotein antibody-associated disorders. Eur J Paediatr Neurol. 2020;29:2-13.
10. Graus F, Titulaer MJ, Balu R, Benseler S, Bien CG, Cellucci T, et al. A clinical approach to diagnosis of autoimmune encephalitis. Lancet Neurol. 2016;15(4):391-404.
11. Bien CG, Bien CI. Autoimmune encephalitis in children and adolescents. Neurol Res Pract. 2020;2:4.
12. Titulaer MJ, McCracken L, Gabilondo I, Armangué T, Glaser C, Iizuka T, et al. Treatment and prognostic factors for long-term outcome in patients with anti-NMDA receptor encephalitis: an observational cohort study. Lancet Neurol. 2013;12(2):157-65.
13. Ursitti F, Roberto D, Papetti L, Moavero R, Ferilli MAN, Fusco L, et al. Diagnosis of pediatric anti-NMDAR encephalitis at the onset: A clinical challenge. Eur J Paediatr Neurol. 2021;30:9-16.
14. Chakrabarty B, Tripathi M, Gulati S, Yoganathan S, Pandit AK, Sinha A, et al. Pediatric anti-N-methyl-D-aspartate (NMDA) receptor encephalitis: experience of a tertiary care teaching center from north India. J Child Neurol. 2014;29(11):1453-9.
15. Raja P, Shamick B, Nitish LK, Holla VV, Pal PK, Mahadevan A, et al. Clinical characteristics, treatment and long-term prognosis in patients with anti-NMDAR encephalitis. Neurol Sci. 2021;42(11):4683-4696.
16. Suthar R, Saini AG, Sankhyan N, Sahu JK, Singhi P. Childhood Anti-NMDA Receptor Encephalitis. Indian J Pediatr. 2016;83(7):628-33.
17. Spatola M, Dalmau J. Seizures and risk of epilepsy in autoimmune and other inflammatory encephalitis. Curr Opin Neurol. 2017;30(3):345-53.
18. Suthar R, Sankhyan N, Singhi P. Hyperkinetic Movement Disorder in a Girl with Anti-NMDA Receptor Encephalitis. Indian Pediatr. 2016;53(1):81.

19. Prüss H. Postviral autoimmune encephalitis: manifestations in children and adults. Curr Opin Neurol. 2017;30(3):327-33.
20. Schein F, Gagneux-Brunon A, Antoine J-C, Lavernhe S, Pillet S, Paul S, et al. Anti-N-methyl-D-aspartate receptor encephalitis after Herpes simplex virus-associated encephalitis: an emerging disease with diagnosis and therapeutic challenges. Infection. 2017;45(4):545-9.
21. Ho ACC, Mohammad SS, Pillai SC, Tantsis E, Jones H, Ho R, et al. High sensitivity and specificity in proposed clinical diagnostic criteria for anti-N-methyl-D-aspartate receptor encephalitis. Dev Med Child Neurol. 2017;59(12):1256-60.
22. Baumann M, Bartels F, Finke C, Adamsbaum C, Hacohen Y, Rostásy K, et al. EU paediatric MOG consortium consensus: Part 2—Neuroimaging features of paediatric myelin oligodendrocyte glycoprotein antibody-associated disorders. Eur J Paediatr Neurol. 2020;29:14-21.
23. Sinmaz N, Nguyen T, Tea F, Dale RC, Brilot F. Mapping autoantigen epitopes: molecular insights into autoantibody-associated disorders of the nervous system. J Neuroinflammation. 2016;13(1):219.
24. Bien CG. Diagnosing autoimmune encephalitis based on clinical features and autoantibody findings. Expert Rev Clin Immunol. 2019;15(5):511-27.
25. Aravamuthan BR, Fernández IS, Zurawski J, Olson H, Gorman M, Takeoka M. Pediatric anti-Hu-associated encephalitis with clinical features of rasmussen encephalitis. Neurol Neuroimmunol Neuroinflamm. 2015;2(5):e150.
26. Dale RC, Gorman MP, Lim M. Autoimmune encephalitis in children: clinical phenomenology, therapeutics, and emerging challenges. Curr Opin Neurol. 2017;30(3):334-44.
27. Abboud H, Probasco JC, Irani S, Ances B, Benavides DR, Bradshaw M, et al. Autoimmune encephalitis: Proposed best practice recommendations for diagnosis and acute management. J Neurol Neurosurg Psychiatry. 2021;92(7):757-68.
28. Steriade C, Moosa ANV, Hantus S, Prayson RA, Alexopoulos A, Rae-Grant A. Electroclinical features of seizures associated with autoimmune encephalitis. Seizure. 2018;60:198-204.
29. Moise AM, Karakis I, Herlopian A, Dhakar M, Hirsch LJ, Cotsonis G, et al. Continuous EEG Findings in Autoimmune Encephalitis. J Clin Neurophysiol. 2021;38(2):124-9.
30. Aydos U, Arhan E, Akdemir ÜÖ, Akbaş Y, Aydin K, Atay LÖ, et al. Utility of brain fluorodeoxyglucose PET in children with possible autoimmune encephalitis. Nucl Med Commun. 2020;41(8):800-9.
31. Turpin S, Martineau P, Levasseur MA, Meijer I, Décarie J-C, Barsalou J, et al. 18F-Flurodeoxyglucose positron emission tomography with computed tomography (FDG PET/CT) findings in children with encephalitis and comparison to conventional imaging. Eur J Nucl Med Mol Imaging. 2019;46(6):1309-24.
32. Nosadini M, Mohammad SS, Ramanathan S, Brilot F, Dale RC. Immune therapy in autoimmune encephalitis: a systematic review. Expert Rev Neurother. 2015;15(12):1391-419.
33. Abboud H, Probasco J, Irani SR, Ances B, Benavides DR, Bradshaw M, et al. Autoimmune encephalitis: proposed recommendations for symptomatic and long-term management. J Neurol Neurosurg Psychiatry. 2021;92(8):897-907.
34. Garg D, Mohammad SS, Sharma S. Autoimmune Encephalitis in Children: An Update. Indian Pediatr. 2020;57(7):662-70.

35. DeSena AD, Noland DK, Matevosyan K, King K, Phillips L, Qureshi SS, et al. Intravenous methylprednisolone versus therapeutic plasma exchange for treatment of anti-N-methyl-D-aspartate receptor antibody encephalitis: A retrospective review. J Clin Apher. 2015;30(4):212-6.
36. Zhang Y, Liu G, Jiang M, Chen W, Su Y. Efficacy of Therapeutic Plasma Exchange in Patients with Severe Refractory Anti-NMDA Receptor Encephalitis. Neurotherapeutics. 2019;16(3):828-37.
37. Lim JA, Lee ST, Moon J, Jun JS, Kim TJ, Shin YW, et al. Development of the clinical assessment scale in autoimmune encephalitis. Ann Neurol. 2019;85(3):352-58.
38. Huang H, Benoist C, Mathis D. Rituximab specifically depletes short-lived autoreactive plasma cells in a mouse model of inflammatory arthritis. Proc Natl Acad Sci USA. 2010;107(10):4658-63.
39. Hachiya Y, Uruha A, Kasai-Yoshida E, Shimoda K, Satoh-Shirai I, Kumada S, et al. Rituximab ameliorates anti-N-methyl-D-aspartate receptor encephalitis by removal of short-lived plasmablasts. J Neuroimmunol. 2013;265(1-2):128-30.
40. Wang BJ, Wang CJ, Zeng ZL, Yang Y, Guo SG. Lower dosages of rituximab used successfully in the treatment of anti-NMDA receptor encephalitis without tumour. J Neurol Sci. 2017;377:127-32.
41. Stingl C, Cardinale K, Van Mater H. An Update on the Treatment of Pediatric Autoimmune Encephalitis. Curr Treat Options Rheumatol. 2018;4(1):14-28.
42. Dale RC, Brilot F, Duffy LV, Twilt M, Waldman AT, Narula S, et al. Utility and safety of rituximab in pediatric autoimmune and inflammatory CNS disease. Neurology. 2014;83(2):142-50.
43. Kadoya M, Onoue H, Kadoya A, Ikewaki K, Kaida K. Refractory status epilepticus caused by anti-NMDA receptor encephalitis that markedly improved following combination therapy with rituximab and cyclophosphamide. Intern Med. 2015;54(2):209-13.
44. Kashyape P, Taylor E, Ng J, Krishnakumar D, Kirkham F, Whitney A. Successful treatment of two paediatric cases of anti-NMDA receptor encephalitis with cyclophosphamide: the need for early aggressive immunotherapy in tumour negative paediatric patients. Eur J Paediatr Neurol. 2012;16(1):74-8.
45. Kanter IC, Huttner HB, Staykov D, Biermann T, Struffert T, Kerling F, et al. Cyclophosphamide for anti-GAD antibody-positive refractory status epilepticus. Epilepsia. 2008;49(5):914-20.
46. Ratuszny D, Skripuletz T, Wegner F, Groß M, Falk C, Jacobs R, et al. Case Report: Daratumumab in a Patient With Severe Refractory Anti-NMDA Receptor Encephalitis. Front Neurol. 2020;11:602102.
47. Feyissa AM, Lamb C, Pittock SJ, Gadoth A, McKeon A, Klein CJ, et al. Antiepileptic drug therapy in autoimmune epilepsy associated with antibodies targeting the leucine-rich glioma-inactivated protein 1. Epilepsia Open. 2018;3(3):348-56.
48. Baizabal-Carvallo JF, Jankovic J. Autoimmune and paraneoplastic movement disorders: An update. J Neurol Sci. 2018;385:175-84.
49. Bruijstens AL, Wendel EM, Lechner C, Bartels F, Finke C, Breu M, et al. EU paediatric MOG consortium consensus: Part 5—Treatment of paediatric myelin oligodendrocyte glycoprotein antibody-associated disorders. Eur J Paediatr Neurol. 2020;29:41-53.
50. de Bruijn MAAM, Aarsen FK, van Oosterhout MP, van der Knoop MM, Catsman-Berrevoets CE, Schreurs MWJ, et al. Long-term neuropsychological outcome following pediatric anti-NMDAR encephalitis. Neurology. 2018;90(22):e1997-e2005.

Neurology

Infantile Spasms

Gouri Rao Passi

■ INTRODUCTION

Infantile spasms, also known as epileptic spasms are a challenge at many levels. It needs an alert parent and a sharp clinician to diagnose it in time. Every day wasted before the diagnosis has disastrous consequences. These seizures are typically seen in West syndrome, which is a triad of epileptic spasms, a bizarre electroencephalogram (EEG) called hypsarrhythmia and significant developmental delay during the critical period of infancy.[1] There are myriad causes which underlie this syndrome and outcomes can be often disappointing if the diagnosis is delayed or inappropriate drugs are used in management.[2,3] Drugs used in this syndrome differ vastly from routine antiepileptics. Pediatricians need to recognize this entity in time since early diagnosis, and appropriate treatment can make a huge difference in outcome.

■ EPIDEMIOLOGY

Like many epilepsy syndromes in childhood, it is age-dependent and begins within the first year in 90% of cases. However, cases with an onset even beyond 2 years of age are well documented.[4]

Onset before 3 months is uncommon. In infancy, it constitutes a big fraction—nearly 25% of all the epilepsies. But only 2% of all childhood epilepsies are epileptic spasms. The estimated incidence is 0.25 per 1,000 live births.[5]

■ ETIOPATHOGENESIS

The pathogenesis of infantile spams is shrouded in mystery. Initially it was hypothesized that it is due to brainstem dysfunction. The evidence in favor was its presence in patients with hydranencephaly, associated sleep disturbances and symmetric nature of spasms. However, isolated cortical lesions have been shown to produce epileptic spasms and have been treated by focal cortical resection.

What is clear is that it is strongly age-dependent. It appears that some neurological dysfunction in certain critical times of development manifest as infantile spasms. Hence, it is hypothesized that temporal desynchronization of simultaneously developing networks in the early brain results in spasms.[6] This explains why a wide variety of neurological insults can result in this stereotyped epileptic pattern.

■ ETIOLOGY

A cause can be identified in up to 60–70% of cases. In the United Kingdom Infantile Spasms Study (UKISS), the etiology was identified in 127 of 207 patients. The most common etiologies are presented in **Table 8.1**. The remaining 32 etiologies were all individually uncommon.[7]

In India, infantile spasms in most patients are mostly due to an underlying structural or metabolic cause. Sadly, the most common cause in India is neonatal hypoglycemic brain injury (36%), something which is eminently preventable.[8] The other causes include perinatal asphyxia, postmeningitis sequelae, intrauterine infections, and structural brain malformations such as lissencephaly. Of the genetic causes, tuberous sclerosis has been the best documented **(Table 8.2)**.

Other genetic causes which have been identified across the world include Down syndrome and rarely pathogenic *de novo* mutations including *ARX, CDKL5, FOXG1, GRIN1, GRIN2A, MAGI2, MEF2C, SLC25A22, SPTAN1,* and *STXBP1*.[9]

Inborn errors of metabolism are rarer causes of epileptic spasms and include disorders such as phenylketonuria, biotinidase deficiency, nonketotic hyperglycinemia, methylmalonic acidemia, propionic acidemia, maple syrup urine disease, and Menkes disease.[9]

■ CLINICAL FEATURES

The characteristic feature of infantile spasms is a cluster of brief flexion, extension or mixed movements of trunk, or sometimes merely the head and neck. The sudden stiffening of the body is associated with the arms flinging outward, the knees pulling up and the body bending forward. They are often seen on awakening but rarely in sleep. They are associated with irritability

TABLE 8.1: The common etiologies of infantile spasms in the UKISS study.[7]	
Etiology of infantile spasms	**No (%)**
Hypoxic ischemic encephalopathy	21 (10%)
Chromosomal	16 (8%)
Malformations	16 (8%)
Stroke	16 (8%)
Tuberous sclerosis complex	15 (7%)
Periventricular leukomalacia (hemorrhage)	11 (5%)

TABLE 8.2: Etiological classification and specific etiology of all infantile spasm patients in an Indian study.[8]

Etiology of Infantile spasms	No
• Genetic	11
– Point mutations	8
– Deletions	3
• Structural	85
– Acquired	77
- Neonatal hypoglycemic brain injury	40
- Asphyxial brain injury	29
- Post-meningitis sequelae	4
- Late hemorrhagic disease of newborn	1
– Genetic	6
- Tuberous sclerosis	5
- Lissencephaly	1
- *Unknown etiology*	2 (bilateral)
• Unknown	17

or expressions of distress. The more ominous feature is a developmental stagnation or regression.

■ DIFFERENTIAL DIAGNOSIS

The common differentials of epileptic spasms include gastroesophageal reflux, benign myoclonus of infancy, hyperekplexia and other benign and severe myoclonic epilepsies of childhood. Infants with gastroesophageal reflux give a history of regurgitation of milk and may be diagnosed using a radionuclide milk scan. Benign myoclonus of infancy is identified by a normal neurological examination, normal development, and normal EEG. They have excellent outcomes.[10] Hyperekplexia starts in the neonatal period unlike infantile spasms which starts after 3 months. Further it is characterized by an exaggerated startle in response to auditory or tactile stimulus followed by a period of persistent generalized stiffness. Tapping the nose can elicit this response. EEG is normal.[11] The characteristic EEG of hypsarrhythmia is absent in the other benign and severe myoclonic epilepsies of childhood.

■ DIAGNOSIS

The diagnosis of infantile spams is often missed both by parents and physicians. It is often brushed aside as a physiological startle. What attracts attention is often the excessive irritability and loss of milestones. Home video recordings are vital for timely diagnosis.

The diagnosis is confirmed by the presence of a characteristic EEG. Electroencephalographic recordings should include at least 30 minutes of sleep recording followed by 10 minutes of an awake record. If it is not confirmatory, a longer duration of video EEG may be planned.[12] The characteristic pattern seen interictally in infantile spasms is called *hypsarrhythmia*. It comprises chaotic high voltage, slow waves with multifocal spikes. This initial chaotic pattern may evolve into a more synchronous and symmetric pattern called atypical or modified hypsarrhythmia. Many hypsarrhythmia variants have also been described. They include an asymmetric pattern with consistent focus, burst suppression-like pattern and predominant slow wave activity with minimal or no spikes.[13]

The next step is to identify the etiology underlying the infantile spasms. A detailed history will help to identify perinatal asphyxia, neonatal hypoglycemia, and a family history must be elicited in patients with suspected tuberous sclerosis or other genetic disorders. Examination may reveal ash leaf dermatosis seen in tuberous sclerosis, alopecia in biotinidase deficiency, or cataract in intrauterine infections or galactosemia.

The most useful first investigation would be a magnetic resonance imaging (MRI) of brain which can help to confirm perinatal hypoxia, neonatal hypoglycemic brain injury, tuberous sclerosis, and malformations of the brain such as lissencephaly or focal cortical dysplasia.

If there is a history to suggest an inborn error of metabolism such as a strong family history, episodic encephalopathy or vomits, and burst-suppression on EEG, one may consider a workup for inborn errors of metabolism. This would include estimations of serum ammonia, lactate, homocysteine, uric acid, tandem mass spectroscopy (which includes amino acids and acyl carnitine), biotinidase levels, urine organic acids, and cerebrospinal fluid (CSF) glucose and glycine.

If an etiological diagnosis is not reached, genetic testing may be considered. In a syndromic child, it may be appropriate to do a chromosomal microarray and in others a whole-exome sequencing (WES) may be ordered.[12]

■ MANAGEMENT

Speed is of essence in the management of epileptic spasms. In India, the median delay between onset of spasms and starting specific antispasm medication has been quite long ranging from 1 to 66 months.[8] There is enough data to show that quick appropriate treatment of infantile spasms leads to better developmental outcomes in patients.

The first line of therapy in infantile spasms is hormonal therapy (either oral prednisolone or intramuscular adrenocorticotropic hormone [ACTH]) or vigabatrin or a combination of the two **(Flowchart 8.1)**. There may be a

Flowchart 8.1: Therapeutic algorithm for infantile spasms.

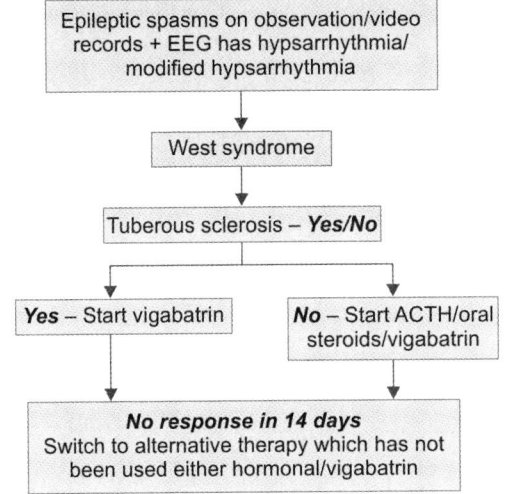

(ACTH: adrenocorticotropic hormone; EEG: electroencephalogram)

slight benefit of hormonal therapy over vigabatrin in the short-term but not in the long-term.[14,15] There is no significant advantage either on seizure control or long-term development outcomes with either of the hormonal therapies.[14] However, vigabatrin has a slight edge over hormonal therapy in children with tuberous sclerosis-related infantile spasms.[16] The combination of vigabatrin and hormonal therapy also has an initial short-term benefit in terms of response.[15] However, this is not translated to any long-term benefits in terms of epilepsy or developmental outcomes.[17]

Hormonal therapy includes high-dose oral steroids or ACTH. Oral steroids have the benefit of cost and ease of usage. The doses recommended are 40–60 mg/day in divided doses for 14 days followed by a taper over 3–4 weeks. For very low-weight children, a dose of 4–8 mg/kg/day may be used for 2 weeks with a taper over 3–4 weeks.

The doses of ACTH range widely. The high-dose protocol which is preferred is 75 U/m^2 12 hourly for 14 days followed by 30 U/m^2 once daily (OD) for 3 days, 15 U/m^2 OD for 3 days, 10 U/m^2 OD for 3 days, and 10 U/m^2 on alternate days for three doses. In the low-dose protocol, 20–30 U/day is used for 2–6 weeks.[18]

Precautions with steroids include no live vaccines for 1 month after stopping therapy, blood pressure measurements weekly, monitoring and treating infections urgently. In high-risk situations, children may be screened for pulmonary tuberculosis. These children are also at risk for adrenal insufficiency for the next 6 months and need to be administered stress doses of hydrocortisone (25–100 mg/m^2 in divided doses) in case of intercurrent illness or surgery.[12]

Vigabatrin is used in a dose of 50 mg/kg per day for 3–5 days and doses may be escalated to 100 mg/kg for 3–5 days and then up to a maximum of 150 mg/kg/day. Precaution includes monitoring for visual side effects by doing a 6-monthly fundus examination and if possible electroretinogram (ERG). If hormonal therapy fails, vigabatrin may be used and vice versa.

Other drugs which have been tried including topiramate, zonisamide, valproate, nitrazepam, pyridoxine, and levetiracetam. An excellent option after failure of hormonal therapy and vigabatrin is the ketogenic diet or modified Atkins diet.[19] Epilepsy surgery is appropriate in certain situations if there is an identifiable epileptogenic region such as focal cortical dysplasia, hemimegalencephaly, or tuberous sclerosis with focal features on clinical semiology, EEG, or positron emission tomography (PET) scan.[20]

■ OUTCOMES

The outcome of epileptic spasms is disappointing. Only one fourth of patients have a good cognitive outcome and only one third become completely seizure-free. Early recognition and treatment with appropriate drugs is key to good long-term outcomes.[15] In a large study from China, patients in whom hormonal therapy or vigabatrin was used as the first or second line of treatment were significantly more likely to be seizure free at 1 year compared to children who had not received these drugs initially.[3]

The effect of delay in starting therapy was studied in 77 children with infantile spasms of the UKISS trial. The lead time to onset of therapy was classified as <7 days, 8–14 days, 15–30 days, 1–2 months, and > 2 months. A delay in starting treatment was associated with a 3.9-point decline in Vineland Adaptive Behavior Scale (VABS) scores at 4 years for each of the subsequent categories.[18]

■ CONCLUSION

Infantile or epileptic spasms are an important group of epileptic encephalopathies of early childhood. They have a signature EEG called hypsarrhythmia. Early treatment with hormonal therapy or vigabatrin results in better epilepsy outcomes and long-term neurodevelopment status.

■ KEY POINTS

- The most common cause of infantile or epileptic spasms is neonatal hypoglycemic brain injury in India and hypoxic-ischemic encephalopathy in Europe.
- A delay in diagnosis by a month results in more than 10-point drop in Vineland Adaptive Behavior Scale Scores.
- Patients who received hormonal therapy or vigabatrin as first- or second-line therapy are more likely to be seizure free at 1 year than those who did not receive therapy.

- A 30-minute sleep EEG and 10-minute awake EEG are necessary to make the diagnosis of hypsarrhythmia seen in infantile spasms.
- Genetic testing may be considered if no etiological diagnosis is confirmed.

REFERENCES

1. Pellock JM, Hrachovy R, Shinnar S, Baram TZ, Bettis D, Dlugos DJ, et al. Infantile spasms: A U.S. consensus report. Epilepsia. 2010;51(10):2175-89.
2. Wirrell EC, Shellhaas RA, Joshi C, Keator C, Kumar S, Mitchell WG, et al. How should children with West syndrome be efficiently and accurately investigated? Results from the National Infantile Spasms Consortium. Epilepsia. 2015;56(4),617-25.
3. Mao L, Kessi M, Peng P, He F, Zhang C, Yang L, et al. The patterns of response of 11 regimens for infantile spasms. Sci Rep. 2020;10(1):11509.
4. Bednarek N, Motte J, Soufflet C, Plouin P, Dulac O. Evidence of late-onset infantile spasms. Epilepsia. 1998;39:55-60.
5. Jia JL, Chen S, Sivarajah V, Stephens D, Cortez MA. Latitudinal differences on the global epidemiology of infantile spasms: systematic review and meta-analysis. Orphanet J Rare Dis. 2018;29;13(1):216.
6. Frost JD, Hrachovy RA. Pathogenesis of infantile spasms: A model based on developmental desynchronization. J Clin Neurophysiol. 2005;22(1):25-36.
7. Osborne JP, Lux AL, Edwards SW, Hancock E, Johnson AL, Kennedy CR, et al. The underlying etiology of infantile spasms (West syndrome): Information from the United Kingdom Infantile Spasms Study (UKISS) on contemporary causes and their classification. Epilepsia. 2010;51(10):2168-74.
8. Surana P, Symonds JD, Srivastava P, Geetha TS, Jain R, Vedant R, et al. Infantile spasms: Etiology, lead time and treatment response in a resource limited setting. Epilepsy Behav Rep. 2020;14:100397.
9. Paciorkowski AR, Thio LL, Dobyns WB. Genetic and biologic classification of infantile spasms. Pediatr Neurol. 2011;45(6):355-67.
10. Maydell BV, Berenson F, Rothner AD, Wyllie E, Kotagal P. Benign myoclonus of early infancy: An imitator of West's syndrome. J Child Neurol. 2001;16(2):109-12.
11. Praveen V, Patole SK, Whitehall JS. Hyperekplexia in neonates. Postgrad Med J. 2001;77:570-2.
12. Sharma S, Kaushik JS, Srivastava K, Goswami JN, Sahu JK, Vinayan KP, et al. Association of Child Neurology (AOCN) – Indian Epilepsy Society (IES) Consensus Guidelines for the diagnosis and management of West syndrome. Indian Pediatr. 2020;58(1):54-66.
13. Koutroumanidis M, Arzimanoglou A, Caraballo R, Goyal S, Kaminska A, Laoprasert P, et al. The role of EEG in the diagnosis and classification of the epilepsy syndromes: A tool for clinical practice by the ILAE neurophysiology task force (part 2). Epileptic Disord. 2017;19(4):385-437.
14. Lux AL, Edwards SW, Hancock E, Johnson AL, Kennedy CR, Newton RW, et al. The United Kingdom Infantile Spasms Study (UKISS) comparing hormone treatment with vigabatrin on developmental and epilepsy outcomes to age 14 months: A multicentre randomised trial. Lancet Neurol. 2005;4(11):712-7.
15. O'Callaghan FJ, Edwards SW, Alber FD, Hancock E, Johnson AL, Kennedy CR, et al. Safety and effectiveness of hormonal treatment versus hormonal treatment

15. with vigabatrin for infantile spasms (ICISS): A randomised, multi- centre, open-label trial. Lancet Neurol. 2017;16(1):33-42.
16. Hancock E, Osborne JP, Milner P. Treatment of infantile spasms. Cochrane Database Syst Rev. 2002;(2):CD001770.
17. O'Callaghan FJK, Edwards SW, Alber FD, Cortina Borja M, Hancock E, et al. International Collaborative Infantile Spasms Study (ICISS) investigators. Vigabatrin with hormonal treatment versus hormonal treatment alone (ICISS) for infantile spasms: 18-month outcomes of an open-label, randomised controlled trial. Lancet Child Adolesc Health. 2018;2(10):715-25.
18. Hrachovy RA, Frost JD Jr, Glaze DG. High-dose, long-duration versus low-dose, short-duration corticotropin therapy for infantile spasms. J Pediatr. 1994;124 (5 Pt 1):803-6.
19. Sharma S, Sankhyan N, Gulati S, Agarwala A. Use of the modified Atkins diet in infantile spasms refractory to first-line treatment. Seizure. 2012;21(1):45-8.
20. Chugani HT, Ilyas M, Kumar A, Juhasz C, Kupsky WJ, Sood S, et al. Surgical treatment for refractory epileptic spasms: The Detroit series. Epilepsia. 2015; 56(12):1941-9.

Cardiology

CHAPTER 9

Cardiac Arrhythmias

Mani Ram Krishna, Balu Vaidyanathan

■ INTRODUCTION

Cardiac arrhythmias are generally perceived to be less common in children compared to adults. Retrospective evaluation of records of visits to pediatric emergency departments (PED) suggests that approximately 0.1% of all PED visits are related to a cardiac rhythm disorder.[1] Pediatric trainees are often not comfortable in interpreting electrocardiograms (ECG) and providing emergency management of children presenting with symptomatic cardiac arrhythmia. In recent decades, there have been several developments in the comprehensive management of children with problems of heart rhythm and most pediatric cardiac centers in our country have the capability to provide high quality management of cardiac arrhythmia comparable with developed countries. However, most pediatricians are not aware of the advances in diagnosis and management of pediatric cardiac arrhythmia. In this chapter, we attempt to elaborate on the recent advances in the diagnosis, pharmacological and nonpharmacological management of pediatric cardiac arrhythmia as well as newer pathways in continuing medical education for pediatricians to improve competency in managing children with arrhythmia. The recognition of genetic arrhythmia syndromes has increased in the recent years and we have dedicated a separate section of the chapter to clinical presentation, evaluation, and management of children with inherited cardiac arrhythmia.

■ DIAGNOSIS OF PEDIATRIC CARDIAC ARRHYTHMIAS

Why a Standardized 12-Lead ECG Recording is Essential?

The ECG is the first investigation in the evaluation of cardiac rhythm disorders. It is an inexpensive investigation and is widely available even in small medical facilities. A standardized 12-lead ECG obtained when the child is experiencing symptoms is the only investigation needed to rule out a potential abnormality of cardiac rhythm. It is often difficult to elucidate the rhythm from a multi-parameter monitor. The ECG channel in the monitor is not standardized to the same level of precision as the ECG machine and is more susceptible to movement artifacts. Hence, it is important to obtain

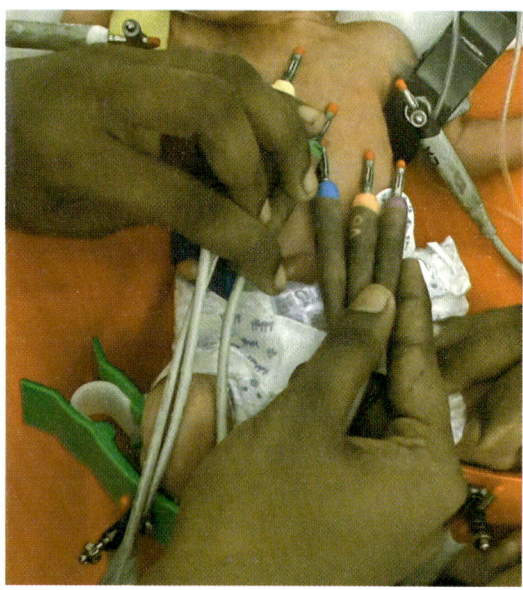

Fig. 9.1: A method to obtain a 12-lead electrocardiogram with all chest leads placed in a preterm very low birth weight baby.

a 12-lead ECG whenever a problem with cardiac rhythm is suspected. A 12-lead ECG in an infant or a young child can be obtained with the same equipment used for adults. Pediatricians and pediatric cardiologists have developed techniques to obtain chest lead tracings in infants overcoming the challenge of small chest surface area to place the six leads **(Fig. 9.1)**.

A *systematic interpretation of the 12-lead ECG* obtained during an episode of arrhythmia often will establish the diagnosis in most children. The logical interpretation should include attention to each of the details mentioned here in an orderly fashion:

1. *ECG standardization*: It is important to ensure that the ECG is standardized. A "standardized" ECG should be obtained at a paper speed of 25 mm/s with the deflections at amplitude of 10 mm/mV. Calculation of the heart rate as well as observations about chamber enlargement would be erroneous if the ECG was not obtained in a standardized fashion.
2. *Calculation of the heart rate*: A simple formula to calculate heart rate would be 300/number of large squares between two consecutive R waves. However, as children have greater heterogeneity in the heart rate, a more accurate heart rate calculation can be obtained by the formula 1,500/number of small squares between two consecutive R waves. An example of calculation of heart rate is illustrated in **Figure 9.2**.
3. *The nature (characteristics) of the QRS complex:* While looking at the QRS complex, the pediatrician should endeavor to look at two important aspects:

Cardiac Arrhythmias

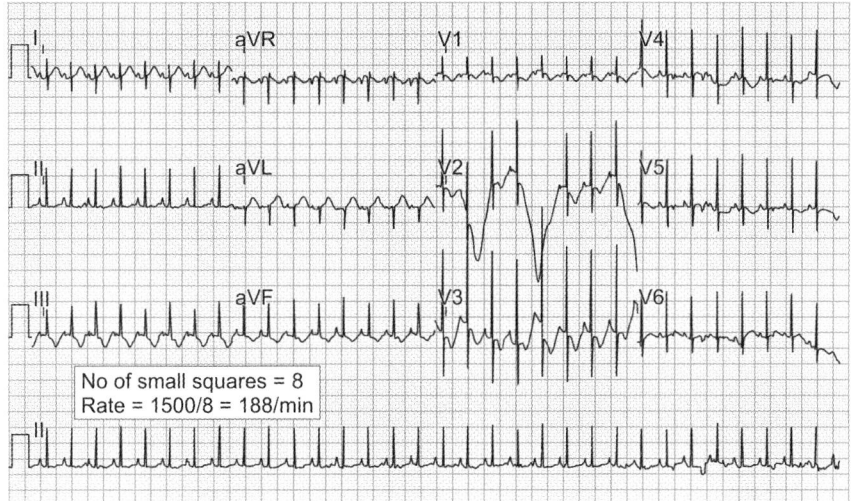

Fig. 9.2: An example of heart rate calculation from a standardized 12-lead ECG. The space between 2 consecutive QRS complexes compromises 8 small squares, and the heart rate is hence 188 per minute.

    a. *Are the QRS complexes narrow or wide?* QRS duration of greater than 90 ms (larger than 2 small squares) is the most commonly accepted definition of a wide QRS complex. A *narrow QRS complex tachycardia* is usually supraventricular in origin. A *wide QRS complex tachycardia* could potentially be ventricular in origin and would hence need urgent management. Similarly in children with bradycardia, the presence of a broad QRS complex should raise the suspicion of a serious rhythm problem and merit urgent referral.

    b. *Are the QRS complexes of similar morphology or varying morphology?* When all the QRS complexes in the ECG are similar, it is referred to as a "monomorphic" tachycardia. When more than one type of QRS complex is visualized, the tachycardia is "polymorphic" and generally considered more ominous and dangerous.

4. *The relationship of the P wave to the QRS complex*: When each QRS complex is preceded or followed by a P wave, the relationship is said to be 1:1. Establishing the relationship between the P wave and the QRS complex provides valuable information about the mechanism of cardiac arrhythmia.

■ COMMON CARDIAC ARRHYTHMIAS IN CHILDREN

The characteristic findings of the "common" cardiac arrhythmias in children as well as the corresponding ECG examples are enumerated below.

1. *Sinus rhythm:* The heart rate is within the normal limits for age. Each QRS complex is preceded by a P wave. The P wave is positive in leads 1 and aVF but negative in aVR. The PR interval remains constant throughout the ECG **(Fig. 9.3A)**.

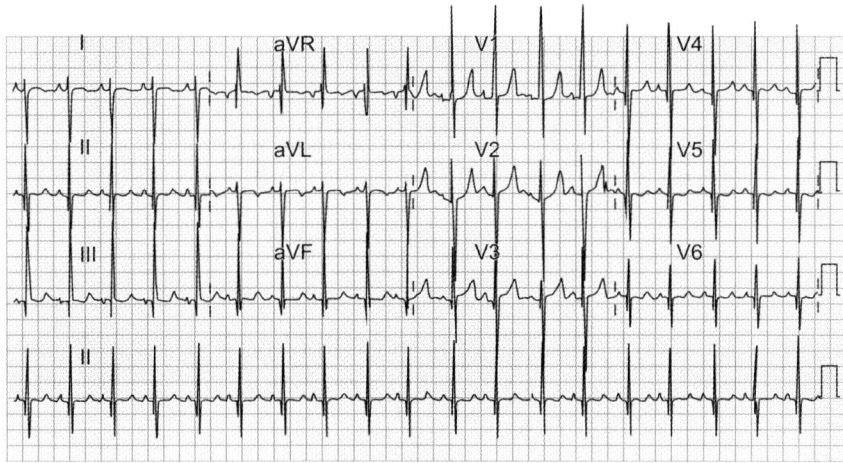

Fig. 9.3A: An example of an ECG in sinus rhythm. The P wave is positive in leads 1 and aVF and the PR interval remains constant.

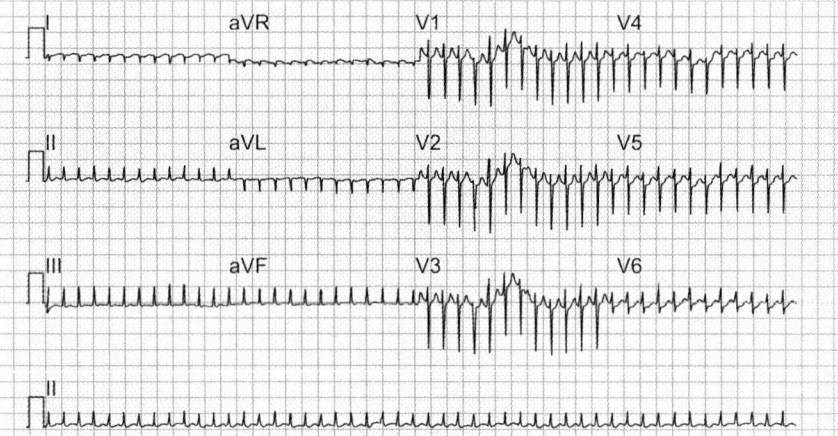

Fig. 9.3B: Standardized 12-lead ECG of a neonate with tachycardia. There is a regular narrow complex tachycardia with a heart rate of close to 300 per minute and a P wave is not readily apparent. The ECG appearance is typical of paroxysmal supraventricular tachycardia.

2. *Paroxysmal supraventricular tachycardia (PSVT)*: This is usually a regular narrow complex tachycardia with a heart rate above 220 per minute. The P waves are usually not readily apparent to the untrained eye. In some cases, the P wave may be seen following the QRS complex, a condition termed 1:1 V-A conduction **(Fig. 9.3B)**.
3. *Atrial flutter*: This is usually a narrow complex regular tachycardia although occasional irregularities can be made out. The P waves outnumber the QRS complexes and the P waves have a characteristic sawtooth pattern **(Fig. 9.3C)**.

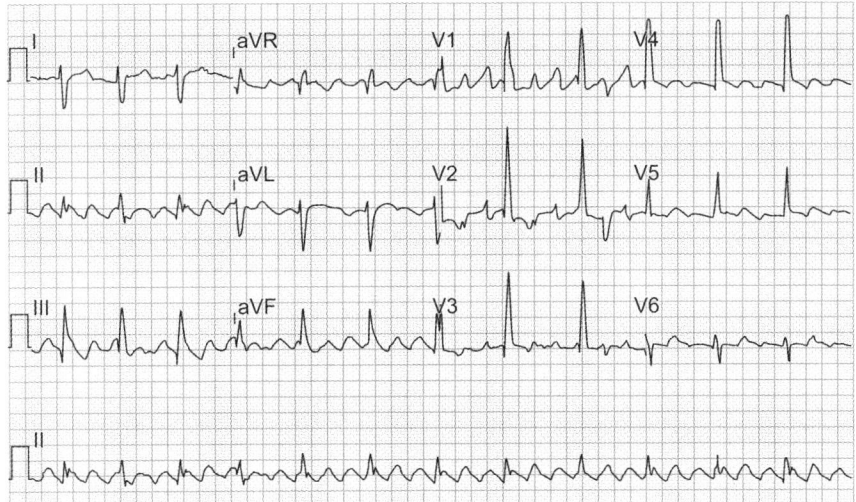

Fig. 9.3C: Standardized 12-lead ECG of a 17-year-old girl with severe valvular pulmonic stenosis. The atrial rate is elevated, and the P waves have a characteristic sawtooth appearance seen in atrial flutter.

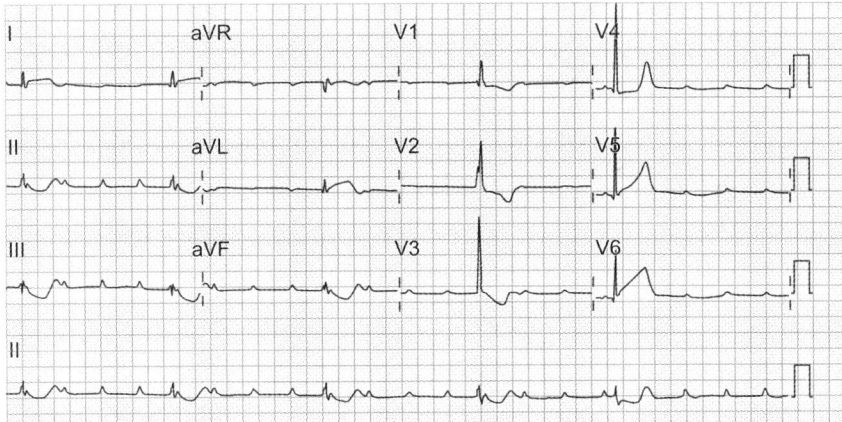

Fig. 9.3D: A standardized 12-lead ECG of an 8-year-old with viral myocarditis. There is bradycardia with no consistent relationship between the P wave and QRS. This is characteristic of complete heart block.

4. *Sinus bradycardia*: The heart rate is lower than normal for age but each QRS complex is preceded by a P wave and the PR interval remains constant.
5. *Complete heart block:* The heart rate is lower than normal for age. There is no consistent relationship between the P wave and the QRS complex and the P waves outnumber the QRS complex **(Fig. 9.3D)**.

A majority of tachyarrhythmias in children are paroxysmal events. It is not unusual for children to present to the medical facility after the symptoms

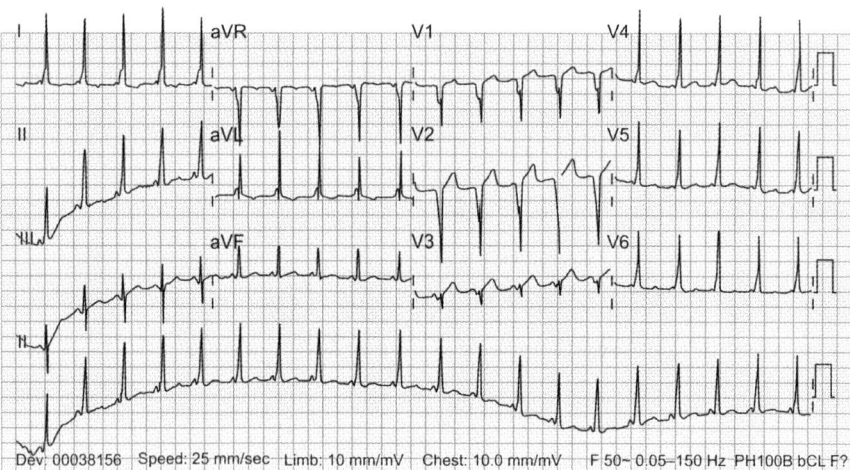

Fig. 9.3E: Standardized 12-lead ECG of a 7-month old boy. This shows sinus rhythm with a short PR interval and a characteristic slurring of the QRS complex (delta wave) typical of Wolff-Parkinson-White (WPW) syndrome.

have subsided. In children with Wolff-Parkinson-White (WPW) syndrome, the 12-lead ECG will show evidence of ventricular preexcitation **(Fig. 9.3E)** characterized by a short PR interval, broad QRS with a characteristic slur on the upstroke of the R wave (delta wave) and reciprocal T wave and other changes. In all other conditions, the baseline ECG will be normal.

■ AMBULATORY ECG MONITORING IN CHILDREN

Pediatric cardiologists sometimes resort to ambulatory ECG (aECG) monitoring to capture the rhythm when symptoms occur. Traditionally, aECG monitoring was obtained by *Holter evaluation.* Holter continues to remain the gold standard for aECG monitoring. It has been utilized for many decades and the quality of recording is not matched by other methods.[2] There are, however, important limitations with Holter for aECG monitoring in children. The Holter monitor can provide recording for only 24–48 hours. A recent retrospective review on aECG monitoring confirmed that a vast majority of positive findings were obtained only beyond 3 days of continuous recording.[3] The wires in the chest can sometimes scare small children and it is often difficult to keep the recorder attached to the hip pocket in active children who run around and play. Holter monitoring also requires families to stay at or close to the medical facility and return the equipment for analysis. This presents an economic and logistic challenge for families from rural areas who need to travel a long distance for specialist consultation.

The advent of technology particularly miniaturization of sensors has allowed for the development of ***patch aECG monitors*** **(Fig. 9.4A)**. These

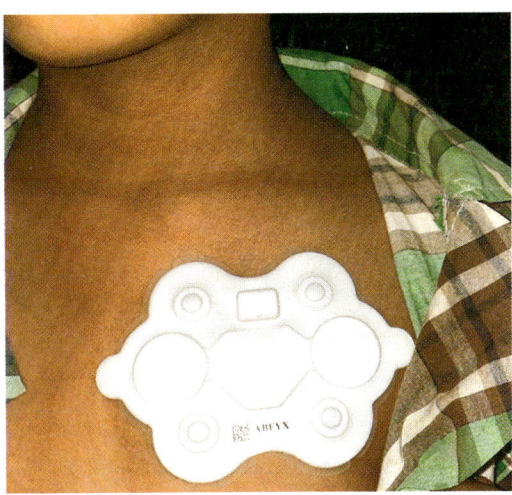

Fig. 9.4A: A commercially available patch ambulatory ECG placed in the chest of a 9-year-old boy with suspected supraventricular tachycardia.

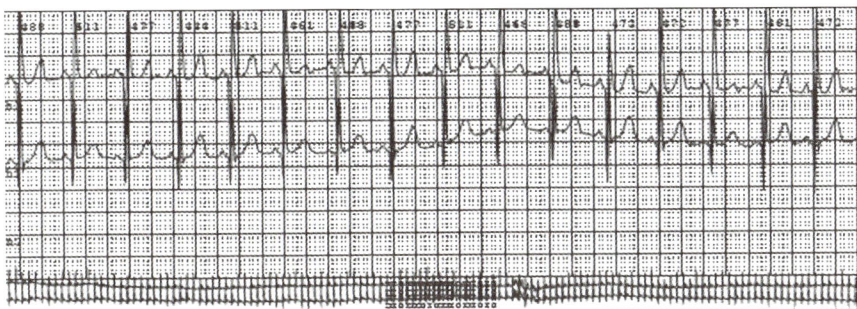

Fig. 9.4B: A 2-channel recording from a commercially available patch ambulatory ECG recording.

monitors contain a microsensor, memory storage segment and a battery with an adhesive patch which can be stuck on the chest wall. These typically provide single or double channel recording **(Fig. 9.4B)** although three channel recording is also available in some devices. These can be used for longer periods ranging from 3 to 30 days. Most such patches are water and shower proof. These practical conveniences have resulted in higher study completions than traditional forms.[4] Most devices transmit the recordings daily to a dedicated server and the analysis is performed either daily or at the end of the recording period depending on the type of device and the vendor. More sophisticated devices permit live analysis of the transmitted recordings. Current commercially available patch aECG monitors in our country provide two-channel recording for periods of 3–7 days. Although recommended for children above 2 years of age, these patches have been used in neonates and young infants with satisfactory recording.[5] Their convenience and ease of use has resulted in greater physician and patient acceptance. These devices can be stored by pediatricians in their office practice and aECG monitoring can be started after the initial consultation without any delay. A major disadvantage of the patch monitor is the dependence on the expertise of the vendor's technician for analysis as well as retrieval of the raw data. It is not unusual in our practice to request for additional data and to make changes in the report due to inappropriate interpretation of data.

The boom in the wearable technology market has provided another option for aECG monitoring. Some of the available devices have received regulatory body approval for detection of atrial fibrillation in adults. At present, none of the available devices are approved for diagnostic use in children. However, there are isolated reports highlighting their utility in the diagnosis of paroxysmal pediatric arrhythmias.

■ ADVANCES IN PHARMACOLOGIC THERAPY OF PEDIATRIC ARRHYTHMIAS

The Vaughan-Williams classification of antiarrhythmic drugs was proposed in the 1970s and there was very little addition to the pharmacological armamentarium till recent years. However, several newer drugs with targeted action on specific channels have been developed in recent years. A modernization of the classification has been proposed to accommodate these drugs with unique mechanisms but is yet to gain wide acceptance.[6] Some of these drugs have percolated into clinical practice.

The current standard of management of the common cardiac arrhythmias is summarized in **Table 9.1**. Pharmacological therapy remains the mainstay of acute and chronic management of pediatric cardiac arrhythmias. The commonly used antiarrhythmic medications in pediatric arrhythmias, their indication, dosage and potential adverse effects are summarized in **Table 9.2**.

Paroxysmal Supraventricular Tachycardia

Paroxysmal supraventricular tachycardia (PSVT) is the most common tachyarrhythmia in the pediatric age group. The arrhythmia is due to an atrioventricular (AV) node-dependent reentrant mechanism. The reentry may be due to an accessory pathway (AVRT) or within the AV node itself (AVNRT). The arrhythmia can be readily terminated by intravenous (IV) administration of *adenosine*. Alternative methods for termination of arrhythmia include vagal maneuvers such as application of ice on the face, carotid massage, and the Valsalva maneuver. These maneuvers have limited efficacy for termination of the arrhythmia.[7] There is currently no safe and effective "non-parenteral" medication for acute termination of PSVT.

Recently, an ultra-short acting nasally administered calcium channel blocker, *etripamil,* has been developed and has undergone early clinical trials. A phase II study showed greater than 95% conversion to sinus rhythm

TABLE 9.1: Common pediatric cardiac arrhythmias: Acute and long-term management options.

Arrhythmia	Acute management	Long-term management
PSVT	IV adenosine for acute termination	Oral beta-blockers
Atrial flutter	Direct current cardioversion (1 J/kg)	• No maintenance therapy is usually needed in neonatal atrial flutter • Oral sotalol is used when recurrence occurs
Atrial tachycardia	IV beta-blockers (metoprolol at a dose of 0.1 mg/kg per dose or esmolol at a dose of 50–300 µg/kg/min)	Oral beta-blockers Sotalol or flecainide
Complete heart block	Temporary transvenous pacing or isoprenaline (at a dose of 0.05–0.5 µg/kg/min)	Oral orciprenaline

(PSVT: paroxysmal supraventricular tachycardia; IV: intravenous)

with high dose etripamil therapy. The drug was well tolerated with most adverse events related to nasal irritation rather than systemic effects.[8] A subsequent larger study including subjects lesser than 18 years is under way. The promising data provides hope that soon, children (and adults) with PSVT can undergo safe and effective self-management of palpitation at their home.

Ivabradine and Automatic Arrhythmias

Ivabradine is a selective inhibitor of the hyperpolarization-activated sodium current (variously termed as the pacemaker current, the funny current or I_f). This current is responsible for the pacemaker activity of the sinus node. Ivabradine was initially approved as a rate-modulating agent in the management of adults with stable coronary artery disease. The drug has an onset of action within 60 minutes and has a favorable safety profile.[9] The only adverse effect of concern with long-term ivabradine use is the visual phenomena referred to as phosphenes. These have been shown to improve with continued use of the drug and discontinuation is not recommended. The drug is also "hemodynamically neutral" and does not result in hypotension.

Recent molecular work has shown that local enhanced pacemaker current is responsible for some of the automatic arrhythmias such as junctional ectopic tachycardia and atrial tachycardia. Congenital junctional ectopic tachycardia (JET) is rare and often difficult to treat in infants. Most infants require a combination pharmacological therapy. Arrhythmia control is suboptimal despite combination therapy. The utility of ivabradine as an

TABLE 9.2: Common antiarrhythmic drugs used in children, their dosage, indications and common adverse effects.

Drug	Dosage	Indications	Adverse effects/ Contraindications
Adenosine	0.1–0.3 mg/kg as rapid IV push	• Treatment of PSVT • Diagnostic tool to understand the mechanism of tachyarrhythmia	• The short half-life of 6 seconds means that the drug does not usually cause any adverse events • Rarely, it may cause atrial fibrillation in older children
Digoxin	5 µg/kg per dose every 12 hours	Additional agent in re-entrant tachyarrhythmias	• Proarrhythmic effects • Contraindicated in WPW syndrome • Anorexia, nausea and vomiting
Propranolol	1–2 mg/kg per dose every 6–8 hours	• PSVT • Atrial tachycardia • Inherited arrhythmias	• Hypoglycemia in neonates and young infants • Fatigability and mood swings in adolescents
Verapamil	2–4 mg/kg per dose every 8 hours	Idiopathic left ventricular (fascicular) tachycardia	• Hypotension • Constipation • Headache and dizziness • Edema
Sotalol	1–2 mg/kg per dose every 8 hours	• Atrial flutter • Atrial tachycardia • Second line management of PSVT	• QTc prolongation and pro-arrhythmic side effects • Fatigue and mood swings • Blurring of vision
Flecainide	0.5–2 mg/kg per dose every 8–12 hours	• Second-line management of PSVT • Atrial tachycardia	• Proarrhythmic side effects – monitored by serial measurement of QRS duration in ECG • Photosensitivity reactions
Amiodarone	5 mg/kg per dose every 12–24 hours	All hemodynamically unstable tachyarrhythmias	• Thyroid function abnormalities • Hypotension • Liver function derangements • Pulmonary fibrosis • QTc prolongation and proarrhythmic effects

(IV: intravenous; PSVT: paroxysmal supraventricular tachycardia; WPW syndrome: Wolff-Parkinson-White syndrome) adjunct therapy was first reported in a small group of infants.[10] Subsequently, the drug has been used with excellent results and reports of its efficacy as a single agent in congenital JET are emerging. Our group used ivabradine in postoperative JET, a very common tachyarrhythmia in the postoperative period and demonstrated its safety and efficacy.[11] Subsequently a larger study has shown ivabradine to be noninferior to the current standard of therapy in postoperative JET.[12] In addition to JET, ivabradine has been shown to be efficacious in other supraventricular automatic tachycardias such as atrial tachycardia.[13] It has also been shown to be effective as a heart rate reduction agent in children with dilated cardiomyopathy with improvement in ejection fraction noted with sustained use.[14] Ivabradine is used in a dose of 0.05–0.2 mg per kg per dose twice daily. It is currently recommended that the drug be initiated in an inpatient setting with monitoring of the heart rate and blood pressure. Although no standard guidelines on monitoring have been published, we typically hospitalize patients for 48 hours during which the drug administration is initiated. The heart rate and blood pressure are monitored hourly in the first 24 hours after the drug is administered.

■ INVASIVE THERAPY FOR PEDIATRIC ARRHYTHMIAS

Pharmacological therapy has a low success rate in children with recurrent tachyarrhythmias.[15] This could potentially be multifactorial. Compliance to drug therapy over a prolonged period is difficult in young children as well as adolescents and young adults. The underlying substrate for arrhythmia is generally more complex in children with congenital heart disease (CHD). The nature of the underlying CHD may also restrict use of certain antiarrhythmic medications. Hence pediatric electrophysiologists are increasingly looking toward a permanent curative solution for children with cardiac arrhythmia. This can be achieved by invasive electrophysiological procedures for catheter ablation.[16]

Radiofrequency Ablation

Over the previous three decades, the safety and efficacy of radiofrequency ablation in re-entrant tachyarrhythmias as well as automatic atrial tachycardias have been established in children weighing greater than 15 kg. Younger age, low weight and association with complex CHD were considered high-risk categories for interventional procedures. With wider availability of smaller hardware required for these procedures, pediatric electrophysiologists are increasingly performing interventional procedures in smaller children with tachyarrhythmias that have not been adequately controlled with pharmacological therapy. Single center analysis of results suggests that the procedural success as well as complication rates in children younger than 4 years is comparable to older children.[17]

During an interventional electrophysiological (EP) study, catheters are advanced from the femoral veins (and occasionally the femoral artery) and advanced to be placed in the atrium, ventricle, bundle of His and coronary sinus. These catheters record the cardiac electrical activity at the site and provide them as electrograms which are interpreted by the cardiologist. This is first performed when the child is in normal sinus rhythm. Once the baseline information is obtained, the cardiologist utilizes provocative therapy (either mechanical or pharmacological) to reproduce the tachyarrhythmia. The site of origin of the arrhythmia as well as the mechanism of arrhythmia can be deduced by studying the difference in the electrical activity recorded at these different sites.

Once this is understood, the cardiologist then places a special catheter capable of providing radiofrequency energy (ablation catheter) at the site of origin of the arrhythmia. The energy emitted increases the temperature of the site and results in localized destruction of tissue (referred to as a *lesion*). One of the major concerns during interventional procedures is clotting of blood at the tips of the ablation catheter which reduces the efficacy of the lesion created. At the turn of the century, irrigated catheters were introduced for use in adults. These catheters were shown to result in wider and deeper tissue destruction and hence greater procedural success. These have become the option of choice in certain arrhythmias in the adult population. However, pediatric electrophysiologists have resisted utilizing irrigated catheters because of a perceived risk of cardiac perforation and injury to the normal conduction system.[18] Recent reports based on small single institute cohorts have shown comparable safety and improved medium-term outcomes of radiofrequency ablation using irrigated catheters in children and have ignited interest in the use of this technology among pediatric electrophysiologists.[19]

Three-Dimensional Mapping Techniques

Electrophysiological studies are among the longest procedures performed in the pediatric cardiac catheterization laboratories and involve the longest fluoroscopy time and radiation dose among pediatric cardiac interventions. This raises the concern about the long-term effects of radiation exposure, as the tissues in children are more vulnerable to ionizing radiation. The concern of increased fluoroscopy exposure in children led to the evolution of non-fluoroscopic techniques of catheter ablation.[20] This method is popularly referred to as three-dimensional (3D) mapping techniques (**Fig. 9.5**). The evolution of 3D mapping has enabled completion of EP studies without the use of fluoroscopy (zero fluoroscopy procedures). In recent years, several prospective studies have confirmed the very high procedural access and near complete absence of complications due to the utilization of 3D mapping in children with tachyarrhythmias.[21,22]

Cardiac Arrhythmias

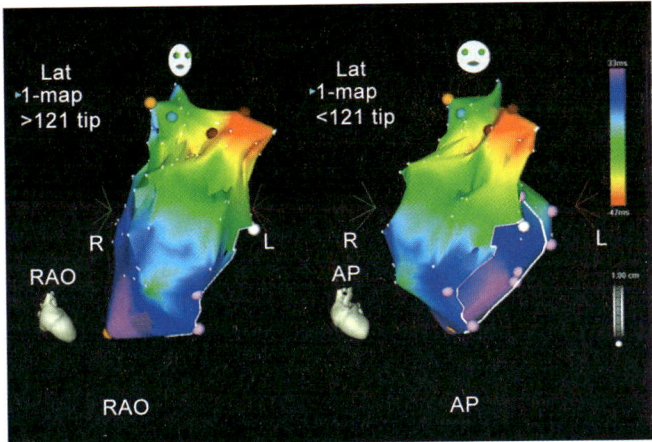

Fig. 9.5: An example of a three-dimensional mapping for radiofrequency ablation for cardiac arrhythmias.
Source: Dr Balaji Seshadri, Pediatric Electrophysiologist, Oregon, USA.

Multi-Center Pediatric and Adult Congenital EP Quality Initiative

To understand the impact of such technological advances in interventional therapies, the Pediatric and Congenital Electrophysiology Society (PACES) created the Multi-Center Pediatric and Adult Congenital EP Quality (MAP-IT) initiative in 2013, to prospectively collect data on EP procedures performed in children.[23] This registry promises to be an important guide to the standards of care in children with tachyarrhythmias in the next few decades.

Implantable Cardiac Devices

Another area of significant advancements in pediatric interventional therapies is the use of implantable cardiac devices. These include permanent pacemakers, implantable cardioverter-defibrillators (ICD) and cardiac resynchronization therapy (CRT).

Pacemakers are the most utilized cardiac devices in children. As the name suggests, these devices provide stimulation of the cardiac electrical activity. The most common indication for pacemaker implantation is heart block. The pacemaker consists of a pulse generator which contains the battery as well as the electronic apparatus necessary for regulating the impulses as well as leads which transmit the electrical stimulus from the device to the heart muscle. The pacemakers can be used to stimulate the atrium or ventricle (single chamber pacemakers) or both (dual chamber pacemakers). In older children, these devices are placed inside the heart through the left subclavian vein (endocardial implantation) **(Fig. 9.6A)**. This results in more stable pacemaker function and longer battery life. However, the subclavian veins

Cardiac Arrhythmias

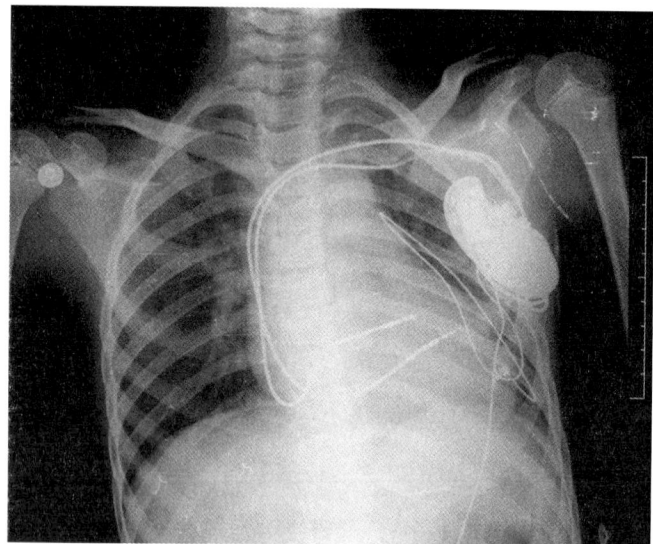

Fig. 9.6A: Chest X-ray of a 9-year-old boy with a single chamber permanent pacemaker. The pacemaker lead has been implanted endocardially through the left subclavian vein.

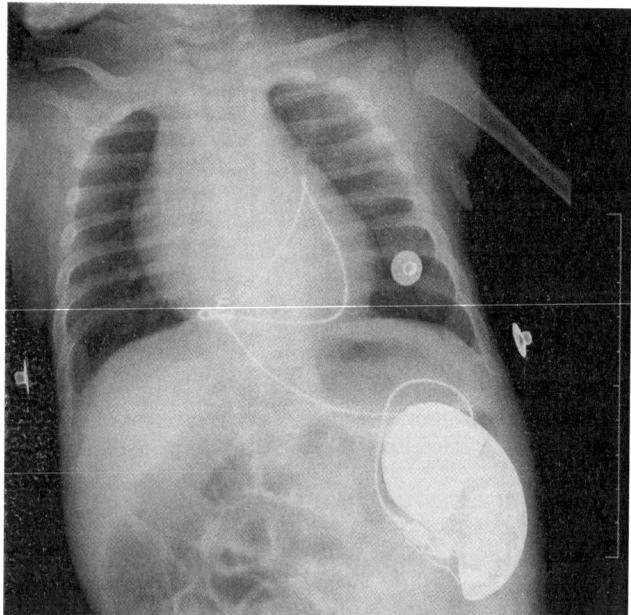

Fig. 9.6B: Chest X-ray of a 1-year-old boy with a permanent pacemaker inserted epicardially by a cardiovascular surgeon.

in infants and young children are too small to accommodate the pacemaker leads. Hence conventionally, these are placed on the epicardial surface of the heart by the cardiac surgeon **(Fig. 9.6B)**.

Current generation batteries last for more than 10 years, and unexpected device failures are exceedingly rare. However, children with implanted pacemakers frequently experience problems related to the lead. The problems include lead migration and lead fracture, both of which can result in loss of pacing. To overcome the problems related to lead malfunction, *leadless pacemakers* have been developed and are available commercially. Its use has been reported in a 4-year old child.[24] However, significant concerns remain about their utility in the pediatric population. Current generation leadless pacemakers are capable of pacing only the ventricles, but dual chamber pacing has been shown to be superior to ventricle only pacing in children over the long-term. The current generation pacemakers are also bulky requiring large delivery sheaths to place them inside the heart. This could result in damage to the femoral veins which are frequently accessed for placement of the devices.[25] Despite the limitations, leadless pacemakers represent a significant advancement in pacing technology, and it is possible that with further refinements in the technology, they could replace traditional pacemakers in children.

A child or an adult implanted with a pacemaker will need to visit his/her cardiologist every 3–6 months to check the function of the pacemaker. Current generation pacemakers and ICD provide the option of remote monitoring of device function. These devices are Bluetooth-enabled and are capable of transmitting information to a dedicated mobile application. This is then transmitted to a secure online server from which it can be reviewed by the cardiologist or cardiac technician. This reduces the need for repeated travel to the healthcare facility. This is especially advantageous in countries such as India where facilities for pacemaker interrogation are available only in larger cities and travel to these centers is expensive and logistically challenging for families from rural areas.

■ THE INHERITED ARRHYTHMIAS

The electrical activity of the heart is regulated by sodium, potassium, and calcium channels. Genetic abnormalities in the functioning of any one of the above channels can result in the inherited arrhythmias—syndromes characterized by an increased propensity for malignant ventricular arrhythmias, syncope, and sudden cardiac deaths. These conditions include long QT syndrome (LQTS), Brugada syndrome (BrS) and catecholaminergic polymorphic ventricular tachycardia (CPVT).[26] Typical ECG examples of some of the inherited arrhythmias are provided in **Figures 9.7A to C**. A less common inherited arrhythmia, short QT syndrome, is unusual in children. The clinical presentation of these disorders includes recurrent syncope, syncope on exertion, seizures, symptoms with specific triggers (fever, loud and shrill noises, swimming, competitive sports, and episodes of

184 Cardiac Arrhythmias

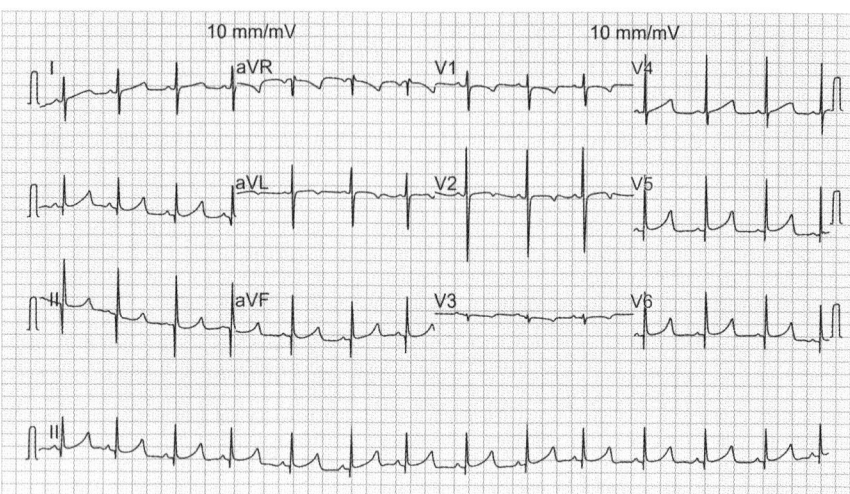

Fig. 9.7A: A standardized 12-lead ECG demonstrating sinus rhythm with an asymmetric T wave and a prolonged QTc measuring 480 milliseconds.

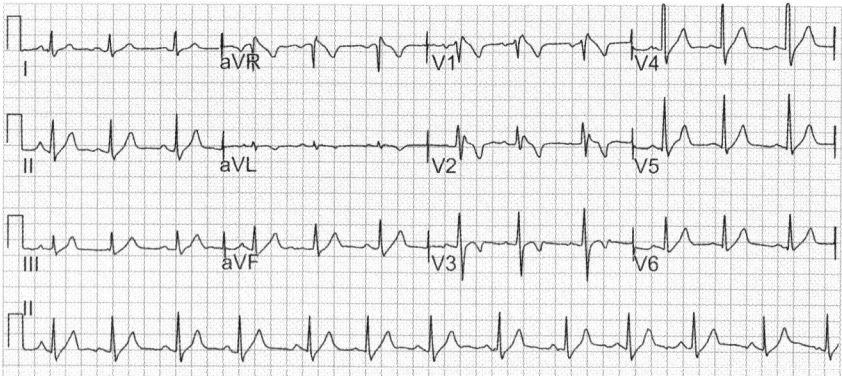

Fig. 9.7B: A standardized 12-lead ECG of a 9-year-old boy with recurrent syncope. There is evidence of right bundle branch block and a typical "cove type ST elevation" in the right precordial lead typical of Brugada syndrome.

gastroenteritis) and family history of sudden unexpected deaths in young members. In addition, channelopathies are implicated in approximately 10% of cases of sudden infant death syndrome (SIDS). The most important evaluation in these patients includes a detailed family history and a 12-lead ECG of the index patient as well as available family members. When a strong suspicion remains after the initial evaluation, provocative testing such as an exercise stress test, adrenaline challenge test or ajmaline challenge test should be considered along with genetic testing. Genetic testing enables genotype specific therapy and permits cascade testing to identify family members who could potentially be at risk for sudden death.[27] The genes implicated in channelopathies are listed in **Table 9.3**.

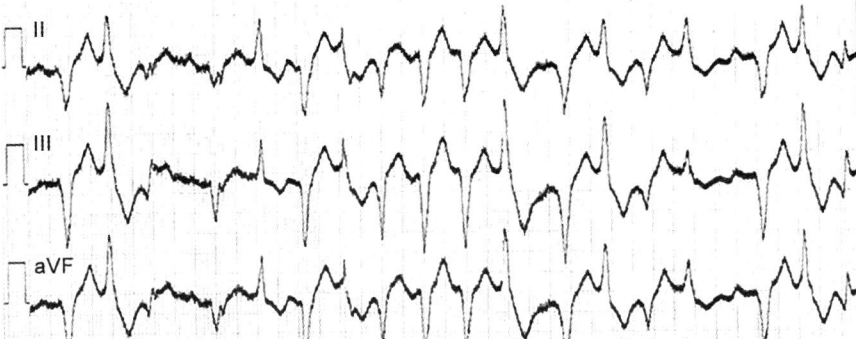

Fig. 9.7C: A three lead telemetry from continuous ECG monitoring of a child with recurrent syncope. There is polymorphic ventricular tachycardia and evidence of a bidirectional ventricular tachycardia which is a diagnostic feature of catecholaminergic polymorphic ventricular tachycardia (CPVT).

TABLE 9.3: The genes implicated in the various inherited arrhythmias.

Inherited arrhythmias	Genes implicated
Classic LQTS	KCNQ1 (LQTS 1) KCNH2 (LQTS 2) SCN5A (LQTS 3)
Atypical LQTS	CALM 1-3 (Calmodulinopathies) TRDN (Triadin knockout syndrome)
Syndromic LQTS	CACNA1C (Timothy syndrome) KCNJ2 (Andersen–Tawil syndrome)
Brugada syndrome	SCN5A
Catecholaminergic polymorphic ventricular tachycardia	RYR2 (Ryanodine receptor 2 – Autosomal dominant) CASQ2 (Calsequestrin – Autosomal recessive) CALM 1-3 (Calmodulinopathy – Autosomal dominant)

(LQTS: long QT syndrome)

A multicenter study on fetuses and neonates with a severe form of LQTS which included Indian children identified LQTS 3 positive genotype to be associated with an increased risk of adverse outcomes including death.[28] Such improved understanding about the genetics and molecular mechanisms of disease has opened avenues for genotype specific therapy in channelopathies (the so called "precision medicine").

Drug Therapy for Inherited Arrhythmias in Children

Mexiletine, a sodium channel blocker has been shown to reduce QTc interval and improve clinical outcomes in LQTS 3. Mexiletine, however, is a non-selective sodium channel blocker. The drug needs to be administered thrice daily and its bitter taste results in a problem with compliance in children. Recently a selective inhibitor of the sodium channel involved in LQTS3, *eleclazine,* has been developed, and has shown promising results in preliminary reports.[27] Similar genotype-specific therapies are in various stages of development for LQTS 2 and CPVT.

Despite improvements in pharmacological therapy, children with inherited arrhythmias remain at high risk for malignant ventricular arrhythmias. Many of them will require ICD to effectively manage their arrhythmias. While endocardial implantation of ICD is preferable, the weight threshold for implantation is usually above 30 kg. Epicardial insertion of ICD is frequently complicated by lead migration **(Fig. 9.8A)**. The recent development of subcutaneously implanted defibrillators **(Fig. 9.8B)** and early evidence of their utility in the pediatric age group provides hope about improved outcomes in this difficult cohort.

Recognizing the challenges related to inherited arrhythmias in the Indian population and the lack of India-specific genetic and clinical data, the Government of India backed Genomics for Understanding Rare Diseases India Alliance Network (GUaRDIAN) has initiated a research network to identify the genetic basis of these diseases in the Indian population. Further information on this project is available at their website https://guardian.genomes.in/research/heart.

■ FUTURE DIRECTIONS

As mentioned in the introduction to the chapter, the expertise for managing pediatric cardiac arrhythmia is lacking among practicing pediatricians

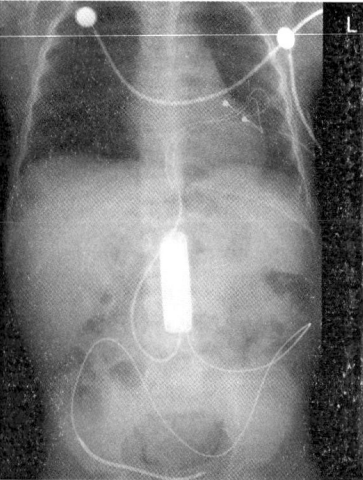

Fig. 9.8A: An abdominal X-ray of a child with an epicardial inserted implantable cardioverter defibrillator with migration of the lead to the pelvis.

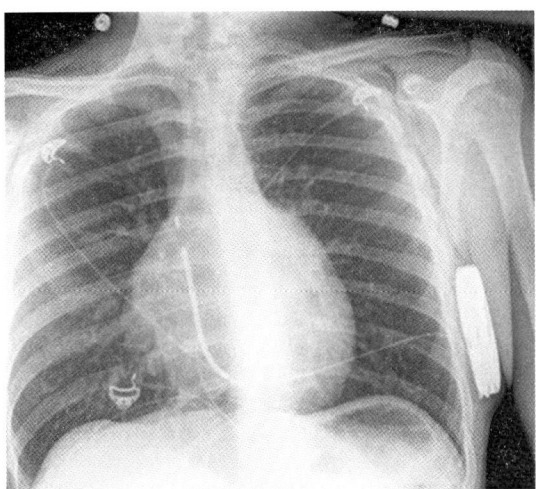

Fig. 9.8B: A chest X-ray of a 14-year-old girl with a subcutaneously inserted implantable cardioverter defibrillator.
Source: Dr Balaji Seshadri, Pediatric Electrophysiologist, Oregon, USA.

and pediatric trainees. With the sole objective of imparting the correct interpretative skills in identifying potentially dangerous cardiac dysrhythmias in children, very informative "hands on experience" workshops for pediatricians with analytical explanatory ECG training modules are being conducted across the country similar to PALS and NALS courses. These have proven to be effective in imparting the essential skills for ECG interpretation and detection to pediatricians to institute the appropriate management protocols to bring about a desirable outcome.

■ KEY POINTS

- Cardiac arrhythmias are not uncommon in children and pediatricians need to be aware of the presenting clinical features as well as basic interpretation of ECG.
- Ambulatory ECG monitoring (aECG) is an important tool for the evaluation of children with suspected rhythm disorders. Advancements in technology has led to the development of patch ECG monitors which are more convenient and offer longer duration of monitoring than the traditional Holter.
- A number of newer antiarrhythmic drugs have been recognized in the recent past. The safety of some of these drugs in children has already been established and the drugs are widely available in our country. It is important that pediatricians remain updated about the utility of these newer agents.
- Children with difficult to control arrhythmias require more invasive therapy including radiofrequency ablation and implantation of cardiac electrical devices. The technology behind both these interventional procedures has evolved over the last few years making them safer and more effective.
- Inherited arrhythmias are not uncommon in the Indian population. Pediatricians need to be aware of the clinical presentation and recognize symptoms early in order to prevent sudden death.

REFERENCES

1. Hanash CR, Crosson JE. Emergency diagnosis and management of pediatric arrhythmias. J Emerg Trauma Shock. 2010;3(3):251-60.
2. Del Mar B. The history of clinical Holter monitoring. Ann Noninvas Electrocardiol. 2005;10(2):226-30.
3. Bolourchi M, Batra AS. Diagnostic yield of patch ambulatory electrocardiogram monitoring in children (from a national registry). Am J Cardiol. 2015;115(5):630-4.
4. Fung E, Jarvelin MR, Doshi RN, Shinbane JS, Carlson SK, Grazette LP, et al. Electrocardiographic patch devices and contemporary wireless cardiac monitoring. Front Physiol. 2015;6:149.
5. Krishna MR, Sennaiyan UN, Ramanathan K. The utility of patch recorders in neonatal ambulatory electrocardiogram recording. Indian Pacing Electrophysiol J. 2021;21(2):128-31.
6. Lei M, Wu L, Terrar DA, Huang CL. Modernized classification of cardiac antiarrhythmic drugs. Circulation. 2018;138(17):1879-96.
7. Faisaluddin M, Ashish K, Hajra A, Mondal S, Bandyopadhyay D. Etripamil: self-management of supraventricular tachycardia is not far away? Int J Cardiol Heart Vasc. 2019;22:82-3.
8. Stambler BS, Dorian P, Sager PT, Wight D, Douville P, Potvin D, et al. Etripamil nasal spray for rapid conversion of supraventricular tachycardia to sinus rhythm. J Am Coll Cardiol. 2018;72(5):489-97.
9. Mason PK, DiMarco JP. New pharmacological agents for arrhythmias. Circ Arrhythm Electrophysiol. 2009;2(5):588-97.
10. Dieks JK, Klehs S, Muller MJ, Paul T, Krause U. Adjunctive ivabradine in combination with amiodarone: A novel therapy for pediatric congenital junctional ectopic tachycardia. Heart Rhythm. 2016;13(6):1297-302.
11. Krishna MR, Kunde MF, Kumar RK, Balaji S. Ivabradine in post-operative junctional ectopic tachycardia (JET): Breaking new ground. Pediatr Cardiol. 2019;40(6):1284-8.
12. Arvind B, Kothari SS, Juneja R, Saxena A, Ramakrishnan S, Gupta SK, et al. Ivabradine versus amiodarone in the management of postoperative junctional ectopic tachycardia: A randomized, open-label, noninferiority study. JACC Clin Electrophysiol. 2021;7(8):1052-60.
13. Janson CM, Tan RB, Iyer VR, Vogel RL, Vetter VL, Shah MJ. Ivabradine for treatment of tachyarrhythmias in children and young adults. Heart Rhythm Case Rep. 2019;5(6):333-7.
14. Bonnet D, Berger F, Jokinen E, Kantor PF, Daubeney PEF. Ivabradine in children with dilated cardiomyopathy and symptomatic chronic heart failure. J Am Coll Cardiol. 2017;70(10):1262-72.
15. Luedtke SA, Kuhn RJ, McCaffrey FM. Pharmacologic management of supraventricular tachycardias in children. Part 1: Wolff-Parkinson-White and atrioventricular nodal reentry. Ann Pharmacother. 1997;31(10):1227-43.
16. Ponnusamy SS, Muthu G, Kumar M, Bopanna D, Anand V, Balasubramanian S. Safety, efficacy, and intermediate-term outcomes of radiofrequency catheter ablation for pediatric arrhythmias. Cureus. 2020;12(9):e10488.
17. An HS, Choi EY, Kwon BS, Kim GB, Bae EJ, Noh CI, et al. Radiofrequency catheter ablation for supraventricular tachycardia: a comparison study of children aged 0-4 and 5-9 years. Pacing Clin Electrophysiol. 2013;36(12):1488-94.

18. Sanatani S, Cunningham T, Khairy P, Cohen MI, Hamilton RM, Ackerman MJ. The current state and future potential of pediatric and congenital electrophysiology. JACC Clin Electrophysiol. 2017;3(3):195-206.
19. Gulletta S, Tsiachris D, Radinovic A, Bisceglia C, Mazzone P, Trevisi N, et al. Safety and efficacy of open irrigated-tip catheter ablation of Wolff-Parkinson-White syndrome in children and adolescents. Pacing Clin Electrophysiol. 2013;36(4):486-90.
20. Drago F, Silvetti MS, Di Pino A, Grutter G, Bevilacqua M, Leibovich S. Exclusion of fluoroscopy during ablation treatment of right accessory pathway in children. J Cardiovasc Electrophysiol. 2002;13(8):778-82.
21. Nagaraju L, Menon D, Aziz PF. Use of 3D electroanatomical navigation (CARTO-3) to Minimize or Eliminate Fluoroscopy Use in the Ablation of Pediatric Supraventricular Tachyarrhythmias. Pacing Clin Electrophysiol. 2016;39(6):574-80.
22. Schoene K, Rolf S, Schloma D, John S, Arya A, Dinov B, et al. Ablation of typical atrial flutter using a non-fluoroscopic catheter tracking system vs. conventional fluoroscopy—results from a prospective randomized study. Europace. 2015;17(7):1117-21.
23. Seslar SP, Kugler J, Batra AS, Collins KK, Crosson J, Dubin AM, et al. The Multicenter Pediatric and Adult Congenital EP Quality (MAP-IT) Initiative-rationale and design: report from the pediatric and congenital electrophysiology society's MAP-IT taskforce. Congenit Heart Dis. 2013;8(5):381-92.
24. Mahendran AK, Bussey S, Chang PM. Leadless Pacemaker Implantation in a Four-year-old, 16-kg Child. J Innov Card Rhythm Manag. 2020;11(10):4257-61.
25. von Alvensleben JC, Collins KK. Leadless Pacemakers in Pediatric Patients: Is Less Actually More? J Innov Card Rhythm Manag. 2020;11(10):4263-4.
26. Behere SP, Weindling SN. Inherited arrhythmias: the cardiac channelopathies. Ann Pediatr Cardiol. 2015;8(3):210-20.
27. Natarajan KU, Krishna MR. Channelopathies: an update 2018. Indian Pacing Electrophysiol J. 2019;19(2):68-71.
28. Moore JP, Gallotti RG, Shannon KM, Bos JM, Sadeghi E, Strasburger JF, et al. Genotype predicts outcomes in fetuses and neonates with severe congenital long QT syndrome. JACC Clin Electrophysiol. 2020;6(12):1561-70.

Pulmonology

CHAPTER 10: Cystic Fibrosis: An Emerging Illness in India

Nitin Dhochak, Sushil Kumar Kabra

■ INTRODUCTION

Cystic fibrosis (CF) is an autosomal recessive multisystem disorder characterized by chronic airway disease and fat malabsorption. It is the most common recessive life-limiting genetic condition in Caucasian population. Most western countries perform routine newborn screening for CF which leads to early diagnosis and optimization of care. Though initially considered to be a disease of western world, more and more children are diagnosed with CF in India since description of earliest cases in 1968.[1] Difference in mutation profile, delayed diagnosis, advanced disease in childhood, frequent malnutrition, and poor affordability to long-term medical care, pose special challenges in management of children with CF in India.[2] In this document, we will discuss the status of CF in India, innovations in diagnostic testing and treatment with special focus on developing world.

■ BURDEN OF DISEASE

Incidence of CF in Canada, United States, Western Europe, and Eastern Europe are approximately 1 in 3,300, 4,000, 4,500, and 6,000 live births respectively. More than 30,000 individuals live with CF in United States alone, while numbers are more than 70,000 worldwide.[3]

Due to gross underdiagnosis and lack of registries, true incidence of CF in India is unknown. Based on epidemiological studies among migrant population of Indian origin in USA and UK, incidence of CF in India was estimated to be 1 in 40,000 and 10,000 live births respectively.[4,5] In a study of cord blood samples from 995 newborns, F508del mutation was detected in 4 samples. Considering frequency of F508del homozygous cases ranging from 19 to 44%, overall incidence of CF was estimated between 1 in 43,321 and 100,323 live births.[6]

■ PATHOPHYSIOLOGY

Cystic fibrosis results from abnormalities in CF transmembrane conductance regulator (CFTR) protein transcribed by *CFTR* gene on long arm of chromosome 7 at position 7q13. CFTR is a cyclic AMP-regulated chloride channel present on apical membrane of airway epithelial cells. CFTR is functionally linked to calcium-dependent chloride channel and epithelial sodium channels (ENaC). In healthy state, extracellular shift of chloride ion maintains hydration of airway epithelial layer surface liquid. Decrease in CFTR function and overactive ENaC lead to dehydration of airway surface liquid. This leads to desiccated and acidic airway secretions and impaired ciliary dysfunction. Poor clearance of thick secretions leads to blockage of small airways leading to hyperinflation. Recurrent infections especially due to *Staphylococcus* and *Pseudomonas*, concentrated inflammatory mediators, and impairment of innate defenses gradually lead to recurrent pneumonia and bronchiectasis.[7] Thick viscid secretions in pancreas lead to blockage of pancreatic ducts, activation of enzymes, and pancreatic injury, eventually progressing to exocrine pancreatic insufficiency initially, followed by endocrine insufficiency. Poor resorption of chloride ions in sweat leads to excessive losses of electrolytes in sweat which can result in hyponatremia, hypochloremia and dehydration in hot weather; renin-angiotensin system activation further leads to hypokalemia and metabolic alkalosis, also known as pseudo-Bartter syndrome.[8]

■ GENETICS

More than 2,000 mutations causing CF have been identified, affecting CFTR expression at different steps. Traditionally *CFTR* mutations are described in five classes, newer classification systems have proposed up to seven classes.[9] Classification of mutations is summarized in **Table 10.1**.

Cystic fibrosis being an autosomal recessive disorder requires *CFTR* gene mutation on both chromosomes for disease manifestations. The mutation can be same on both chromosomes (homozygous) or different (compound heterozygote). Class I, II, III and VII usually have severe defects and are associated with severe lung disease and pancreatic exocrine insufficiency. Class IV, V and VI have some residual CFTR activity, hence less severe lung disease and may have residual pancreatic exocrine function, but are predisposed for recurrent pancreatitis.[9]

Profile of CFTR Mutations

Worldwide, F508del is the most common mutation with varying frequency across regions. In UK, F508del constitute approximately 76% of all *CFTR* gene mutations; *G542X* and *G551D* are the other common mutations. Overall F508del constituted 65% of all *CFTR* mutation alleles in Europe; few countries had low frequency of the mutation (e.g., Turkey 27%, Tunisia 18%).[10] In USA, F508del constitutes nearly 65% of all *CFTR* mutations (44.2% homozygous and 40.5% heterozygous for F508del among all CF patients).[11]

TABLE 10.1: *CFTR* mutation classification.

Class	Defect	Examples	Potential therapies
I	Immature stop codon, no protein synthesis	Gly542X, Trp1282X	Read through agents
II	Misfolded protein, retained and destroyed at endoplasmic reticulum	Phe508del, Asn1303Lys, Ala561Glu	Correctors + Potentiators
III	Impaired gating	Gly551Asp, Ser549Arg, Gly1349Asp	Potentiators
IV	Impaired conductance	Arg117His, Arg334Trp, Ala455Glu	Potentiators
V	Reduction in surface CFTR concentration, usually splice variants	Ala455Glu, 3272-26A→G, 3849+10 kb C→T	Antisense oligonucleotides, correctors, potentiators
VI	Unstable CFTR, increased endocytosis	c.120del23, rPhe508del	Stabilizers
VII	Large deletions, no mRNA production	dele2,3(21 kb), 1717-1G→A	Unrescuable

Source: De Boeck K, Amaral MD. Progress in therapies for cystic fibrosis. Lancet Respir Med. 2016;4(8):662-74.

In Indian population, mutation profile is very different from western population as well as in different regions across India. Proportion of F508del among *CFTR* mutations varies between 19 and 44% in different studies.[12-16] Other common mutations included 1161delC, 3849+10kbC-T and S549N.[13,16] Children from Indian states of Jammu and Kashmir, Punjab, and Gujarat, had higher proportion of F508del mutation. Among children whose ancestors could be traced to Pakistan, 56% had F508del mutations compared to 12% in rest of the children.[12]

■ CLINICAL FEATURES

As most developed countries have newborn screening for CF, most of the patients are diagnosed in neonatal period and early infancy. These children are frequently asymptomatic at the time of diagnosis and early instillation of treatment delays the progression of pulmonary morbidity. Due to lack of newborn screening, relative rarity of disease, lack of awareness among pediatric physicians and lack of methods for diagnosis of CF, children are frequently diagnosed late when there is advanced pulmonary disease with bronchiectasis and *Pseudomonas* colonization along with malnutrition.[17] In studies performed between 2002 and 2003 in India, median age of diagnosis

TABLE 10.2: Clinical manifestation of cystic fibrosis in India.

Clinical features	n = 120[12]	n = 18[19]
Symptoms		
Recurrent/persistent pneumonia	118 (98%)	13 (73%)
Chronic cough		14 (77.8%)
Recurrent wheezing		10 (55.6%)
Failure to thrive	108 (90%)	17 (94%)
Malabsorption	96 (80%)	9 (50%)
Recurrent sinusitis		5 (28%)
Dehydration	16 (13%)	
Rectal prolapse	16 (13%)	1 (5.6%)
Meconium ileus	10 (8%)	
Salty taste	5 (5%)	
Salt craving	5 (5%)	
Skin rashes	5 (5%)	
Vitamin D deficiency	4 (4%)	
Vitamin A deficiency	10 (8%)	
Pneumothorax/empyema	3 (3%)	
Meconium ileus equivalent	2 (2%)	
Deafness	2 (2%)	
Examination		
Severe malnutrition	50 (42%)	
Z-score for weight for age*	−2.59 (−3.01, −2.32)	
Clubbing	80 (75%)	13 (72%)
Chest hyperinflation	100 (83%)	
Crepitations	110 (92%)	
Rhonchi	40 (33%)	
Bronchial breathing	20 (17%)	
Nasal polyposis	5 (4%)	
CF score*	51 (20, 80)	

*Mean (95% confidence interval)
Source: References 12 and 19.

was 4.8 years and 30 months respectively.[12,18] More recently in 2019, though the median age of diagnosis has improved to 22 months, there is still gap of nearly 20 months between onset of symptoms and diagnosis (median age of onset of symptoms being 2.7 months).[2] Disease manifestations vary as per time of diagnosis in children. A summary of studies on clinical features in children with CF in India is presented in **Table 10.2**.

Clinical features also vary with age of the child. Age-specific manifestations of CF are summarized in **Table 10.3**.

Due to acidic secretion and thick dehydrated mucus, meconium is hardened and can cause obstruction at ileocecal junction antenatally or at birth. This is known as *meconium ileus*. Meconium ileus is seen in approximately 20% of neonates with CF. Neonates with meconium ileus have CF in 80–90% cases, necessitating evaluation for CF in all neonates with

TABLE 10.3: Clinical features of cystic fibrosis according to age of child.

Age group	Clinical features
Neonatal period	• Meconium ileus, meconium peritonitis, bowel perforation • Prolonged neonatal jaundice • Persistent cough, hyperinflation, lung collapse
Infants	• Prolonged jaundice • Persistent cough, recurrent wheezing, recurrent pneumonia • Steatorrhea (may present once weaning feed is started) • Micronutrient deficiency (hemolytic anemia due to vitamin E deficiency, acrodermatitis enteropathica) • Hypoalbuminemia • Dehydration with electrolyte disturbances, especially in summer months (Hyponatremia, hypochloremia, hypokalemia, metabolic alkalosis; also known as Pseudo-Bartter syndrome) • Rectal prolapse
Toddlers and preschool children	• Recurrent and persistent pneumonia, chronic wet cough • Steatorrhea, malnutrition • Dehydration and electrolyte abnormalities • Micronutrient deficiency, especially fat-soluble vitamin deficiency • Distal intestinal obstruction syndrome (Meconium ileus equivalent) • CF-related liver disease • Rectal prolapse
School-going children	• Productive cough • Recurrent pneumonia • Bronchiectasis • ABPA • Steatorrhea • Distal intestinal obstruction syndrome (meconium ileus equivalent) • CF-related liver disease • Failure to thrive
Adolescents	• Chronic bronchiectasis and recurrent pneumonia • ABPA • CF-related diabetes • CF-related liver disease • Azoospermia • Depression and psychosocial abnormality • Hypertrophic pulmonary osteoarthropathy • Decreased bone mineral density

(ABPA: allergic bronchopulmonary aspergillosis; CF: cystic fibrosis) meconium ileus.[19] In childhood, similar presentation of intestinal obstruction is seen due to collection of hardened stools in ileocecal region, known as distal intestinal obstruction syndrome (DIOS).

At birth, airways are sterile in children with CF. Different organisms predominate in different age groups. *Haemophilus influenzae* and *Staphylococcus aureus* appear early in life (infants and children) while *Pseudomonas aeruginosa* infection occurs later (adolescents and adults) in developed countries.[20,21] Series from India suggest that *Pseudomonas* is frequently seen in infants and young children with CF.[22,23] In studies from India, *Pseudomonas* is the commonest agent isolated followed by *Burkholderia cepacia*, *Staphylococcus* species and *Acinetobacter*.[22] Other colonizing agents include fungi (*Aspergillus fumigatus*, *Candida* species, and *Mycobacterium tuberculosis*). Non-tubercular mycobacteria were not identified in any of the 104 children in an Indian study.[22]

Infants and toddlers may develop rectal prolapse; common contributing factors being constipation and straining, fat malabsorption, uncontrolled pulmonary disease and chronic cough, and malnutrition.[24] Rectal prolapse usually improves by correcting these factors.

During summer months, excessive water, and electrolyte loss due to excessive sweating with poor oral replenishment in infants and young children leads to dehydration with dyselectrolytemia (hyponatremia and hypochloremia). Renin-angiotensin axis-mediated water and sodium reabsorption and potassium excretion in kidney and sweat lead to hypokalemia. Metabolic alkalosis is due to contraction of extracellular fluid, hypochloremia, and secretion of hydrogen ion in kidneys.[25] In a few infants such episodes may be the presenting feature of CF.[8,25] These are frequently confused with Bartter syndrome.

As children grow older, bystander injury and progressive loss of beta cell in pancreatic islets lead to insulin deficiency. This is initially apparent in periods of high glucose loads (post-meal hyperglycemia with normal fasting blood glucose), which gradually progress to severe insulin insufficiency, known as CF-related diabetes (CFRD).[26] Other hypotheses point toward dysfunctional insulin and glucagon release by pancreatic islet cells due to primary dysfunction of CFTR channels. CFRD is present in 2% of children and 19% of adolescents. In adults, CFRD is seen in 40% of individuals in their 20s, and 45–50% of those aged ≥30 years.[27] In a study of Indian children with CF, 23% had abnormal glucose tolerance test (mean age 11 years).[28] Children with CFRD may present with typical diabetic manifestations of polyuria, polydipsia, weight loss or poor weight gain, and frequent pulmonary exacerbations.

Flowchart 10.1: Diagnostic algorithm of cystic fibrosis.

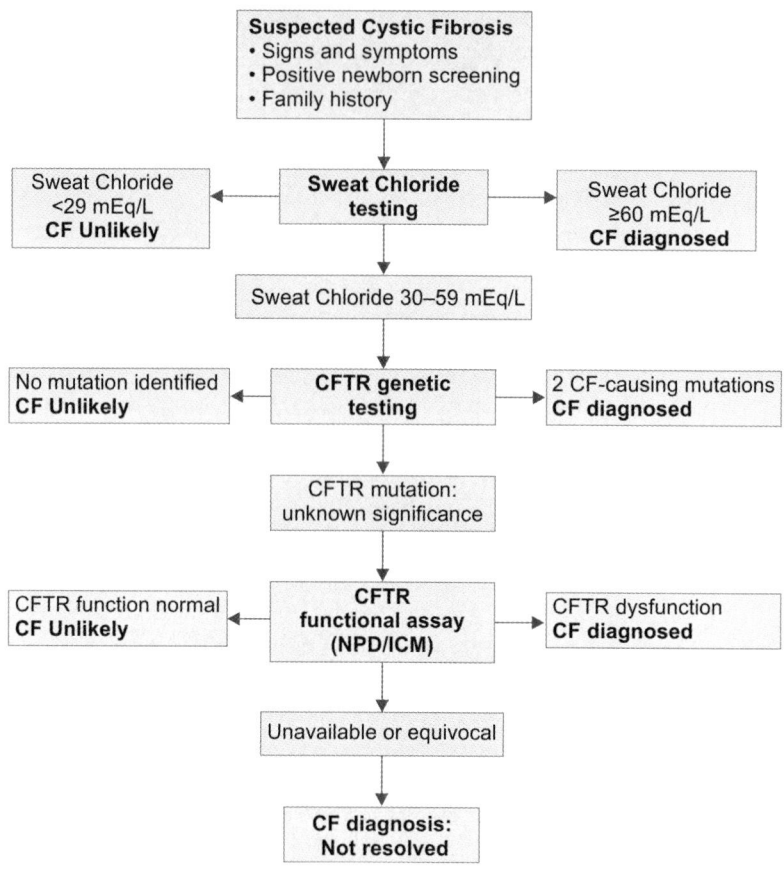

DIAGNOSIS OF CYSTIC FIBROSIS

Diagnostic tests for CF include sweat chloride estimation, *CFTR* mutation analysis, and CFTR physiological testing [nasal potential difference (NPD) or intestinal current measurement (ICM)], preferably done sequentially in that order. Diagnostic algorithm based on Consensus Guidelines from the Cystic Fibrosis Foundation is described in **Flowchart 10.1**.[29]

Sweat Chloride Estimation

Sweat chloride estimation is first-line investigation in the diagnosis of CF. Elevated sweat chloride ($\geq$ 60 mEq/L) is highly sensitive (99%) and specific (93%) for the diagnosis of CF.[30] The test includes two steps: (1) collection of sweat by pilocarpine iontophoresis, and (2) estimation of sweat chloride. Sweat chloride estimation should be performed in neonates > 36 weeks corrected for gestational age and > 2 kg weight, after 48 hours of life—preferably after 10 days of life, ideally by 28 days. Sweat chloride may be falsely elevated in the first 24 hours of life.[29]

Sweat testing can be done using Gibson and Cooke method or Macroduct sweat test system. In Gibson and Cooke method, sweat production is stimulated by pilocarpine iontophoresis by passing current through a pilocarpine-soaked filter paper/gauze for 5 minutes. The stimulated area must be 2 inches by 2 inches (4 inches^2) and electrode must cover at least 2 inches.[2] Thereafter, a dry filter paper is applied to the stimulated area for up to 30 minutes for sweat collection. The minimum acceptable sweat weight is 75 mg. Sweat chloride estimation can be performed by chemical titration of chloride ions.[29] A commercially available Macroduct sweat testing system uses coil for collecting sweat (minimum required sweat amount is 15 µL) and automated chloridometer for estimation of chloride concentration.[30] Sweat chloride values of ≥ 60 mEq/L are considered as positive test, 30–59 mEq/L as intermediate and ≤ 29 mEq/L are considered as negative.

Availability of sweat chloride estimation system is scarce in India and is available only in limited centers. An indigenously made sweat collection system based on Gibson and Cooke method was devised which significantly reduced the cost of sweat chloride test **(Figs. 10.1A and B)**. Cost of this equipment was 7 US$ (500 rupees) and cost of each test was 0.5 US$ (35 rupees). The method had excellent repeatability (intraobserver variability of 2.5 ± 4.24 mEq/L, and interobserver variability of 1.12 ± 4.34 mEq/L).[31]

Causes of elevated sweat chloride other than CF may be untreated adrenal insufficiency, atopic dermatitis, hereditary nephrogenic diabetes insipidus, malnutrition, mucopolysaccharidosis, hypothyroidism, and glycogen storage disorder.

Mutation Analysis

Identification of two disease-causing mutations can be considered diagnostic of CF. Mutation analysis is useful in children with consistently borderline sweat chloride estimations. More than 2,000 mutations have been identified

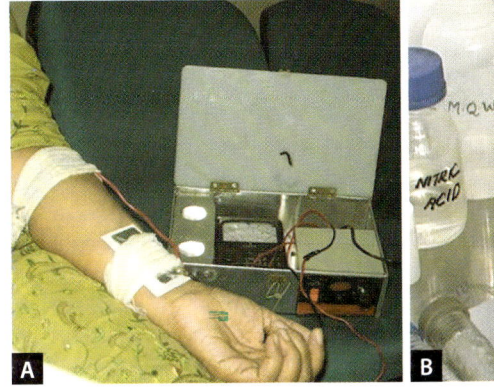
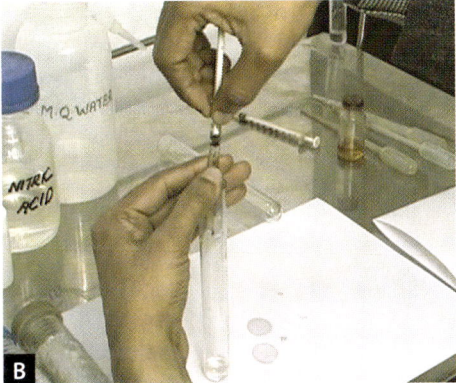

Figs. 10.1A and B: (A) Indigenous sweat collection system; (B) Chloride titration by mercuric nitrate.

in patients with CF. In Caucasian population, a small number of mutations identify large number of CFTR mutations. A panel of four most common mutations including F508del, G551D, G542X and 621+1G>T identify >80% of disease-causing CFTR mutations. Extended panels further increase the sensitivity.[32] Pathogenicity of CFTR mutations identified can be checked on online repository (https://www.cftr2.org/index.php). Due to very low frequency of F508del and wide variability in mutation profile in India, these mutation panels are not useful.[6]

Sequencing of *CFTR* gene can identify mutations in children where common mutations are not present and in areas where sweat testing is not available. But it is costly and frequently identifies mutations of unknown significance.

Apart from diagnosis, identification of CFTR mutations has significance in genetic counseling and antenatal screening of CF in future pregnancies, and eligibility for newer targeted therapies. It should be offered to all patients with diagnosed CF, especially when parents plan for further pregnancies.

CFTR Physiological Testing

Nasal potential difference (NPD) and intestinal current measurement (ICM) are tests to assess functional status of CFTR channels. In patients with intermediate sweat chloride and less than 2 disease-causing mutations, physiological testing can help in the diagnosis of CF.[33] Currently these tests are not available in India.

Basal NPD is more negative in children with CF. A larger change in potential is seen on blocking of Na channels by amiloride (representing hyperfunctioning of ENaC) in children with CF, and no change in potential is seen in response to CFTR stimulation by zero chloride solution and isoproterenol. Stimulation of other chloride channels by ATP shows normal response in both children with CF and healthy subjects. Limitations of NPD include lack of wide availability, and large variability in cut-offs (vary between labs) and intrasubject variability.

Intestinal current measurement is an ex vivo test, performed on rectal biopsy tissue sample. Response to stimulation by carbachol and histamine has two components: positive current by potassium efflux and negative current by chloride efflux through CFTR channel. In healthy subjects, chloride efflux masks potassium efflux, while in CF, current is reverse due to only potassium efflux.

Cystic Fibrosis Newborn Screening

In most developed countries, routine newborn screening is performed for CF. In most places, tiered screening approach is used. First tier test for CF screen is immunoreactive trypsinogen (IRT) by heal prick blood sample within

24–72 hours (marker of pancreatic injury). If IRT is elevated, child undergoes second tier screen, which varies in different places; could be repeat IRT (at 2–4 weeks), mutation panel or pancreatic-associated-protein. Patients with positive screen have to be confirmed for diagnosis by a confirmatory test (most commonly sweat chloride).[33]

In India, CF newborn screening is not a routine. As the sensitivity and specificity of IRT test is not very good, it cannot be used for making a diagnosis of CF. Confirmatory test is necessary for those positive on IRT screening. Patients with meconium ileus may have low IRT levels even with CF; so all children with meconium ileus should be evaluated by CF diagnostic tests. As CFTR mutations are highly variable in India, use of a panel of mutations is not a preferred second tier test.

If sweat test facility is not available, children with symptomatic disease and multiple suggestive features of CF including recurrent/persistent pneumonia with malabsorption, family history of CF, positive aquagenic wrinkling (see below), biochemical profile (metabolic alkalosis, hypochloremia, hyponatremia and hypokalemia) and *Pseudomonas* colonization in sputum, should receive treatment for CF pending confirmatory test as and when available.

Other Tests

Children with CF are predisposed to the development of early skin wrinkling on exposure to water. Aquagenic wrinkling of skin of palm and fingers on dipping of hand in room temperature water can be used as a screening diagnostic test in children with CF **(Figs. 10.2A and B)**. Using a cut-off of 3 minutes, aquagenic wrinkling has modest diagnostic accuracy for CF (sensitivity = 81% and specificity = 57%).[34]

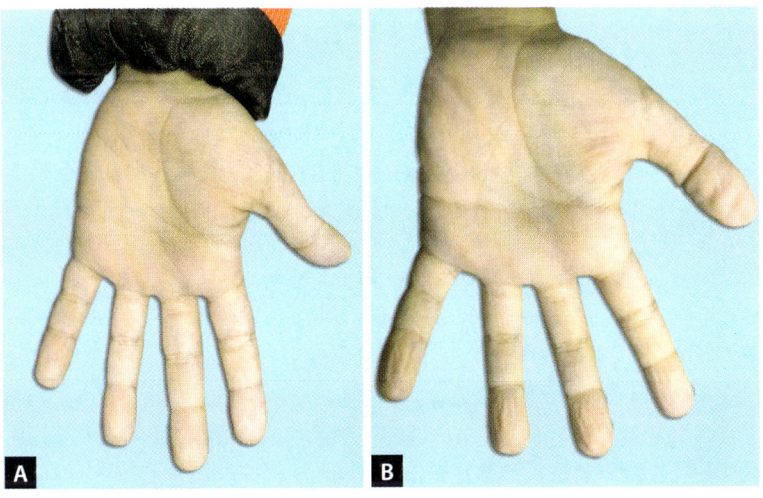

Figs. 10.2A and B: Aquagenic wrinkling demonstrated in a child with cystic fibrosis. (A) Picture of hand before test; (B) Wrinkling seen after 3 minutes of immersion in water.

Other tests are aimed for the following:
- *Estimation of disease severity:* For example, pulmonary function tests and chest imaging.
- *Detection of complications of CF:* These include—(1) total IgE and aspergillus-specific IgE for allergic bronchopulmonary aspergillosis; (2) oral glucose tolerance test and HbA1c for CFRD; (3) liver function tests and ultrasound abdomen for CF-related liver disease; and (4) echocardiography for pulmonary arterial hypertension.
- *Tests for airway colonization*: Sputum or cough swab bacterial culture should be routinely done; sputum for fungus and non-tubercular mycobacteria in selected cases with high suspicion.
- *Tests for pancreatic function:* Fecal elastase, fecal fat estimation, and stool for fat globules.

Spirometry (FEV1) is traditionally used to monitor pulmonary function. Lung clearance index (LCI) based on multiple breath washout technique, which is calculated as cumulative expired volume at the point where end-tidal inert gas concentration falls below 1/40th of the original concentration, divided by the functional residual capacity (FRC). LCI has been shown to be a more sensitive test for identification of pulmonary involvement in CF, especially due to its ability to better evaluate lower airway disease.[35]

Imaging findings vary with age and disease severity. Infants may present with hyperinflation and peribronchial thickening, especially in upper zones **(Fig. 10.3A)**. Older patients may show typical bronchiectasis, mucous plugging, with or without pulmonary hypertension **(Fig. 10.3B)**.

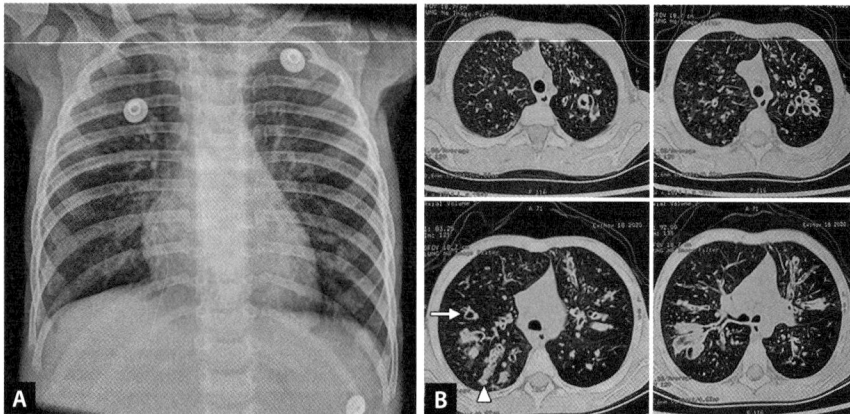

Figs. 10.3A and B: (A) Chest X-ray of an infant with cystic fibrosis showing hyperinflation (flattened diaphragm) and increased bronchial markings; (B) Older child contrast-enhanced CT scan of chest showing diffuse bronchiectasis (arrow mark pointed to typical signet ring sign), and mucus plugging (arrowhead).

MANAGEMENT

Management of children with CF can be divided into respiratory and nonrespiratory therapies. Respiratory therapies include airway clearance therapy, management of pulmonary exacerbations and airway colonization, and complications such as ABPA, pulmonary hemorrhage. Nonrespiratory therapies include pancreatic enzyme replacement, fat-soluble vitamin and micronutrient supplementations, and management of complications such as DIOS/meconium ileus, CFRD, and CF-related liver injury.

Respiratory Management

Airway Clearance Therapy

The secretions in children with CF are thick, dry, and viscid. These are difficult to clear without specific efforts. Airway clearance therapies have two main objectives—(1) thinning of airway secretions, and (2) clearance of secretions from airways. The sequence followed is administration of a bronchodilator followed by inhaled mucolytic medications followed by chest physiotherapy to remove the thinned secretions. Adequate water and salt intake also helps in maintaining hydration of respiratory secretions.

Mucolytic agents: Commonly used mucolytic agents include recombinant human DNase, hypertonic saline (HS), inhaled mannitol, and N-acetyl cysteine (inhaled or oral).

Recombinant human DNase: Children with CF have high DNA content in respiratory secretions due to disintegration of neutrophils and inflammatory cells. Use of DNase is associated with improved lung clearance, decrease in pulmonary exacerbations, and decrease in lung function deterioration.[36] Dose of inhaled DNase is 2.5 mg (2.5 mL solution) by nebulization once daily (may be given twice daily in selected patients). Side effects include airway irritation, hypersensitivity, rash, chest pain, and conjunctivitis. It is not routinely available in India.

Hypertonic saline (HS): HS (3% saline and 7% saline) is used by nebulization to stimulate mucociliary clearance, increase hydration, and hence loosening of respiratory secretions. Though mechanism of DNase is different and there are no randomized control trials to compare HS and DNase, the relatively inexpensive HS can be used to enhance airway clearance. HS may cause bronchoconstriction and excessive coughing in some patients; hence salbutamol inhalation [by metered dose inhaler (MDI) or nebulization] is given before HS nebulization. Clinical trials between 3% and 7% HS showed slightly better lung function after 3% saline use.[37] HS nebulization should be given twice daily (usually 3–5 mL nebulization, may be given more frequently as needed) 15–30 minutes before chest physiotherapy session.

Inhaled N-acetyl cysteine and inhaled mannitol (dry powder inhalation): These are not as well studied but can be utilized as add-on therapies if needed.

Inhaled steroids are given in children with features of reactive airway disease following chest physiotherapy and expectoration.

Chest physiotherapy: Aim of chest physiotherapy is movement of respiratory secretion from peripheral to central airways followed by huffing and coughing to expectorate the secretions. Deep inspiration and inspiratory hold (deep breathing, active cycle breathing, and autogenic drainage) help to accumulate air beyond secretions in peripheral airways, which then push these secretions out during exhalation. Positive airway pressure applied by various devices such as acapella, positive expiratory pressure (PEP) device and flutter help in splinting and opening of airways for facilitating air accumulation beyond secretions as well as separation of secretions from airway walls. Vibrations produced by chest percussions, acapella, flutter and high frequency chest wall oscillation vest also help in separation of secretions from airway wall. Different chest physiotherapy techniques are detailed below:[38]

- *Postural drainage and chest percussion*: This can be performed at any age even during exacerbations. As per CF Foundation recommendations, head down position should not be used for percussion and postural drainage.[39]
- *Positive expiratory pressure devices*: These include acapella, PEP device, flutter, starting from 5 to 6 years. They may be difficult to use during severe exacerbation.
- *Breathing exercises:* These include active cycle breathing (beyond 5 years), and autogenic drainage (beyond 8–10 years). These are difficult to perform during exacerbations.
- *High frequency chest wall oscillation*: These can be used at any age and during exacerbations.

Playful activity involving jumping (such as trampoline and skipping), inflating balloons, making soap bubbles, and tickling can also be incorporated in the chest physiotherapy routine to make it more acceptable to children. Postural drainage and chest percussion is dependent on care taken. Use of devices and breathing exercises enable older children to have independence on caretakers, making them more independent and simultaneously decreasing work for caretakers and parents.

Management of Pulmonary Exacerbations

Pulmonary exacerbations are defined as acute worsening of respiratory symptoms requiring medical treatment. For the sake of research, pulmonary exacerbations are commonly defined as the need for new antibiotic therapy along with combination of respiratory symptoms (change in sputum, increased cough, breathing difficulty, new oxygen requirement, hemoptysis or sinus pain), nonpulmonary symptoms (fever, decreased appetite or weight loss), change in chest examination, reduced pulmonary function and radiographic changes. The definition by Fuchs et al. included 4 (out of 12) signs/symptoms and use of new parenteral antibiotics.[36]

Treatment of pulmonary exacerbations requires *antibiotic therapy*. Choice of antibiotics is decided by culture of respiratory samples (sputum or cough swab), organisms isolated on last surveillance culture, and clinical clues (e.g., green sputum points toward *Pseudomonas* infection). As sputum culture in current exacerbation takes 48–72 hours to report, it is less helpful in deciding initial choice of antibiotics but is helpful in modification of antibiotic regimen. In developing countries, *Pseudomonas* colonization is very common in infancy and hence empirical antibiotics regimen should cover for *Pseudomonas* infection. For treatment of *Pseudomonas* and other gram-negative infection (e.g., *Burkholderia* and *Stenotrophomonas*), combination of two sensitive antibiotics is preferred over monotherapy and higher doses of antibiotics should be used.[40] Usual empirical regimen includes an antipseudomonal beta-lactam (cefoperazone-sulbactum, ceftazidime, cefepime or piperacillin-tazobactam) along with an aminoglycoside (amikacin). Multiple sputum/cough swab cultures (usually daily for initial 3 days, and later if not improving clinically) should be sent. Regimen may be modified as per culture sensitivity or lack of clinical improvement. Other choices of antibiotics for action against *Pseudomonas* include carbapenems (meropenem and imipenem), aztreonam, fluoroquinolones, cotrimoxazole, and polymyxin B/colistin.

Staphylococcal infection can be treated by a single antibiotic regimen. Antibiotics should be given for a duration of 10–21 days (usually 2 weeks). An ongoing trial (STOP 2) is studying the difference among various antibiotics durations (10 days vs. 14 days vs. 21 days).[41]

Reasons of nonimprovement in pulmonary exacerbations may be due to:
- Poor lung clearance therapies
- Lower antibiotic dosage
- Presence of multiple strains of *Pseudomonas* (selection of antibiotic-resistant strains)
- Atypical organism (*Burkholderia*, *Stenotrophomonas*, and nontubercular mycobacterium)
- Poor glycemic control or new onset CFRD
- Mimickers such as ABPA exacerbation.

Mild pulmonary exacerbation (no significant breathing difficulty and no oxygen requirement) may be treated with combinations of oral antibiotics if the organism is sensitive or no organism is isolated. The typical antibiotic regimen includes a fluoroquinolone (ciprofloxacin, ofloxacin or levofloxacin) and cotrimoxazole. For children with staphylococcal colonization, single oral sensitive antibiotic may be given.

Viral infection can also cause significant pulmonary symptoms. Viral infections can disturb bacterial microbiome and predispose for bacterial infections. Also, viral infection may cause wheezing in children with hyper-reactive airways. Viral infections are managed with appropriate antiviral (oseltamivir for influenza) and supportive care. Annual influenza vaccination is recommended for all children with CF.[40] It is observed that children with viral infection may have a long-term adverse outcome in the form of greater worsening of Shwachman-Kulczycki clinical score, number of pulmonary exacerbations requiring antibiotic usage and hospitalization and mortality (30.4% vs. 4.7% respectively).[42]

Prevention of Pulmonary Exacerbations

Pulmonary exacerbations cause significant pulmonary morbidity and decline in lung health. In various studies, 25–50% of individuals with pulmonary exacerbations did not achieve lung function to pre-exacerbation levels. Various therapies for prevention of pulmonary exacerbations aim at suppression of long-term colonizing organisms (mainly *Pseudomonas*).

Long-term azithromycin therapy has been associated with a decrease in pulmonary exacerbation in CF patients, especially with *Pseudomonas* colonization.[43] Azithromycin works by decreasing inflammation, decreasing mucoid transformation and pathogenicity of *Pseudomonas* and by antiviral effects. Typically, azithromycin is given as 3 days a week regimen (5–10 mg/kg/day). Daily regimen (5 mg/kg/day) may also be given.[44]

Inhaled antibiotics are recommended for children with *Pseudomonas* colonization. Commonly recommended antibiotics are tobramycin (300 mg twice daily), colistin (1–2 megaunit twice daily) or aztreonam. Traditionally inhaled antibiotics are given as alternate month regimen (1 month on and 1 month off regimen). More recently, continuous regimens with single antibiotic or continuous alternating regimen (alternating between two antibiotics every month) are the preferred approaches, especially if there are low lung functions and frequent exacerbations.[45]

Eradication Therapies for Bacterial Colonization

Pseudomonas aeruginosa is difficult to eradicate in children with CF. Intense antibiotic regimen is given at the time of first isolation of *Pseudomonas* irrespective of symptoms. The typical regimen includes:
- IV/oral sensitive antibiotic (usually oral fluoroquinolone) for 4 weeks, and
- Inhaled antibiotics for 4 weeks (some regimens recommend continuing inhaled antibiotics till sequential respiratory specimen culture is negative for *Pseudomonas*).

Repeat culture is performed at 4–6 weeks to demonstrate negative results. Regrowth may be treated with repeat systemic antibiotics or long-term inhaled antibiotic therapy.

Methicillin-resistant *Staphylococcus aureus* colonization should be treated with following regimen:
- Two oral antistaphylococcal antibiotics for 4 weeks.[46]
- Mupirocin local application for 4 weeks.
- Inhaled vancomycin for 4 weeks (optional, may be associated with bronchospasm).

Routine eradications therapy is not recommended for asymptomatic carriage of methicillin-sensitive *Staphylococcus aureus* and other gram-negative organisms.[46]

Allergic Bronchopulmonary Aspergillosis

Allergic bronchopulmonary aspergillosis (ABPA) is a serious complication of CF, which should be suspected in children with blackish granules in sputum, frequent wheezing, and recurrent exacerbations. Sometimes it may be diagnosed in annual surveillance investigations of hemogram, IgE and chest imaging. Indian children with CF are at increased risk of developing ABPA and risk factors include older age and poor clinical scores.[47,48] The diagnostic criteria for ABPA (ISHAM 2013) include the following:[49]
- *Major criteria (both should be present)*
  - Total serum IgE > 1,000 kU/L (> 500 kU/L may be taken as positive)
  - Aspergillus specific IgE > 0.35 kUA/L, or positive skin prick test for *Aspergillus fumigatus*
- *Minor criteria (2 out of 3 should be present)*
  - Compatible imaging finding (e.g., central bronchiectasis, high-attenuation mucus)
  - Eosinophilia (absolute eosinophil count > 500/mm^3)
  - IgG positivity for *Aspergillus fumigatus* (> 27 mgA/L)

Treatment for ABPA includes steroids with/without antifungal agents. Commonly combination of steroids and antifungals is preferred. Oral prednisolone 1–2 mg/kg/day for 2 weeks followed by tapering over 6 months is given. Antifungal therapy includes voriconazole or itraconazole for 6 months. Total IgE levels are done for monitoring for evaluating response to therapy.

Pulmonary Complications

Pulmonary complications include hemoptysis, pneumothorax and pulmonary arterial hypertension. Children with small hemoptysis are treated for coexistent bacterial infection. Compliance to vitamin K therapy and coagulation function should be assessed. Aggressive physiotherapy is avoided. Antifibrinolytic therapeutic agents (aminocaproic acid and tranexamic acid) should be given. Long-term antifibrinolytic therapy has been associated with 50% reduction in hemoptysis-related hospitalization and bleeding episodes in adults with CF.[50] Massive pulmonary hemorrhage requires urgent therapies by bronchial arterial embolization, endobronchial therapies (glue or bronchial blockers) and lung resection.

Pneumothorax is managed appropriately by drainage (pigtail or intercostal tube drainage). Recurrent pneumothorax should be treated by chemical or surgical pleurodesis. Pulmonary arterial hypertension is treated initially by diuretics (furosemide or furosemide-spironolactone combination); further therapy with sildenafil, endothelin receptor antagonists, etc., may be required in nonresponsive patients.

Nonrespiratory Therapies

Pancreatic Enzyme Replacement Therapy

Pancreatic enzyme replacement therapy (PERT) is administered as capsules containing enteric-coated spherules of pancreatic enzymes (lipase, amylase, and protease combinations). Common available preparation strengths include 10,000, 25,000 and 40,000 IU lipase content in capsule form. Small children may not be able to swallow capsule, and some may require lesser dose; capsule may be opened in such situation and appropriate dose may be swallowed (without chewing) after mixing in jam, juice, or curd (acidic food). PERT is administered immediately before meal. Usual dose of PERT is 500–1,000 U/kg/meal. Dose may be adjusted by monitoring clinical steatorrhea, growth, and stool fat content. Typically, daily PERT dose should be less than 6,500 U/kg/day. Doses higher than 10,000 U/kg/day may lead to fibrosing colonopathy.[51]

Nutritional Management of Cystic Fibrosis

Children with CF are at risk of malnutrition due to higher energy requirement, fat and micronutrients malabsorption, frequent infections, and delayed diagnosis. Malnutrition is associated with worse lung health and improved nutrition has been associated with longer life.

ESPEN-ESPGHAN-ECFS guidelines of nutritional management of CF recommend 110–120% of energy requirement for the age directed to achieve 50th centile of weight and height for the age (< 1 year age) and BMI for age (older than 1 year).[52] Diet plan should not be rigid and should be modified to suit child's preferences and socially appropriate food. If calorie targets are not achieved, nasogastric or gastrostomy feeding may be required. Nutritional status should be assessed on every visit and plotted to view trends.

Breastfed infants should be supplemented for sodium 1–2 mEq/kg/day. Infants in high ambient temperature may require sodium supplementation up to 4 mEq/kg/day. Potassium supplement (1–2 mEq/kg/day) should be done in hot months (typically April to September in India). Fat-soluble vitamins (A, D, E, and K) should be supplemented to twice-recommended dietary allowance. Fat-soluble vitamin supplements should be administered with food after taking PERT for better absorption.

Management of GI Complications

Distal intestinal obstruction syndrome (DIOS, meconium ileus equivalent): DIOS can be an incomplete or complete obstruction. Incomplete DIOS is associated with intermittent pain abdomen, constipation, vomiting, and abdominal distension. Complete DIOS is associated with persistent symptoms such as bilious vomiting and abdominal distension. DIOS with complete obstruction is seen in 5–12 per 1,000 children per year. Palpable mass in the right lower quadrant and X-ray showing right lower quadrant loading with multiple air-fluid levels support a diagnosis of DIOS.

Incomplete DIOS is managed with oral hydration and stool softening therapies. Polyethylene glycol can be administered orally or by nasogastric (NG) tube at dose of 2 g/kg/day. Other agents include sodium meglumine diatrizoate (gastrografin), N-acetyl cysteine and lactulose. Complete DIOS should be managed with IV hydration, NG aspiration, and enema by gastrografin (diluted four times with water). Gastrografin enema may cause dehydration, shock, perforation, or enterocolitis; these should be monitored. Colonoscopy-guided instillation of diatrizoate in the cecum may also be tried. Surgery is seldom required. Washout via enterostomy is preferred over resection.[53]

Meconium ileus: Neonates with complex meconium ileus (associated with prenatal volvulus, ischemic necrosis, intestinal atresia, or perforation and extrusion of meconium into the peritoneum) require surgical intervention. Simple meconium ileus is managed with osmotic enema (diluted gastrografin, or undiluted omnipaque or cysto-conray II). If persistent, surgical intervention is required.[20]

Cystic Fibrosis-related Liver Disease

Incidence of CF-related liver disease (CFLD) is approximately 2.5 per 100 children per year during first 10 years of life, declining sharply during second decade. Cumulative incidence range is 27–35%. Indian reports suggest that almost one-third of children with CF surviving adolescent and beyond may develop liver dysfunction.[48] Common patterns include focal biliary cirrhosis (20–30%), multifocal biliary cirrhosis (10%) and portal hypertension (2–5%). CFLD is diagnosed by the presence of any two of the following:[54]
1. Hepatomegaly on examination and/or splenomegaly on ultrasound.

2. Elevated liver enzymes—aspartate aminotransferase (AST) and alanine aminotransferase (ALT), or gamma-glutamyl transferase (GGT) above normal upper limit on three occasions over 12 months.
3. Ultrasound evidence of liver involvement or portal hypertension.
4. Liver biopsy.

Ursodeoxycholic acid (UDCA) is the recommended therapy at dose 20 mg/kg/day in two divided doses. Administration of UDCA in early stage may reduce progression of disease.

Cystic Fibrosis-related Diabetes Mellitus

Cystic fibrosis-related diabetes (CFRD) is an important cause of morbidity and develops with increasing age. It is desirable to test all children every year for early identification of impaired glucose tolerance test and CFRD.[24,48] During a period of stable baseline health, the diagnosis of CFRD can be made in CF patients according to standard American Diabetes Association (ADA) criteria summarized here:
1. Fasting plasma glucose ≥ 126 mg/dL.
2. 2-hour oral glucose tolerance test—plasma glucose ≥ 200 mg/dL.
3. HbA1c ≥ 6.5%—HbA1c below this does not exclude CFRD.
4. Random glucose ≥ 200 mg/dL with symptoms.

The diagnosis of CFRD can be made in CF patients with acute illness (on IV antibiotics in the hospital or at home or systemic glucocorticoid therapy) when fasting plasma glucose levels are ≥ 126 mg/dL or 2-hour postprandial plasma glucose levels ≥ 200 mg/dL persist for more than 48 hours.[55]

Children with CFRD are treated with insulin therapy. Daily insulin dose is typically 0.5–0.8 U/kg/day. In early stages without fasting hyperglycemia, premeal rapid-acting insulin is administered. For children with fasting hyperglycemia and frequent carbohydrate meals, basal-bolus therapy is a preferred approach. Oral hypoglycemic agents have no role in CFRD.[55]

Dehydration with Metabolic Abnormalities

Children with CF can present with dehydration with metabolic derangements including hyponatremia, hypochloremia, hypokalemia, normal anion gap metabolic alkalosis, especially during summer months. Parents are advised to increase salt and potassium supplementation during summer months. Oral rehydrating solution (ORS) should be used for water losses instead of plain water at home. In hospital, these children should be treated by rehydration with isotonic solutions like normal saline.

Targeted Therapies

Over the past 10 years, targeted therapies for improving the function of CFTR channel have been approved for use in CF. These molecules can be classified as potentiators (improving gating function of CFTR channel, e.g., ivacaftor) and

TABLE 10.4: Overview of CFTR channel targeted molecular therapies.

Drug	Age range	Mutations	Efficacy
Ivacaftor	≥6 months	G511D, R117H, S125N, and class IV and V mutations	FEV1: +10% Exacerbation: −55%
Lumacaftor/ Ivacaftor	≥2 years	Homozygous F508del	FEV1: +2.6% Exacerbation: −30%
Tezacaftor/ Ivacaftor	≥6 years	Homozygous F508del Heterozygous F508del with a class IV or V mutation	FEV1: +6.8% Exacerbations: −35%
Elexacaftor/ Tezacaftor/ Ivacaftor	≥12 years	At least one F508del allele	FEV1: +13.8% Exacerbations: −63%

(FEV1: forced expiratory volume in 1 second)

correctors (stabilizing CFTR folding and increasing membrane levels of CFTR channel, e.g., lumacaftor, tezacaftor and elexacaftor).[56,57] A brief description of these medications is summarized in **Table 10.4**. Triple combination of elexacaftor/tezacaftor/ivacaftor has significantly higher efficacy compared to two-drug combinations of lumacaftor/ivacaftor or tezacaftor/ivacaftor. Cost of these medications is prohibitive for use in developing countries. Monthly cost of these drugs ranges from 20–50 lakh rupees per month. These need to be imported for clinical use.

Other targeted therapies include read-through agents and gene therapy. ENaC channel inhibitors and calcium-activated chloride channel stimulators are under development but do not have proven clinical efficacy yet.

Follow-up

Children with CF should be followed regularly (usually every 3 months) in a special CF clinic. CF clinic should have support staff consisting of clinical expert, physiotherapist, nutritionist, trained nurse, and psychologist. On every visit, evaluation of clinical features, anthropometry, dietary assessment, compliance to drugs and physiotherapy, pulmonary function and respiratory specimen culture should be performed. Annual evaluation should be performed for development of complications: blood counts, liver function test, serum electrolytes, chest X-ray, total IgE and specific IgE for *Aspergillus fumigatus*, and if available levels of fat-soluble vitamins. Older children (> 10 years) should also be annually screened for CFRD (oral glucose tolerance test) and pulmonary hypertension (echocardiography).

■ PROGNOSIS

Based on the 2019 registry data, median life expectancy of children born with CF between 2015 and 2019 is predicted to be 46 years. With rapidly developing molecular therapies, the life expectancy is expected to improve with time. Life expectancy data is not available for children with CF form India.[58] Advanced pulmonary disease at diagnosis, malnutrition, economic burden of chronic CF therapies and infections contribute to lower life expectancy of CF in India. Nonaffordability or nonavailability of highly effective molecular agents has made these therapies out of reach of children in developing countries.

■ KEY POINTS

- Cystic fibrosis (CF) is an autosomal recessive multisystem disorder characterized by chronic airway disease and fat malabsorption. Its true incidence in India is not known.
- CF results from abnormalities in CF transmembrane conductance regulator (CFTR) protein transcribed by *CFTR* gene, which is functionally linked to calcium-dependent chloride channel and epithelial sodium channels (ENaC).
- Decrease in CFTR function and overactive ENaC lead to dehydration of airway epithelial secretions leading to small airway obstruction (hyperinflation) followed by pneumonia and bronchiectasis. Thick viscid secretions result in blockage of pancreatic ducts and pancreatic exocrine and endocrine insufficiency.
- Poor resorption of chloride ions in sweat leads to hyponatremia, hypochloremia, dehydration, hypokalemia and metabolic acidosis.
- Worldwide, F508del is the most common mutation of the *CFTR* gene constituting >65% of the mutations; it much less reported from India.
- The clinical profile in India is different due to late diagnosis in the absence of newborn screening, and lack of awareness among pediatricians, with median age of diagnosis around 22 months.
- Recurrent or persistent pneumonia, failure to thrive and malabsorption are the common symptoms with hyperinflation of chest the most common clinical sign.
- Elevated sweat chloride ($\geq$ 60 mEq/L) is highly sensitive and specific for the diagnosis of CF.
- Due to very low frequency of F508del and wide variability in mutation profile, the mutation panels of four commonest mutations including F508del, G551D, G542X and 621+1G>T are not useful in diagnosis of CF in India.
- Newborn screening involves screening of immunoreactive trypsinogen (IRT) by heel prick blood sample at 24–72 hours followed by either repeat IRT test, mutation panel or estimation of pancreatic-associated protein.
- Respiratory therapies include airway clearance therapies, management of pulmonary exacerbations and eradication of airway colonization, and treatment of pulmonary complications such as ABPA and pulmonary hemorrhage.
- In developing countries, *Pseudomonas* colonization is common in infancy and hence empirical antibiotics regimen should cover for *Pseudomonas* infection.
- Long-term azithromycin therapy has been associated with a decrease in pulmonary exacerbation in CF patients, especially with *Pseudomonas* colonization.
- Nonrespiratory therapies include pancreatic enzyme replacement, fat-soluble vitamin and micronutrient supplementations, and management of complications such as distal intestinal obstruction syndrome/meconium ileus, CFRD, CF-related liver injury, etc.
- Targeted therapies for improving the function of CFTR channel include potentiators (improving gating function of CFTR channel) and correctors (stabilizing CFTR folding and increasing membrane levels of CFTR channel).

REFERENCES

1. Bhakoo ON, Kumar R, Walia BN. Mucoviscidosis of the lung. Report of a case. Indian J Pediatr. 1968;35(243):183-5.
2. Dhochak N, Jat KR, Sankar J, Lodha R, Kabra SK. Predictors of malnutrition in children with cystic fibrosis. Indian Pediatr. 2019;56(10):825-30.
3. Scotet V, L'Hostis C, Férec C. The changing epidemiology of cystic fibrosis: Incidence, survival and impact of the CFTR gene discovery. Genes. 2020;11(6):E589.
4. Powers CA, Potter EM, Wessel HU, Lloyd-Still JD. Cystic fibrosis in Asian Indians. Arch Pediatr Adolesc Med. 1996;150(5):554-5.
5. Spencer DA, Venkataraman M, Higgins S, Stevenson K, Weller PH. Cystic fibrosis in children from ethnic minorities in the West Midlands. Respir Med. 1994;88(9):671-5.
6. Kapoor V, Shastri SS, Kabra M, Kabra SK, Ramachandran V, Arora S, et al. Carrier frequency of F508del mutation of cystic fibrosis in Indian population. J Cyst Fibros. 2006;5(1):43-6.
7. Elborn JS. Cystic fibrosis. Lancet. 2016;388(10059):2519-31.
8. Mantoo MR, Kabra M, Kabra SK. Cystic fibrosis presenting as pseudo-Bartter syndrome: an important diagnosis that is missed! Indian J Pediatr. 2020;87(9):726-32.
9. De Boeck K, Amaral MD. Progress in therapies for cystic fibrosis. Lancet Respir Med. 2016;4(8):662-74.
10. Lao O, Andrés AM, Mateu E, Bertranpetit J, Calafell F. Spatial patterns of cystic fibrosis mutation spectra in European populations. Eur J Hum Genet. 2003;11(5):385-94.
11. Patient Registry Annual Data Report (2018). Available at https://www.cff.org/Research/Researcher-Resources/Patient-Registry/2018-Patient-Registry-Annual-Data-Report.pdf.
12. Kabra SK, Kabra M, Lodha R, Shastri S, Ghosh M, Pandey RM, et al. Clinical profile and frequency of delta f508 mutation in Indian children with cystic fibrosis. Indian Pediatr. 2003;40(7):612-9.
13. Shastri SS, Kabra M, Kabra SK, Pandey RM, Menon PSN. Characterisation of mutations and genotype-phenotype correlation in cystic fibrosis: experience from India. J Cyst Fibros. 2008;7(2):110-5.
14. Prasad R, Sharma H, Kaur G. Molecular basis of cystic fibrosis disease: an Indian perspective. Indian J Clin Biochem. 2010;25(4):335-41.
15. Sharma N, Singh M, Acharya N, Singh SK, Thapa BR, Kaur G, et al. Implication of the cystic fibrosis transmembrane conductance regulator gene in infertile family members of Indian CF patients. Biochem Genet. 2008;46(11-12):847-56.
16. Sharma N, Singh M, Kaur G, Thapa BR, Prasad R. Identification and characterization of CFTR gene mutations in Indian CF patients. Ann Hum Genet. 2009;73(1):26-33.
17. Kabra SK, Kabra M, Lodha R, Shastri S. Cystic fibrosis in India. Pediatr Pulmonol. 200;42(12):1087-94.
18. Singh M, Prasad R, Kumar L. Cystic fibrosis in North Indian children. Indian J Pediatr. 2002;69(7):627-9.

19. Kawoosa MS, Bhat MA, Ali SW, Hafeez I, Shastri S. Clinical and mutation profile of children with cystic fibrosis in Jammu and Kashmir. Indian Pediatr. 2014;51(3):185-9.
20. Sathe M, Houwen R. Meconium ileus in cystic fibrosis. J Cyst Fibros. 2017;16(Suppl 2):S32-9.
21. Tang AC, Turvey SE, Alves MP, Regamey N, Tümmler B, Hartl D. Current concepts: host-pathogen interactions in cystic fibrosis airways disease. Eur Respir Rev. 2014;23(133):320-32.
22. Arvind B, Medigeshi GR, Kapil A, Xess I, Singh U, Lodha R, et al. Aetiological agents for pulmonary exacerbations in children with cystic fibrosis: an observational study from a tertiary care centre in northern India. Indian J Med Res. 2020;151(1):65-70.
23. Gautam V, Kaza P, Mathew JL, Kaur V, Sharma M, Ray P. Review of a 7-year record of the bacteriological profile of airway secretions of children with cystic fibrosis in North India. Indian J Med Microbiol. 2019;37(2):203-9.
24. El-Chammas KI, Rumman N, Goh VL, Quintero D, Goday PS. Rectal prolapse and cystic fibrosis. J Pediatr Gastroenterol Nutr. 2015;60(1):110-2.
25. Marah MA. Pseudo-Bartter as an initial presentation of cystic fibrosis. A case report and review of the literature. East Mediterr Health J. 2010;16(6):699-701.
26. Prentice BJ, Jaffe A, Hameed S, Verge CF, Waters S, Widger J. Cystic fibrosis-related diabetes and lung disease: an update. Eur Respir Rev. 2021;30(159):200-93.
27. Moran A, Dunitz J, Nathan B, Saeed A, Holme B, Thomas W. Cystic fibrosis-related diabetes: current trends in prevalence, incidence, and mortality. Diabetes Care. 2009;32(9):1626-31.
28. Jain V, Kumar S, Vikram NK, Kalaivani M, Bhatt SP, Sharma R, et al. Glucose tolerance and insulin secretion and sensitivity characteristics in Indian children with cystic fibrosis: A pilot study. Indian J Med Res. 2017;146(4):483-8.
29. Farrell PM, White TB, Ren CL, Hempstead SE, Accurso F, Derichs N, et al. Diagnosis of Cystic Fibrosis: Consensus Guidelines from the Cystic Fibrosis Foundation. J Pediatr. 2017;181S:S4-S15.
30. Rueegg CS, Kuehni CE, Gallati S, Jurca M, Jung A, Casaulta C, et al. Comparison of two sweat test systems for the diagnosis of cystic fibrosis in newborns. Pediatr Pulmonol. 2019;54(3):264-72.
31. Kabra SK, Kabra M, Gera S, Lodha R, Sreedevi KN, Chacko S, et al. An indigenously developed method for sweat collection and estimation of chloride for diagnosis of cystic fibrosis. Indian Pediatr. 2002;39(11):1039-43.
32. McCormick J, Green MW, Mehta G, Culross F, Mehta A. Demographics of the UK cystic fibrosis population: implications for neonatal screening. Eur J Hum Genet. 2002;10(10):583-90.
33. De Boeck K, Vermeulen F, Dupont L. The diagnosis of cystic fibrosis. Presse Med. 2017;46(6 Pt 2):e97-e108.
34. Singh A, Lodha R, Shastri S, Sethuraman G, Sreedevi KN, Kabra M, et al. Aquagenic wrinkling of skin: A screening test for cystic fibrosis. Indian Pediatr. 2019;56(2):109-13.
35. Horsley A. Lung clearance index in the assessment of airways disease. Respir Med. 2009;103(6):793-9.

36. Fuchs HJ, Borowitz DS, Christiansen DH, Morris EM, Nash ML, Ramsey BW, et al. Effect of aerosolized recombinant human DNase on exacerbations of respiratory symptoms and on pulmonary function in patients with cystic fibrosis. The Pulmozyme Study Group. N Engl J Med. 1994;331(10):637-42.
37. Gupta S, Ahmed F, Lodha R, Gupta YK, Kabra SK. Comparison of effects of 3 and 7% hypertonic saline nebulization on lung function in children with cystic fibrosis: a double-blind randomized, controlled trial. J Trop Pediatr. 2012;58(5):375-81.
38. Chaudary N, Balasa G. Airway clearance therapy in cystic fibrosis patients insights from a clinician providing cystic fibrosis care. Int J Gen Med. 2021;14: 2513-21.
39. Cystic Fibrosis Foundation; Borowitz D, Robinson KA, Rosenfeld M, Davis SD, Sabadosa KA, et al. Cystic Fibrosis Foundation evidence-based guidelines for management of infants with cystic fibrosis. J Pediatr. 2009;155(6 Suppl): S73-93.
40. Ng C, Nadig T, Smyth AR, Flume P. Treatment of pulmonary exacerbations in cystic fibrosis. Curr Opin Pulm Med. 2020;26(6):679-84.
41. Heltshe SL, West NE, VanDevanter DR, Sanders DB, Beckett VV, Flume PA, et al. Study design considerations for the Standardized Treatment of Pulmonary Exacerbations 2 (STOP2): a trial to compare intravenous antibiotic treatment durations in CF. Contemp Clin Trials. 2018;64:35--40.
42. Gulla KM, Balaji A, Mukherjee A, Jat KR, Sankar J, Lodha R, et al. Course of illness after viral infection in Indian children with cystic fibrosis. J Trop Pediatr. 2019;65(2):176-82.
43. Mayer-Hamblett N, Retsch-Bogart G, Kloster M, Accurso F, Rosenfeld M, Albers G, et al. Azithromycin for early pseudomonas infection in cystic fibrosis. The OPTIMIZE Randomized Trial. Am J Respir Crit Care Med. 2018; 198(9):1177-87.
44. Kabra SK, Pawaiya R, Lodha R, Kapil A, Kabra M, Vani AS, et al. Long-term daily high and low doses of azithromycin in children with cystic fibrosis: a randomized controlled trial. J Cyst Fibros. 2010;9(1):17-23.
45. Flume PA, Clancy JP, Retsch-Bogart GZ, Tullis DE, Bresnik M, Derchak PA, et al. Continuous alternating inhaled antibiotics for chronic pseudomonal infection in cystic fibrosis. J Cyst Fibros. 2016;15(6):809-15.
46. Kabra S, Lodha R. AIIMS Pediatric Pulmonology Protocols. New Delhi: AIIMS; 2017. pp. 26-58.
47. Sharma VK, Raj D, Xess I, Lodha R, Kabra SK. Prevalence and risk factors for allergic bronchopulmonary aspergillosis in Indian children with cystic fibrosis. Indian Pediatr. 2014;51(4):295-7.
48. Kumar A, Aggarwal B, Bamal P, Jat KR, Lodha R, Kabra SK. Clinical profile of children with cystic fibrosis surviving through adolescence and beyond. Indian Pediatr. 2021;S097475591600362.
49. Agarwal R, Chakrabarti A, Shah A, Gupta D, Meis JF, Guleria R, et al. Allergic bronchopulmonary aspergillosis: review of literature and proposal of new diagnostic and classification criteria. Clin Exp Allergy J. 2013;43(8):850-73.
50. Al-Samkari H, Shin K, Cardoni L, Pighetti EH, Rits S, McMahon L, et al. Antifibrinolytic agents for hemoptysis management in adults with cystic fibrosis. Chest. 2019;155(6):1226-33.

51. Ng C, Major G, Smyth AR. Dosing regimens for pancreatic enzyme replacement therapy (PERT) in cystic fibrosis. Cochrane Database Syst Rev. 2019;2019(12): CD013488.
52. Turck D, Braegger CP, Colombo C, Declercq D, Morton A, Pancheva R, et al. ESPEN-ESPGHAN-ECFS guidelines on nutrition care for infants, children, and adults with cystic fibrosis. Clin Nutr Edinb Scotl. 2016;35(3):557-77.
53. Colombo C, Ellemunter H, Houwen R, Munck A, Taylor C, Wilschanski M, et al. Guidelines for the diagnosis and management of distal intestinal obstruction syndrome in cystic fibrosis patients. J Cyst Fibros. 2011;10(Suppl 2):S24-28.
54. Debray D, Kelly D, Houwen R, Strandvik B, Colombo C. Best practice guidance for the diagnosis and management of cystic fibrosis-associated liver disease. J Cyst Fibros. 2011;10(Suppl 2):S29-36.
55. Moran A, Pillay K, Becker D, Granados A, Hameed S, Acerini CL. ISPAD Clinical Practice Consensus Guidelines 2018: Management of cystic fibrosis-related diabetes in children and adolescents. Pediatr Diabetes. 2018;(19 Suppl 27):64-74.
56. Ridley K, Condren M. Elexacaftor-Tezacaftor-Ivacaftor: The first triple-combination cystic fibrosis transmembrane conductance regulator modulating therapy. J Pediatr Pharmacol Ther. 2020;25(3):192-7.
57. Mall MA, Mayer-Hamblett N, Rowe SM. Cystic fibrosis: emergence of highly effective targeted therapeutics and potential clinical implications. Am J Respir Crit Care Med. 2020;201(10):1193-208.
58. Cystic Fibrosis Foundation. Understanding Changes in Life Expectancy. [online] Available from: https://www.cff.org/Research/Researcher-Resources/Patient-Registry/Understanding-Changes-in-Life-Expectancy/. [Last Accessed January, 2022].

Gastroenterology

CHAPTER 11

Cow's Milk Protein Allergy

John Matthai

■ INTRODUCTION

Many parents report that their infants have food allergy after the introduction of new foods, based on nonspecific gastrointestinal symptoms. However, the true incidence is much lower, because the term allergy is often loosely applied in the community. Globally, cow's milk, taken here as representative of all mammalian milk except the human milk, is the most common cause of food allergy in children below 2 years of age, followed by egg protein. Allergy to soy protein, peanuts, walnuts, almonds, and shellfish (shrimp, crabs, and lobster) is not uncommon. Food additives (dyes, thickeners, and preservatives) are also being increasingly implicated in food allergy. One-third of patients have allergy to multiple foods.[1]

Food allergy is an immune-mediated adverse response to a food component, usually a protein. Accordingly, a diagnosis of cow's milk protein allergy (CMPA) can be made only if there is a compatible clinical history as well as positive in vitro/in vivo test proving an underlying immune etiology. Positive test alone should not be used for diagnosis because many children are sensitized (positive tests alone) but are not allergic (no clinical reaction). In contrast, *food intolerance* is nonimmune and nonallergenic food hypersensitivity. It is a response of the digestive system to food components and hence symptoms are limited to the gastrointestinal tract (GIT). Lactose intolerance (LI) and salicylate or food additive sensitivity are examples. *Food aversion* is a strong feeling of dislike for a particular food, which is psychologically mediated. Symptoms may therefore include nausea or retching, even before the food is ingested.

■ EPIDEMIOLOGY

In a survey of 89 countries, Prescot et al. found that around half the countries had no data on food allergies, while only 10% reported prevalence based on the oral food challenge (OFC) test, which is the gold standard for diagnosis. In addition, most data was based on self- or parent-reported questionnaires, which generally are an overestimate of the prevalence.[2] In western studies, the incidence of CMPA is 2–3% during infancy, declining to <0.7% by 6 years of age.[3] About 10–15% of children with CMPA are also allergic to soy and the risk of cross allergy is higher if the first symptoms are seen below 6 months of age.[4] Infants with food protein-induced enterocolitis syndrome (FPIES) to cow's milk also have a higher frequency of FPIES to soy. There are no published data on the prevalence in the community of food allergy and CMPA in Indian children. In hospital-based studies, CMPA was reported as a cause of chronic diarrhea in 13% of children below 2 years of age in one study and in 35% of toddler's diarrhea in another study.[5]

■ PATHOGENESIS

Symptoms of CMPA may be immunoglobulin E (IgE)-mediated, non-IgE-mediated, or a combination of both. The incidence of IgE and non-IgE reactions is almost equal in the West, but in developing countries, non-IgE reaction is believed to be more common. Cow's milk when digested by rennin in acidic pH separates into two fractions—lactoserum or whey (20%) and coagulum or casein (80%). Whey is composed mostly of globular proteins such as β-lactoglobulin, α-lactalbumin, bovine serum albumin, and lactoferrin. The major allergenic proteins are casein, β-lactoglobulin, and α-lactalbumin. While 26% patients are sensitized to only one protein, the rest get sensitized to two or more proteins.

■ CLINICAL FEATURES

A detailed history is mandatory to establish any temporal association between the introduction of animal milk and the onset of symptoms. History of atopic disorders in the child and family members is helpful. Examination should focus on the presence of growth faltering, anemia, and edema suggestive of intestinal mucosal disease. Common skin manifestations include eczema, atopic dermatitis, angioedema, and urticaria, while respiratory symptoms include wheezing, rhinoconjunctivitis, serous otitis media, and laryngeal edema.[6] Approximately 40–50% of infants with CMPA have atopic dermatitis while 30% of children with atopic dermatitis may have food allergy.

Presenting symptoms in infants depend on the mechanism of allergy. In IgE-mediated allergy, symptoms usually start within minutes after exposure to cow's milk, making the diagnosis easy. However, in non-IgE-mediated reactions, symptoms may be delayed by a few days or even weeks and this makes it more difficult to identify the association. Clinical manifestations of CMPA and their probable mechanisms are shown in **Table 11.1**. While 50–60% report predominant gastrointestinal or cutaneous symptoms, 20–30% have respiratory symptoms. However, most children have symptoms related to two or more organs.[7]

Cow's milk protein allergy can rarely occur in exclusively breastfed infants. It is caused by transfer of the allergenic proteins through breast milk. Many of

Cow's Milk Protein Allergy

TABLE 11.1: Clinical manifestations of CMPA.

Non-IgE-mediated (onset > 24 hours, usually after 5–7 days)	• *Proctocolitis*:
	  – Fresh bleeding per rectum
	• *Enteropathy*:
	  – Watery diarrhea
	  – Failure to thrive
	• *Protein-losing enteropathy*:
	  – Occult gastrointestinal bleeding
	• *Enterocolitis*:
	  – Dysentery
	  – Unexplained anemia
	  – Hypoalbuminemia
	• *Gastroesophagitis*:
	  – Hematemesis
	  – Gastroesophageal reflux
	  – Feed refusal (infants)
	• *Skin*:
	  – Atopic dermatitis

IgE-mediated (onset < 1 hour)	• Anaphylaxis/angioedema • Perioral urticaria/erythema • Generalized rash • Vomiting • Rhinoconjunctivitis • Wheezing/cough
Mixed (onset 1 hour to < 24 hours)	• *FPIES*: Vomiting/diarrhea/colitis • Shock-like state

(FPIES: food protein-induced enterocolitis syndrome)

these infants may have been exposed and sensitized when formulas are supplemented in newborn intensive care units soon after birth. In infants, CMPA has been reported to cause regurgitation of feeds with feed refusal, atopic dermatitis unresponsive to topical therapy and severe unremitting colic. However, it is important to stress that CMPA is not a common cause for these symptoms and should be considered only in those with persistent symptoms after other common causes have been ruled out. Among gastrointestinal manifestations, persistent diarrhea, or dysentery in otherwise well infants, is most common.[8] CMPA may be subjectively classified as mild, moderate, or severe. Presence of symptoms (e.g., anaphylaxis) or failure to thrive (FTT) along with gastrointestinal symptoms is taken as severe disease. Presence of gastrointestinal symptoms without FTT is classified as mild-to-moderate disease.[9] The red flags in CMPA are shown in **Box 11.1**.

A particularly dramatic presentation of CMPA is FPIES. Typically seen below 2 years of age, the child presents with unexplained vomiting and signs of shock mimicking sepsis within a few hours of ingestion of the offending food.[10] Bloody diarrhea may be seen in infants below 2 months with cow's

Cow's Milk Protein Allergy

> **BOX 11.1:** Red flag signs in cow's milk protein allergy (CMPA).
> - Systemic reactions
> - Severe atopy/eczema
> - Failure to thrive
> - Multiple food allergies
> - No response to exclusion diet
> - Eosinophilic gastrointestinal syndromes
> - Food protein-induced enterocolitis syndrome (FPIES)

milk-related FPIES. Absence of fever, prompt resolution of symptoms with supportive therapy, and recurrence of similar episodes are pointers to the diagnosis of FPIES. While cow's milk, soy, rice, and chicken are the common offenders, some children also react to fruits or vegetables. FPIES has been classified as mild, moderate or severe. Presence of any of the following features such as altered consciousness or lethargy, hypothermia, hypotension, abdominal distension, or the need of intravenous fluids is taken as severe disease. The controversy regarding the association between food protein allergy and eosinophilic gastrointestinal syndromes of infancy is still unsettled.[11]

Cow's Milk Protein Allergy and Lactose Intolerance

Cow's milk protein allergy, which is an allergy to proteins in milk, should be differentiated from lactose intolerance (LI), which is an inability to digest lactose, the sugar in milk. It is due to deficiency of the intestinal brush border enzyme, lactase. LI may be congenital, primary (decline in lactase enzyme with age), or secondary (mucosal damage after severe gastroenteritis or other causes), which is the most common. It is quantity-dependent, and symptoms are exclusively gastrointestinal (diarrhea, abdominal pain, and flatulence). In congenital and primary LI, the intolerance is permanent, while in secondary LI, complete recovery occurs in a few days to weeks, depending on the underlying cause. The main differences are given in **Table 11.2**.

■ DIAGNOSIS

Empirical exclusion diet without confirmation of diagnosis should be discouraged. A reliable detailed history focusing on the allergy in the child and family as well as a good clinical examination are important in arriving at a diagnosis. Non-IgE-mediated disease, which is more common in India manifests with only gastrointestinal symptoms. Important differential diagnosis to keep in mind includes *Shigella dysentery*, celiac disease, persistent diarrhea, and immune deficiency. Skin and/or respiratory tract symptoms in addition to those in the GIT are pointers to IgE-mediated disease. Other important differential diagnosis includes gastroesophageal reflux disease and swallowing disorders.

TABLE 11.2: Differences between cow's milk protein allergy (CMPA) and lactose intolerance.

	Lactose intolerance	CMPA
Cause	Deficiency of the enzyme lactase in intestinal brush border	Immune-mediated adverse reaction
Component in milk responsible	Disaccharide lactose	Proteins (Casein, β-lactoglobulin, and α-lactalbumin)
Types	Secondary (common), congenital, and primary (rare)	IgE- and non-IgE-mediated
Symptoms	Only gastrointestinal (diarrhea, flatulence)	Gastrointestinal, respiratory and skin
Treatment	Lactose-free diet/formula	Milk protein free diet or Extensively hydrolyzed formula
Outcome	Resolves in days if secondary type	Recovers by 6 years of age in 90%

Screening Score

The cow's milk-related symptom score (CoMiSS) is the most popular scoring system used in making a diagnosis. The score ranges from 0 to 33 and cut-off values of >12 are considered a positive score for CMPA in western settings. However, it has poor sensitivity and specificity and there are no studies on its utility from the developing countries, where breastfeeding is much more common.[12] Hence CoMiSS cannot be recommended as a screening tool in our setting.

Specific IgE Antibodies to Cow's Milk

Cow's milk specific serum IgE ≥0.35 kU/L is used as supporting evidence for IgE-mediated CMPA.[13] However, positive levels do not differentiate between sensitization and clinically significant allergy and thus may lead to overdiagnosis. Specific IgE tests are not useful in the diagnosis of non-IgE-mediated CMPA.[14]

Skin Prick Test

Skin prick tests (SPT) detect the presence of tissue-bound IgE antibodies. It can be considered in IgE-mediated disease and a wheal size of ≥5 mm (≥2 mm in an infant ≤ 2 years) has high specificity. More importantly, a negative skin test rules out IgE-mediated reactions.[15] The lower the wheal size, the higher the chances of the child outgrowing CMPA. SPT has no role in non-IgE-mediated CMPA.

Diagnostic Elimination and Oral Challenge

The Indian Society of Pediatric Gastroenterology, Hepatology, and Nutrition (ISPGHAN) practice guidelines recommend that the diagnosis of CMPA should be based on the clinical response to milk protein elimination diet followed by an oral food challenge (OFC).[16] Elimination should be total and particular attention should be paid to hidden sources of antigen (biscuits, cake, bread etc.). In IgE-mediated disease, response to withdrawal is noticed within 3–5 days, while in those with non-IgE-mediated disease with symptoms such as chronic diarrhea and/or FTT, it may be 2–4 weeks. If symptoms do not improve during this time frame, the diagnosis of CMPA is unlikely in most cases.

For infants who are exclusively breastfed, elimination requires the mother to exclude milk and milk products from her diet. This is because milk proteins are excreted in breast milk. Non-infants should be started on an extensively hydrolyzed formula (eHF) after stopping all forms of milk protein. Soy formula may be used beyond 6 months of age. Older children do not need formulas and milk can be substituted with other proteins.

It is important to make sure that the child is not allergic to the milk protein substitutes (soy/eHF) that are given during the CMP exclusion period. If multiple food allergies (egg, wheat, or nuts) are suspected, all of them should be stopped and an amino acid-based formulation (AAF) should be used during the allergen elimination. If symptoms still persist, then CMPA cannot be the cause for the child's symptoms. Children whose symptoms improve with allergen elimination should have an oral milk challenge after 2–4 weeks of CMP-free diet to confirm the diagnosis.[17]

Food challenge should be done under observation in a hospital particularly in those with IgE-mediated symptoms. In those with only gastrointestinal manifestations, cow's milk-protein either pasteurized milk or formula is administered beginning with 1 mL and gradually increased to 3, 10, 30, and 100 mL every 30 minutes. If the child is asymptomatic after food challenge, the child is sent home after another 2 hours, with an advice to give 200 mL of the formula daily, observe for recurrence of symptoms and review after 2 weeks. For those with IgE-mediated symptoms at the initial presentation, milk challenge is done using even smaller increments (0.1, 0.3, 1, 3, 10, 30, and 100 mL given every 30 minutes) in an in-patient setting with resuscitation facilities. If no reactions are reported, 200 mL/day of milk may be continued for 2 weeks while observing for any delayed manifestations. Reappearance of symptoms anytime during the challenge, confirms the diagnosis of CMPA.[18]

Sigmoidoscopy

Sigmoidoscopy and rectal biopsy have very high diagnostic value in patients with any gastrointestinal manifestations of CMPA. The most common endoscopic findings are focal erythema, erosions, and nodular lymphoid hyperplasia. The presence of >15–20 eosinophils per high power field and/or >60 eosinophils in six high power fields is considered significant.[19] However, the endoscopic and histological changes are not specific for cow's milk, but similar in all food allergies. Therefore, they should be considered diagnostic only in an appropriate clinical setting.

In India, gastrointestinal symptoms seem to be the most common manifestation of CMPA. The ISPGHAN guidelines recommend that sigmoidoscopy and rectal biopsy can also be considered for confirmation of diagnosis in children whose parents do not give consent for OFC.[16]

■ MANAGEMENT

The clinical approach to a child with suspected CMPA is shown in **Flowchart 11.1**. The suggested protocol for the management of infants with non-IgE mediated CMPA is given in **Flowchart 11.2**. The singular step in the

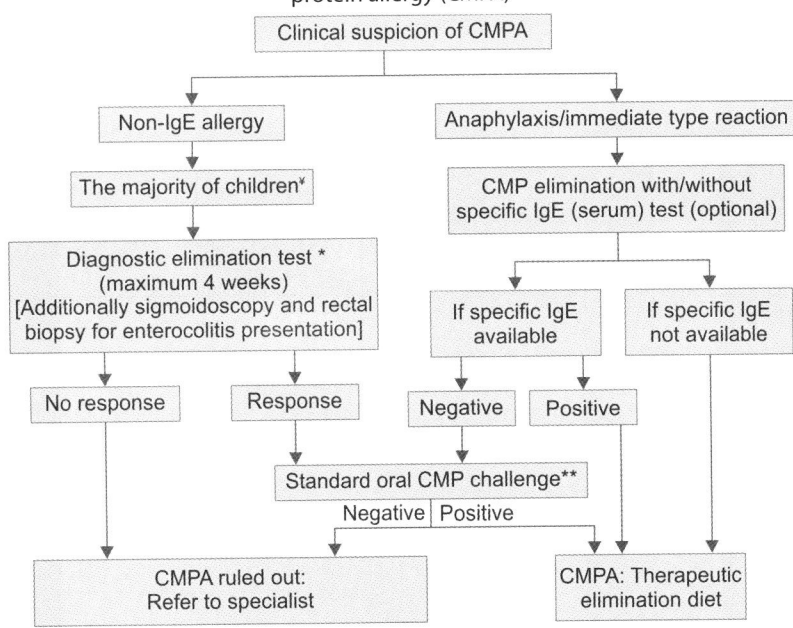

Flowchart 11.1: Approach to a child with suspected Cow's milk protein allergy (CMPA)

¥ *Subset of patients with enterocolitis*: Sigmoidoscopy and rectal biopsy are useful
* *Exclusively breastfeeding (EBF) infant*: Eliminate all CMP containing food in mother; *Mixed/formula fed*: eliminate all CMP food/formula in mother and infant and eHF/soy trial; *Symptoms with first CMP feeds*: return to EBF (maternal restriction of milk protein not required). (Elimination duration: 1–2 weeks for most, 2–4 weeks for chronic symptoms)
** *Exclusively breastfed*: Mother returns to normal CMP diet; *Mixed/formula fed*: Home challenge with CMP formula/milk
Source: Matthai J, Sathiasekharan M, Poddar U, Sibal A, Srivastava A, Waikar Y, et al. Guidelines on diagnosis and management of cow's milk protein allergy. Indian Pediatr. 2020;57(8):723-9.

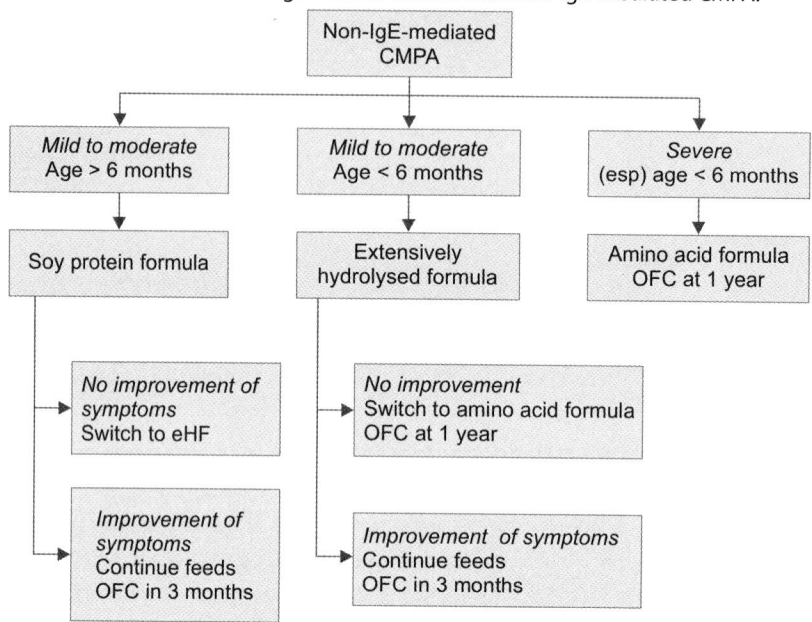

Flowchart 11.2: Management of infants with non-IgE-mediated CMPA.

(eHF: extensively hydrolyzed formula; OFC: oral food challenge)
Source: Matthai J, Sathiasekharan M, Poddar U, Sibal A, Srivastava A, Waikar Y, et al. Guidelines on diagnosis and management of cow's milk protein allergy. Indian Pediatr. 2020;57(8):723-9.

management is the total avoidance of CMP for a defined length of time.[17] It is vital to stress at the time of diagnosis that exclusion is not lifelong and most children will outgrow it before schoolgoing age. The most common issue today is overdiagnosis of CMPA by parents, and older members in the family. This leads to unnecessary diet restrictions, reduced protein intake, and increased risk of rickets in growing children, not to mention the economic burden of alternative foods. Pediatricians, who believe that the costly hypoallergenic formulas are nutritionally superior to milk, often endorse the diagnosis.

In an Exclusively Breastfed Infant

The gastrointestinal manifestations of CMPA in exclusively breastfed infants are mild and they have normal growth. A plausible explanation is that the quantity of CMP in breast milk is 100,000 times lower than that in cow's milk. In addition, it is in the form of peptides and not as intact protein, since breast milk also contains proteases that digest protein. The mother is advised to exclude bovine milk and all dairy products from her diet and exclusive breastfeeding is continued till at least 6 months. It takes a few days to observe clinical response, since antigens continue to be secreted in breast milk for 72 hours.[20] Complete resolution takes much longer, the duration of which depends on the mechanism of allergy. In those with IgE-mediated allergy, it is 3–6 days, while in non-IgE-mediated it is 2–4 weeks. If symptoms persist beyond this period, other etiologies should be considered. If symptoms improve, milk should be reintroduced in the maternal diet after a few weeks. If the same symptoms recur, the diagnosis of CMPA is confirmed and the mother should avoid milk and milk products as long as she breastfeeds. Protein, calcium (1,000 mg per day) and vitamin D (600 IU per day) supplementation is essential for the mother during the period of elimination. There is no scientific basis to recommend avoidance of other potentially allergenic foods like fish, egg, soy, wheat, and gluten products in the mother, since it results in nutritional deficiencies and reduced milk secretion.[21]

In Infants on Exclusive Formula Feeds

If breastfeeds have been stopped only recently, it must be restarted. Not only CMP but also other animal milk (buffalo, goat, and sheep) should be immediately stopped. Infants below 6 months of age should be started on eHF. In view of the safety concerns with the use of soy protein, and the chances of cross allergy in up to 15% of infants, soy preparations are best avoided in infants <6 months of age.[22] However, soy is cheaper and more palatable than eHF and these should be discussed with the parents before the decision is made. In infants >6 months, soy protein formula can be safely used instead of eHF if there are financial constraints. If the diagnosis is certain, but there is no improvement after 2 weeks of eHF, then amino acid formula (AAF) should be started.[23] In infants who are sick or have severe symptoms it is better to straight away give AAF rather than eHF.

In Infants on Mixed Feeds

Breastfeeding should be continued and there is no need for any elimination in the maternal diet. All mammalian milk and milk products should be completely withdrawn. Rest of the management is similar to that of infants who are exclusively artificially fed.

In IgE-Mediated CMPA

Angioedema, urticaria, and anaphylaxis are features suggestive of IgE-mediated allergy and require appropriate care as for any allergy. In mild-to-moderate allergy, eHF is sufficient. Only those whose symptoms persist should be switched to AAF.[24] Those with severe symptoms should be hospitalized for emergency care and should be given only AAF once they are ready to take feeds. The OFC should be done with caution in a hospital setting after 12–18 months of asymptomatic period. In those with mild-to-moderate symptoms, challenge is done with intact cow's milk protein (CMP), while those with severe IgE-mediated allergy it should be done only with eHF.

Choice of Alternate Feed

Choosing an appropriate substitute for milk is crucial to ensure that nutritional requirements are adequately met. The following variables should be considered before a decision is made:[25]
- Age and existing feeding pattern
- Type of allergy (IgE-mediated or not)
- Severity of reaction
- Financial aspect (alternative formulas are expensive).

Hypoallergenic Formula

The allergenicity of the milk protein decreases with decreasing the chain length of the protein. Milk proteins are hydrolyzed by enzymes and such formulas are classified based on the degree of hydrolysis. Those with 5–10 kDa are called "partially hydrolyzed formula (pHF)", those with <3 kDa are referred to as "eHF" and those with only amino acids as "elemental formula (AAF or EF)". More the hydrolysis, better is the immune tolerance, but higher the cost and poorer is the taste. pHF should not be used for treatment of CMPA. More than 90% of infants with CMPA will respond to eHF.[26] AAF is recommended only in the following situations:
- Infants below 6 months with severe disease (FTT and abundant blood in stools)
- Multiple food allergies
- Exclusively breastfed infants with associated severe atopic eczema
- Severe forms of non-IgE-mediated CMPA (eosinophilic esophagitis, enteropathies, and FPIES)
- Infants not responding to eHF

Rice-based Feeds or Hydrolyzed Formula

Rice is one of the least allergenic foods with reactions in <1% of children. Rice-based feeds or hydrolyzed formula (RHF) is currently not available in India, but cooked rice is a good alternative in older infants. They do not contain lactose and are poor in lysine, threonine, and tryptophan, which will need supplementation. RHF is safe in children allergic to milk and soy. Growth parameters in children on RHF have been found to be similar to eHF.[27] RHF is recommended by ESPGHAN for infants refusing or not tolerating eHF and for strict vegan families.[17]

Soy Protein Formula

Allergy to soy protein is seen in 10–15% of infants with CMPA. This is because of the presence of the allergens—conglycinin and glycinin. Soy is, however, cheaper, and the taste is more acceptable than eHF. It contains essential fatty acids that can be easily absorbed, but being a vegetable protein, the bioavailability is lower. There are concerns regarding the use of soy protein below 6 months of age due to high concentration of aluminum (600–1,300 ng/mL vs. 4–65 ng/mL in human milk) and excess of phytoestrogens. Children with IgE-mediated CMPA tolerate soy protein better than non-IgE-mediated CMPA.[28] ISPGHAN practice guidelines recommend its use below 6 months only if there are financial considerations.[16] NASPGHAN and ESPGHAN do not recommend soy formula under 6 months of age.[17]

Natural History

The milk protein elimination diet should be continued for a minimum of one year. Reevaluation should be done every 6 months subsequently. The prognosis of infants and children with CMPA is good. Around 50% will tolerate CMP by 1 year, 75% by 3 years, and 90% by 6 years of age.[29] Inappropriately prolonged restriction should be avoided since it impairs the quality of life of the child, causes nutritional deficiency, and imposes significant health costs on the family. Only around 5% of children continue to have allergy into adulthood. Those with high total IgE and specific IgE levels, more serious clinical manifestations and multiple allergies are less likely to outgrow their disease.[30]

Pharmacotherapy

In hypersensitivity reactions, epinephrine is the drug of choice. H2 receptor antagonists and corticosteroids are used in minor reactions. They provide only symptomatic relief and do not modify the natural course of the disease. Probiotics have been studied for their beneficial effects in food allergy. The World Allergy Organization in its position paper has concluded that currently no probiotic supplement has shown any significant influence on allergic manifestations or demonstrated any long-term benefits.[31] There is also no recommendation for the use of immunotherapy in CMPA.

■ PREVENTION

The main strategy for prevention of CMPA is avoidance of the offending proteins. In primary prevention, exposure to CMP is delayed in all infants, while in secondary prevention, atopic infants are not exposed to the antigen. Early inadvertent exposure occurs when neonates receive intact cows' milk formula in the hospital or newborn intensive care unit (NICU).

Exclusively Breastfed Infants

Exclusive breastfeeding for 4–6 months is the best means to prevent CMPA. The incidence of CMPA (0.5%) in exclusively breastfed infants is much lower than in formula-fed or mixed-fed infants (2–7.5%). The reproducible clinical reactions to CMP are mild-to-moderate in the majority. This is because the amount of CMP in breast milk is 100,000 times lower than that in cow's milk and are in the form of peptides and not as intact protein due to the proteases in breast milk.[32] There is no evidence that modification of maternal diet during pregnancy or lactation has any protective effect against allergy in at-risk infants.[33] Allergen avoidance should be advised in the mother only when the breastfed infant has proven CMPA.

There is also no evidence to suggest that delaying the introduction of solid foods, even potentially allergenic foods, beyond age 4–6 months offers any protective effect against allergy. Complementary foods should be introduced in small quantities, while the mother is still breastfeeding after at least 17 weeks of age in children who are at high risk of food allergies.

Infants not Exclusively Breastfed

The choice of formula for infants at risk for allergy due to a positive family history is contentious. Infants are categorized as low risk if there is no family history of atopic disease. If one parent has atopic disease, it increases the likelihood of allergy to 20–40%, and if both have, it becomes 40–50%. The usefulness of hydrolyzed formulae (both partial and extensively) in the prevention of CMPA is still debated. If both parents have severe allergic disease, there may be some justification in using hydrolyzed formula with whey protein as starter formula. However, a recent meta-analysis failed to demonstrate any benefit in using hydrolyzed formula to prevent CMPA.[34] Soy is not recommended for prevention based on a Cochrane review that showed no difference in the incidence of eczema between infants fed soy and cow's milk. Available data do not support use of probiotics, prebiotics, or synbiotics in the prevention of allergy.

■ SUMMARY

Cow's milk protein allergy is most commonly seen in infancy and its incidence is increasing. In IgE-mediated CMPA, symptoms occur early and are multisystemic, while in non–IgE-mediated CMPA symptoms are delayed and usually limited to the GIT. The response to elimination of diet and reappearance of symptoms on food challenge is the gold standard in diagnosis. In children with persistent diarrhea and colitis, sigmoidoscopy and biopsy are diagnostic. Continuing breastfeeding, withdrawal of all forms of CMP, and substitution with an age-appropriate formula are recommended. Most children outgrow the allergy by 6 years.

■ KEY POINTS

- Cow's milk protein is the most common cause of food allergy in young children.
- The GIT is most commonly involved in non-IgE-mediated allergy and presents with colitis or chronic diarrhea.
- There is a strong association between CMPA and atopic dermatitis.
- The response to elimination of diet and the recurrence of symptoms on a food challenge is pathognomonic. Eosinophilic infiltration in a rectal biopsy is diagnostic in those with colitis, but the histological changes are similar in all types of food protein allergies.
- Treatment includes withdrawal of all forms of milk protein, continuation of breastfeeding, and substitution with either an eHF or soy formula.
- Milk protein elimination should be continued for a minimum of 1 year and rechallenge should be done under supervision in appropriate cases.
- Over 90% of children will outgrow the allergy by 6 years.

■ REFERENCES

1. Hossny E, Ebisawa M, El-Gamal Y, Arasi S, Dahdah L, El-Owaidy R, et al. Challenges of managing food allergy in the developing world. World Allergy Organ J. 2019;12(11):100089.
2. Prescott SL, Pawankar R, Allen KJ, Campbell DE, Sinn JKh, Fiocchi A, et al. A global survey of changing patterns of food allergy burden in children. World Allergy Organ J. 2013;6;(1):21.
3. Schoemaker AA, Sprikkelman AB, Grimshaw KE, Roberts G, Grabenhenrich L, Rosenfeld L, et al. Incidence and natural history of challenge-proven cow's milk allergy in European children—Euro Prevall birth cohort. Allergy. 2015;70(8):963-72.
4. Klemola T, Vanto T, Juntunen-Backman K, Kalimo K, Korpela R, Varjonen E. Allergy to soy formula and to extensively hydrolyzed whey formula in infants with cow's milk allergy: a prospective, randomized study with a follow-up to the age of 2 years. J Pediatr. 2002;140(2):219-24.
5. Poddar U, Agarwal J, Yachha SK, Srivastava A. Toddler's diarrhea: is it an under-recognized entity in developing countries? J Trop Pediatr. 2013;59(6):470-5.
6. Høst A. Frequency of cow's milk allergy in childhood. Ann Allergy Asthma Immunol. 2002;89(6 Suppl 1):33-7.
7. Burks AW, Tang M, Sicherer S, Muraro A, Eigenmann PA, Ebisawa M, et al. ICON: Food allergy. J Allergy Clin Immunol. 2012;129(4):906-20.
8. Allen KJ, Hill DJ, Heine RG. Food allergy in childhood. Med J Aust. 2006;185(7):394-400.
9. Vandenplas Y, Koletzko S, Isolauri E, Hill D, Oranje AP, Brueton M, et al. Guidelines for the diagnosis and management of cow's milk protein allergy in infants. Arch Dis Child. 2007;92(10):902-8.
10. Nowak-Węgrzyn A, Chehade M, Groetch ME, Spergel JM, Wood RA, Allen K, et al. International consensus guidelines for the diagnosis and management of food protein-induced enterocolitis syndrome. J Allergy Clin Immunol. 2017;139(4):1111-26.e4

11. Rothenberg ME. Eosinophilic gastrointestinal disorders (EGID). J Allergy Clin Immunol. 2004;113:11-28.
12. Prasad R, Venkata RSA, Ghokale P, Chakravarty P, Anwar F. Cow's milk-related symptom score as a predictive tool for cow's milk allergy in Indian children aged 0-24 months. Asia Pac Allergy. 2018;8(4):e36.
13. Martorell-Aragonés A, Echeverría-Zudaire L, Alonso-Lebrero E, Boné-Calvo J, Martín-Muñoz MF, Nevot-Falcó S, et al. Position document: IgE-mediated cow's milk allergy. Allergol Immunopathol (Madr). 2015;43(5):507-26.
14. Muraro A, Werfel T, Hoffmann-Sommergruber K, Roberts G, Beyer K, Bindslev-Jensen C, et al. EAACI food allergy and anaphylaxis guidelines: diagnosis and management of food allergy. Allergy. 2014;69(8):1008-25.
15. Boyce JA, Assa'ad A, Burks AW, Jones SM, Sampson HA, Wood RA, et al. Guidelines for the diagnosis and management of food allergy in the United States: summary of the NIAID-sponsored expert panel report. Nutr Res. 2011;31(1):61-75.
16. Matthai J, Sathiasekharan M, Poddar U, Sibal A, Srivastava A, Waikar Y, et al. Guidelines on diagnosis and management of cow's milk protein allergy. Indian Pediatr. 2020;57(8):723-9.
17. Koletzko S, Niggemann B, Arato A, Dias JA, Heuschkel R, Husby S, et al. Diagnostic approach and management of cow's-milk protein allergy in infants and children: ESPGHAN GI Committee practical guideline. J Pediatr Gastroenterol Nutr. 2012;55(2):221-9.
18. Niggemann B, Beyer K. Diagnosis of food allergy in children: Towards a standardization of food challenge. J Pediatr Gastroenterol Nutr. 2007;45(4):399-404.
19. Tataranu E, Diaconescu S, Ivanescu CG. Clinical and pathological profile of infants suffering from cow's milk protein allergy. Rom J Morphol Embryol. 2016;57:1031-5.
20. Lifschitz C, Szajewska H. Cow's milk allergy: evidence-based diagnosis and management for the practitioner. Eur J Pediatr. 2015;174(2):141-50.
21. Kneepkens CMF, Yolanda M. Clinical practice. Diagnosis and treatment of cow's milk allergy. Eur J Pediatr. 2009;168(8):891-6.
22. Vandenplas Y, Abuabat A, Al-Hammadi S, Aly GS, Miqdady MS, Shaaban SY, et al. Middle East consensus statement on the prevention, diagnosis, and management of cow's milk protein allergy. Pediatr Gastroenterol Hepatol Nutr. 2014;17(2):61-73.
23. Høst A, Koletzko B, Dreborg S, Muraro A, Wahn U, Aggett P, et al. Dietary products used in infants for treatment and prevention of food allergy. Arch Dis Child. 1999;81(1):80-4.
24. Fiocchi A, Schünemann HJ, Brozek J, Restani P, Beyer K, Troncone R, et al. Diagnosis and rationale for action against cow's milk allergy (DRACMA): a summary report. J Allergy Clin Immunol. 2010;126(6):1119-28.e12.
25. Fiocchi A, Brozek J, Schünemann H, Bahna SL, von Berg A, Beyer K, et al; World Allergy Organization (WAO) Diagnosis and Rationale for Action against Cow's Milk Allergy (DRACMA) guidelines. Pediatr Allergy Immunol. 2010;21(Suppl 21):1-125
26. Greer FR, Scott H, Sicherer SH, Burks W. Effects of early nutritional interventions on the development of atopic disease in infants and children: the role of maternal dietary restriction, breastfeeding, timing of introduction of complementary foods, and hydrolyzed formulas. Pediatrics. 2008;121:183-91.

27. Fiocchi A, Dahda L, Dupont C, Campoy C, Fierro V, Nietto A. Cow's milk allergy: towards an update of DRACMA guidelines. World Allergy Organ J. 2016;9(1):35.
28. Osborn DA, Sinn J. Soy formula for prevention of allergy and food intolerance in infants. Cochrane Database Syst Rev. 2006;(4):CD003741.
29. Høst A, Halken S, Jacobsen HP, Christensen AE, Herskind AM, Plesner K. Clinical course of cow's milk protein allergy/intolerance and atopic diseases in childhood. Pediatr Allergy Immunol. 2002;13(s15):23-8.
30. Skripak JM, Matsui EC, Mudd K, Wood RA. The natural history of IgE-mediated cow's milk allergy. J Allergy Clin Immunol. 2007;120(5):1172-7.
31. Fiocchi A, Burks W, Bahna SL, Bielory L, Boyle RJ, Cocco R, et al. Clinical use of probiotics in pediatric allergy (CUPPA): A World Allergy Organization position paper. World Allergy Organ J. 2012;5(11):148-67.
32. Vandenplas Y. Prevention and management of cow's milk allergy in non-exclusively breastfed infants. Nutrients. 2017;9(7):731.
33. Kramer MS, Kakuma R. Maternal dietary antigen avoidance during pregnancy or Lactation, or both, for preventing or treating atopic disease in the child. Cochrane Database Syst Rev. 2012;(9):CD000133.
34. Osborn DA, Sinn JK, Jones LJ. Infant formulas containing hydrolyzed protein of allergic disease. Cochrane Database Syst Rev. 2018;(10):CD003664.

Hepatology

CHAPTER 12

Nonalcoholic Fatty Liver Disease

Yogesh Waikar

■ INTRODUCTION

Nonalcoholic fatty liver disease (NAFLD) is an accumulation of excessive fat in the liver. It may progress to inflammation and cirrhosis. Hence, NAFLD includes a spectrum of clinical presentations, from isolated hepatic steatosis, to nonalcoholic steatohepatitis (NASH) with hepatic inflammation and fibrosis. Sometimes, it may lead to cirrhosis and end-stage liver disease (ESLD). Ethnic differences and clinical heterogeneity regarding NAFLD are well known. More children are getting diagnosed with NAFLD. Multiple factors are involved in the pathological process of NAFLD. This chapter focuses on the diagnosis of NAFLD in children based on available guidelines and literature. Clinical approach to NAFLD is suggested.

■ IS IT NONALCOHOLIC FATTY LIVER DISEASE?

Nonalcoholic fatty liver (NAFL) is rare in children <3 years. In children between 3 and 10 years, other causes of fatty liver should be ruled out prior to considering a diagnosis of NAFLD. In children above 10 years, the classical setting for the diagnosis of NAFLD includes the presence of central adiposity, elevated body mass index (BMI), clinical signs of insulin resistance, and positive family history of comorbid metabolic pathology. Sedentary lifestyles do contribute to its development. Obvious liver failure, neonatal conjugated hyperbilirubinemia, or large hepatosplenomegaly is indicative of liver diseases other than NAFLD.[1]

Metabolic diseases such as ornithine transcarbamylase deficiency may present as microvesicular steatosis.[1] Citrin deficiency, hepatic forms of glycogenosis, hereditary fructose intolerance, congenital disorders of glycosylation, and cholesterol ester storage disease should be suspected in the differential diagnosis. The nonclassical presentation of clinical signs and atypical age group would help in their diagnosis. Children with abetalipoproteinemia and hypobetalipoproteinemia may develop abnormal accumulation of fat in liver. Other differential diagnoses include cystic fibrosis, celiac disease, and malnutrition, which may present as fatty liver or hepatic steatosis. Endocrinopathies such as hypothyroidism and hypothalamic diseases are suspected in the presence of associated clinical signs and symptoms.[1] Genetic disorders such as Down syndrome and Turner syndrome have NAFL as a frequent comorbidity. Autoimmune hepatitis may present with steatohepatitis. Human immunodeficiency virus (HIV)-infected children may have hepatic steatosis. Long-term use of drugs including steroids, methotrexate, tetracycline, amiodarone, nucleoside analogs, aspirin, and antiretroviral drugs is an important cause of fatty liver.[1] Diagnosis of NAFLD needs thorough clinical evaluation, ruling out comorbid clinical conditions, and appropriate drug history.

Secondary NAFLD is suspected in nonobese children with elevated alanine transaminase (ALT >2 times the upper limit), which is persistent for 6 months even after lifestyle intervention.[2] Secondary NAFLD sometimes is called as lean NAFLD. Lipodystrophy and alternative diagnosis due to genetic and congenital conditions should be ruled out. Monogenic causes of chronic liver disease such as fatty acid oxidation defects, peroxisomal disorders, and lysosomal storage diseases should be considered in nonoverweight and very young children as per the American Association for the Study of Liver Diseases (AASLD) guideline.[3] North American Society of Pediatric Gastroenterology, Hepatology and Nutrition (NASPGHAN) guideline gives the strength of recommendations as "strong (1)" and "weak (2)", and the level of evidence as "high (A), moderate (B), and low (C)" for recommending or excluding alternative etiologies for evaluating hepatic steatosis.[4]

■ DIAGNOSIS OF NONALCOHOLIC FATTY LIVER DISEASE

Clinical Diagnosis of Nonalcoholic Fatty Liver Disease

Most children with hepatic steatosis are asymptomatic. There may be nonspecific abdominal pain, malaise, or fatigue. Mild hepatomegaly may be appreciated. Acanthosis nigricans and raised waist circumference are the accompanying clinical signs in some cases with NAFLD.[5-7] Waist circumference and waist to height ratio provide an estimate for adiposity. Clinical history of obstructive sleep apnea (OSA) should raise a suspicion of lean NAFLD.[8]

Spectrum of Disease

- *Hepatic steatosis or NAFL:* >5% hepatic fatty changes without necroinflammatory or fibrotic changes.
- *Nonalcoholic steatohepatitis:* Fatty liver with inflammation and hepatocellular injury, with or without fibrosis.

Biochemical Investigations

The best screening test recommended by NASPGHN for the diagnosis NAFLD is the liver enzyme, *alanine aminotransferase (ALT)* (strength 1, evidence B), but it has limitations.[4] ALT may be elevated in many other hepatic disorders also. Persistently elevated ALT of twice the upper limit of normal for >3 months should direct one to investigate for NAFLD or other causes (strength 1, evidence C). Furthermore, if ALT > 80 U/L, the likelihood of significant liver disease is higher (strength 2, evidence C). Normal ALT does not exclude liver steatosis or its progression to cirrhosis as per the European Society of Pediatric Gastroenterology, Hepatology and Nutrition (ESPGHAN) guideline.[5] The aspartate aminotransferase (AST) to ALT ratio > 1 directs toward increasing fibrosis.[9]

Serum uric acid is an important investigation in considering the diagnosis of NAFLD. Higher serum uric acid is noted with hepatic steatosis in children.[10]

The risk of developing NAFLD increases with increase in gamma-glutamyl transferase (GGT) levels.[11] High GGT in NAFLD is associated with liver fibrosis.[12]

One of the best independent predictive risk factors for diagnosis NAFLD in obese children is fasting serum insulin >18.9 U/mL.[13] Insulin resistance and high serum triglyceride levels are additional risk factors for NAFLD.[5] Homeostatic model assessment for insulin resistance (HOMA-IR) provides an estimate for insulin resistance. It has its limitation in metabolic conditions.[14] The cut-off value for HOMA-IR of 4.9 is associated with severe steatosis in obese children with a 100% negative predictive value and a 33% positive predictive value in studies.[14]

Other noninvasive biomarkers have also been studied in children with NAFLD.[15] More validation studies are required as per AASLD and NASPGHAN as well as ESPGHAN guidelines. In atypical, lean or secondary NAFLD cases, other causes for hepatic steatosis should be ruled out by doing the following investigations—hepatitis B surface antigen (HbsAg), GGT, immunoglobulin A (IgA), tissue transglutaminase IgA (tTg-IgA), serum creatine phosphokinase (CPK), serum ceruloplasmin, and autoimmune markers.[2] Serum thyroid stimulating hormone (TSH) should be done to rule out hypothyroidism. Lipid profile would rule out comorbid dyslipidemia.

Mean ALT of the child over follow-up of 96 weeks and percentage of change of ALT from baseline to 96 weeks are noted to be significant predictors of NAFLD. In children with ALT > 60 U/L at baseline, a mean ALT at or <62–77 U/L overtime predicted improvement in NASH.[16]

UK National Institute for Health and Care Excellence (NICE) guideline considered using enhanced liver fibrosis (ELF) test in children diagnosed with NAFLD. An ELF score > 10.50 suggests advanced liver fibrosis and early referral to specialist. If ELF is <10.51, children should be retested every 2 years.[17] During follow-up, HOMA-IR might help to identify patient at risk of fibrosis progression.

Genetic Signature of NAFLD

Patatin-like phospholipase domain-containing protein 3 (PNPLA3) single nucleotide polymorphism is associated with portal pattern of steatosis, inflammation, and fibrosis.[18] Another study identified that PNPLA3, and TM6SF2T (transmembrane 6 superfamily member 2) alleles have more than threefold higher risk of NAFLD than noncarriers.[19] The mutated PNPLA3 1148M variant attached to the surface of lipid droplets reduces the cleavage of triglyceride leading to lipid retention in hepatocyte and hepatic steatosis.[20] The genetic risk score based on a combination of variants and clinical risk factors improves the prediction of NAFLD in obese children by 5.2% as compared to clinical factor alone.[21]

Metabolic Signature of NAFLD

The lipid lipoprotein profile in NAFLD is characterized by increased amounts of extremely large to small very low-density lipoprotein (VLDL). Triglyceride remnant cholesterol and saturated fatty acid concentrates of glycoprotein acetyls are also increased which suggest a chronic inflammation.[22] Saturated fatty acids, palmitic acid, and myristic acid in salvia are increased in pediatric obesity-related liver disease. Higher level of salivary pyroglutamic acid is a suggested biomarker of increasing severity of NALFD.[23]

Steroid metabolites are also altered in nonsyndromic childhood obesity. Urine 5-alpha-reductase and 21-hydroxylase activities are increased while 11-beta-hydroxysteroid dehydrogenase-1 (11BHSD1) activity and dehydroepiandrosterone (DHEA) are reduced in NAFLD. These findings reflected lesser hepatic recycling of cortisone to cortisol, which is compensated by increased adrenal cortisol leading to higher glucocorticoid metabolites and lower mineralocorticoid metabolites.[24] It is also called as steroid metabolic signature of liver disease in childhood obesity.

Microbiome Signature of NAFLD

Children with NAFLD have altered intestinal flora. The proportion of actinomycetes is lower and proportion of thermus is higher in NAFLD group at the level of phylum. At the level of genus, the proportion of bacteroid and bifidobacterium in children with NAFLD is lower while the proportion of prevotella is higher. This is supposed to alter lipid metabolic pathway leading to NAFLD.[25]

Intestinal dysbiosis is also confirmed in analysis of fecal microbiomes of children with NAFLD. Children with NAFLD have lower diversity of microbiome in the gut. High prevotella is associated with fibrosis. Genes involved in flagellar assembly are enriched in patients with fibrosis.[26] Small intestinal bacterial overgrowth also affects the insulin level and NAFLD.[27]

Genetic, metabolic, and microbiome signatures of NAFLD are newer approaches to study and diagnose NAFLD. There is a need for studies across different ethnicity for further validation.

Newer Biomarkers of NAFLD

The various scores for steatosis prediction such as NAFLD liver fat score, fatty liver index, and hepatic steatosis index need further validation.[4] Combined pediatric NAFLD fibrosis index and ELF score are found to be accurate in assessing fibrosis in children with NAFLD.[4,5] ESPGHAN, NASPGHAN, and AASLD recommend more studies to confirm the role of biomarkers in children with NAFLD. NICE guideline considers ELF test for NAFLD liver fibrosis. A brief overview of clinically significant tests is described here.

Pediatric NAFLD fibrosis index (PNFI) using age, waist circumference, and triglyceride can be used in place of liver biopsy to rule in liver fibrosis.[28] A PNFI score of >9 has positive predictive value of 98.5%. ELF test is proposed for screening progressive fibrosis.[29] It uses hyaluronic acid, procollagen III N-terminal peptide (P3NP), and tissue inhibitor of metalloproteinase (TIMP-1). The combination of PNFI and ELF is also used to predict presence of fibrosis.[30] PNFI < 3.47 rules out liver fibrosis. PNFI > 9 can rule in liver fibrosis. If PNFI is 3.47–9 then ELF score is used. ELF < 8.49 can rule out fibrosis.

Pediatric study for validation for fibrosis-4 (FIB-4) index calculated as [(age in years) × AST in U/L) / platelet count in 10^9/L × $\sqrt{ALT\ in\ U/L}$] is noted to be insensitive.[31] AST to ALT (AST/ALT) ratio, AST to platelet ratio index (APRI), and NAFLD fibrosis score (NFS) also have poor accuracy. BARD score (BMI, AST/ALT ratio, and diabetes) is not evaluated for detecting mild-to-moderate fibrosis. It has also poor accuracy. ELF is the test with high accuracy, but it is costly and needs a kit from the manufactures, which makes it difficult to assess. PNFI is complex with poor to moderate accuracy.[32]

Low neuregulin 4 levels and adipokine in NAFLD are diagnostic. Elevated neuregulin 4 is associated with decreased risk of NAFLD.[33] Another adipokines, chemerin is noted be a suitable biomarker of liver steatosis.[34] Leptin to adiponectin ratio is also raised in children with NAFLD.[35] Hepatokines are functional proteins produced by liver regulating glucose and lipid metabolism similar to fibroblast growth factor-21 (FGF-21) and are significantly higher in NAFLD.[36]

Liver Biopsy

As per AASLD guideline, liver biopsy should be done in children with suspected NAFLD in whom diagnosis is unclear and there is a possibility of multiple diagnosis, or before starting hepatotoxic medical therapy. While NASPGHAN guideline considered liver biopsy in a patient with increased risk of NASH and/or advanced fibrosis, ALT > 80 U/L, splenomegaly and AST/ALT > 1, panhypopituitarism, type 2 diabetes mellitus (strength 1, evidence B), and ESPGHAN guidelines accepted the indication to do liver biopsy as follows:

- To exclude other treatable diseases
- In case of clinically advanced disease
- Before pharmacological or surgical treatment
- As a part of intervention protocol or clinical research trial
- <10 years of age
- Family history of severe NAFLD.

Histopathology of liver biopsy in children, particularly prepubertal boys show more steatosis, less ballooning and more portal-based inflammation and fibrosis, commonly described as type II NASH.[32] The diagnosis of NAFLD is established when at least 5% of hepatocytes present with micro- or macrovesicular steatosis.[37] Two widely accepted and validation methods for scoring and staging the pathologic changes of NAFLD are NASH-Clinical Research Network (NASH-CRN) proposed "NAFLD activity score (NAS)" and the European fatty liver inhibition of progression (FLIP) proposed "Steatosis, Activity, and Fibrosis (SAF) score".[38,39] Another "Pediatric NAFLD histological score (PNHS)" based on steatosis, lobular inflammation, ballooning, and portal inflammation strongly correlates with the presence of NASH.[40]

Imaging for NAFLD

Ultrasonography

It is the first-line imaging modality for NAFLD. Ultrasonography (USG) for fatty liver is a safe and inexpensive test, but plain ultrasound cannot quantify steatosis or fibrosis. It is useful mainly to rule out other pathologies, as it has poor specificity for NAFLD as per NASPGHAN and ESPGHAN guidelines. NICE guideline uses USG for screening purpose. Increased brightness of the liver compared to adjacent right kidney or spleen indicates hepatic steatosis.[41] USG score ≥2 by Saverymuttu score has high pool specificity of 96% and sensitivity of 52%.[42] The mean sensitivity of USG for steatosis identification ranges from 73–90%.[43] "Controlled attenuation parameter (CAP)" is used to assess presence of hepatic steatosis by using shear wave propagation. It is used in transient elastography; fibroscan CAP value > 241 dB/m suggests steatosis.[44] CAP value estimation has limitation in obese children.[44] Liver stiffness measurement by fibroscan > 5.5 kilopascal (kPa) is useful to diagnose hepatic fibrosis.[45] More validation studies are needed.

Magnetic Resonance Imaging (MRI)

It is not cost effective but can help in diagnosing steatosis and fibrosis. Proton density fat fraction (PDFF) assessed by MRI is an objective test for quantification of liver steatosis.[46] MRI-PDFF allows fat mapping of entire liver. Nuclear magnetic resonance (NMR) spectroscopy measures concentration of lipids in a small area of interest in liver.[47] More pediatric specific research is indicated.

Newer Imaging Modalities

Newer tests such as noninvasive semiquantitative USG fatty liver indicator (USFLI) are studied in pediatric NAFLD. USFLI score > 2 is diagnostic of NAFLD.[48] USFLI score > 6 has positive predicative value of 71%, sensitivity of 75% and specificity of 63% for predicting hepatitis in children with NAFLD.[49]

Field of artificial intelligence integrating radiologic bioimages with genomic data and its correlation with liver biopsy would improve diagnosing NAFLD in future.

A systematic approach to assessment and diagnosis of NAFLD is given in **Flowchart 12.1**.

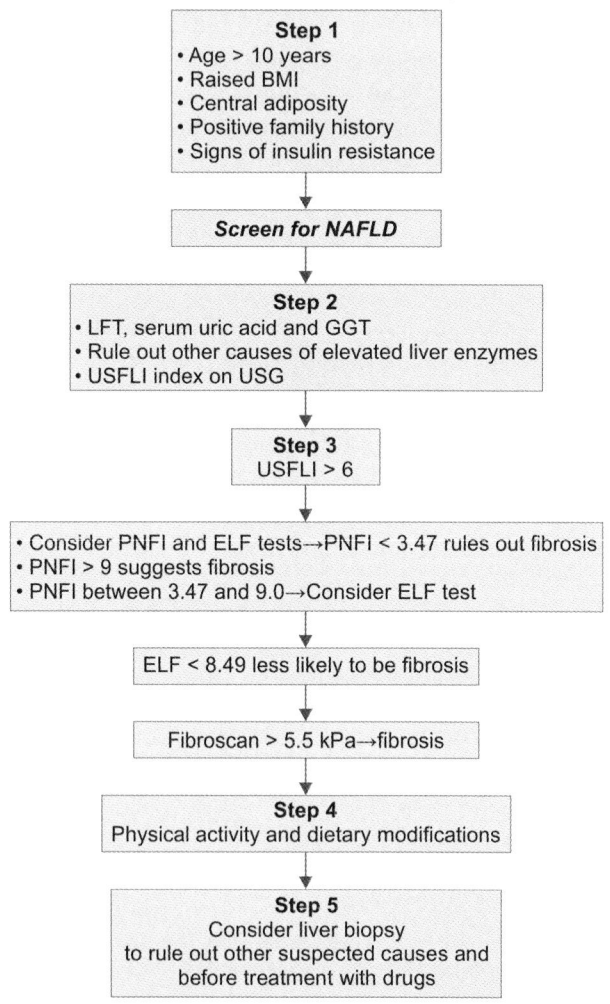

Flowchart 12.1: Stepwise approach for the diagnosis of NAFLD.

(BMI: body mass index; ELF: enhanced liver fibrosis; GGT: gamma-glutamyl transferase; LFT: liver function test; NAFLD: Nonalcoholic fatty liver disease; PNFI: pediatric NAFLD fibrosis index; USG: ultrasonography; USFLI: ultrasonography fatty liver indicator)

MANAGEMENT

NICE 2016 guidelines stresses on physical activity and dietary modifications. Vitamin E can be considered only with advanced fibrosis. There is no role of ursodeoxycholic acid (UDCA).[17] As per NASPGHAN 2017 guidelines, proper diet consultation, increase in physical activity, avoiding sugar-sweetened beverages, and screen time activities to < 2 hours per day are the cornerstones in the management of NAFLD. No medications or drugs are recommended. Bariatric surgery can be considered with BMI > 35 kg/m^2 who have noncirrhotic NAFLD and other associated comorbidities in adolescents.[4] AASLD 2018 guideline advocates intensive lifestyle modifications and no role of metformin.[3] Vitamin E 800 IU/day may be considered after one-to-one discussion with parents. Histological benefits in some children are noted with vitamin E. Long-term safety of high dose of vitamin E is unknown.

The common suggested goals for management include the following:[50]
- Weight reduction of 5–7% of initial weight in first 6 months
- Reduction in carbohydrate intake particularly simple sugars like fructose
- Reduction in dietary fat to less than 7%
- Avoiding high consumption of transfat (bakery fat, fried fast food, margarine, instant meals, and cakes).

A randomized controlled clinical trial on children with biopsy-proven NASH of lifestyle modification plus a mix containing docosahexaenoic acid, choline, and vitamin E (DHA-CHO-VE) suggested improving hepatic steatosis and reduced ALT and glucose levels in children with NASH.[51] But more data is needed before recommending such a therapy.

TONIC trial was a large, randomized, placebo-controlled study involving children (aged 8–17 years) with biopsy-proven NAFLD comparing metformin, vitamin E, and placebo. It revealed that neither vitamin E nor metformin was superior to placebo in attaining the primary outcome of sustained reduction in ALT level in patients with pediatric NAFLD.[38] There was improvement in hepatocyte ballooning of the children taking metformin (500 mg twice daily). But there was no difference in steatosis, inflammation, or fibrosis compared with placebo.[52] Side effects such as nausea or lactic acidosis with renal impairment should be discussed with the family and the patient before considering metformin treatment. Studies on omega-3 fatty acids in NAFLD have shown variable results.[53]

Results of the randomized study over the period of 1 year have demonstrated the positive effects of diet plus n-3 PUFA (polyunsaturated fats) in NAFLD. PUFA in a dose of 1,000 mg was given daily to children in this study.[54] More studies are needed. 500 mg of docosahexaenoic acid and 800 IU of vitamin D in children with vitamin D deficiency improved insulin-resistance, lipid profile, ALT, and NAS.[55]

Randomized controlled trials with a larger sample size, long-term follow-up, and assessment of efficacy based on liver histology are required before the use of probiotics for NAFLD.[53] Antioxidant such as cysteamine bitartrate was studied for NAFLD, but efficacy is limited due to isolated trial.[56] Interesting study of fecal microbiota transplantation (FMT) in mice suggested that FMT might be effective in attenuating high-fat diet (HFD)-induced steatohepatitis.[57]

Obeticholic acid (OCA), elafibranor, selonsertib, cenicriviroc, aramchol, and liraglutide are drugs in pipeline for NAFLD.[53] Plasminogen activator inhibitor-1 (PAI-1) is elevated in children with NAFLD. It is associated with increased disease severity. Losartan is an angiotensin II receptor blocker (ARB). It was studied for 8 weeks using a dose of 50 mg daily orally in 12 normotensive children. Reducing trend of liver enzymes was confirmed.[58] Most studies on pharmacological aspects of NAFLD need more evidence-based support and larger randomized trials before their widespread use.

■ KEY POINTS

- Children above 10 years with central adiposity should be considered for assessment of NAFLD.
- In secondary NAFLD in nonobese children, the underlying metabolic or monogenic disease should be ruled out.
- Elevated ALT is suggested as the screening test for NAFLD. Elevated serum uric acid points to significant hepatic steatosis. High GGT points toward increasing fibrosis. All these parameters are sensitive but not specific and need more studies for correlation.
- *PNPLA3* gene, lipid lipoprotein profile, and stool flora assessment for association with NAFLD are the emerging research tools.
- Various tests individually or in combination, based on the anthropometry, biochemical values and other parameters, may help in ruling out liver fibrosis.
- Physical activity, weight loss with long-term dietary modification, and lifestyle management are the cornerstones in management of NAFLD.
- Liver biopsy remains gold standard to diagnose and prognosticate NAFLD; it is indicated whenever the diagnosis is uncertain and before starting drug treatment.
- Drug treatment is not routinely recommended and is still under trials.

■ REFERENCES

1. Alfani R, Vassallo E, De Anseris AG, Nazzaro L, D'Acunzo I, Porfito C, et al. Pediatric fatty liver and obesity: Not always just a matter of non-alcoholic fatty liver disease. Children (Basel). 2018;5(12):169.
2. Di Sessa A, Marzuillo P, Guarino S, Cirillo G, del Giudice EM. When a secondary form of pediatric non-alcoholic fatty liver disease should be suspected? Expert Rev Gastroenterol Hepatol. 2019;13(6):519-21.
3. Chalasani N, Younossi Z, Lavine JE, Charlton M, Cusi K, Rinella M, et al. The diagnosis and management of nonalcoholic fatty liver disease: Practice guidance from the American Association for the Study of Liver Diseases. Hepatology. 2018;67(1):328-57.

4. Vos MB, Abrams SH, Barlow SE, Caprio S, Daniels SR, Kohli R, et al. NASPGHAN clinical practice guideline for the diagnosis and treatment of nonalcoholic fatty liver disease in children: Recommendations from the expert committee on NAFLD (ECON) and the North American Society of Pediatric Gastroenterology, Hepatology and Nutrition (NASPGHAN). J Pediatr Gastroenterol Nutr. 2017;64(2):319-34.
5. Vajro P, Lenta S, Socha P, Dhawan A, McKiernan P, Baumann U, et al. Diagnosis of nonalcoholic fatty liver disease in children and adolescents: position paper of the ESPGHAN Hepatology Committee. J Pediatr Gastroenterol Nutr. 2012;54(5):700-13.
6. Eng K, Lopez R, Liccardo D, Nobili V, Alkhouri N. A noninvasive prediction model for non-alcoholic steatohepatitis in paediatric patients with non-alcoholic fatty liver disease. Dig Liver Dis. 201;46(11):1008-13.
7. Bacopoulou F, Efthymiou V, Landis G, Rentoumis A, Chrousos GP. Waist circumference, waist-to-hip ratio and waist-to height ratio reference percentiles for abdominal obesity among Greek adolescents. BMC Pediatr. 2015;15:50.
8. Nobili V, Cutrera R, Liccardo D, Pavone M, Devito R, Giorgio V, et al. Obstructive sleep apnea syndrome affects liver histology and inflammatory cell activation in pediatric nonalcoholic fatty liver disease, regardless of obesity/insulin resistance. Am J Respir Crit Care Med. 2014;189(1):66-76.
9. Patton HM, Lavine JE, Van Natta ML, Schwimmer JB, Kleiner D, Molleston J. Nonalcoholic Steatohepatitis Clinical Research Network. Clinical correlates of histopathology in pediatric nonalcoholic steatohepatitis. Gastroenterology. 2008;135(6):1961-71.
10. Zhao K, Ju H, Wang H. Metabolic characteristics of obese children with fatty liver: A STROBE-compliant article. Medicine (Baltimore). 2019;98(16):e14939.
11. Kim JY, Cho J, Yang HR. Biochemical predictors of early onset non-alcoholic fatty liver disease in young children with obesity. J Korean Med Sci. 2018;33(16):e122.
12. Molleston JP, Schwimmer JB, Yates KP, Murray KF, Cummings OW, Lavine JE, et al; NASH clinical research network. Histological abnormalities in children with nonalcoholic fatty liver disease and normal or mildly elevated alanine aminotransferase levels. J Pediatr. 2014;164(4):707-13.
13. Prokopowicz Z, Malecka-Tendera E, Matusik P. Predictive value of adiposity level, metabolic syndrome, and insulin resistance for the risk of nonalcoholic fatty liver disease diagnosis in obese children. Can J Gastroenterol Hepatol. 2018;2018:9465784.
14. Ubiña-Aznar E, Tapia-Ceballos L, Rosales-Zabal JM, Prcel-Chacon R, Poveda-Gomez F, Lozano-Cuevas C, et al. Insulin resistance and the metabolic syndrome are related to the severity of steatosis in the pediatric population with obesity. Rev Esp Enferm Dig. 2017;109(11):772-7.
15. He L, Deng L, Zhang Q, Guo J, Zhou J, Song W, et al. Diagnostic Value of CK-18, FGF-21, and related biomarker panel in nonalcoholic fatty liver disease: A systematic review and meta-analysis. Biomed Res Int. 2017:2017:9729107.
16. Arsik I, Frediani JK, Frezza D, Chen W, Ayer T, Keskinocak P, et al. Alanine aminotransferase as a monitoring biomarker in children with nonalcoholic fatty liver disease: A secondary analysis using TONIC trial data. Children (Basel). 2018;5(6):64.

17. UK National Institute for Health and Care Excellence (NICE). (2016). Non-alcoholic fatty liver disease (NAFLD): assessment and management. [online] Available from: https://www.nice.org.uk/guidance/ng49. [Last accessed December, 2021].
18. Hudert CA, Selinski S, Rudolph B, Blaker H, Loddenkemper C, Thielhorn R, et al. Genetic determinants of steatosis and fibrosis progression in paediatric non-alcoholic fatty liver disease. Liver Int. 2019;39(3):540-56.
19. Di Costanzo A, Pacifico L, Chiesa C, Perla FM, Ceci F, Angeloni A, et al. Genetic and metabolic predictors of hepatic fat content in a cohort of Italian children with obesity. Pediatr Res. 2019;85(5):671-7.
20. Mosca A, De Cosmi V, Parazzini F, Raponi M, Alisi A, Agostoni C, et al. The role of genetic predisposition, programing during fetal life, family conditions, and post-natal diet in the development of pediatric fatty liver disease. J Pediatr. 2019;211:72-7.
21. Zusi C, Mantovani A, Olivieri F, Morandi A, Corradi M, Del Giudice EM, et al. Contribution of a genetic risk score to clinical prediction of hepatic steatosis in obese children and adolescents. Dig Liver Dis. 2019;51(11):1586-92.
22. Hartley A, Santos Ferreira DL, Anderson EL, Lawlor DA. Metabolic profiling of adolescent non-alcoholic fatty liver disease. Wellcome Open Res. 2018;3:166.
23. Troisi J, Belmonte F, Bisogno A, Pierri L, Colucci A, Scala G, et al. Metabolomic salivary signature of pediatric obesity related liver disease and metabolic syndrome. Nutrients. 2019;11(2):274.
24. Gawlik A, Shmoish M, Hartmann MF, Wudy SA, Olczak Z, Gruszczynska K, et al. Steroid metabolomic signature of liver disease in nonsyndromic childhood obesity. Endocr Connect. 2019;8(6):764-71.
25. Jianrong L, Yinjie Z, Zhihui Z, et al. Intestinal flora specific changes in children with nonalcoholic fatty liver disease. Chinese J Pediatr. 2018;56(11):850-5.
26. Schwimmer JB, Johnson JS, Angeles JE, Behling C, Belt PH, Borecki I, et al. Microbiome signatures associated with steatohepatitis and moderate to severe fibrosis in children with nonalcoholic fatty liver disease. Gastroenterology. 2019;157(4):1109-22.
27. Stepanov YM, Zavhorodnia NY, Yagmur VB, Lukianenko OY, Zygalo EV. Association of nonalcoholic fatty liver disease with small intestine bacterial overgrowth in obese children. Wiad Lek. 2019;72(3):350-6.
28. Nobili V, Alisi A, Vania A, Tiribeli C, Pietrobattista A, Bedogni G. The pediatric NAFLD fibrosis index: a predictor of liver fibrosis in children with non-alcoholic fatty liver disease. BMC Med. 2009;7:21.
29. Nobili V, Parkes J, Bottazzo G, Marcellini M, Cross R, Newman D, et al. Performance of ELF serum markers in predicting fibrosis stage in pediatric non-alcoholic fatty liver disease. Gastroenterology. 2009;136(1):160-7.
30. Alkhouri N, Carter-Kent C, Lopez R, Rosenberg WM, Pinzani M, Bedogni G, et al. A combination of the pediatric NAFLD fibrosis index and enhanced liver fibrosis test identifies children with fibrosis. Clin Gastroenterol Hepatol. 2011;9(2,):150-5.
31. Jackson JA, Konomi JV, Mendoza MV, Krasinskas A, Jin R, Caltharp S, et al. Performance of fibrosis prediction scores in paediatric non-alcoholic fatty liver disease. J Paediatr Child Health. 2018;54(2):172-6.

32. Draijer L, Benninga M, Koot B. Pediatric NAFLD: an overview and recent developments in diagnostics and treatment. Expert Rev Gastroenterol Hepatol. 2019;13(5):447-61.
33. Wang R, Yang F, Qing L, Huang R, Liu Q, Li X. Decreased serum neuregulin 4 levels associated with non-alcoholic fatty liver disease in children with obesity. Clin Obes. 2019;9(1):e12289.
34. Mohamed AA, Sabry S, Abdallah AM, Elazeem NAA, Refaey D, Algebaly HAF, et al. Circulating adipokines in children with nonalcoholic fatty liver disease: possible noninvasive diagnostic markers. Ann Gastroenterol. 2017;30(4):457-63.
35. Angin Y, Arslan N, Kuralay F. Leptin-to-adiponectin ratio in obese adolescents with nonalcoholic fatty liver disease. Turk J Pediatr. 2014;56(3):259-66.
36. Flisiak-Jackiewicz M, Bobrus-Chociej A, Wasilewska N, Tarasow E, Wojtkowska M, Lebensztejn, et al. Can hepatokines be regarded as novel non-invasive serum biomarkers of intrahepatic lipid content in obese children? Adv Med Sci. 2019;64(2):280-4.
37. Brunt EM, Janney CG, Di Bisceglie AM, Neuschwander-Tetri BA, Bacon BR. Nonalcoholic steatohepatitis: a proposal for grading and staging the histological lesions. Am J Gastroenterol. 1999;94(9):2467-74.
38. Kleiner DE, Brunt EM, Van Natta M, Behling C, Contos MJ, Cummings OW, et al. Design and validation of a histological scoring system for nonalcoholic fatty liver disease. Hepatology. 2005;41(6):1313-21.
39. Bedossa P, FLOP Pathology Consortium. Utility and appropriateness of the fatty liver inhibition of progression (FLIP) algorithm and steatosis, activity, and fibrosis (SAF) score in the evaluation of biopsies of nonalcoholic fatty liver disease. Hepatology. 2014;60(2):565-75.
40. Alkhouri N, De Vito R, Alisi A, Yerian L, Lopez R, Feldstein AE, et al. Development and validation of a new histological score for pediatric non-alcoholic fatty liver disease. J Hepatol. 2012;57(6):1312-8.
41. Koot BGP, Nobili V. Screening for non-alcoholic fatty liver disease in children: do guidelines provide enough guidance? Obes Rev. 2017;18(9):1050-60.
42. Saverymuttu SH, Joseph AE, Maxwell JD. Ultrasound scanning in the detection of hepatic fibrosis and steatosis. Br Med J (Clin Res Ed). 1986;292(6512):13-5.
43. Bohte AE, van Werven JR, Bipat S, Stoker J. The diagnostic accuracy of US, CT, MRI and ^{1}H-MRS for the evaluation of hepatic steatosis compared with liver biopsy: a meta-analysis. Eur Radiol. 2011;21(1):87-97.
44. Shin J, Kim MJ, Shin HJ, Yoon H, Kim S, Koh H, et al. Quick assessment with controlled attenuation parameter for hepatic steatosis in children based on MRI-PDFF as the gold standard. BMC Pediatr. 2019;19(1):112.
45. Kwon YD, Ko KO, Lim JW, Cheon EJ, Song YH, Yoon JM. Usefulness of transient elastography for non-invasive diagnosis of liver fibrosis in pediatric non-alcoholic steatohepatitis. J Korean Med Sci. 2019;34(23):e165.
46. Middleton MS, Van Natta ML, Heba ER, Alazraki A, Trout AT, Masand P, et al. Diagnostic accuracy of magnetic resonance imaging hepatic proton density fat fraction in pediatric nonalcoholic fatty liver disease. Hepatology. 2018;67(3):858-72.
47. Di Martino M, Pacifico L, Bezzi M, Di Miscio R, Sacconi B, Chiesa C, et al. Comparison of magnetic resonance spectroscopy, proton density fat fraction

and histological analysis in the quantification of liver steatosis in children and adolescents. World J Gastroenterol. 2016;22(39):8812-9.
48. Ballestri S, Lonardo A, Romagnoli D, Carulli L, Losi L, Day CP, et al. Ultrasonographic fatty liver indicator, a novel score which rules out NASH and is correlated with metabolic parameters in NAFLD. Liver Int. 2012;32:1242-52.
49. Liu HK, Yang MC, Su YT, Tai CM, Wei YF, Lin IC, et al. Novel ultrasonographic fatty liver indicator can predict hepatitis in children with non-alcoholic fatty liver disease. Front Pediatr. 2019;6:416.
50. Jeznach-Steinhagen A, Ostrowska J, Czerwonogrodzka-Senczyna A, Boniecka I, Shahnazaryan U, Kuryłowicz A. Dietary and pharmacological treatment of nonalcoholic fatty liver disease. Medicina (Kaunas). 2019;55(5):166.
51. Zöhrer E, Alisi A, Jahnel J, Mosca A, Corte CD, Crudele A, et al. Efficacy of docosahexaenoic acid-choline-vitamin E in paediatric NASH: a randomized controlled clinical trial. Appl Physiol Nutr Metab. 2017;42(9):948-54.
52. Lavine JE, Schwimmer JB, Van Natta ML, Molleston JP, Murray KF, Rosenthal P, et al; Nonalcoholic Steatohepatitis Clinical Research Network. Effect of vitamin E or metformin for treatment of nonalcoholic fatty liver disease in children and adolescents: the TONIC randomized controlled trial. JAMA. 2011;305(16):1659-68.
53. Selvakumar PKC, Kabbany MN, Alkhouri N. Nonalcoholic fatty liver disease in children: Not a small matter. Paediatr Drugs. 2018;20(4):315-29.
54. Boyraz M, Pirgon Ö, Dündar B, Çekmez F, Hatipoğlu N. Long-term treatment with n-3 polyunsaturated fatty acids as a monotherapy in children with nonalcoholic fatty liver disease. J Clin Res Pediatr Endocrinol. 2015;7(2):121-7.
55. Corte CD, Carpino G, De Vito R, De Stefanis C, Alisi A, Cianfarani S, et al. Docosahexanoic acid plus vitamin D treatment improves features of NAFLD in children with serum vitamin D deficiency: Results from a single centre trial. PLoS One. 2016;11(12):e0168216.
56. Mann JP, Tang GY, Nobili V, Armstrong MJ. Evaluations of lifestyle, dietary, and pharmacologic treatments for pediatric nonalcoholic fatty liver disease: A systematic review. Clin Gastroenterol Hepatol. 2019;17(8):1457-1476.e7.
57. Zhou D, Pan Q, Shen F, Cao HX, Ding WJ, Chen YW, Fan JG. Total fecal microbiota transplantation alleviates high-fat diet-induced steatohepatitis in mice via beneficial regulation of gut microbiota. Sci Rep. 2017;7(1):1529.
58. Vos MB, Jin R, Konomi JV, Cleeton R, Cruz J, Karpen S, et al. A randomized, controlled, crossover pilot study of losartan for pediatric nonalcoholic fatty liver disease. Pilot Feasibility Stud. 2018;4:109.

Nephrology

CHAPTER 13 — Renal Tubular Disorders

Priyanka Khandelwal, Arvind Bagga

■ INTRODUCTION

Renal tubular disorders are heterogeneous disorders chiefly causing abnormalities in electrolytes, acid-base and fluid balance. Each tubular segment has a characteristic transport function. Specialized tubular segments allow the following:
- Secretion of protons
- Tubular reabsorption of several solutes coupled to the electrochemical gradient generated by the basolateral sodium-potassium ATPase, such as cotransport of glucose, phosphate, and amino acids
- Paracellular uptake of calcium and magnesium
- Vasopressin-induced reabsorption of water.

Tubular disorders are frequently inherited, and they either cause an isolated transport defect (nephrogenic diabetes insipidus or renal glucosuria) or generalized tubular dysfunction (Fanconi syndrome). **Table 13.1** lists the common disorders of tubular function.

Tubular disorders can present with varied clinical manifestations such as growth impairment, refractory rickets, polyuria and unexplained hypertension (**Box 13.1**). Features of the inherited diseases causing Fanconi syndrome might be prominent at presentation, including photophobia and blond hair in cystinosis or cataract, buphthalmos, hypotonia and developmental delay in Lowe syndrome. Patients present with biochemical patterns that indicate dysfunction of specific tubular segments (**Box 13.1**). These patterns are specific to a set of disorders affecting a particular tubular segment, and therefore act as diagnostic fingerprints.[1] An overview of these biochemical patterns with associated inherited defects is given in **Table 13.2**. Careful clinical examination and evaluation of blood and urinary biochemistry reports will enable diagnosis, guide genetic testing, and specific management.

Patients with suspected tubulopathy should be screened with the following blood and urine investigations:
- Serum sodium, potassium, pH, bicarbonate, chloride, calcium, and phosphate

TABLE 13.1: Function of various segments of the renal tubule and associated disorders.

Tubular segment	Function	Disorder
Proximal tubule	Phosphate absorption	Hypophosphatemic rickets
	Glucose absorption	Renal glucosuria
	Amino acid absorption	Cystinuria, generalized aminoaciduria
	Bicarbonate absorption	Proximal renal tubular acidosis
	Low molecular weight protein absorption	Dent disease
	Generalized proximal tubular function	Fanconi syndrome, primary or secondary to systemic disorders (e.g., cystinosis, galactosemia, Lowe syndrome)
Thick ascending limb	Sodium, potassium, chloride transport	Bartter syndrome
	Paracellular magnesium and calcium reabsorption	Hypomagnesemia and hypercalciuria
Distal tubule	Proton (H^+) secretion	Distal renal tubular acidosis
	Sodium, chloride transport	Pseudohypoaldosteronism type 2 Gitelman syndrome
	Magnesium reabsorption	Isolated hypomagnesemia Hypomagnesemia with hypocalcemia
Collecting duct	Sodium, potassium transport	Pseudohypoaldosteronism type 1 Liddle syndrome
	Water transport	Nephrogenic diabetes insipidus

- Urine pH, protein, sugar and osmolality
- Estimation of 24-hour urine calcium and creatinine
- Ultrasonography for medullary nephrocalcinosis and renal stones.

Depending on the abnormal screening test, specific tubular function tests and genetic sequencing for the underlying diagnosis should be done.[2]

■ PATTERNS OF TUBULAR DYSFUNCTION

Hyperchloremic Metabolic Acidosis with Hypokalemia

Bicarbonate losses causing metabolic acidosis and potassium loss leading to hypokalemia are chiefly from the gastrointestinal tract (diarrhea, intestinal fistula and ureterosigmoidostomy) or from the renal tubules. The characteristic biochemical abnormality in renal tubular acidosis (RTA) is

> **BOX 13.1:** Clinical and biochemical features of tubular disorders.
>
> *Clinical*
> - Growth retardation, failure to thrive
> - Polyuria, excessive thirst
> - Recurrent episodes of dehydration, vomiting, fever
> - Refractory rickets
> - Episodic weakness
> - Preference for salty and savory food
> - Delayed gross motor milestones
> - Seizures, tetany
> - Renal calculi, nephrocalcinosis
> - Unexplained hypertension
>
> *Biochemical patterns*
> - Hyperchloremic metabolic acidosis with hypokalemia
> - Hypokalemic metabolic alkalosis, with normal blood pressure or hypertension
> - Hypomagnesemia, with or without hypercalciuria
> - Hyperkalemia, with hyponatremia or hypertension
> - Polyuria, with or without hypernatremia

hyperchloremic metabolic acidosis, due to decreased capacity for excretion of net acid despite normal glomerular function. **Figures 13.1A to C** show the mechanisms of acid base homeostasis in the kidney, with channels affected in patients with RTA. *Hypokalemia* classically accompanies hyperchloremic metabolic acidosis in RTA; *hyperkalemia* may occur rarely from a voltage-defect in the cortical collecting duct.

Distal RTA is caused either by impaired distal secretion of protons, due to an inherited defect in the apical vacuolar-type H^+-ATPase or basolateral HCO_3^-/Cl^- exchanger in the intercalated cells of the cortical collecting duct **(Table 13.2)**, or by a permeability defect causing back leak of secreted protons.[3] Defective reabsorption of bicarbonate causes *proximal RTA*. Isolated proximal RTA is rare and bicarbonaturia typically occurs as a part of generalized tubular dysfunction in the context of Fanconi syndrome. Inherited systemic diseases such as cystinosis, tyrosinemia, Dent disease or Lowe syndrome are the chief causes of Fanconi syndrome that presents with variable degrees of aminoaciduria, low molecular weight proteinuria, phosphaturia, glucosuria and bicarbonaturia **(Table 13.2)**.

Evaluation

Stepwise evaluation of patients with hyperchloremic metabolic acidosis is shown in **Table 13.3**. The initial steps are estimations of the plasma and urine anion gap. While plasma anion gap is normal (8–12 mEq/L) in both RTA and extrarenal (gastrointestinal) bicarbonate loss, their differentiation is possible by clinical findings and a negative urine anion gap in extrarenal

TABLE 13.2: Genetic causes of common tubular disorders.

Pattern	Etiology	Gene, protein	Additional features
Hyperchloremic metabolic acidosis with hypokalemia	Distal renal tubular acidosis[a]	SCL4A1, anion exchanger 1 (Cl⁻/HCO3⁻ exchanger)	Hemolytic anemia
		ATP6V1B1, H⁺-ATPase (B1 subunit); FOXL1, forkhead transcription factor L1	Early onset deafness
		ATP6V0A4, H⁺-ATPase (A4 subunit)	Normal hearing or delayed hearing loss
		WDR72, tryptophan-aspartate repeat domain 72	Amelogenesis imperfecta
	Isolated proximal renal tubular acidosis	SLC4A4, sodium bicarbonate cotransporter 1	Band keratopathy, cataract; defective enamel; mental impairment, basal ganglia calcification
	Fanconi syndrome[a]	CTNS, cystinosin	*Cystinosis:* Corneal cystine deposits, progression to kidney failure
		CLCN5, chloride channel OCRL, phosphatidylinositol bisphosphate phosphatase	*Dent disease:* Nephrocalcinosis, hypercalciuria, night blindness *Lowe syndrome:* Congenital glaucoma, cataract, Intellectual disability
		SLC2A2, Na-glucose transporter	*Fanconi Bickel syndrome:* Hypoglycemia, hepatomegaly
		FAH, Fumarylacetoacetate hydrolase	Tyrosinemia type 1

Contd...

Contd...

Pattern	Etiology	Gene, protein	Additional features
Hypokalemic metabolic alkalosis, normal blood pressure	Bartter syndrome Type I[a]	SLC12A1, NKCC2 transporter	Neonatal-onset, polyhydramnios, prematurity, nephrocalcinosis
	Type II[a]	KCNJ1, potassium (ROMK) channel	Usually early infantile onset, transient hyperkalemia, nephrocalcinosis
	Type III[a]	CLCKNB, chloride channel	Childhood-onset, growth retardation, hypomagnesemia
	Type IV	BSND, Barttin; CLCKNB + CLCKNA, chloride channels	Variable age of onset, sensorineural deafness, hypomagnesemia
	Type V[a]	MAGED2, Maged2	Infantile-onset, transient
	Gitelman syndrome	SLC12A3, NCC transporter	Later onset, muscle cramps, tetany, hypomagnesemia, hypocalciuria
	EAST/SeSAME syndrome	KCNJ10, KCNJ10/Kir4.1	Seizures, deafness, ataxia, hypomagnesemia
Hypokalemic metabolic alkalosis, hypertension	Apparent mineralocorticoid excess[a]	HSD11B2, 11β-hydroxysteroid dehydrogenase-2	Low birth weight, growth failure, polyuria, nephrocalcinosis
	Liddle syndrome	SCNN1B, SCNN1G, SCNN1A, epithelial sodium channel (ENaC)	Late onset, familial hypertension
	Familial hyperaldosteronism types I–IV	Chimeric CYP11B1/CYP11B2, CLCN2, KCNJ5, CACNA1H; all affecting aldosterone synthase enzyme	Variable age of onset and severity; early onset stroke and intracranial aneurysm in type I; adrenal hyperplasia in type III
	Congenital adrenal hyperplasia	CYP17A1, 17α-hydroxylase CYP11B1, 11β-hydroxylase	Delayed puberty in CYP17A1 defect; ambiguous genitalia, precocious puberty in CYP11B1 defect

Contd...

Contd...

Pattern	Etiology	Gene, protein	Additional features
Hypomagnesemia with hypercalciuria	Hypomagnesemia type 3 and 5[a]	CLDN16 and CLDN19, claudin 16 and 19	Nephrocalcinosis, hypercalciuria, deranged kidney function. High myopia in CLDN19 defect
	Autosomal dominant hypocalcemia[a]	CASR, calcium sensing receptor	Hypocalcemia
Hypomagnesemia without hypercalciuria	HNF1B-related kidney disease	HNF1B, hepatocyte nuclear factor 1 homeobox B	Maturity onset diabetes of the young, renal cyst
	Hypomagnesemia type 1	TRPM6, transient receptor potential channel M6	Neonatal onset, severe hypomagnesemia, and hypocalcemia
	Autosomal dominant hypomagnesemia	KCNA1, potassium channel Kv1.1	Episodic myokymia
Hyperkalemia with hyponatremia	Pseudohypoaldosteronism type I	SCNN1A, SCNN1B, SCNN1G (ENaC subunits)	Autosomal recessive, generalized salt wasting, pulmonary and skin manifestations
		NR3C2 mineralocorticoid receptor	Autosomal dominant, urinary salt wasting
Hyperkalemia with hypertension	Pseudohypoaldosteronism type II	WNK4, WNK1, KLHL3, CUL3; With no lysine kinase 1 and 4, Kelch-like, Cullin 3	Thiazide responsive hypertension, variable age of onset
Polyuria	Nephrogenic diabetes insipidus	AVPR2, vasopressin receptor	X-linked inheritance (90%)
		AQP2, aquaporin 2	Autosomal recessive inheritance (10%)
Nephrolithiasis or nephrocalcinosis (without hypercalciuria)	Primary hyperoxaluria type 1	AGXT, Alanine-glyoxylate aminotransferase	Dense nephrocalcinosis, kidney failure
	Cystinuria	SLC3A1, SLC7A9, cystine transporter	Positive nitroprusside test, abnormal aminoacidogram or hexagonal crystals in urine support the diagnosis
	Xanthinuria	XDH, xanthine dehydrogenase	Radiolucent stones, low serum, and urine uric acid
		MOCOS, Molybdenum cofactor sulfurase	

[a]Conditions associated with nephrocalcinosis, other than primary hyperoxaluria, cystinuria and xanthinuria

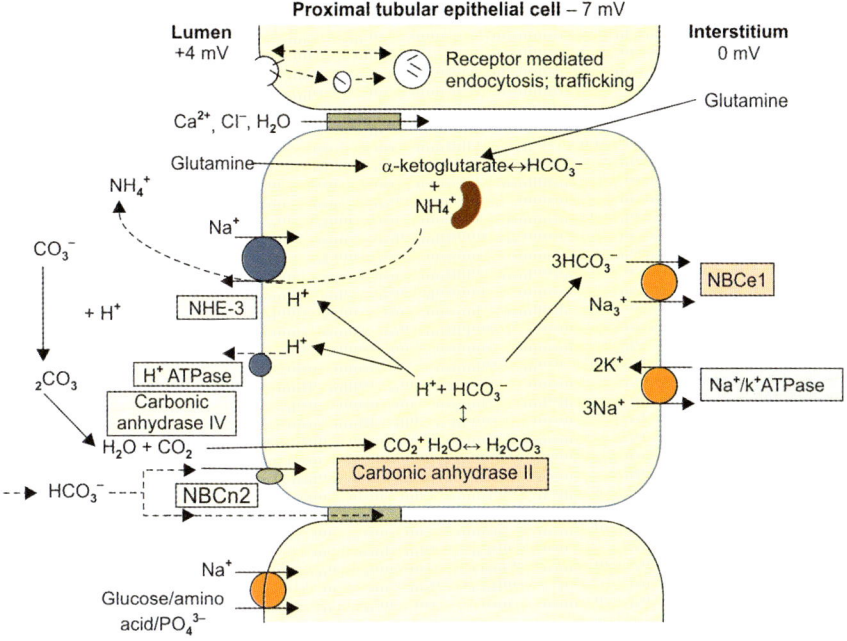

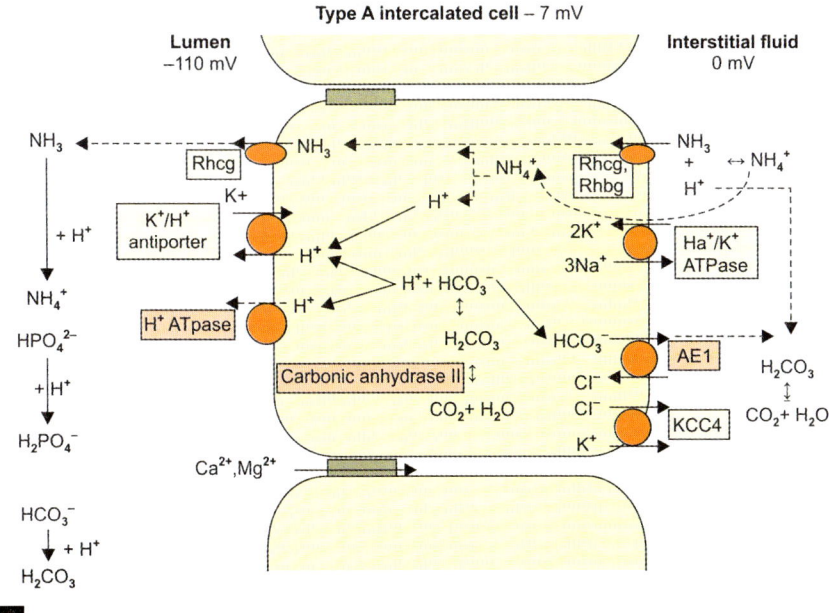

Figs. 13.1 and B

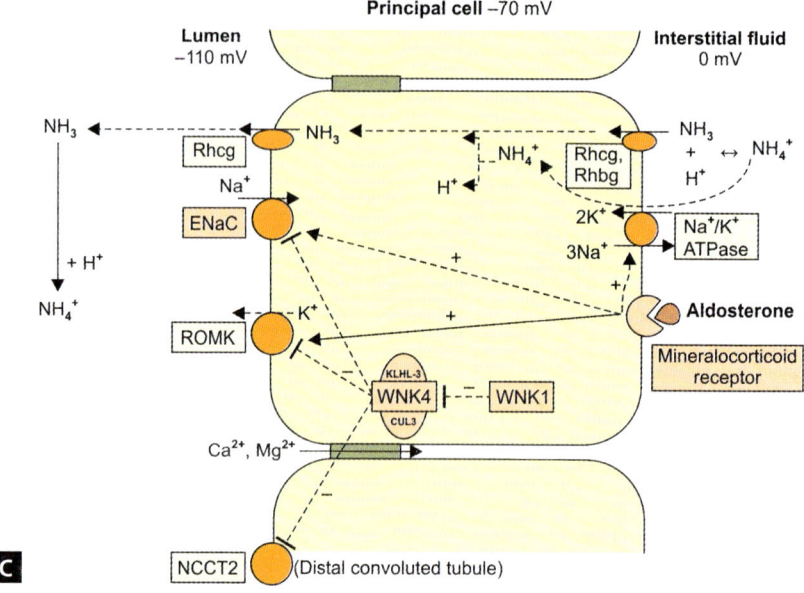

Figs. 13.1A to C: Mechanisms of acid base homeostasis in the kidney. Colored text boxes indicate the channels or proteins affected in patients with renal tubular acidosis (RTA). (A) *Bicarbonate absorption and ammoniagenesis in proximal tubule.* H^+ is secreted into the lumen by the sodium (Na^+)-hydrogen (H^+)-exchanger-3 (NHE-3). Secreted H^+ combines with filtered luminal HCO_3^- to form H_2CO_3, which dissociates to H_2O and CO_2, which then diffuses into the cell to form H_2CO_3. HCO_3^- and Na^+ cross the basolateral membrane using Na^+/HCO_3^- cotransporter/exchanger 1 (NBCe1). Na^+ exits the cell via active transport by Na^+/K^+-ATPase. Electrogenic H^+ secretion generates a small lumen-positive voltage promoting paracellular flow of cations. NH_4^+ is generated in the mitochondria, and utilizes NHE-3 for exit to the luminal aspect. Luminal NH_4^+ is partly reabsorbed in the thick ascending limb of loop of Henle and accumulates in the interstitium. Proximal tubular cells are also the site of Na^+ coupled reabsorption of glucose, amino acids and PO_4^{3-}; (B) *Distal acidification in cortical collecting ducts.* α-intercalated cells actively secrete H^+, through the H^+ ATPase and H^+/K^+ antiporter. HCO_3^- ions generated intracellularly exit the cell by the HCO_3^-/Cl^- exchanger [anion exchanger 1 (AE1)]. Ammonia (NH_3) enters the intercalated and principal cells through Rhesus glycoproteins (Rhbg, Rhcg) and is secreted into the lumen through Rhcg. Secreted H^+ is buffered by HPO_4^{2-} to $H_2PO_4^-$ (titratable acidity) and by luminal ammonia to NH_4^+; (C) *H^+ and K^+ secretion in collecting ducts.* Principal cells mediate Na^+ absorption and K^+ secretion. The apical membrane has the amiloride sensitive epithelial sodium channel (ENaC); Na^+ exits basolaterally via Na^+/K^+ ATPase. Aldosterone binding to its receptor (MR) enhances Na^+ absorption by ENaC and basolateral exchange by Na^+/K^+-ATPase, K^+ secretion through renal outer medullary potassium (ROMK) channels and H^+ secretion by H^+-ATPase. WNK-kinase 4 (WNK4) interacts with sodium chloride symporter (NCCT), ENaC and ROMK channels in an inhibitory manner; WNK 1 inhibits WNK 4. Kelch-like 3 (KLHL3) and cullin 3 (CUL3) proteins promote degradation of WNK 4.
(NBCn2: sodium bicarbonate cotransporter-2)
Source: Adopted with permission from Bagga A, Sinha A. Renal tubular acidosis. Indian J Pediatr. 2020;87(9):733-44.

TABLE 13.3: Steps for diagnosis and characterization of renal tubular acidosis (RTA).

Step	Remarks
1. Plasma anion gap, calculated as: $Na^+ - (Cl^- + HCO_3^-)$	Normal 8–12 mEq/L in patients with RTA and diarrhea
2. Urine anion gap (UAG, net charge) estimates urine ammonium excretion, and is calculated as: $Na^+ + K^+ - Cl^-$	Urinary ammonium excretion = 80 – UAG. UAG is positive normally, and in RTA. Extrarenal bicarbonate losses (diarrhea) causes increased ammonium excretion causing negative UAG
3. Urine pH is measured on fresh voided specimen with pH meter. Furosemide test involves administration of furosemide at 2 mg/kg with fludrocortisone (1 mg), either simultaneously or 2 hours prior to testing. Urine pH is checked hourly for maximum 6 hours	pH > 5.5 during metabolic acidosis suggests distal RTA; value <5.5 suggests proximal RTA. Furosemide test assesses the ability to lower urine pH maximally provided distal sodium delivery is adequate, especially in patients without metabolic acidosis. In patients with distal RTA the urine pH remains >5.3
4. Bicarbonate loading with oral or intravenous sodium bicarbonate till urine pH >7.5 and blood bicarbonate >22 mEq/L, to estimate: • Fractional excretion of bicarbonate (FEHCO$_3$)[a] • Urine to blood pCO$_2$ gradient (U-B CO$_2$)[b]	• FEHCO$_3$ >15% suggests proximal RTA. Level is normal in distal RTA (<5%) • Urine pCO$_2$ reflects distal H$^+$ secretion. U-B CO$_2$ <10 mm Hg suggests distal RTA. Level is normal in proximal RTA (>20 mm Hg)
5. Additional evaluation: • Calculation of fractional excretion of phosphate[c] on a timed (6-h, 12-h) void, to estimate tubular reabsorption of phosphate (TRP)[d] and tubular maximum for phosphate corrected for GFR (TmP/GFR) • Urinary aminoacidogram, beta-2-microglobulin, glucose • 24-hour urine calcium, ultrasound for nephrocalcinosis, hearing assessment • Slit lamp examination for cystine crystals	• About 88–95% of phosphate is reabsorbed in the proximal tubule. The threshold for urinary phosphate excretion is expressed as TmP/GFR, derived using Bijvoet nomogram to index for plasma phosphorus and kidney function. TmP/GFR <2.8 reflects phosphaturia • Markers of proximal tubular dysfunction • Patients with distal RTA may have hypercalciuria (urine calcium >4 mg/kg/day), nephrocalcinosis and hearing loss • Corneal cystine crystals, a diagnostic marker of cystinosis, is found in patients older than 2-years
6. Clinical exome sequencing for variations in implicated genes (common causes listed in **Table 13.2**).	Genetic studies enables diagnosis, prognostication, and prenatal diagnosis

[a]$FEHCO_3 (\%) = \dfrac{\text{Urine bicarbonate} \times \text{serum creatinine}}{\text{Serum bicarbonate} \times \text{urine creatinine}} \times 100$

[b]U-B CO$_2$ = urine pCO$_2$ – blood pCO$_2$

[c]$FEPO_4 (\%) = \dfrac{\text{Urine phosphate} \times \text{plasma creatinine}}{\text{Plasma phosphate} \times \text{urine creatinine}} \times 100$

[d]TRP (%) = 100 – FEPO4 (%)

causes, indicating elevated ammonium excretion.[4] Further classification of RTA requires loading with sodium bicarbonate and estimations of urine to blood CO_2 gradient and fractional excretion of bicarbonate (*see* **Table 13.3**).[3] Additional evaluation includes assessment of aminoaciduria, glucosuria, low molecular weight proteinuria, and tubular maximum for phosphate corrected for GFR (TmP/GFR) (*see* **Table 13.3**).[3]

Evaluation for hypercalciuria and medullary nephrocalcinosis is essential in patients with distal RTA. Early hearing screening with at least one diagnostic audiology assessment by 24–30 months of age is recommended in patients with distal RTA.[4] Eye examination for cystine crystals should be done in all patients with Fanconi syndrome, with additional evaluation for Dent disease, Lowe syndrome, tyrosinemia, Fanconi–Bickel syndrome, galactosemia and Wilson disease, where clinically relevant. Genetic studies are required for confirmation of the underlying molecular defect.

Management

Treatment of RTA involves replacement of urinary losses of solutes and bicarbonate. The requirement of bicarbonate is lower in distal RTA (2–3 mEq/kg/day) compared to proximal RTA (4–15 mEq/kg/day). Administration of potassium citrate corrects both hypokalemia and acidosis.[4] A new prolonged-release formulation of potassium citrate and potassium bicarbonate, ADV7103, has been shown to be effective in distal RTA.[5] Sodium and water replacement is required for volume depletion. Rickets and hypophosphatemia require supplementation of phosphate (50–75 mg/kg/day in 3–6 divided doses), with or without supplementation of calcium and/or vitamin D, targeted to their respective blood levels.

Growth failure despite adequate nutrition and electrolyte supplementation is a major concern;[6] administration of recombinant growth hormone might be useful in patients with cystinosis.[7] Specific therapies include the following: cysteamine for cystinosis,[8] nitisinone for tyrosinemia, lactose-free diet for galactosemia and penicillamine for Wilson disease.

Patients with distal RTA usually have a good clinical prognosis in childhood, however recent longitudinal cohort studies suggest deterioration of kidney function in adulthood, particularly after puberty, in 30–40% of patients.[6,9,10]

Metabolic Alkalosis and Hypokalemia

Bartter, Gitelman and EAST (epilepsy, ataxia, sensorineural deafness and tubulopathy)/SeSAME (seizures, sensorineural deafness, ataxia, mental retardation and electrolyte disturbances) syndromes are salt-wasting disorders, characterized by increased excretion of chloride accompanied by

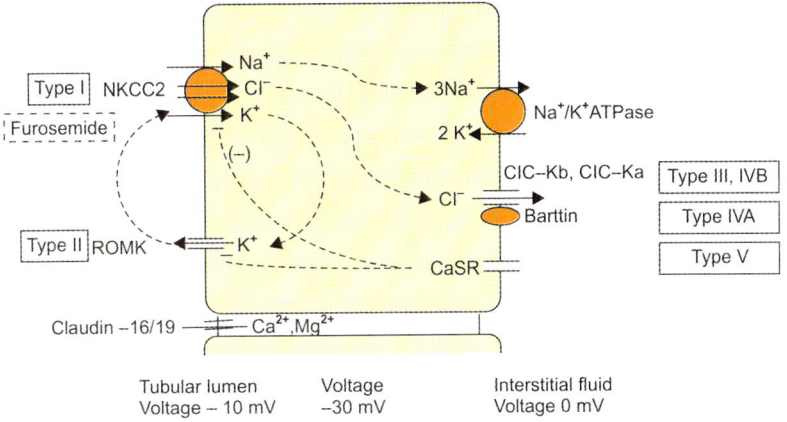

Fig. 13.2: Mechanism of absorption of sodium and chloride ions in thick ascending limb of loop of Henle. Transepithelial sodium chloride absorption is facilitated through coordinated activity of the apical furosemide-sensitive sodium (Na^+) potassium (K^+) chloride (Cl^-) cotransporter (NKCC2), renal outer membrane potassium (ROMK) channel, basolateral Na^+/K^+-ATPase and basolateral ClC-Kb (in the thick ascending limb and distal convoluted tubule) or ClC-Ka (in the thin and thick ascending limbs). While the NKCC2 is the predominant channel for sodium chloride reabsorption, the luminal exit of potassium through apical ROMK channels is essential to replenish urinary potassium to ensure activity of the NKCC2 along the thick ascending limb, and provides the driving force for paracellular absorption of calcium and magnesium. The basolateral calcium sensing receptor (CaSR) inhibits ROMK1 activity. The exit of chloride from the basolateral side is mediated through Cl^- channels ClC-Ka and ClC-Kb that require a functioning beta subunit called Barttin for their proper membrane localization. The calcium sensing receptor (CaSR) inhibits ROMK activity, thus affecting salt reabsorption. Recently, identified MAGED2 protein is essential for fetal expression of NKCC2. Patients with Bartter syndrome have defective transepithelial transport of Na^+ and Cl^- due to a variety of defects in transport of these ions, as depicted in textboxes.

sodium in the thick ascending limb of Henle and distal convoluted tubule, respectively. Sodium is reclaimed in the collecting duct accompanied by excretion of proton and potassium in the urine to maintain electroneutrality, thus causing hypochloremic metabolic alkalosis **(Fig. 13.2)**. Patients have a genotype-phenotype correlation with severe neonatal-onset, prematurity, nephrocalcinosis and hypercalciuria in Bartter syndromes type I and II, infantile to childhood onset with hypomagnesemia and hypocalciuria in type III, Gitelman and EAST/SeSAME syndromes, and a combination of the above, severe early-onset disease and deafness in Bartter type IV.[11]

Patients with increased mineralocorticoid action, such as renal artery stenosis and monogenic disorders of hypertension also present with a similar biochemical pattern. Monogenic disorders of hypertension can be classified as causing excessive aldosterone synthesis (familial hyperaldosteronism), dysregulated adrenal steroid metabolism and action (congenital adrenal hyperplasia and apparent mineralocorticoid excess,) or hyperactivity of sodium and chloride transporters in the distal tubule (Liddle syndrome, **Table 13.2**). The final common pathway is plasma volume expansion and catecholamine excess that causes urinary potassium wasting; hypokalemia and early-onset refractory hypertension are characteristic.[12]

Evaluation

Tubulopathies causing metabolic alkalosis and hypokalemia should be differentiated from extrarenal causes such as cystic fibrosis, vomiting and chloride diarrhea by appropriate history; diuretic use should be excluded.[13] The level of urine chloride on a spot sample can distinguish renal (>20 mEq/L) from extrarenal causes (<20 mEq/L). Measurement of blood pressure differentiates Bartter/Gitelman syndrome from monogenic causes of hypertension, that is further characterized by determining plasma aldosterone and renin levels (**Flowchart 13.1**).[12] While clinical phenotype might enable the diagnosis of subtypes of these disorders, genetic studies for demonstration of the molecular defect are confirmatory.

Flowchart 13.1: Approach to a patient with metabolic alkalosis and hypokalemia. Level of urine chloride differentiates renal and extrarenal causes. Patients with Bartter/Gitelman syndrome have a normal blood pressure that differentiates from monogenic causes of hypertension.

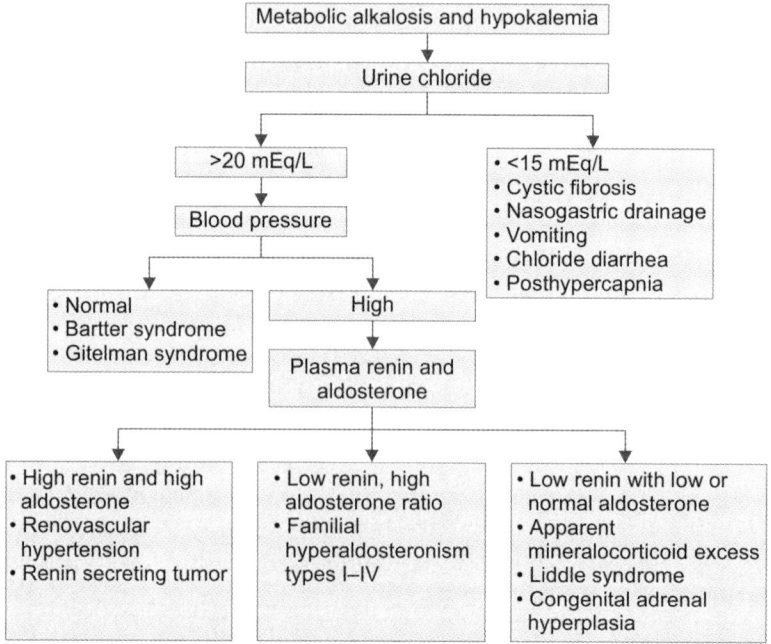

Management

Treatment of Bartter and Gitelman syndromes includes adequate hydration and potassium chloride supplementation (1–3 mEq/kg/day). Patients with Bartter syndrome benefit from therapy with indomethacin (2–3 mg/kg/day) or ibuprofen (30 mg/kg/day) that reduces prostaglandin levels and polyuria.[11,14] Administration of magnesium (50–100 mg/kg/day, as oral magnesium chloride, gluconate, or oxide) is required in patients with hypomagnesemia due to Bartter type III, EAST and Gitelman syndromes.[14] Specific therapies for monogenic disorders of hypertension include dexamethasone (familial hyperaldosteronism type I), spironolactone (apparent mineralocorticoid excess) and amiloride (Liddle syndrome).[12]

Hypomagnesemia

Hypomagnesemia causes neuromuscular manifestations such as muscle cramps, tremors, tetany, paresthesia, seizures and arrhythmia, depending on the severity of hypomagnesemia. The most important tool to differentiate renal from extrarenal magnesium wasting is estimation of fractional excretion of magnesium (FEMg), calculated as:[15]

$$\text{FEMg (\%)} = \frac{\text{Urine magnesium} \times \text{serum creatinine} \times 100}{0.7 \times \text{serum magnesium} \times \text{urine creatinine}}$$

In the presence of hypomagnesemia FEMg > 4% indicates renal magnesium wasting **(Flowchart 13.2)**.[15] Renal magnesium wasting occurs in various genetically heterogeneous disorders. These are classified into four groups: (1) hypercalciuric hypomagnesemia, (2) Gitelman-like hypomagnesemia (with hypokalemia and hypocalciuria), (3) mitochondrial hypomagnesemia and (4) other isolated hypomagnesemia.[15] Recessive mutations in genes encoding claudin-16 and 19 are the most common causes of hypercalciuric hypomagnesemia.[16] Patients have dense nephrocalcinosis and progress to end stage kidney failure in adolescence or young adulthood; patients with *CLDN19* mutations have high myopia.[16] The approach to a patient with hypomagnesemia is shown in **Flowchart 13.2**, common diseases are described in **Table 13.2**.

Polyuria

Polyuria occurs in several tubulopathies, and, other renal and extrarenal causes. The clinical and biochemical assessment should be focused to differentiate nephrogenic diabetes insipidus [due to resistance to antidiuretic hormone (ADH); **Fig. 13.3**] from other tubulopathies causing polyuria, especially those causing chronic hypokalemia or hypercalciuria, structural renal diseases (renal dysplasia, nephronophthisis) and other nonrenal

Flowchart 13.2: Common tubular diseases causing hypomagnesemia. A high fractional excretion of magnesium in the presence of hypomagnesemia indicates urinary wasting. Level of calcium excretion allows differentiation between various categories: hypercalciuric hypomagnesemia, Gitelman-like hypomagnesemia, and other isolated hypomagnesemia. Corresponding genetic defect is enclosed within brackets.

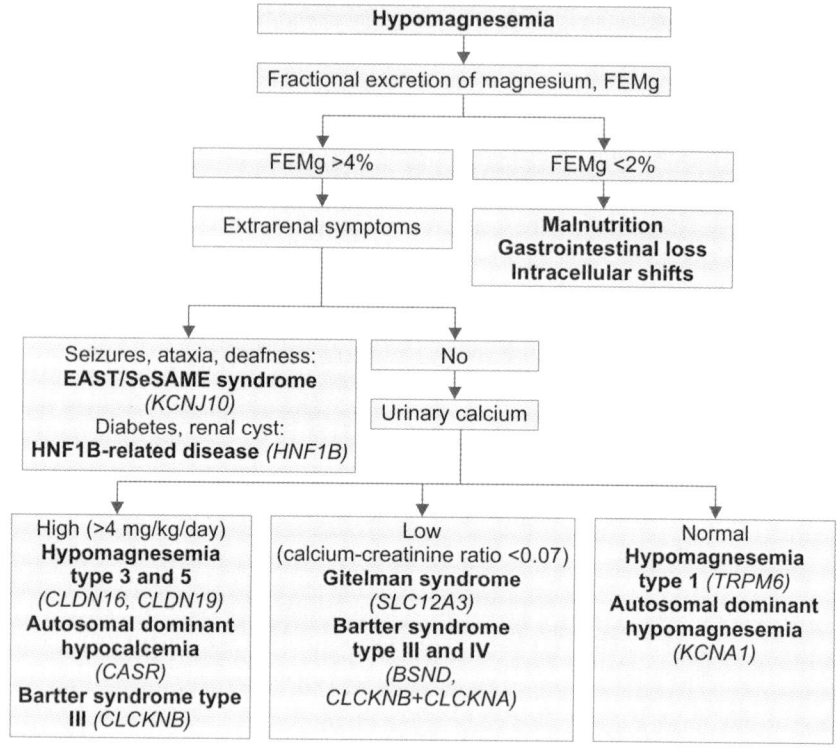

causes, such as central diabetes insipidus, diabetes mellitus, and adrenal insufficiency.[17] X-linked recessive defects in the *AVPR2* gene causes 90% of the cases of nephrogenic diabetes insipidus, autosomal recessive *AQP2* mutations account for 10%.[17]

Evaluation

Polyuria is confirmed measuring urine output that should exceed 2 L/m^2/day; 150 mL/kg/24 hr at birth, 100–110 mL/kg/24 hr till the age of 2 years and 40–50 mL/kg/24 hr in older children and adults. Initial investigations include blood levels of creatinine, pH, bicarbonate, electrolytes, glucose, calcium, along with early morning osmolality, urine osmolality (on the first morning void), urine microscopy, and ultrasonography. Urine osmolality <200 mOsm/kg and blood osmolality >300 mOsm/kg suggest diabetes insipidus. Further classification as central (deficiency of ADH) or nephrogenic diabetes insipidus (resistance to ADH) is based on the response to vasopressin/ADH (vasopressin test, **Flowchart 13.3**). Diabetes insipidus is ruled out if urine osmolality exceeds 750 mOsm/kg or blood osmolality is below 270 mOsm/

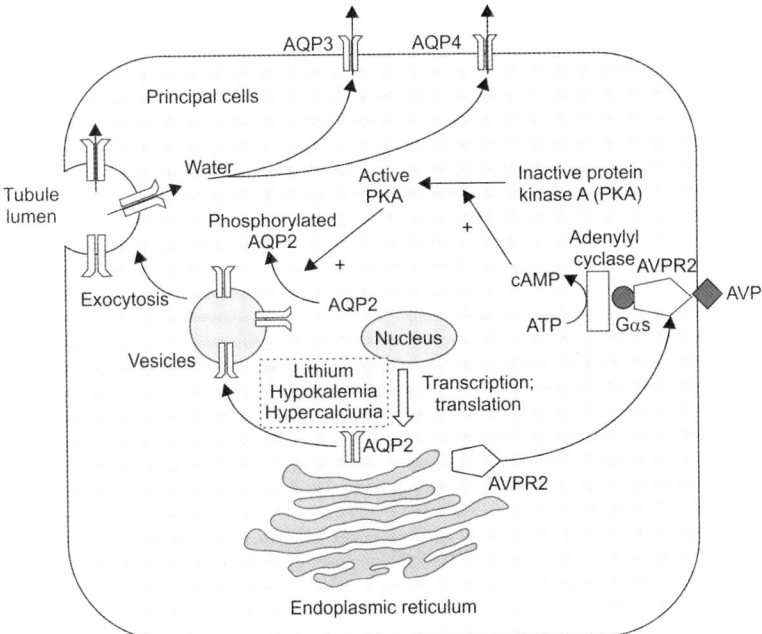

Fig. 13.3: Nephrogenic diabetes insipidus. Arginine vasopressin (ADH) binds to vasopressin receptor type 2 (AVPR2), a G protein-coupled receptor on the basolateral side of principal cells of the collecting duct. Activation of cytosolic G protein (GαS) activates adenylate cyclase, leading to increased cyclic AMP, protein kinase A (PKA) activation, phosphorylation of water channel aquaporin-2 (AQP2) and movement of vesicles containing the channels to the apical surface of principal cells. At the apical plasma membrane, AQP2 mediates water reabsorption along an osmotic gradient. Water entering the principal cell via AQP2 exits via AQP3 and AQP4 in the basolateral plasma membrane. Mutations in *AVPR2 gene*, underlying X-linked recessive NDI, most commonly cause misfolding of the receptor and its retention in the endoplasmic reticulum, but may also affect the receptor's interaction with vasopressin or G protein or cause it to localize to another cellular compartment. Mutations in *AQP2* gene underlying autosomal recessive NDI cause misfolding of AQP2 causing retention in the endoplasmic reticulum and rapid degradation. Patients with autosomal dominant NDI form heterotetramers of AQP2 monomers containing both wild type and mutated proteins such that AQP2 is misrouted, retained in the endoplasmic reticulum or sorted to late endosome, lysosomes or basolateral plasma membrane, manifesting a dominant negative mechanism. However, these patients may behave as partial NDI since some functional homotetramers are formed that contain only wild type protein. Polyuria in patients treated with lithium is secondary to decreased AQP2 transcription; hypokalemia and hypercalciuria have the same effect.

kg; blood osmolality between 280 and 300 mOsm/kg is an indication to perform water deprivation test to differentiate between diabetes insipidus and psychogenic polydipsia **(Flowchart 13.3)**.[18]

Management

Patients with nephrogenic diabetes insipidus require free access to water to avoid dehydration. Administration thiazide diuretics (2–3 mg/kg/day) and

Flowchart 13.3: Approach to a patient with polyuria defined as urine output that exceeds 2 L/m²/day. Diabetes insipidus is diagnosed in patients with low urine osmolality coupled with high blood sodium or osmolality. Water deprivation test differentiates between diabetes insipidus and psychogenic polydipsia. Further classification as central or nephrogenic diabetes insipidus is based on response to vasopressin.

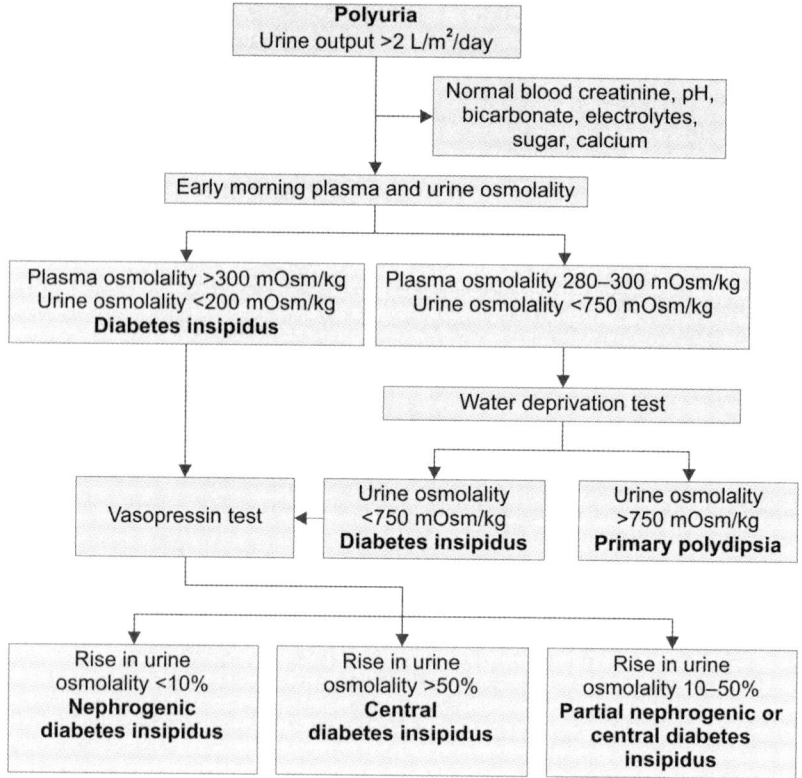

indomethacin (0.25–3 mg/kg/day) is beneficial particularly during infancy.[18] Adequate nutrition, with minimal osmolar load, is essential for growth.

Refractory Rickets

Refractory rickets is defined as failure of radiological healing and normalization of biochemical abnormalities, despite adequate therapy with vitamin D. Refractory rickets is caused by chronic kidney disease, renal tubular acidosis, calcipenic rickets or hypophosphatemic rickets **(Flowchart 13.4)**.[19] Metaphyseal dysplasia should be considered in patients with features of refractory rickets with normal biochemistry.

Calcipenic rickets [vitamin D dependent rickets (VDDR)] results from either inability to generate 25-hydroxyvitamin D (VDDR type 1b) or 1,25 hydroxyvitamin D (VDDR type 1a), resistance to 1,25 hydroxyvitamin D due to mutations in the vitamin D receptor (VDDR type 2a) or excessive inactivation of vitamin D metabolites (VDDR type 3).[19,20] Calcipenic rickets

Flowchart 13.4: Biochemical evaluation of patients with refractory rickets. Evaluation of renal tubular acidosis is detailed in **Table 13.3**. Patients with vitamin D dependent rickets show elevated levels of parathyroid hormone (PTH) and 1.25 dihydroxyvitamin D; type 2a has severe manifestations including alopecia and ectodermal defects. Elevated levels of fibroblast growth factor-23 (FGF-23) are characteristic of X-linked hypophosphatemic rickets.

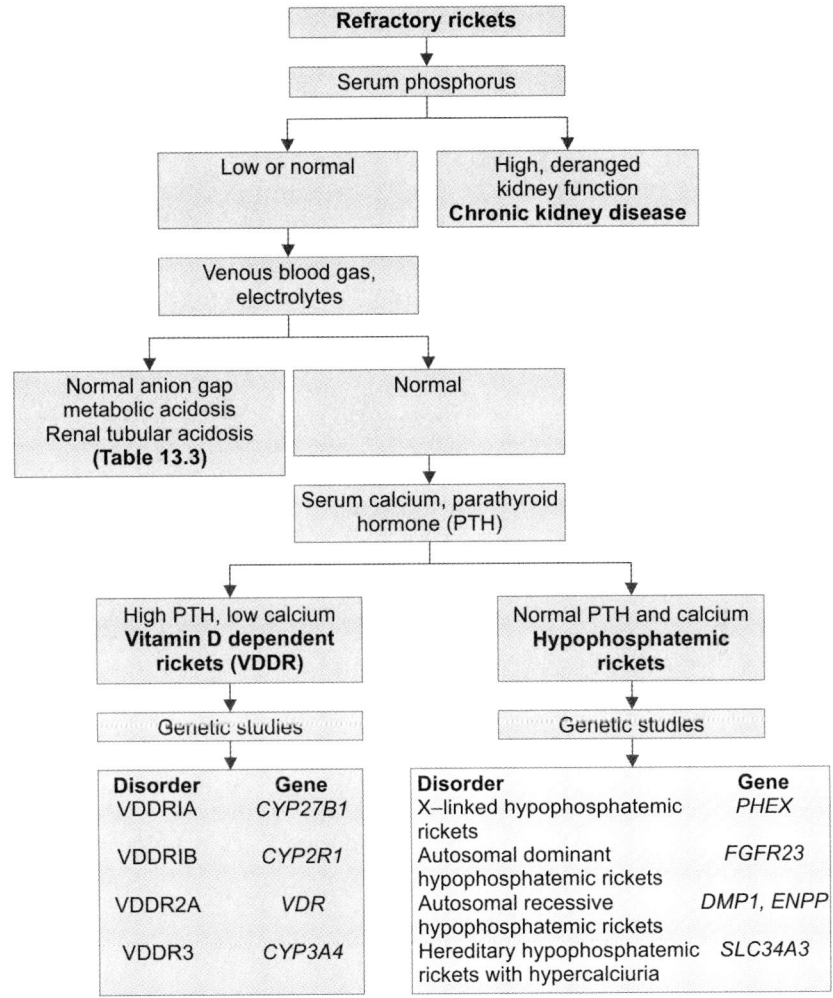

is characterized by infantile onset, with tetany or seizures due to severe hypocalcemia, aminoaciduria, and high parathyroid hormone (PTH); enamel hypoplasia (VDDR type 1) or alopecia and ectodermal defects (VDDR type 2a) might be found.[20]

Hypophosphatemic rickets, with normal serum calcium and PTH, is most commonly due to impaired tubular reabsorption of phosphate reflected by low TmP/GFR. Dent disease, Fanconi syndrome, and X-linked dominant defect in the *PHEX* gene are the most common causes of hypophosphatemic rickets.[21] An approach to evaluation is outlined in **Flowchart 13.4**. The diagnosis should be confirmed by molecular genetic analysis; elevated levels of fibroblast growth factor-23 (FGF-23) are supportive for diagnosis of X-linked hypophosphatemic rickets.[21,22] Patients with X-linked hypophosphatemic rickets present with lower limb deformities causing short stature, and dental abnormalities (pulp deformities, abscess).[22]

Management

Therapy of calcipenic rickets is with calcium and phosphate supplements, with active vitamin D (calcitriol) at a dose of 1–2 μg/day in VDDR type 1 or 0.05–0.2 μg/kg/day in VDDR type 2.[19,20] Therapy of hypophosphatemic rickets is with oral phosphorus (20–60 mg/kg/day) and calcitriol (20–30 ng/kg/day), while monitoring for hypercalcemia, hyperparathyroidism and nephrocalcinosis.[19] Burosumab, a monoclonal antibody targeting FGF-23, is recommended for use beyond infancy in patients with refractory disease, complications with or noncompliance to conventional therapy.[22] Holistic care of the musculoskeletal system, growth, hearing, and dentition is required.

Nephrolithiasis or Nephrocalcinosis

Patients might present with hematuria, frequency, dysuria, and abdominal pain, or be asymptomatic. An underlying metabolic cause is detected in 70–80% patients with nephrolithiasis or nephrocalcinosis.[23] Conditions that predispose to nephrolithiasis in children include hypercalciuria, hyperoxaluria, hypocitraturia, hyperuricosuria, urinary tract anomalies and infection, cystinuria and xanthinuria. Hypercalciuria (RTA, Dent disease, hypomagnesemia) and primary hyperoxaluria are the most common causes of nephrocalcinosis.

Evaluation

Metabolic evaluation should be done in all cases of nephrolithiasis including those with suspected anatomic obstruction and/or urinary tract infection since more than one condition may be present. Solute measurement in urine is preferably done on multiple, 24-hour urine specimens. **Box 13.2** lists the steps in evaluation. Hypercalciuria (calcium excretion >4 mg/kg/day) is the most common abnormality detected and is caused by tubulopathies such as distal RTA, Dent disease, hypomagnesemia, and Bartter syndrome; vitamin D excess, hyperparathyroidism and hyperthyroidism are also associated with hypercalcemia. Primary hyperoxaluria is an inherited disorder of glyoxylate metabolism, causing recurrent nephrolithiasis or nephrocalcinosis and eventual progression to kidney failure. Accurate diagnosis requires testing for oxalate in 24-hour urine and genetic studies.[24]

> **BOX 13.2:** Evaluation for nephrolithiasis or nephrocalcinosis.
>
> *Step 1*
> - Ultrasonography to confirm nephrolithiasis
> - Urinalysis, urinary crystals, and urine pH; urine culture in suspected urinary tract infection
> - Two or more estimations of 24-hour urine collection for volume, calcium, oxalate, citrate, uric acid, protein, and creatinine
> - Blood urea, creatinine, calcium, phosphate, alkaline phosphate, pH, bicarbonate, sodium, potassium, uric acid, magnesium
> - Stone analysis by infrared spectroscopy, if retrieved
>
> *Step 2*
> - Urine aminoacidogram, sodium nitroprusside test; quantitative 24-hour urinary cystine excretion
> - If hypercalciuria:
>   - Thyroid function test, parathyroid hormone, vitamin D levels
>   - Urine beta-2 microglobulin
>   - Fludrocortisone furosemide test
>   - Fractional excretion of magnesium if hypomagnesemia
>   - Tubular maximum for phosphate corrected for GFR (TmP/GFR) if hypophosphatemia
>   - Clinical exome sequencing (common genetic etiology listed in **Table 13.2**)

Management

Therapy of the underlying condition (RTA, Bartter and hypomagnesemia) is required. Patients should be advised a high fluid intake and ensure adequate calcium intake. Dietary sodium should be restricted below 2 g/day. Potassium citrate (1–2 mEq/kg/day) is administered to target urine pH 6.2–7.4 for uric acid and calcium oxalate stones and above 8 for cystine stones. Thiazides (0.5–1 mg/kg) may be useful for persistent hypercalciuria. Specific therapy includes penicillamine, tiopronin or captopril for cystinuria, allopurinol for hyperuricosuria and pyridoxine for primary hyperoxaluria (limited benefit). An important milestone in drug development in primary hyperoxaluria is small interfering RNA (siRNA) agents (lumasiran and nedosiran) targeting silencing of genes involved in glyoxylate metabolism, thereby reducing hepatic oxalate production. Subcutaneous lumasiran was recently approved for treatment of primary hyperoxaluria in all age groups based on a phase 3 trial showing clinically significant decline in 24-hour urinary oxalate excretion at 6-month follow-up.[25]

■ KEY POINTS

- Tubular disorders may present with varied clinical manifestations such as growth impairment, refractory rickets, polyuria, and hypertension. Patients need long-term follow-up for monitoring adequacy of growth and renal function.

- Their biochemical patterns indicate dysfunction of specific tubular segments and act as diagnostic fingerprints.
- Bicarbonate losses causing hyperchloremic metabolic acidosis and potassium loss leading to hypokalemia are usually from the gastrointestinal tract or from the renal tubules.
- Estimations of plasma and urine anion gap are the initial steps in diagnosis of hyperchloremic metabolic acidosis.
- Treatment of RTA involves replacement of urinary losses of solutes and bicarbonate. Rickets and hypophosphatemia require supplementation of phosphate.
- Bartter, Gitelman and EAST/SeSAME syndromes are characterized by increased excretion of chloride accompanied by sodium in the thick ascending limb of Henle and distal convoluted tubule respectively, resulting in hypochloremic metabolic alkalosis with hypokalemia.
- Estimation of fractional excretion of magnesium (FEMg) is the most important tool to differentiate renal from extrarenal magnesium wasting.
- Polyuria is confirmed when urine output exceeds $2 L/m^2/day$—150 mL/kg/24 hr at birth, 100–110 mL/kg/24 hr till the age of 2 years and 40–50 mL/kg/24 hr in older children.
- Calcipenic rickets usually have an infantile onset, with tetany or seizures due to severe hypocalcemia, aminoaciduria, and high PTH. Enamel hypoplasia (VDDR type 1) or alopecia and ectodermal defects (VDDR type 2a) are often seen.
- Therapy of calcipenic rickets is with calcium and phosphate supplements, with active vitamin D (calcitriol).
- Hypophosphatemic rickets, with normal serum calcium and PTH, is most commonly due to impaired tubular reabsorption of phosphate.
- Short stature and dental abnormalities are the common manifestations of X-linked hypophosphatemic rickets.
- Therapy of hypophosphatemic rickets is with oral phosphorus and calcitriol, while monitoring for hypercalcemia, hyperparathyroidism and nephrocalcinosis.
- Patients with nephrolithiasis and nephrocalcinosis are often asymptomatic or present with hematuria, frequency, dysuria, and abdominal pain. An underlying metabolic cause is detected in 70–80%.

■ REFERENCES

1. Bockenhauer D, Kleta R. Tubulopathy meets Sherlock Holmes: biochemical fingerprinting of disorders of altered kidney tubular salt handling. Pediatr Nephrol. 2021;36(8):2553-61.
2. Downie ML, Lopez Garcia SC, Kleta R, Bockenhauer D. Inherited tubulopathies of the kidney: Insights from genetics. Clin J Am Soc Nephrol. 2021;16(4):620-30.
3. Bagga A, Sinha A. Renal tubular acidosis. Indian J Pediatr. 2020;87(9):733-44.
4. Trepiccione F, Walsh SB, Ariceta G, Boyer O, Emma F, Camilla R, et al. Distal renal tubular acidosis: ERKNet/ESPN clinical practice points. Nephrol Dial Transplant. 2021;36(9):1585-96.
5. Bertholet-Thomas A, Guittet C, Manso-Silvan MA, Joukoff S, Navas-Serrano V, Baudouin V, et al. Safety, efficacy, and acceptability of ADV7103 during 24 months of treatment: an open-label study in pediatric and adult patients with distal renal tubular acidosis. Pediatr Nephrol. 2021;36(7):1765-74.
6. Gomez-Conde S, Garcia-Castano A, Aguirre M, Herrero M, Gondra L, Garcia-Perez N, et al. Molecular aspects and long-term outcome of patients with primary distal renal tubular acidosis. Pediatr Nephrol. 2021;36(10):3133-42.

7. Hohenfellner K, Rauch F, Ariceta G, Awan A, Bacchetta J, Bergmann C, et al. Management of bone disease in cystinosis: statement from an international conference. J Inherit Metab Dis. 2019;42(5):1019-29.
8. van Stein C, Klank S, Gruneberg M, Ottolenghi C, Grebe J, Reunert J, et al. A comparison of immediate release and delayed release cysteamine in 17 patients with nephropathic cystinosis. Orphanet J Rare Dis. 2021;16(1):387.
9. Atmis B, Cevizli D, Melek E, Bisgin A, Unal I, Anarat A, et al. Evaluation of phenotypic and genotypic features of children with distal kidney tubular acidosis. Pediatr Nephrol. 2020;35(12):2297-306.
10. Besouw MTP, Bienias M, Walsh P, Kleta R, Van't Hoff WG, Ashton E, et al. Clinical and molecular aspects of distal renal tubular acidosis in children. Pediatr Nephrol. 2017;32(6):987-96.
11. Nunez-Gonzalez L, Carrera N, Garcia-Gonzalez MA. Molecular basis, diagnostic challenges and therapeutic approaches of Bartter and Gitelman syndromes: a primer for clinicians. Int J Mol Sci. 2021;22(21):11414.
12. Khandelwal P, Deinum J. Monogenic forms of low-renin hypertension: clinical and molecular insights. Pediatr Nephrol. 2021.
13. Bamgbola OF, Ahmed Y. Differential diagnosis of perinatal Bartter, Bartter and Gitelman syndromes. Clin Kidney J. 2021;14(1):36-48.
14. Konrad M, Nijenhuis T, Ariceta G, Bertholet-Thomas A, Calo LA, Capasso G, et al. Diagnosis and management of Bartter syndrome: executive summary of the consensus and recommendations from the European Rare Kidney Disease Reference Network Working Group for Tubular Disorders. Kidney Int. 2021;99(2):324-35.
15. Tseng MH, Konrad M, Ding JJ, Lin SH. Clinical and genetic approach to renal hypomagnesemia. Biomed J. 2021.
16. Vall-Palomar M, Madariaga L, Ariceta G. Familial hypomagnesemia with hypercalciuria and nephrocalcinosis. Pediatr Nephrol. 2021;36(10):3045-55.
17. Duicu C, Pitea AM, Sasaran OM, Cozea I, Man L, Banescu C. Nephrogenic diabetes insipidus in children (Review). Exp Ther Med. 2021;22(1):746.
18. Mutter CM, Smith T, Menze O, Zakharia M, Nguyen H. Diabetes insipidus: Pathogenesis, diagnosis, and clinical management. Cureus. 2021;13(2):e13523.
19. Chanchlani R, Nemer P, Sinha R, Nemer L, Krishnappa V, Sochett E, et al. An overview of rickets in children. Kidney Int Rep. 2020;5(7):980-90.
20. Levine MA. Diagnosis and management of vitamin D dependent rickets. Front Pediatr. 2020;8:315.
21. Bharati J, Bhatia D, Khandelwal P, Gupta N, Sinha A, Khadgawat R, et al. C-Terminal Fibroblast growth factor-23 levels in non-nutritional hypophosphatemic rickets. Indian J Pediatr. 2019;86(6):555-7.
22. Haffner D, Emma F, Eastwood DM, Duplan MB, Bacchetta J, Schnabel D, et al. Clinical practice recommendations for the diagnosis and management of X-linked hypophosphataemia. Nat Rev Nephrol. 2019;15(7):435-55.
23. Sas DJ. An update on the changing epidemiology and metabolic risk factors in pediatric kidney stone disease. Clin J Am Soc Nephrol. 2011;6(8):2062-8.
24. Daga A, Majmundar AJ, Braun DA, Gee HY, Lawson JA, Shril S, et al. Whole exome sequencing frequently detects a monogenic cause in early onset nephrolithiasis and nephrocalcinosis. Kidney Int. 2018;93(1):204-13.
25. Forbes TA, Brown BD, Lai C. Therapeutic RNA interference: A novel approach to the treatment of primary hyperoxaluria. Br J Clin Pharmacol. 2021.

Endocrinology

Ambulatory Management of Type 1 Diabetes Mellitus

Sapna Nayak, Vijayalakshmi Bhatia

■ INTRODUCTION

Diabetes mellitus is a chronic metabolic disorder resulting in hyperglycemia due to defective insulin secretion or action. Type 1 diabetes mellitus (T1DM) is the predominant form of diabetes in children and is the second most common chronic disease affecting children, after bronchial asthma. The increasing disease burden emphasizes the need for all pediatricians to be aware of the appropriate management of the condition and provide standard care and education to the child and family to ensure a good quality of life. Furthermore, adequate control of blood glucose prevents or delays the development of long-term microvascular and macrovascular complications.

Type 1 diabetes mellitus occurs due to immune-mediated destruction of the pancreatic β-cells of islets of Langerhans resulting in insulin deficiency. Various environmental factors play a role to trigger autoimmunity in a genetically predisposed individual. This chapter highlights the current standard of care in ambulatory management of T1DM in children.

■ CLINICAL FEATURES OF TYPE 1 DIABETES MELLITUS

Type 1 diabetes mellitus can occur at any age from late infancy to adolescence. Absolute insulin deficiency results in a catabolic state manifesting as weight loss despite increased appetite and polyphagia. Generalized weakness and easy fatigability ensue along with osmotic symptoms, viz. polyuria, polydipsia and nocturnal enuresis. The presentation is insidious with symptoms progressing over a few days to months. Some patients complain of blurring of vision, recurrent infections of eye, skin, or vaginal candidiasis, and noticing ants around spilled urine. When these manifestations go unnoticed, the child lands in an acute life-threatening condition called diabetic ketoacidosis (DKA), marked by acute onset of abdominal pain, vomiting, fast breathing, drowsiness, and altered consciousness. Varying severity of dehydration leads to signs of volume depletion such as tachycardia, delayed capillary refill time, cold extremities, and dry tongue. Rapid and deep respiration (Kussmaul breathing) with a fruity odor to breath results from acidosis and ketosis, respectively. Hypotension is rare and urine output is high until late in the course despite dehydration. The presentation in DKA can mimic other acute conditions such as asthma, pneumonia, acute abdomen, or encephalopathy.

■ DIAGNOSIS

Diagnosis of all types of diabetes in children and adolescents should be based on laboratory measurement of plasma glucose (PG) and the presence or absence of symptoms. The American Diabetes Association (ADA) has laid down criteria for the diagnosis of diabetes mellitus **(Box 14.1)**.[1]

■ AMBULATORY MANAGEMENT OF TYPE 1 DIABETES MELLITUS

After recovery from DKA, the child is switched from intravenous (IV) to subcutaneous (SC) insulin, and all the aspects of ambulatory management are gradually put in place.

Goals of Management

Regardless of the presentation of the child, lifelong insulin replacement remains the mainstay of treatment of T1DM. The management entails a multidisciplinary approach through a team comprising of the pediatric

---

BOX 14.1: Criteria for diagnosis of diabetes mellitus.

- A random PG of ≥ 200 mg/dL in presence of overt symptoms or hyperglycemic crisis

    Or

- Fasting PG of ≥126 mg/dL (fasting defined as no caloric intake for at least 8 hours)*

    Or

- An OGTT, performed as described by the WHO, showing a PG ≥ 200 mg/dL post-2-hour glucose load after intake of 75 g (1.75 g/kg) anhydrous glucose dissolved in water*

    Or

- A HbA1c of >6.5%, performed in a laboratory using an NGSP certified method and standardized to the DCCT assay*,#

(PG: plasma glucose; OGTT: oral glucose tolerance test; WHO: World Health Organization; HbA1c: glycosylated hemoglobin; NGSP: national glycohemoglobin standardization program; DCCT: diabetes control and complications trial)

*The diagnosis using these criteria must be confirmed using repeat tests in the absence of unequivocal hyperglycemia.

#The use of HbA1c alone in establishing the diagnosis of T1DM in children is not clear.

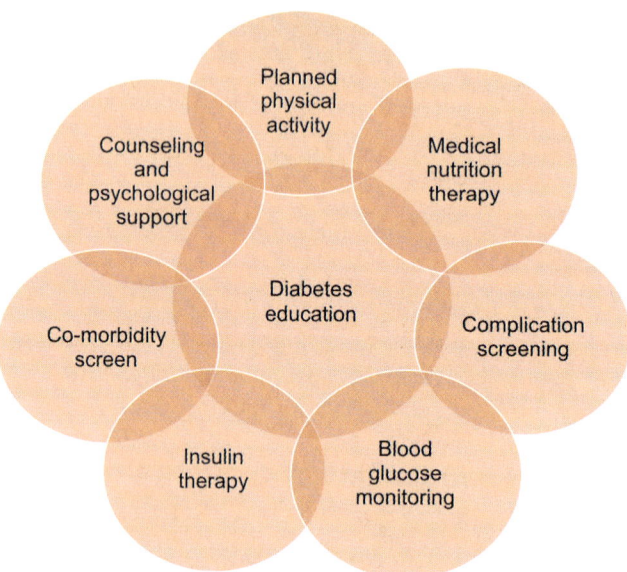

Fig. 14.1: Components of management of type 1 diabetes mellitus (T1DM).

endocrinologist, pediatrician, diabetes nurse educator, dietician, child psychologist, and medical social worker, with the child and family having the central role. The therapy aims to ensure that the child achieves the glycemic targets, remains symptom-free, is capable of carrying out routine schooling and extracurricular activities, has normal physical growth and mental and psychological development, leads a life free of acute and long-term complications of diabetes, and lives a good quality of life with social interactions at par with his/her peers. Treatment incorporates various components as shown in **Figure 14.1**.[2]

Insulin Therapy

Type 1 diabetes mellitus was a fatal disease before 1922, when Professor John Macleod, Friedrich Banting, Charles Best, and James Collip, demonstrated the role of injected animal insulin in the treatment of an adolescent with T1DM. Today, almost a hundred years since then, insulin remains inevitable for the survival of an individual with T1DM. The use of insulin has seen major developments over the years, evolving from insulin derived from animal extract (porcine or bovine insulin) to recombinant human insulin since the 1980s to insulin analogs introduced in 1996.[3] This is accompanied by continued progress in the mode of insulin delivery, with the incorporation of technology in diabetes care.

A child diagnosed with T1DM should be immediately started on insulin. A stable child with no or mild DKA can be started on insulin via SC route,

TABLE 14.1: Types of insulin with their action profile.

Type	Examples	Onset of action (hours)	Peak action (hours)	Duration of action (hours)
Ultra-rapid-acting analog	Faster Aspart (Fiasp)	0.1–0.2	1–3	3–5
Rapid-acting	• Lispro • Aspart • Glulisine	0.15–0.35	1–3	3–5
Short-acting	Regular	0.5–1	2–4	5–8
Intermediate-acting	NPH	2–4	4–12	12–24
Long-acting	• Detemir • Glargine	1–2 2–4	• 4–7 • No pronounced peak	20–24 22–24
	• Glargine U300	2–6	• No pronounced peak	30–36
Ultra-long-acting	Degludec	0.5–1.5	No pronounced peak	>42

(NPH: neutral protamine Hagedorn)

while IV insulin is used in the treatment of a child with moderate and severe DKA; SC insulin to be started after resolution of acidosis.

Insulins Available for Use

The insulins currently in use are classified based on their action profile **(Table 14.1)**.[3,4] Regular insulin (natural insulin secreted by the human pancreas and manufactured by recombinant DNA technology) and insulin NPH (neutral protamine Hagedorn, structurally a laboratory modification of regular insulin that renders it long-acting) are the *conventional insulins*. Rapid and long-acting analogs of insulin are developed by slightly modifying the molecular structure of human insulin to alter the pharmacokinetics thereby affecting its absorption from the SC tissue and hence the onset of action. These have a better action profile than the conventional insulins but are costlier.

The choice of the insulin prescribed for a given child is decided after discussion with the family and depends upon factors such as age, lifestyle and eating pattern of child, current glycemic control and targets of therapy, availability of insulin, and affordability.

Newer Insulins and Their Relevance in Children

The newer analog, fast-acting Aspart insulin has a faster onset than Aspart insulin by virtue of the presence of niacinamide and L-arginine that increases the speed of breakdown of stable hexamers to dissociate into monomers. The quick onset of action is useful in toddlers and preschool children who have erratic and unpredictable eating patterns. Degludec, another novel insulin analog forms soluble multi-hexamers after SC injection leading to a slow and steady release of monomers with the effect lasting for up to 40 hours. Similarly, glargine U300, with its slow and protracted release from the injection site, has been recently approved for use in children over 6 years of age.

Principles of Insulin Therapy/Insulin Regimen

Physiologically the insulin secretion in the human body continues at a low level in the fasting state as well as in between meals, with levels rising sharply with food intake. The aim of any insulin therapy should be to mimic the physiology as closely as possible.

Split Mix Regimen

A large dose of intermediate-acting insulin (NPH insulin) with short-acting insulin (regular insulin) is given at breakfast and the remaining dose at night (two-thirds of the total insulin dose in the morning and one-third at night. At each dose, the intermediate-acting insulin comprises two-thirds of that dose while the remaining one-third is given as short-acting insulin). Despite only two injections per day, this regimen is not ideal for a child. There is rigidity with respect to the timing and the carbohydrate content of meals. The large dose of the intermediate-acting insulin leads to an increased risk of hypoglycemia around mid-day and midnight and hyperglycemia when the effect of insulin starts waning off, as during the early morning hours.

Premixed insulins are preformed mixtures of short and intermediate-acting insulins in ratios of 30:70 or 50:50, prescribed as twice-daily injections. They do not offer the flexibility of dosage adjustment for individual insulin components. Therefore, the use of premixed insulin is not advocated in children except in the presence of poor adherence to treatment or barriers to diabetes education.

Basal Bolus Regimen

This is closer to physiology and has become the standard of care. It consists of an intensive insulin regimen delivered either through multiple daily injections (MDI) or an insulin pump (continuous SC insulin infusion, CSII). MDI incorporates insulin dosing with basal insulin in the form of single or twice-daily doses of long-acting insulin (example: glargine) or a twice-daily (or once, at night) dose of intermediate-acting insulin (NPH insulin) combined with rapid or short-acting insulin accompanying each major meal and snack which form the boluses. Details about insulin pumps can be found in a separate section later. The basal bolus regimen

TABLE 14.2: Insulin dosing according to the age of patient and stage of T1DM.*

Age/stage of disease	Daily dose of insulin (unit/kg)
Younger child	0.7–1
Pubertal child	1–1.2 or up to 2
Post DKA or at onset of diabetes (for 1–2 months)	1.5–2
Honeymoon phase of diabetes	<0.5

*The doses are a guide to initiate therapy. Further dose adjustment should be based on SMBG/CGM and carbohydrate intake.
(DKA: diabetic ketoacidosis; SMBG: self-monitoring of blood glucose; CGM: continuous glucose monitoring)

offers flexibility in the timing and content of meals and better glycemic control.

Insulin Dosing

The dose of insulin depends upon various factors such as the stage of diabetes after diagnosis, the age, weight, and pubertal status of the patient **(Table 14.2)**. The dose is higher at the onset of illness when the child has increased appetite to make up for the weight loss since the onset of clinical illness. Insulin resistance occurs due to the phenomenon of glucose toxicity. Gradually the requirement decreases, and some children may require very low doses that may last for a few months to a year (honeymoon phase). Importantly, the caregivers must be educated that this is a temporary phase and in no instance should insulin be stopped without expert medical advice. Other variables affecting the dose include the eating pattern, daily physical activity, glucose levels, and presence of illness.

Basal insulin forms 30–50% of the total daily dose (TDD) of insulin and the rest is divided into multiple bolus doses. When regular insulin is the prandial (bolus) insulin used, it can make up to 70% of the TDD as it has some basal effect, while a rapid-acting analog makes up to 50% of the TDD. Further fine-tuning of the insulin doses for better glycemic control can be achieved using the insulin carbohydrate ratio and the insulin sensitivity factor **(Boxes 14.2 and 14.3)**.

Insulin Injection Technique

Conventional insulins are available in vials in two strengths, 40 units/mL and 100 units/mL. The caregiver must ensure the usage of the correct syringe with the insulin vial of appropriate strength. Insulin analogs, on the other hand, are available in vials or cartridges with a strength of 100 units/mL only. Insulin injection can be given at various sites, viz. outer aspect of arms, the anterolateral aspect of thighs, upper outer quadrant of the buttocks, the flanks, and on the front of abdomen away from the

> **BOX 14.2:** Insulin carbohydrate ratio (ICR).
>
> - The dose of the bolus depends predominantly on the carbohydrate intake in the succeeding meal and on the protein and fat content, to some extent. Insulin dose can be adjusted for the amount of carbohydrate to be consumed in the food using the ICR calculated as under:
>
> $$ICR = 500/TDD\ [300/TDD\ in\ toddlers]$$
>
> - The value of ICR obtained is the amount of carbohydrate that would be covered by 1 unit of prandial insulin.
>   *Example:* If a child is on 15 units of glargine and lispro insulin in a dose of 5–5–1–4 units before breakfast, lunch, evening snack, and dinner respectively, then the TDD would be 15 + 5 + 5 + 1 + 4 = 30. The ICR is 500/30 = 16.6. This means that 1 unit of lispro insulin could cover approximately 16 g of carbohydrate for the child.
> - This dose is a guide, to begin with. Doses are further fine-tuned based on the SMBG readings.
>
> (TDD: total daily dose; SMBG: self-monitoring of blood glucose)

> **BOX 14.3:** Insulin sensitivity factor (ISF) and prandial insulin adjustment according to premeal blood glucose (BG).
>
> - The insulin sensitivity factor is the amount of blood glucose (BG) that is expected to fall with 1 unit of regular or rapid-acting insulin. It is calculated as follows:
>
> $$ISF = 1800/TDD\ (for\ rapid\text{-}acting\ analog)$$
> $$or\ 1500/TDD\ (for\ regular\ insulin)$$
>
> - The value obtained can be used to adjust the dose of the bolus when the premeal sugars are above the target range (90–130 mg/dL).
>   For example, if the child is on 10 units of glargine and 5–4–8 units of regular insulin before the 3 main meals and 2–1 units before mid-morning and evening snacks, the TDD would be 30 units.
>
> $$Insulin\ sensitivity\ factor = 1500/TDD\ (for\ regular\ insulin) = 1500/30 = 50$$
>
> - Accordingly, if the child's premeal BG at breakfast is high, the child must be advised additional insulin as follows:
>
> | Premeal BG (mg/dL) | Dose of regular insulin to be taken (units) |
> |---|---|
> | 90–130 | 5 |
> | 130–180 | 5 + 1 = 6 |
> | 180–230 | 5 + 2 = 7 |
> | 230–280 | 5 + 3 = 8 |
> | >280 | 5 + 4 = 9 |
>
> (BG: blood glucose; TDD: total daily dose)

umbilicus. Insulin must be stored between 2–8°C and never be frozen. The sharps generated from treatment (lancets, syringes, and pen needles) should be safely collected in puncture-proof containers and disposed of at the nearest health center.[4]

Modes of Insulin Delivery

Syringes: Disposable syringes have been the traditional way of injecting insulin. Syringes of 40 units/mL and 100 units/mL with finer needles of 4–6 mm are used, which give virtually painless pricks.

Pen devices: Conventional and analog insulins are available as disposable prefilled pens and also as 100 units/mL cartridges for use in reusable pens. These are easier for transport and administration, with finer needles, but are costlier than the insulin vials.

Injection port (i-Port): The potential pain and fear associated with injections, in the child or the family member taking care can compromise the number of doses the child receives and thus the glycemic control. The i-port device is kept inserted into the SC space which enables multiple SC injections through the port and can be used for up to three days. High cost prohibits its regular use.

Insulin Pumps or Continuous Subcutaneous Insulin Infusion (CSII)

Ever since the discovery of insulin, the aim has been to match the insulin delivery as close to physiology as possible, where insulin level autoregulates according to the blood glucose (BG). Insulin pump with its recent advances brings us closer to mimicking the normal pancreatic function.

Insulin pumps are new electronic devices of the size of a small mobile phone for continuous administration of insulin. It consists of an insulin reservoir that stores rapid-acting insulin. Insulin is delivered through a tubing ending in a subcutaneously inserted catheter that requires to be changed every 2–3 days **(Fig. 14.2)**. The basal needs are met by a continuous

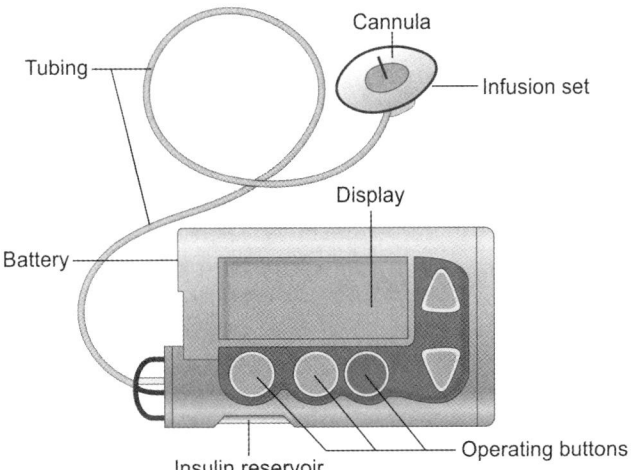

Fig. 14.2: Schematic diagram of an insulin pump set.

flow of the rapid-acting insulin throughout the day (basal rate) and the bolus doses are administered by the patient/parent along with meals and snacks (boluses).

Although any child with T1DM irrespective of age and duration of diabetes can be initiated on insulin pump therapy, it is particularly useful in and should be offered to infants and toddlers with unpredictable meal patterns, children with poor glycemic control despite intensive regimen with MDI, children with recurrent hypoglycemia especially in presence of hypoglycemic unawareness.[5]

Starting a Child on an Insulin Pump

The diabetes team must assess the suitability of a child and family for insulin pump therapy and intensive education is required before initiating the insulin pump to achieve target glycemic control. Basic understanding of diabetes, insulin action, management of hypoglycemia and hyperglycemia along with motivation and willingness to carry out self-monitoring of blood glucose (SMBG) multiple times every day and carbohydrate counting is a must. Newer pumps are integrated with continuous glucose monitoring (CGM) devices for glucose monitoring (see later), thus needing fewer pricks for SMBG.

- The choice of the insulin pump model is determined by the availability and the family preferences. The family must afford the pump as well as the monthly consumables.
- Initial doses are determined by the TDD of insulin.
- If transition is being made from MDI, the dose is reduced by 20–30%, due to better insulin absorption with pump therapy.
- The basal insulin is administered at an hourly rate and different basal rates can be set for different segments of the day in contrast to the once or twice-daily administered fixed dose of long-acting insulin analog through injections. For example, a lower basal rate can be set during the time of planned exercise and a higher basal rate to account for hyperglycemia in the early morning (dawn phenomenon) or hyperglycemia in the early night in preschool children (reverse dawn phenomenon) or during illness to prevent glucose excursions.
- The bolus doses are administered by the patient along with meal intake or to correct high BG levels. The dose is determined depending upon the premeal BG, the carbohydrate one plans to eat, and the active insulin or the insulin on board, from the previous bolus dose. The pump software makes these calculations if one gives the input of the number of carbohydrates to be consumed.
- The family must have round the clock access to the diabetes care provider for help in case of pump failure.

Advantages of Insulin Pump

- There is no need for multiple pricks each day, encouraging the use of boluses with each meal and snack.
- Different basal rates can be set throughout the day depending upon the activity level and the school hours and temporary basal rates at the time of exercise or illness.
- The delivery of the bolus can be the full dose at a time (normal or standard bolus), prolonged over a certain duration of time (square wave or an extended bolus), or a combination of both (combo or dual wave bolus) depending upon the content of the meal being taken (protein and fat deliver late BG rise).
- Very small and precise doses of insulin up to 0.025 units can be ensured.
- Insulin delivery can be suspended during episodes of hypoglycemia.

Problems Associated with Pump Usage

Insulin pump malfunctions and infusion set failures can interrupt the insulin delivery, putting the patients at risk of DKA, as there is no long-acting insulin action in the body. Lipodystrophy and skin reactions can occur at the infusion site.

With the appropriate use of insulin pump therapy, there are lower rates of hypoglycemia, less glycemic variability with improved glycosylated hemoglobin (HbA1c). Flexibility in lifestyle leads to better patient satisfaction. However, in India, cost remains an impediment.

Advances in the Insulin Pumps including Artificial Pancreas

Sensor augmented pump with low glucose suspend or predictive low glucose management: These devices are linked to the CGM and the insulin delivery is cut off when the sensor glucose values fall below a preset threshold value (low glucose suspend) or when the glucose level is rapidly falling with impending hypoglycemia [sensor augmented pump (SAP) with predictive low glucose management] **(Table 14.3)**.

Insulin-only artificial pancreas
- *Hybrid-closed loop (HCL) pump*: These are the latest insulin delivery devices commercially available. BG values in real-time from the CGM device are fed directly into the pump which delivers the dose of basal insulin based on inbuilt algorithms. The basal rate automatically changes when upward excursions occur beyond a pre-set threshold. Thus, such a device is called an "artificial pancreas". However, the mealtime boluses need to be fed in by the patient, hence it is called a "hybrid" closed-loop system. The first commercially available HCL device is the MiniMed 670G and its most advanced version, the MiniMed 780G has just become available in India.

TABLE 14.3: Some models of insulin pumps currently available in India.

Name	Type	CGM integration
MiniMed Paradigm 715	Basic	No
MiniMed Paradigm Real-time 722	Basic	No
MiniMed 620G	Alarms to hypoglycemia	Yes
MiniMed 640G (with smart guard technology)	SAP with predictive low glucose suspend*	Yes
MiniMed 780G	Hybrid closed-loop	Yes
My life YpsoPump	Basic	No

(CGMS: continuous glucose monitoring system; SAP: sensor augmented pump)
*The MiniMed Paradigm Veo, an insulin pump with low glucose suspend has been withdrawn from the market after the launch of MiniMed 640G.

- *Fully closed-loop system*: In addition to the features of the HCL system, this provides the meal bolus also automatically. At present, they are under investigative trials.

Dual hormone artificial pancreas: This aims to reduce the rates of hypoglycemia by incorporating glucagon in the system. The need for two infusion sets and a stable liquid glucagon formulation are the limitations.[6,7]

Adverse Effects of Insulin

Exogenous insulin use can be associated with immediate-type local or systemic *hypersensitivity reaction* which is IgE-mediated or delayed IgG-mediated allergic reaction that may lead to insulin resistance. However, with the use of purified recombinant insulins, allergic reactions are extremely rare. Insulin-mediated *lipodystrophy* includes lipohypertrophy, owing to the trophic effect of insulin, resulting from repeated injections at the same site and lipoatrophy, an immune-mediated loss of fat at the site of injections. The family must be educated to practice site rotation to avoid the occurrence of lipohypertrophy which leads to erratic insulin absorption and poor glycemic control.[4] *Insulin edema* is another rare side effect seen with the initiation of intensive insulin therapy, which usually is self-limiting. Some cases may develop pleural effusion or anasarca. Treatment consists of fluid restriction and the use of diuretics in severe cases. Rarely, *insulin neuritis* or *treatment-induced neuritis in diabetes (TIND)* can result in pain and paresthesia after therapy initiation. Evidence suggests no increased risk of malignancy among glargine-treated patients, as was previously thought.

Monitoring of Glycemic Control

The levels of BG in an individual with T1DM vary throughout the day. Frequent monitoring of BG is therefore required to titrate the doses of insulin with the diet and physical activity so that normoglycemia is achieved at most times.

The Diabetes Control and Complications Trial (DCCT, 1982–93), a multicenter randomized clinical trial compared the outcome of intensive insulin treatment (with ideal BG targets) against the conventional treatment (with liberal targets) in adolescents and young adults with T1DM. An intensified treatment with the basal-bolus regimen and SMBG multiple times a day resulted in lower HbA1c. *The study provided evidence that the rate of development and progression of long-term complications of nephropathy, retinopathy, and neuropathy was much lower with the intensive treatment.*[8] The Epidemiology of Diabetes Interventions and Complications (EDIC, 1994 onward) trial showed that the effects of the interventions of the DCCT trial continued much after the study period irrespective of whether the intensive therapy was continued or not.[9-11] *Thus, it is worth the effort, time, and costs involved to carry out good quality monitoring and achieve as tight a BG control as possible.*

Self-monitoring of Blood Glucose at Home

About 6–10 readings of BG daily are recommended as per the convenience, lifestyle, affordability, and education of the patient viz. premeal, 2 hours post-meal, and occasional midnight BG. The readings must be recorded in a logbook/diary or cloud-based program, along with the respective insulin doses, adjustments, and carbohydrate intake. The post-meal BG reflects the action of prandial insulin; the others reflect that of the basal insulin. Importantly, diet and exercise affect all the BG readings.

Newer glucometers with Bluetooth connectivity and data transfer options are now available that enable sharing the glucose values with a remote care provider.

Apart from a regular review of the records with the health care provider, the family should be taught to identify the glycemic patterns and make necessary changes at home frequently. The dose adjustments are aimed to achieve the BG within the target levels at most times **(Table 14.4)**.[12] The readings obtained are used to fine-tune the insulin dosage as follows:

- The premeal BG allows an immediate increase of the dose of prandial insulin (for that meal only) according to the insulin sensitivity factor (*see* **Box 14.3**).

TABLE 14.4: Targets of blood glucose control (International Society of Pediatric and Adolescent Diabetes, ISPAD 2018).

Time	Target values
Fasting/premeal	70–130 mg/dL
Postprandial	90–180 mg/dL
Bedtime	80–140 mg/dL
HbA1c	<7%

(HbA1c: Glycosylated hemoglobin).

- BG patterns recorded over a few days help to make necessary changes in the basal and bolus dosing.

However, the limitations of the SMBG include repeated pricks that the child may not comply with, and the cost involved. The readings provide a snapshot of the glucose levels; the direction in which the glucose value changes and the rate of change cannot be identified. Periods of hyperglycemia and asymptomatic hypoglycemia, especially nocturnal may not be picked up if frequent testing is not done. These lacunae are addressed by the CGM system (see later).

Ketone Testing

When there is a relative deficiency of insulin in a child with T1DM, at times of stress and sickness or due to chronic insulin deficiency resulting from poor compliance, lipolysis begins to produce ketones as a source of energy. The ketones produced, acetoacetic acid and β-hydroxybutyrate are acidic and decrease the pH of the blood. If untreated with adjustments in insulin doses, DKA is precipitated. The presence of persistent high BG beyond 250 mg/dL should alert the parents to test for urine ketone levels. Lately, blood ketones can also be tested using a glucometer and are advantageous over urine ketones as a rise in blood ketones can be detected much earlier than urine ketones and depicts β-hydroxybutyrate, the major ketone, rather than acetone. Normal blood ketone is < 0.6 mmol/L.

Monitoring at the Diabetes Center

Apart from the daily SMBG, 3-6 monthly visits at the diabetes center enable monitoring for growth, weight, height, growth velocity, and pubertal status. The clinical evaluation must include assessment of injection sites, feet and thyroid examination. The knowledge of the child and the family about insulin, hypoglycemia, and other aspects of diabetes management must be assessed and reinforced regularly.

HbA1c: This is the conventional method to assess glycemic control over many years. HbA1c is the measure of glycemic control over the past 2-3 months and correlates with the risk of long-term complications.[13] However, the use of HbA1c alone is fraught with limitations. The value of HbA1c reflects an acceptable or poor glycemic control but fails to provide details of day-to-day glucose variability. It does not provide details of periods of hypoglycemia or postprandial hyperglycemia and thus fails to yield the care provider with the necessary information to make changes in the insulin regimen.

Continuous Glucose Monitoring System

The Continuous glucose monitoring system (CGM) devices are in place since 1999 and have overcome certain disadvantages of HbA1c and SMBG.

A CGM device consists of a sensor that is inserted into the subcutaneous tissue and measures the interstitial glucose every 5–15 minutes. There are three categories of CGM:
- *Blinded/retrospective CGM*: The data recorded in the sensor is transmitted onto a reader, downloaded onto a computer and the results obtained in the form of graphs depict the daily trends of BG levels over the past 7–14 days. The diabetes care provider in conjunction with the family uses the retrospective data to identify specific patterns of BG and take necessary steps for rectification. *Example:* Abbott Freestyle Libre Pro.
- *Real-time CGM (rtCGM):* This provides a numerical value of glucose in real-time and graphical trend of BG change. It utilizes real-time alarms for thresholds and predictions of hypo- and hyperglycemia, as well as the rate of change alarms for rapid glucose excursions. The device requires calibration with capillary glucose reading twice a day. The rtCGM linked to insulin pumps has made closed-loop systems possible. *Example:* Enlite Glucose sensor (works with the MiniMed 640G insulin pump) and Dexcom G6.
- *Intermittently scanned/viewed CGM (isCGM) (Flash glucose monitoring):* It provides readings when the sensor is scanned by holding a reader or smartphone close to the sensor. The readings displayed include the BG value in the present time and a trend over 8 hours. The currently available flash device in India is factory calibrated and lasts for 14 days. *Example:* Abbott Freestyle Libre.

Both rtCGM and *is*CGM help in monitoring the time spent in the target glucose range termed as "time in range (TIR)". The TIR and the glycemic patterns obtained from the CGM data can be utilized to make necessary changes in the insulin, diet, and activity levels. It is recommended that CGM must be used in concert with capillary SMBG and with HbA1c.[14]

Complication and Comorbidity Screen

Type 1 diabetes mellitus can be associated with other autoimmune conditions. Autoimmune thyroid disease is common with a prevalence of 3–8% in children with T1DM and increases with age, with the majority manifesting with hypothyroidism. Celiac disease is another associated autoimmune condition, with a prevalence ranging from 1 to 10% in children and adolescents with T1DM. Screening for thyroid dysfunction with anti-thyroid peroxidase (TPO) antibodies and thyroid-stimulating hormone (TSH) at diagnosis and every 2 yearly thereafter with TSH is recommended in asymptomatic children. More frequent monitoring of TSH is required in the presence of antibody positivity or symptoms.

Similarly, screening for celiac disease with anti-tissue transglutaminase (anti-tTG) antibody is recommended at diagnosis and 2 and 5 years thereafter.

TABLE 14.5: Screening recommendations for long-term complications (ISPAD 2018). (Screening must begin at 11 years of age in a child with diabetes of 2–5 years duration)

Complication	Screening methods
Nephropathy	Spot urine albumin/creatinine ratio on a first-morning urine sample
Retinopathy	Fundus evaluation by direct ophthalmoscopy on dilated pupil by a retina specialist
Neuropathy	Clinical history and examination yearly during clinic visit
Macrovascular disease	• Lipid profile every 2 years* • Blood pressure at least annually

(ISPAD: International Society of Pediatric and Adolescent Diabetes)
*In presence of a family history of hypercholesterolemia or early cardiovascular disease, screening for dyslipidemia should begin by 2 years of age.

More frequent monitoring is needed in presence of symptoms or a first-degree relative with celiac disease.[15] Other vitiligo, autoimmune conditions, viz. adrenal insufficiency, Graves' disease, vitiligo and pernicious anemia have lower prevalence and thus do not require routine screening.

Poor glycemic control is associated with long-term microvascular and macrovascular complications.[16] Screening for complications must begin at 11 years of age in a child with diabetes of 2–5 years duration **(Table 14.5)**.[17]

Medical Nutrition Therapy

Diet is an essential component of diabetes management and largely influences the outcome. The dietary habits and the meal composition vary from one region to another even within a country owing to the differences in the culture, traditions, agricultural, and cooking practices. Therefore, the interventions in the nutrition and meal plan must be individualized based on the eating patterns and lifestyle of the child. The choice of insulin and its schedule is tailored to this dietary pattern, among other things. Further, dietary recommendations for a child with diabetes should be based on the daily routine and nutritional needs of the child and must take into consideration the family background and socioeconomic status. It is important to note that there is no special diet or "diabetic diet". A child with diabetes should consume the same amount of calories as is recommended for any healthy child of a particular age and gender. The child should not be treated differently and the entire family must be encouraged to make appropriate changes to consume a healthy diet. Imposing stringent restrictions on intake of certain foods or eating out can be counterproductive and lead to poor compliance and psychological distress to the child.

The diet must be composed of all essential nutrients in required amounts to ensure optimum growth and development without excessive weight gain, along with maintaining target glycemic control with reduced rates of hypoglycemia. Carbohydrates should comprise 45–50% of the total calories consumed and should include whole grain products, cereals, legumes, low-fat dairy products, fruits, and vegetables. High dietary fiber intake must be encouraged. Sucrose must be limited to 10% of the total energy intake. Fat intake should not be more than 30 to 35% of total daily energy intake with no more than 10% from saturated fat. Proteins should make up 15–20 % of daily calories.

Simple sugars are not totally restricted. Non-nutritive sweeteners such as aspartame, stevia, and sucralose can be safely used while avoiding nutritive sweeteners such as sorbitol. Diabetic snacks contain nutritive sweeteners, and are high in calories and saturated fats. Therefore, their use in T1DM management is not recommended. Glycemic index (GI) is a measure of the postprandial rise in the BG to constant amounts of different carbohydrate-containing foods. Foods with low GI cause a lower rise in BG post 2-3 hours of their ingestion. Low GI instead of high GI foods will prevent postprandial hyperglycemia and are therefore preferred.[18]

The post-meal BG variability can be controlled by keeping a check on the carbohydrate consumed in the meals using the principles of food exchanges and carbohydrate counting.

A list of foods similar in the number of calories and carbohydrates should be provided to families so that a variety of foods with a constant carbohydrate content can be included in the meal plan without monotony in the diet. This basic carbohydrate counting (BCC) is particularly useful for those on split mix regimen or families that are not adequately motivated to do advanced carbohydrate counting (ACC) as described later. The use of food exchange lists prevents major excursions in BG in such patients. Using BCC, the bolus dose of insulin for a particular meal stays the same from day to day, whereas using ACC, the bolus dose can be changed to match the grams of carbohydrate to be ingested in the coming meal.

Carbohydrate Counting

The concept of ACC can be taught to motivated families. This consists of matching the bolus insulin dose in the basal bolus regimen to the carbohydrate intake allowing greater flexibility in the meal pattern. The ICR is calculated as previously described and the amount of insulin required to cover a particular meal is determined by measuring the carbohydrate content in the planned meal. The method includes weighing the foods (cooked and uncooked) that the patient commonly consumes and calculating the required prandial insulin using the ICR, which can vary for each meal of the day. Patients are usually taught to measure and recognize portion sizes of 15 grams of carbohydrates. Resources that provide the carbohydrate content of different foods are available and should be given to the patients. Standardized measures (weighing scale, bowls, cups and spoons) are used and with time and training, the family learns the visual impression of the portion size without the need for weighing.

The child and the family should have frequent (at least 6 monthly) visits with the dietitian to revise the diet plan according to the changing nutritional requirements of the child, as per growth and puberty. This also helps in the reinforcement of knowledge about carbohydrate counting and insulin adjustments.

Special Days and Parties

Intake of high-energy calorie-dense foods and deep-fried foods on a regular basis must be avoided. However, on occasions like birthday parties of family and close friends and important festivals, the child may be allowed to consume foods of his/her choice, albeit judiciously. Attempts at adjusting insulin according to the intended meal are desirable on these occasions.

Hypoglycemia

A BG value of <70 mg/dL is termed hypoglycemia and is used as a cut-off for treatment. Prompt recognition and management of low BG are crucial to prevent brain injury **(Flowchart 14.1)**.[19] Hypoglycemia occurs as a complication of insulin treatment and is a major barrier to achieving target BG values. It results from a mismatch between the timing and dose of insulin,

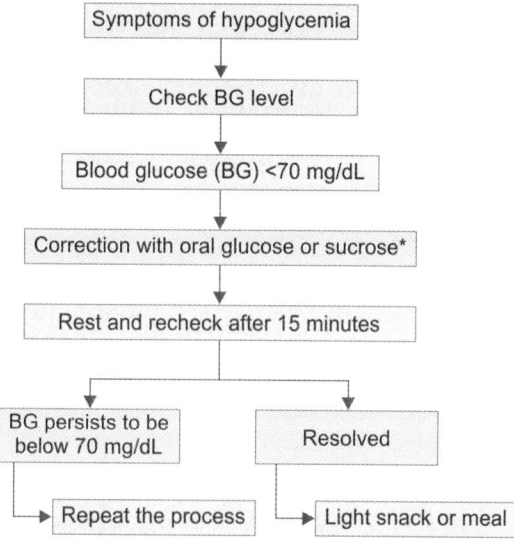

Flowchart 14.1: Management of hypoglycemia.

*Glucose about 0.3 g/kg i.e., 5 g for a 15 kg children and 15 g for 50 kg child.

meal and quantum of physical activity. Manifestations include autonomic symptoms such as tremors, palpitations, sweating and hunger, as well as neuroglycopenic symptoms such as headache, blurring of vision, and dizziness.

Severe Hypoglycemia

Hypoglycemia is termed severe if an individual requires assistance in managing the event. There is no cut-off level of BG to define severe hypoglycemia. However, since most children usually need help for managing any level of low BG, severe hypoglycemia in children refers to low glucose levels resulting in seizures or loss of consciousness, or any event requiring emergency medical care and hospitalization.

The immediate caregivers of a child with diabetes must be taught the technique of preparation and administration of injection glucagon in case of severe hypoglycemia. The dose of glucagon is 0.5 mg for children weighing <25 kg and 1 mg for children >25 kg and adults. BG rises in 10–15 minutes. Nasal glucagon has recently become available internationally.[20]

Planned Physical Activity

A child with diabetes is entitled to play and participate in any age-appropriate physical activity, viz. sports, dance, swimming etc. Exercise enhances physical and psychological well-being and helps in maintaining ideal body weight. Regular physical activity improves insulin sensitivity, thereby lowering the dose of insulin required. It decreases the risk of obesity, hypertension, dyslipidemia, and cardiovascular morbidity. Daily physical activity for at least 60 minutes of moderate to vigorous intensity is recommended for children between 6 and 18 years of age, as in non-diabetic children. However, as the BG is determined by a balance between calorie intake and energy expenditure, an individual with diabetes must carefully plan a physical activity to prevent undue glucose excursions. Exercise can lead to hypoglycemia in a child with diabetes who is well controlled or may increase the risk of precipitation of DKA if BG is not well controlled. Precautions while undertaking physical activity include monitoring of BG, adjustments in insulin doses and food consumed, before and after exercise.

In the case of planned activity lasting for >30 minutes, especially to be undertaken at the peak of insulin action, the dose of the rapid or short-acting insulin before the activity must be reduced. In the case of CSII users, the pump may be disconnected, or a lower temporary basal rate can be set. To prevent hypoglycemia, children must be instructed not to inject insulin into the exercising limb. Exercise leads to increased insulin sensitivity immediately after and the resulting post-exercise hypoglycemia can be prevented by taking an appropriate carbohydrate-containing meal within 1–2 hours of the activity, along with a reduction in the dose of the insulin bolus that follows. However, the risk of hypoglycemia can last up to 24 hours after physical activity and should be anticipated and monitored. Delayed nocturnal hypoglycemia can occur with exercise performed in the afternoon. To prevent this, the dose of the basal insulin must be reduced by 20% on the day of exercise along with monitoring the BG at bedtime and midnight. In addition, extra bedtime carbohydrates (0.4 g/kg) should be consumed.

BG can also be regulated by carbohydrate intake before, during, or after exercise, especially if the physical activity is unplanned. In the case of moderate physical activity of short duration (<30 minutes), with BG in the target range, no additional carbohydrate may be needed. However, for low to moderate-intensity exercise of duration >30 minutes, carbohydrate intake of 0.2–0.5 g/kg/h is recommended.

Fear of hypoglycemia should not hinder the child's participation in physical activities of any kind. The child must always carry simple sugar such as glucose powder or tablets or candy along with high GI snacks, to the sporting area. The physical instructor must be aware of the child's diabetes and well versed in the management of hypoglycemia. Injection glucagon must be readily available to handle a severe hypoglycemic episode.

Intense exercise can result in hyperglycemia during or after the activity. Exercise is contraindicated when BG is more than 250 mg/dL, especially with the presence of ketones, as it may precipitate DKA. Additional insulin dosing may be required, and exercise must be postponed until clearance of ketonemia. Similarly, it is not advisable to exercise during sick days. Children and adolescents should carry a diabetes ID card, especially when not accompanied by an adult.[21]

Diabetes Education

Diabetes is a chronic disease with no cure currently. Since insulin injections and other components of therapy become a lifelong daily affair, the family members should be well versed with all aspects of treatment over time. Various factors such as the socioeconomic status, cultural background, educational status of parents, their motivation and state of mind while coping with the diagnosis of diabetes, access to healthcare facilities affect diabetes management and hence glycemic control.[22] Thus, diabetes education plays a central role in the management and must be individualized in a manner the family can comprehend. The initial education must be slow, stepwise, detailed and continuous, and delivered considering the above factors. Initial teaching includes information on insulin, injection techniques, SMBG, and prevention and management of hypoglycemia. Further diabetes education must include sick day management, carbohydrate counting, insulin dose adjustments, etc., along with reinforcement of the basic knowledge from time to time.

> **BOX 14.4:** Sick day management guidelines in T1DM.
> - Monitor BG every 3 to 4 hourly
> - Ketone testing in urine or blood on sick days is of utmost importance. The methods of testing must be taught to the family. Having the testing kits/strips at home helps timely identification, treatment, and decreases the need for hospitalization
> - Insulin doses are not to be missed, despite reduced oral intake; simple carbohydrate-containing foods can be used to prevent hypoglycemia. Insulin doses may need to be increased when BG is >180 mg/dL (5–20% of TDD) and is guided by the level of ketones
> - Ensure adequate carbohydrate intake. A semisolid or liquid diet must be given if the child is unable to eat well. Adequate intake of salted fluid prevents dehydration. If vomiting precludes any oral intake, hospitalization is necessary

Sick Day Management Education

During times of illness, the body requires a higher amount of insulin. Therefore, if in a child with T1DM, the doses are not appropriately titrated, there can be precipitation of DKA due to increased lipolysis and ketogenesis to serve as an alternate energy source. **Box 14.4** outlines the guidelines for care during times of illness, viz. fever, diarrhea, toothache, etc., in T1DM.[23]

Immediate hospitalization is necessary in case of persistent vomiting, rapid breathing, and drowsiness, or if ketones continue to rise despite extra insulin doses.

Management at School

Children spend a major part of their time in school. It is important to ensure the child maintains normoglycemia at school which demands the involvement of the school authorities, teachers, and the staff. The family should inform the teachers and a few friends about the child's condition and handouts and supplies for management of acute hypoglycemia are made available. It is also important to ensure that the child gets equal opportunities to participate in sports and extracurricular activities at school without being bullied or treated differently due to his/her condition.

Psychosocial Aspects

The diagnosis of diabetes is distressing to the child and family. Various questions, doubts about the illness along with feelings of grief, anger, and guilt invade their minds and many families find it hard to accept the facts. At the onset, the parents may not be receptive to the knowledge about insulin imparted by the team. However, with the help of the diabetes team, most parents cope up with the situation. Affected children may develop an anxiety disorder, depression, and eating disorders, and hence should be screened for the same. Psychological support and counseling by a trained psychologist experienced in childhood diabetes prove rewarding. Group meetings and interaction with families and patients living with diabetes strengthen their spirit and belief in dealing with the situation.

■ CHILDHOOD DIABETES WHICH MAY NOT BE TYPE 1 DIABETES MELLITUS

With the advancement of genetic diagnostic techniques, various monogenic causes of childhood-onset diabetes are being identified. Since some of these differ in treatment and prognosis, it is important to correctly identify these rare variants. Usually, the monogenic forms of diabetes occur in the first 6 months of life, termed neonatal diabetes mellitus (NDM). Nevertheless, in certain situations, the onset can be during or after late infancy. One should question the diagnosis of T1DM in an older child in the following situations:

- *Absence of autoantibodies associated with T1DM.* However, a significant proportion of Indian children and adolescents are islet antibody-negative at diagnosis (idiopathic T1DM).[24]
- *Presence of other associated features* such as anemia, hearing loss, liver or kidney involvement, skeletal dysplasia, cardiac involvement, exocrine pancreatic insufficiency, intestinal atresia, and neurological manifestations.
- *Presence of family history of NDM or maturity-onset diabetes of young (MODY).*
- *History of hyperglycemia or hypoglycemia in the neonatal period.* Transient NDM may remit soon after onset to recur during adolescence or early. MODY due to *HNF-4α* mutation may have hyperinsulinemic hypoglycemia in infancy.
- *Obesity, acanthosis, PCOS, Turner syndrome, and Klinefelter syndrome.*
- *Low insulin requirement and detectable C-peptide levels beyond extended partial remission phase,* i.e., 5 years beyond the diagnosis of diabetes.[25,26]

■ WHAT DOES THE FUTURE HOLD?

Inhaled Insulin

Inhaled insulins are powdered formulations for delivery into the lower airways. Exubera® was the first inhaled insulin available in 2006, used as prandial insulin, but was withdrawn for several reasons. Another inhalable insulin Afreeza® approved in 2014 remains unpopular due to the respiratory side effects and commercial reasons.[27]

Transplantation

Approaches toward finding a cure for T1DM include pancreas transplantation, islet cell transplantation, and stem cell transplantation. At present, these are in the experimental stage, due to drawbacks such as the need for prolonged immunosuppression, and difficulty in procuring sufficient donor cells, among others.[28]

Disease Prevention Interventions

Of the interventions for disease prevention, anti-CD3 monoclonal antibody teplizumab has shown success in delaying the onset of clinical disease and insulin dependence by about two years following a single course of 14-day infusion versus placebo in at-risk individuals (relatives of T1DM patients with two or more islet antibody positivity and dysglycemia). Further studies are underway.

Other immunomodulatory agents being tried include 'cytotoxic T-lymphocyte associated protein-4' (CTLA4) inhibitor abatacept, anti-CD20 rituximab, anti-thymocyte globulin, etc.[29]

■ CONCLUSION

Type 1 diabetes mellitus is a common chronic condition of childhood with an increasing incidence. The management comprises of multiple daily insulin injections, self-monitoring of blood glucose and regulation of diet and physical activity. Insulin injections given multiple times a day in basal bolus regimen (or as insulin pump) form the standard of care. Glycemic control within the target range can be achieved through such intensive insulin regimen and is shown to decrease the rates of long-term microvascular and macrovascular complications. This, however, may be limited by the fear of hypoglycemia and its consequences. Comprehensive diabetic education of the child and family has a central role in management. Holistic care delivered through multidisciplinary team ensures a child with T1DM remains free of symptoms and complications, and leads a good quality of life.

■ KEY POINTS

- Advances in knowledge and technology have improved ease of care and long-term prognosis. Individualized treatment regimen must be chosen, to suit the child and family socially, economically and medically.
- Intensive insulin therapy delivered through multiple daily injections (MDI) or continuous SC insulin infusion (CSII)/insulin pumps is the standard of care in children with T1DM.
- Calculations, viz. insulin carbohydrate ratio and insulin sensitivity factor further help to fine tune the insulin doses according to the carbohydrate content of the meal and the premeal BG values, respectively.
- Advances in insulin pump that include integration with continuous glucose monitoring system (CGMS) are bringing us closer to mimicking the physiology. Low glucose suspend and predictive low glucose suspend devices help in achieving tight glucose control with decreased rates of hypoglycemia.

- Self-monitoring of blood glucose is required multiple times every day. Use of CGMS is recommended and real-time CGMS has enabled the integration with insulin pump into hybrid closed loop system.
- Carbohydrate counting and insulin dosing matched according to the carbohydrate content allows for greater flexibility in the meal pattern. Regular review with the dietitian is required to adjust for the changing nutritional requirements of the child.
- Atypical features and negative autoantibodies in a child diagnosed with T1DM should raise suspicion and prompt investigation for monogenic forms of diabetes.
- Insulin remains the mainstay of treatment even after a century of its discovery. Advances toward finding a cure include pancreas transplantation, islet cell transplantation and stem cell transplantation, all of which have major limitations and hence are still experimental in children.
- Trials are underway evaluating the use of immunomodulatory agents for the prevention of T1DM in at-risk individuals.

■ REFERENCES

1. American Diabetes Association. 2. Classification and diagnosis of diabetes: standards of medical care in diabetes—2021. Diabetes Care. 2021;44(Suppl 1): S15-33.
2. American Diabetes Association. 13. Children and adolescents: standards of medical care in diabetes—2021. Diabetes Care. 2021;44(Suppl 1):S180-99.
3. Hirsch IB, Juneja R, Beals JM, Antalis CJ, Wright EE. The evolution of insulin and how it informs therapy and treatment choices. Endocr Rev. 2020;41(5):733-5.
4. Danne T, Phillip M, Buckingham BA, Jarosz-Chobot P, Saboo B, Urakami T, et al. ISPAD Clinical Practice Consensus Guidelines 2018: Insulin treatment in children and adolescents with diabetes. Pediatr Diabetes. 2018;19 (Suppl 27):115-35.
5. Sherr JL, Tauschmann M, Battelino T, de Bock M, Forlenza G, Roman R, et al. ISPAD Clinical Practice Consensus Guidelines 2018: Diabetes technologies. Pediatr Diabetes. 2018;19 (Suppl 27):302-25.
6. Lal RA, Ekhlaspour L, Hood K, Buckingham B. Realizing a closed-loop (artificial pancreas) system for the treatment of type 1 diabetes. Endocr Rev. 2019;40(6):1521-46.
7. Ramli R, Reddy M, Oliver N. Artificial pancreas: current progress and future outlook in the treatment of type 1 diabetes. Drugs. 2019;79(10):1089-101.
8. Diabetes Control and Complications Trial Research Group, Nathan DM, Genuth S, Lachin J, Cleary P, Crofford O, et al. The effect of intensive treatment of diabetes on the development and progression of long-term complications in insulin-dependent diabetes mellitus. N Engl J Med. 1993;329(14):977-86.
9. Diabetes Control and Complications Trial/Epidemiology of Diabetes Interventions and Complications (DCCT/EDIC) Study Research Group. Intensive diabetes treatment and cardiovascular disease in patients with type 1 diabetes. N Engl J Med. 2005;353(25):2643-53.
10. Nathan DM, Group for the DR. The Diabetes Control and Complications Trial/ Epidemiology of Diabetes Interventions and Complications Study at 30 Years: Overview. Diabetes Care. 2014;37(1):9-16.

11. Diabetes Control and Complications Trial (DCCT)/Epidemiology of Diabetes Interventions and Complications (EDIC) Study Research Group. Intensive diabetes treatment and cardiovascular outcomes in type 1 diabetes: the DCCT/EDIC study 30-Year follow-up. Diabetes Care. 2016;39(5):686-93.
12. DiMeglio LA, Acerini CL, Codner E, Craig ME, Hofer SE, Pillay K, et al. ISPAD Clinical Practice Consensus Guidelines 2018: glycemic control targets and glucose monitoring for children, adolescents, and young adults with diabetes. Pediatr Diabetes. 2018;19 (Suppl 27):105-14.
13. Lind M, Pivodic A, Svensson AM, Ólafsdóttir AF, Wedel H, Ludvigsson J. HbA1c level as a risk factor for retinopathy and nephropathy in children and adults with type 1 diabetes: Swedish population based cohort study. Br Med J. 2019;366: l4894.
14. Battelino T, Danne T, Bergenstal RM, Amiel SA, Beck R, Biester T, et al. Clinical targets for continuous glucose monitoring data interpretation: recommendations from the international consensus on time in range. Diabetes Care. 2019;42(8):1593-603.
15. Pham-Short A, Donaghue KC, Ambler G, Phelan H, Twigg S, Craig ME. Screening for celiac disease in type 1 diabetes: a systematic review. Pediatrics. 2015;136(1):e170-6.
16. Sudhanshu S, Nair VV, Godbole T, Reddy SVB, Bhatia E, Dabadghao P, et al. Glycemic control and long-term complications in pediatric onset type 1 diabetes mellitus: a single-center experience from northern India. Indian Pediatr. 2019;56(3):191-5.
17. Donaghue KC, Marcovecchio ML, Wadwa RP, Chew EY, Wong TY, Calliari LE, et al. ISPAD Clinical Practice Consensus Guidelines 2018: Microvascular and macrovascular complications in children and adolescents. Pediatr Diabetes. 2018;19 (Suppl 27):262-74.
18. Salis S, Joseph M, Agarwala A, Sharma R, Kapoor N, Irani AJ. Medical nutrition therapy of pediatric type 1 diabetes mellitus in India: Unique aspects and challenges. Pediatr Diabetes. 2021;22(1):93-100.
19. Abraham MB, Jones TW, Naranjo D, Karges B, Oduwole A, Tauschmann M, et al. ISPAD Clinical Practice Consensus Guidelines 2018: assessment and management of hypoglycemia in children and adolescents with diabetes. Pediatr Diabetes. 2018;19(Suppl 27):178-92.
20. Singh-Franco D, Moreau C, Levin AD, Rosa DDL, Johnson M. Efficacy and usability of intranasal glucagon for the management of hypoglycemia in patients with diabetes: a systematic review. Clin Ther. 2020;42(9):e177-208.
21. Adolfsson P, Riddell MC, Taplin CE, Davis EA, Fournier PA, Annan F, et al. ISPAD Clinical Practice Consensus Guidelines 2018: Exercise in children and adolescents with diabetes. Pediatr Diabetes. 2018;19 (Suppl 27):205-26.
22. Mangla P, Gupta S, Chopra A, Bhatia V, Vishwakarma R, Asthana P. Influence of socio-economic and cultural factors on type 1 diabetes management: report from a tertiary care multidisciplinary diabetes management center in India. Indian J Pediatr. 2020;87(7):520-5.
23. Laffel LM, Limbert C, Phelan H, Virmani A, Wood J, Hofer SE. ISPAD Clinical Practice Consensus Guidelines 2018: sick day management in children and adolescents with diabetes. Pediatr Diabetes. 2018;19(Suppl 27):193-204.

24. Vipin VP, Zaidi G, Watson K, G Colman P, Prakash S, Agrawal S, et al. High prevalence of idiopathic (islet antibody-negative) type 1 diabetes among Indian children and adolescents. Pediatr Diabetes. 2021;22(1):47-51.
25. Hattersley AT, Greeley SAW, Polak M, Rubio-Cabezas O, Njølstad PR, Mlynarski W, et al. ISPAD Clinical Practice Consensus Guidelines 2018: the diagnosis and management of monogenic diabetes in children and adolescents. Pediatr Diabetes. 2018;19 (Suppl 27):47-63.
26. Riddle MC, Philipson LH, Rich SS, Carlsson A, Franks PW, Greeley SAW, et al. Monogenic diabetes: from genetic insights to population-based precision in care. reflections from a diabetes care editors' expert forum. Diabetes Care. 2020;43(12):3117-28.
27. Heinemann L. Inhaled Insulin: dead horse or rising phoenix? J Diabetes Sci Technol. 2017;12(2):239-42.
28. Verhoeff K, Marfil-Garza BA, Shapiro AMJ. Update on islet cell transplantation. Curr Opin Organ Transplant. 2021;26(4):397-404.
29. Rapini N, Schiaffini R, Fierabracci A. Immunotherapy strategies for the prevention and treatment of distinct stages of type 1 diabetes: an overview. Int J Mol Sci. 2020;21(6):2103.

Pediatric Hematology

Autoimmune Hemolytic Anemia

Richa Jain, Deepak Bansal

■ INTRODUCTION

Autoimmune hemolytic anemia (AIHA) is the most common acquired hemolytic anemia in children. It occurs due to autoantibody formation against red blood cell (RBC) membrane antigens leading to cell lysis. It is considered an extrinsic rather than an intrinsic disorder of the RBC, as the antibodies attach to the surface of an intrinsically normal red cell, leading to hemolysis. AIHA can be classified based on the thermal reactivity and the type of the autoantibodies generated by the body into warm antibody AIHA (warm AIHA), cold agglutinin disease (cold AIHA), paroxysmal cold hemoglobinuria (PCH), and mixed AIHA **(Table 15.1)**. Direct Coombs test (DCT) is typically positive in most patients. AIHA can also be classified into primary and secondary AIHA based on the presence of a recognizable underlying disease. The diseases which are known to have an association with AIHA are listed in **Table 15.2**.

TABLE 15.1: Classification of autoimmune hemolytic anemia based on thermal reactivity of antibodies.

Type of AIHA	Frequency	Type of antibody	Antigen specificity	Temperature of maximal reactivity (°C)	DCT result
Warm AIHA	60–90%	IgG	Anti-Rh	34–37	IgG (± C3d)
Cold autoimmune hemolytic anemia (Cold AIHA)	10–25%	IgM	Anti-I/i	4–30	C3d (>1:64)
Paroxysmal cold hemoglobinuria (PCH)	5–12%	IgG	Anti-P	Fixing: 4–30 Lysis: 34–37	± C3d (Donath-Landsteiner antibody+)
Mixed AIHA	<5%	IgG and IgM	Anti-Rh (IgG) Anti-I/i (IgM)	IgG: 34–37 IgM: 4–30	IgG and C3d (>1:64)

(AIHA: autoimmune hemolytic anemia; DCT: direct Coombs test; IgG: immunoglobulin G; IgM: immunoglobulin M; Rh: rhesus)

TABLE 15.2: Causes of secondary AIHA and initial screening investigations.

Causes	Investigations
Autoimmune diseases: • Evans syndrome • Systemic lupus erythematosus • Juvenile idiopathic arthritis • APLA • Autoimmune hepatitis • Nephritis • Primary sclerosing cholangitis • Thyroiditis	Antinuclear antibodies, anti-double stranded DNA (anti-dsDNA) antibodies
Immunodeficiency disorders: • CVID • ALPS • Combined immunodeficiency • ADA deficiency	• Immunoglobulin profile, lymphocyte subset analysis • Screening for ALPS
Infections: • Epstein-Barr virus • Mycoplasma pneumoniae • Human immunodeficiency virus (HIV) • Cytomegalovirus • Parvovirus B19 • Varicella • SARS-CoV-2 • Hepatitis C • Rubella	• Mycoplasma serology • ELISA for HIV • Screening for other infections to be done if clinically suspected
Malignancy: • Acute leukemia • Non-Hodgkin lymphoma • CML • Myelodysplastic syndrome	CBC, with peripheral smear; bone marrow examination if clinical suspicion
Drugs: • Penicillins, piperacillin • Cephalosporins • Erythromycin • Tetracycline • Acetaminophen • Ibuprofen	

(ADA: adenosine deaminase; ALPS: autoimmune lymphoproliferative syndrome; APLA: antiphospholipid syndrome; CBC: complete blood count; CML: chronic myeloid leukemia; CVID: common variable immunodeficiency; ELISA: enzyme-linked immunosorbent assay)

Autoimmune hemolytic anemia is more common in adults than in children. There is no sex predilection in children. Population-based data is not available from our country; however, western registry data estimates the incidence of pediatric AIHA to be around 1 in 80,000–100,000.[1,2] AIHA peaks in young children <4 years of age, with another peak in adolescents. It is a disease associated with significant morbidity and mortality, especially in the presence of secondary causes. Increased recognition of underlying genetics of the secondary causes, more readily available diagnostics, and improvement of care have helped to improve the outcome of this disease. While mortality of up to 10% has been reported from older data, the mortality has decreased to 4% in recent years.[3,4] However, several patients may have a recurrent or persistent disease, leading to long-term morbidity. In a nationwide study from France, more than one-fourth of the children remained dependent on immunosuppressive agents at 3 years of diagnosis.[3]

■ CLINICAL FEATURES

Anemia is present in all patients. It ranges from mild to severe. The symptoms in a patient with AIHA depend on the rapidity of development and the severity of anemia. The usual presentation is of rapid-onset progressive anemia, evolving within days to a few weeks. Fatigue and low-grade fever are present and attributable to anemia. Congestive cardiac failure is rare, despite severe anemia, and children are usually well compensated. Abdominal pain may be present more often with intravascular hemolysis than with extravascular hemolysis. Jaundice is often evident on clinical examination. Urine may be discolored due to jaundice or because of intravascular hemolysis leading to cola-colored urine. A preceding history of viral infections, ingestion of drugs, and vaccinations should be sought. History suggestive of autoimmune disorders, primary immunodeficiency, or malignancy, is crucial as it points towards secondary AIHA.

Examination confirms the presence of anemia, which may be mild to severe. Jaundice may be present and is typically mild; deep icterus is uncommon and points toward an alternative diagnosis. A cardiac examination is required to assess hemodynamic compromise. Flow murmur and features of cardiac failure, though uncommon, should be looked for. Mild-to-moderate splenomegaly is typically present in most patients with AIHA. Hepatomegaly is less prominent than splenomegaly. Other systems are generally normal in a primary AIHA. These findings are common to all forms of AIHA. The presence of massive organomegaly or significant/generalized lymphadenopathy are findings inconsistent with primary AIHA. They may be present in secondary AIHA associated with leukemia, lymphoma, autoimmune diseases, immunodeficiency diseases, including common variable immunodeficiency, human immunodeficiency virus (HIV) infection, and autoimmune lymphoproliferative syndrome (ALPS). These diseases may have anemia due to multiple causes and may also be associated with secondary AIHA, with DCT positivity.

BOX 15.1: Markers of hemolysis common to both intravascular and extravascular hemolysis.

↑ Unconjugated bilirubin (and total bilirubin)
↑ Aspartate aminotransferase
↑ Absolute and corrected reticulocyte count
↓ Hemoglobin
↓ Plasma haptoglobin level

TABLE 15.3: Differentiation between intravascular and extravascular hemolysis.

Feature	Intravascular hemolysis	Extravascular hemolysis
Site of hemolysis	Circulation	Reticuloendothelial system (spleen, liver, and bone marrow)
Jaundice	+/–	++
Cola-colored urine	Yes	No
Serum LDH	Elevated	Normal
Hemoglobinemia	+	–
Hemoglobinuria	+	–
Hemosiderinuria	+	–
Iron overload	–	Yes (with chronicity)
Examples	Malaria, G6PD deficiency, MAHA, and PCH	Thalassemia, HS, warm AIHA

(AIHA: autoimmune hemolytic anemia; G6PD: glucose-6-phosphate dehydrogenase; HS: hereditary spherocytosis; LDH: lactic dehydrogenase; MAHA: microangiopathic hemolytic anemia; PCH: paroxysmal cold hemoglobinuria)

The goal of a detailed history and examination in the pediatric emergency is to enable the physician to make a provisional diagnosis of hemolytic anemia and direct the investigations accordingly. The laboratory investigations that further help to confirm hemolytic anemia and differentiate between intravascular versus extravascular hemolysis are listed in **Box 15.1** and **Table 15.3**.

■ WARM AUTOIMMUNE HEMOLYTIC ANEMIA
Case Vignette

A 4-year-old girl presented to the emergency with a history of low-grade fever and fatigability for the last 3 days. The parents had also noted yellowish discoloration of eyes for 5–6 days. There was no history of cola-colored urine. She had a history of low-grade fever with upper respiratory tract infection 3 weeks ago. On examination, there was tachycardia with a flow murmur. She had severe pallor with mild icterus. There was no lymphadenopathy. Systemic examination was remarkable for the presence of soft hepatomegaly (liver 2 cm

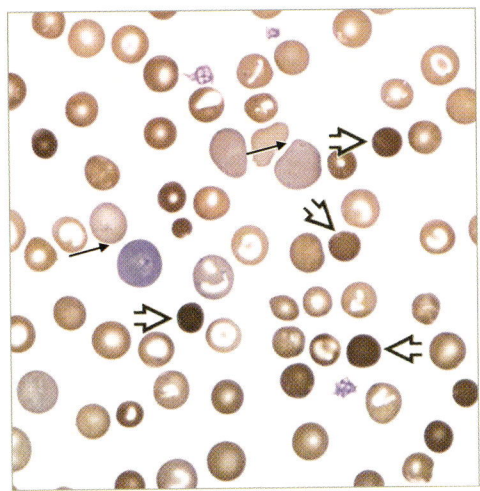

Fig. 15.1: Warm autoimmune hemolytic anemia; high power (100×; Giemsa stain). Peripheral smear showing spherocytes (open arrows) and polychromatic cells (black arrows) in a 4-year-old girl, with sudden onset severe pallor and abdominal pain. There was a preceding viral infection. Hemoglobin 4.5 g/dL, MCV 115 fl and reticulocyte count 16%. DCT was positive for IgG.
(MCV: mean corpuscular volume; DCT: direct Coombs test)
(*Courtesy*: Dr Prateek Bhatia)

below the costal margin, with a span of 9 cm) and splenomegaly (2 cm below the costal margin). A complete blood count (CBC) confirmed severe anemia, with a hemoglobin of 4.5 g/dL, while the other cell lines were preserved. The mean corpuscular volume (MCV) was elevated at 115 fl. The reticulocyte count was also high at 16%. The peripheral smear can be seen in **Figure 15.1**. A transfusion request was sent to the blood bank. The blood bank alerted the pediatric emergency that they had significant difficulty in cross matching a packed RBC unit for the patient. A DCT was done with the clinical and laboratory suspicion of AIHA, which was positive for immunoglobulin G (IgG). Prednisolone at a dose of 2 mg/kg/day was initiated along with folic acid. A blood transfusion was administered urgently after the initiation of steroids. Further transfusions were not indicated, as the hemolysis stopped after 4 days of steroid initiation. Following 2 weeks, a complete response was obtained, and steroids could be tapered over 6 months, with a plan for regular monitoring for relapse.

Clinical Features and Diagnosis of Warm AIHA

Warm AIHA is the most common form of AIHA in children, accounting for 60–80% of all cases of AIHA.[5,6] It is typically abrupt in onset and presents with severe anemia. Primary warm AIHA constitutes 50–60% of cases. The DCT is positive for IgG but may at times be weakly positive for complement C3d as well. It can be differentiated from mixed AIHA, where the C3d positivity is stronger. Rarely, the DCT may be negative when the antibodies causing hemolysis are immunoglobulin A (IgA) or immunoglobulin M (IgM). The hemolysis in warm AIHA is almost exclusively extravascular, and splenomegaly is almost always present. Hepatomegaly may be present as well. The urine is either clear or yellow due to jaundice, with the passage of urobilinogen.

Investigations in the case of warm AIHA are directed toward recognizing and quantifying anemia. The evaluation of CBC and peripheral smear helps to assess the degree of anemia and the other cell lines. At times, thrombocytopenia or leukopenia may be present. More frequently, a child with AIHA may have mild neutrophilia. The presence of concomitant thrombocytopenia or leukopenia indicates Evans syndrome, which is discussed later. A peripheral smear evaluation by an experienced pathologist can confirm the presence of hemolysis (*see* **Fig. 15.1**). The reticulocyte count is elevated in most patients; however, it may be normal or low in up to 39% of patients, particularly in the initial few days.[3]

Direct Coombs Test

The DCT, also known as the direct antiglobulin test, forms the basis of diagnosis and classification of AIHA. It detects antibodies or complement on the surface of the RBC to confirm the immune-mediated nature of hemolysis. IgG antibodies are present on the surface of RBC in patients with AIHA. The Coombs reagent, consisting of antihuman globulin, binds these antibodies and leads to RBC agglutination. A polyspecific Coomb's reagent consists of both anti-IgG and anticomplement antibodies and does not differentiate between various subtypes of AIHA. A monospecific Coombs reagent is used to classify the type of AIHA further. **Table 15.1** includes the DCT finding in various types of AIHA. A diagnostic algorithm for AIHA is provided in **Flowchart 15.1**.

Oddities in Warm AIHA: When Investigations and Clinical Diagnosis Differ from Each Other

Direct Coombs Test False Negativity

This may be observed in up to 10% of cases of AIHA. It is more common with the tube technique of DCT. A lower incidence of false negativity is observed when the DCT is carried out by alternative techniques, including gel cards analysis, enzyme-linked immunosorbent assay (ELISA), and flow cytometry-based detection of RBC-bound IgG. Most of the laboratories prefer the gel card technique, and false negativity is observed in <5% of cases. False negative DCT may also be observed when the antibody causing AIHA is a low-affinity antibody that is removed during the washing procedure of the test. This may be prevented by using a low ionic strength solution or normal saline at low temperatures instead of room temperature normal saline. Low ionic strength solution is now commonly used by most of the laboratories performing this test and is readily available.

Flowchart 15.1: Diagnostic algorithm for autoimmune hemolytic anemia.

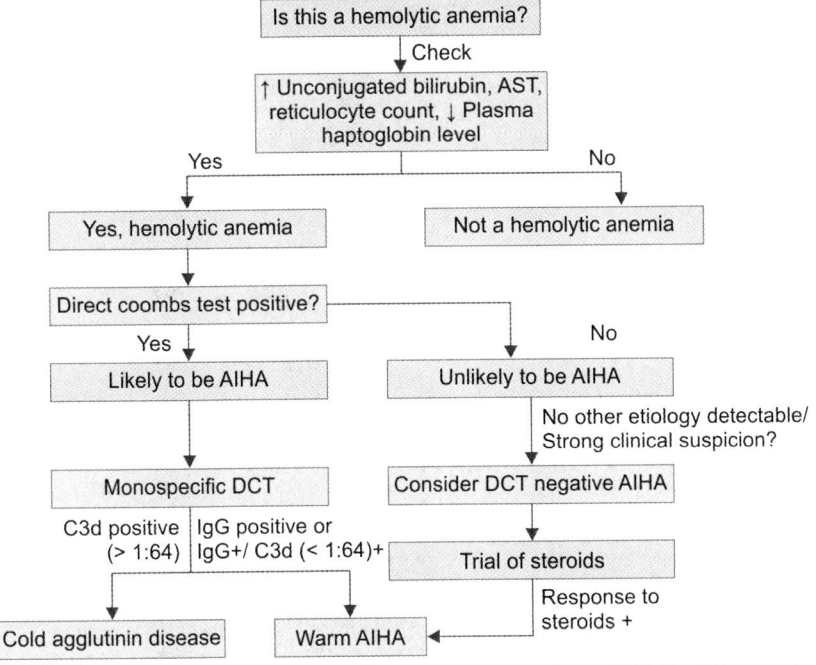

(AIHA: autoimmune hemolytic anemia; AST: aspartate transaminase; DCT: direct Coombs test)

Another reason for a false negative DCT is the presence of non-IgG antibodies. In such cases, which account for 0.2–2.7% of warm AIHA cases, the antibody leading to hemolysis is IgM or IgA not detectable by the DCT. Paroxysmal cold hemoglobinuria (PCH) is caused by IgG, which fixes at low temperatures. A DCT is frequently negative in cases of PCH.

The diagnosis of DCT-negative AIHA is difficult. It is typically made after one has excluded alternative causes of hemolysis and evaluated in detail for hemolytic anemias. Confirmation by a sensitive technique, where available, is helpful. Response to steroid therapy supports the diagnosis of AIHA.

False Positive Direct Coombs Test

The DCT can at times be falsely positive due to several causes, listed in **Box 15.2**. In infancy, hemolysis due to ABO or Rh incompatibility is a common cause of DCT positivity. The anemia, as well as the DCT positivity, may persist from weeks to months. These infants can be mistaken to have an infantile form of AIHA if birth details are not available to the treating pediatrician.

Reticulocytopenia in Autoimmune Hemolytic Anemia

A corrected reticulocyte count should be >1.5% to be considered high, but most of the cases of AIHA may have a significant rise in reticulocyte count,

> **BOX 15.2:** Causes of false-positive direct Coombs test.
> - Liver disease
> - Chronic infection
> - Malignancy
> - Systemic lupus erythematosus
> - Renal disorders
> - Drug-induced immune hemolytic anemia (e.g., intravenous immunoglobulin (IVIg) or antithymocyte globulin)
> - Delayed hemolytic reaction after a transfusion (up to 3 months after a transfusion)
> - ABO mismatched stem cell transplant
> - Passenger lymphocyte syndrome in a solid organ transplant recipient

reaching 10–20%. Reticulocytopenia is defined as an absolute reticulocyte count <120 × 10^9/L or a corrected reticulocyte count of <1.5%. It may occur in up to 30–40% of children with warm AIHA and is transient in the majority. It typically occurs in the initial period of the illness, and after about a week, the reticulocyte count rises in most of the patients.[3] The lag period may be significantly prolonged if the autoantibodies leading to AIHA act against the reticulocyte membrane antigens as well, leading to premature destruction of the reticulocyte within the bone marrow. Reticulocytopenia may also be due to direct suppression of the bone marrow in cases of postinfectious AIHA, primarily due to parvovirus B19 infection. In secondary AIHA, due to marrow infiltration by leukemia or lymphoma, the reticulocyte count is typically suboptimal.

Secondary Autoimmune Hemolytic Anemia

Secondary AIHA is an increasingly recognized entity and contributes to a large percentage of warm AIHA. In a recent nationwide study from France, secondary causes accounted for 40% of warm AIHA.[3] In multiple other studies, secondary causes were noted in one-third to two-thirds of all children with warm AIHA.[6,7] The causes of secondary AIHA and the first-line investigations required for diagnosis are detailed in **Table 15.2**. Immune dysregulation is now considered to be the most frequent secondary cause of AIHA. Evans syndrome, autoimmune disorders, and various infections account for 10% of cases. The clinical presentation of primary or secondary AIHA is similar. Investigating for the common secondary causes of AIHA is essential in all patients.

Treatment of Warm Autoimmune Hemolytic Anemia

Flowchart 15.2 provides an overview of the treatment for warm AIHA. Typically, patients who develop warm AIHA have a protracted course in comparison to cold AIHA. Steroids are the front-line therapy. The drug of choice is prednisolone. The starting dose is 2–4 mg/kg/day in two to three

Flowchart 15.2: Treatment algorithm for warm autoimmune hemolytic anemia.

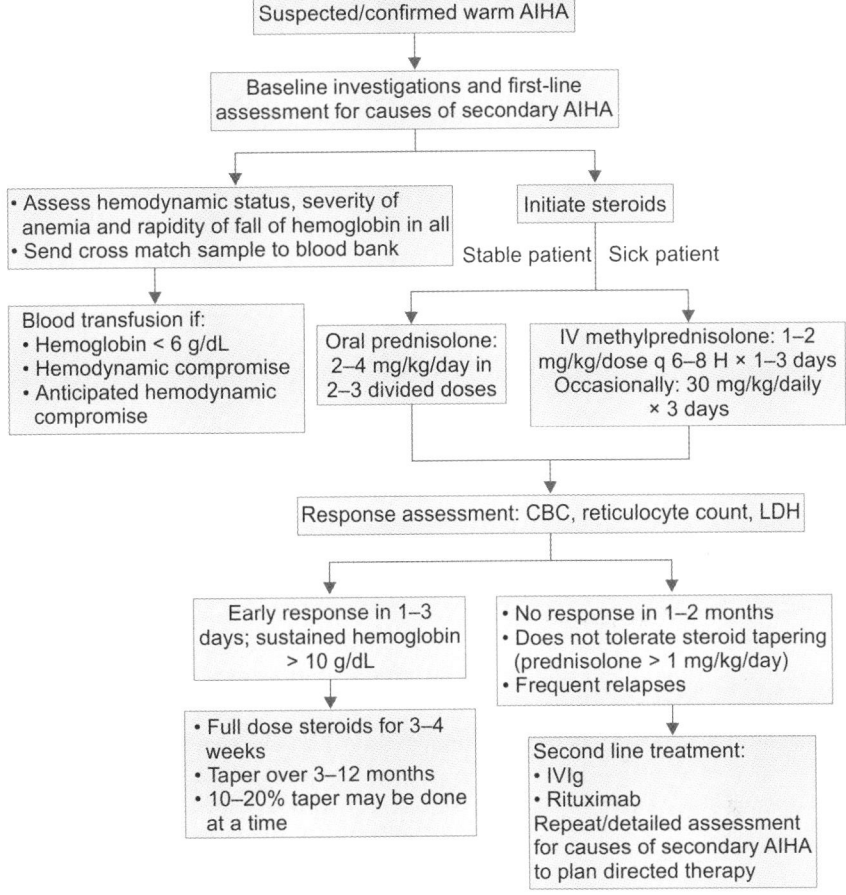

(AIHA: autoimmune hemolytic anemia; CBC: complete blood count; LDH: lactate dehydrogenase)

divided doses. Rarely, higher doses of up to 6-8 mg/kg per day have also been described.[2,8] Alternatively, methylprednisolone may be used intravenously in sick patients, at a dose of 1-2 mg/kg every 6-hourly for 1-3 days, before converting to oral prednisolone. This high dose of steroids is required for 3-4 weeks before tapering is attempted. The tapering must be slow and over 3-12 months to prevent relapses. Typically, 10-20% taper may be done at a time. It is prudent to change to once-daily doses followed by every alternate day dosing while tapering the dose to minimize adverse effects.

A goal of therapy is to stabilize the patient, minimize blood transfusion requirements acutely, and attain a long-term remission. The monitoring of response is by CBC and reticulocyte count. Repeating the DCT does not help to assess response in newly diagnosed cases; however, it is helpful in cases of relapsed or refractory AIHA.

An initial remission with steroid monotherapy is attained in approximately 80% of patients. However, durable long-term remissions are noted in only 20–40% of children. Second-line agents are required when there is nonresponse, with persistent severe hemolysis and transfusion dependence after 1–3 days of full-dose of steroids. They are also required in cases of refractory disease, steroid dependence, or recurrent disease. The preferred second-line agent is intravenous immunoglobulin (IVIg) at a dose of 1 g/kg/day for 2 days, though the response may not be long-lasting. Failing this, or in the presence of refractory disease, rituximab at a dose of 375 mg/m^2 weekly for 4 weeks can be initiated. Rituximab leads to an early response in 60–85% of patients and a sustained response in 25–75% of patients.

Blood Transfusion in Warm Autoimmune Hemolytic Anemia

The warm autoantibodies present in the patient's serum are directed against the Rh antigen present on all red cells and prevent any true cross-matched units from being available for transfusion. The inherent risk with a blood transfusion is precipitating a hemolytic transfusion reaction. On the other hand, a fear of hemolytic reaction should not prevent transfusion in patients with severe anemia or a rapid rate of hemoglobin fall. Transfusion is recommended, if the hemoglobin is below 6 g/dL or the rapid fall leads to hemodynamic compromise. The blood bank should be requested to issue the least incompatible packed red cell unit with the patient's serum which should be transfused under cover of steroids. If multiple transfusions are required, the patient will be at risk for the development of alloantibodies. Alloantibodies may be prevented by blood grouping for the significant blood groups, including Rh, Kidd, Kell, Duffy, and providing phenotypically matched blood units.

Supportive Care

Supportive care is essential in all children with AIHA. Folic acid should be prescribed to all patients to support the high turnover occurring in the bone marrow. Children on long-term steroids require monitoring for adverse effects, including hypertension, osteoporosis, hyperglycemia, impaired height gain, and excessive weight gain. Screening for cataracts is required in children on long-term steroids. Regular monitoring of blood pressure is required in the outpatient clinic visits. Patients on prolonged steroid treatment should be supplemented with vitamin D and calcium. Diet and lifestyle modifications should be advised to prevent obesity and improve bone health.

Refractory Autoimmune Hemolytic Anemia

Refractory AIHA is a term that is not very well defined. The disease may be called refractory if hemoglobin does not stabilize despite 3–4 weeks of appropriate therapy. The hemoglobin should be at least above 10 g/dL,

> **BOX 15.3:** Treatment options in warm autoimmune hemolytic anemia.
>
> *First-line treatment*:
> - Prednisolone
> - Methylprednisolone
>
> *Second-line treatment*:
> - Intravenous immunoglobulin (IVIg)
> - Rituximab
> - Sirolimus
> - Splenectomy
>
> *Third-line treatment*:
> - Mycophenolate mofetil
> - Azathioprine
> - Cyclosporin
> - Low dose prednisolone along with a steroid-sparing agent
> - Cyclophosphamide
> - Alemtuzumab
>
> *Other modalities, including experimental drugs*:
> - Hematopoietic stem cell transplant
> - Abatacept
> - Syk inhibitors

without transfusion support to be called stable. The treatment options for refractory and chronic AIHA are listed in **Box 15.3**.

Splenectomy has long been considered an option for relapsed and refractory AIHA. However, it is not a preferred treatment option any longer. This is because of increasing recognition of the secondary causes of AIHA, with several less invasive treatment options becoming available. Moreover, while splenectomy leads to an initial response rate is 60–70% of patients with refractory AIHA, the long-term remission is maintained in only 20% of children.

■ EVANS SYNDROME

Evans syndrome accounts for nearly 10–30% of cases of pediatric AIHA.[3] It is diagnosed in the presence of immune-mediated cytopenia involving any two cell lines. Previously, the presence of AIHA was mandatory for the diagnosis of Evans syndrome; however, currently, any two of autoimmune cytopenia, among neutropenia, thrombocytopenia, or anemia, may be present to qualify as Evans syndrome. The most frequent combination of cytopenia is anemia and thrombocytopenia, and they may develop sequentially or simultaneously. It is not necessary for both the cell lines to be affected simultaneously, and AIHA may predate or occur after developing the other cell line involvement. Underlying genetic causes may be present in more than half of the cases.[3,8,9] Hence, it is vital to evaluate the genetic causes of Evans syndrome in all cases of AIHA.

Evans syndrome may be diagnosed as early as infancy. It is estimated to occur at a frequency of 0.4 per 100,000 children per year. Mortality in

Evans syndrome is higher than in AIHA, and in some series, up to 10% of the patients may succumb to the disease or treatment-related complications.[3] Evans syndrome is often secondary and may develop in association with an underlying immunodeficiency disorder, infection, malignancy, or other disorders **(Box 15.4)**.

Children with primary immunodeficiency are at an 80–120-fold risk of developing autoimmune cytopenia compared to an age-matched cohort. Mutations that have been associated with Evans syndrome include various monogenic immunodeficiency disorders. Common mutations are in genes causing *ALPS* (Fas apoptotic pathway), *LRBA* deficiency, *TNFRSF6* mutation, *STAT3* mutation, *RAG1* mutations, and *CTLA4* deficiency. In a nationwide cohort of children with Evans syndrome, pathogenic or potentially pathogenic mutations were observed in 65% of patients, while 35% were not detected to have mutations.[9] Mutation-positive Evans syndrome patients may develop lymphoproliferation, hypogammaglobulinemia, and infections

---

BOX 15.4: Disorders causing Evans syndrome.

Immunodeficiency disorders:
- Autoimmune lymphoproliferative syndrome
- Common variable immunodeficiency
- Severe combined immunodeficiency
- *LRBA* deficiency
- *CTLA4* deficiency
- *TNFRSF6* mutation
- *RAG1* mutation
- *STAT3* mutation
- DiGeorge syndrome

Infections:
- Epstein-Barr virus
- Cytomegalovirus
- Human immunodeficiency virus
- *Helicobacter pylori*
- Hepatitis C virus
- *Mycoplasma pneumoniae*
- Parvovirus B19

Rheumatological disorders:
- Systemic lupus erythematosus
- Anti-phospholipid syndrome
- Rheumatoid arthritis
- Giant-cell hepatitis

Malignancies:
- Lymphoma
- Leukemia
- Myelodysplasia

Others:
- Castleman disease
- Post-stem cell transplantation

more frequently than mutation-negative patients. At times, there may be an apparent infectious trigger for AIHA; however, the patient may develop immune dysregulation and Evans syndrome on follow-up. Therefore, it is recommended that all children who develop warm or mixed AIHA be assessed for an underlying immunodeficiency disorder.

When AIHA is present, the DCT is typically positive for IgG. Infrequently, AIHA may be mediated by IgM antibodies and be positive for C3d, or both IgG and C3d positivity may be present. Assessment and evaluation of patients are initially performed as for AIHA and include a CBC, reticulocyte count, and a peripheral smear evaluation. Reticulocytopenia is more common in Evans syndrome than in AIHA and may be observed in up to 40% of patients. Evaluation for underlying etiology should be undertaken at the earliest, as Evans syndrome is associated with more morbidity and higher mortality than simple AIHA. The treatment may be directed toward an underlying genetic cause, if detected. First-line diagnostic evaluation should include assessment for various viral infections, anti-nuclear antibodies (ANA), anti-double strand DNA antibodies (anti-dsDNA), immunoglobulin profile, lymphocyte subset analysis, and assessment for ALPS. Subsequent evaluation, including for monogenic immunodeficiency disorders, may be done as per the availability. They should be carried out if the initial evaluation does not yield an etiology, and the patient has recurrent or persistent symptoms or develops new-onset symptoms pointing to an underlying immunodeficiency.

Treatment of Evans Syndrome

Steroids are the first-line treatment of choice for Evans syndrome. The dose used is the same as the dose used in AIHA. In case of treatment failure, or steroid dependence, rituximab is the preferred second-line treatment. In children who develop Evans syndrome secondary to ALPS, sirolimus is the preferred second-line agent. Mycophenolate mofetil may also be effective in these patients.

COLD AIHA, COLD AGGLUTININ DISEASE, AND COLD AGGLUTININ SYNDROME

The term cold AIHA includes cold agglutinin disease, cold agglutinin syndrome, and PCH. While PCH is discussed in more detail in the next section, cold agglutinin disease and cold agglutinin syndrome are discussed in this section.

The two terms, cold agglutinin disease and cold agglutinin syndrome are often used interchangeably and may lead to confusion. Cold agglutinin disease is used to define cold AIHA in adults caused by primary IgM-mediated complement-dependent hemolysis. This chronic condition is typically associated with lymphoproliferative disorders including, chronic lymphoid leukemia. The IgM antibody causing the hemolysis is monoclonal. In contrast, cold agglutinin syndrome occurs in children and is typically secondary to an infection. The IgM antibodies leading to hemolysis are acute in onset and polyclonal in nature. The frequently implicated infections leading to cold agglutinin syndrome in children are *Mycoplasma pneumoniae* and Epstein-Barr virus (EBV). However, several other bacterial and viral infections may lead to the development of cold agglutinins and include varicella, adenovirus, hepatitis C, rubella, parvovirus, mumps, and cytomegalovirus.

Cold agglutinin syndrome occurs with infections but has also been associated with common variable immunodeficiency and systemic lupus erythematosus (SLE) uncommonly.[6] The onset is typically after 2–3 weeks of the infection. The primary presentation is rapidly developing anemia and jaundice, often with tender splenomegaly and abdominal pain. Acrocyanosis and hemoglobinuria are uncommon. Anemia is typically not severe enough to lead to congestive cardiac failure. Confirmation of the diagnosis is by the presence of a monospecific DCT positivity for C3d. The cold agglutinin titer should be ≥64 at a temperature of 4°C. Peripheral smear evaluation may show clumping of RBC **(Fig. 15.2)**.

Pathophysiology of Cold Agglutinin Syndrome

Immunoglobulin M autoantibodies active against RBC membrane I/i antigen develop a few days to weeks after mycoplasma or EBV infection.

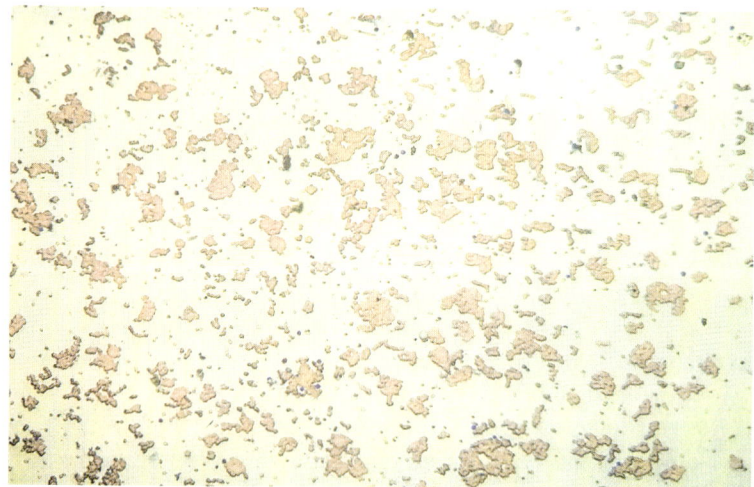

Fig. 15.2: Cold agglutinin syndrome; low power (20×; Giemsa stain). Peripheral smear showing a large number of RBC clumps in a 6-year-old boy who presented with fever and fatigue. On examination, he had severe pallor and mild hepatomegaly. CBC showed anemia with MCV of 130 fl.

(CBC: complete blood count; MCV: mean corpuscular volume)
(*Courtesy*: Dr Prateek Bhatia).

Hemolysis occurs due to these IgM antibodies and is complement-mediated and predominantly extravascular, with a small degree of an intravascular component. As these antibodies are cold reactive and active between 4 and 30°C, the symptoms are more notable in the winter season. Due to the cold temperature, the peripheries, including fingertips, toes, and ear lobes, become cold with the cooling of the blood. This allows binding of pentameric IgM antibodies to RBCs I/i antigen, with agglutination of the RBCs. The antigen-antibody complex, which is formed, activates the classical complement pathway, and leads to the formation of C3 convertase. C3 convertase triggers the cleavage of C3 and the formation of C3a and C3b, which binds to the RBC. Once the antibody-coated RBCs reach the central circulation, they are warmed, and the cold antibodies detach from the RBC. However, the C3b remains bound to the cells and marks them for phagocytosis in the liver and splenic macrophages, leading to predominant extravascular hemolysis. The intravascular component is minor and occurs due to the formation of a membrane attack complex. This leads to elevated plasma hemoglobin, hemoglobinuria, and hemosiderinuria. The C3b molecule is cleaved from the residual RBCs leaving behind C3d, which the DCT then detects.

Treatment of Cold Agglutinin Syndrome

The disease is typically self-limited and nonrecurrent. The treatment is supportive and includes avoiding cold exposure and keeping the extremities warm. A blood transfusion, if required, should warrant the use of blood warmer to ensure that the transfused blood is at body temperature. This prevents further hemolysis. IgM antibodies of cold AIHA do not interfere in cross-matching, and there is no difficulty in obtaining a compatible RBC unit for transfusion. Treatment with macrolide antibiotics may improve AIHA in cases secondary to *Mycoplasma pneumoniae* infection.

While steroids do not have a defined role in treating IgM-mediated cold AIHA, they may be tried in cases where there is severe or life-threatening hemolysis not controlled by supportive care. In a series of pediatric cases, cold agglutinin syndrome was responsive to steroids in 75% of cases.[6] Plasma exchange is an alternative first-line therapy, which can be attempted in life-threatening hemolysis despite supportive care. In clinical practice, plasma exchange and steroids are rarely required. An alternative second-line treatment option is exchange transfusion, which reduces antibody load and removes presensitized RBCs from the circulation, thereby decreasing the hemolysis. Any exchange procedure must also be performed with the use of in-line blood warmer. Rituximab can be tried in cases of refractory and uncontrolled disease.[5] A standard dose of 375 mg/m^2 weekly for four doses may be used. There is no clear evidence for the use of other immunosuppressants in children with cold agglutinin syndrome. Overall, the disease has a good prognosis, with 70–75% of children achieving a long-term remission.[3,6]

■ PAROXYSMAL COLD HEMOGLOBINURIA

Paroxysmal cold hemoglobinuria (PCH) is less common than warm and cold AIHA and contributes to 5–12% of pediatric AIHA.[5,6] It is caused by cold reacting IgG autoantibodies, known as Donath Landsteiner antibodies, directed against the P-antigen on the RBC membrane. The hemolysis is caused by complement activation and is primarily intravascular. Like cold agglutinin syndrome, PCH in children is typically postinfectious. There may be a history of viral fever or an upper respiratory tract infection in the preceding weeks before developing hemolysis. The hemolysis is abrupt in onset and predominantly intravascular. Anemia may be severe in some children and may be accompanied by abdominal pain. Reticulocytosis is frequent, but viral-induced reticulocytopenia may be present in a minority of patients. Spherocytes are uncommonly seen on the peripheral smear. Organomegaly is less common than in warm AIHA. The cold agglutinin syndrome due to the intravascular nature of hemolysis is reported in up to 25% of patients.[10] While cold exposure may aggravate the symptoms, it is not essential for the development of hemolysis.

The Donath Landsteiner antibodies bind to RBC and fix complement at a lower temperature, but the complement-mediated lysis occurs at a temperature of 30–37°C. Markers for hemolysis are positive in the form of anemia, reticulocytosis, decreased haptoglobin, and elevated LDH. In addition, the DCT is negative in most patients as the cold-reacting IgG antibodies dissociate from the surface of RBC at room temperature. DCT may be positive for C3d in a minority of patients. Confirmation of the diagnosis is with a positive Donath Landsteiner antibody test, which can be performed only in specific reference laboratories, and is not freely available. PCH is underreported in children due to the difficulty in establishing the diagnosis and the self-limited nature of the disease. Limited laboratories have the facility of testing for Donath Landsteiner antibody. The antibodies become undetectable after the episode of acute hemolysis is resolved.

Treatment of Paroxysmal Cold Hemoglobinuria

Paroxysmal cold hemoglobinuria is a nonrecurring disease. Supportive care is the mainstay of therapy and includes keeping the patient warm and using in-line blood warmer for RBC transfusion. Blood transfusion should be given in cases of severe anemia and impending hemodynamic compromise. Finding a compatible blood product is typically not difficult because the cold antibodies do not interfere in routine pretransfusion screening and compatibility testing. This is secondary to the low thermal amplitude of the antibodies, which do not bind to the RBC at temperatures above 20°C. The use of P negative RBCs is not required for transfusion support, and adequate hematocrit can be obtained using P positive RBCs.

The condition is self-resolving in most of the cases. Urine output should be monitored as intravascular hemolysis may lead to kidney injury, and adequate hydration should be ensured. Treatment of any specific infection that may be associated with PCH should be done simultaneously. While steroids do not have a significant role in PCH treatment, they may be initiated in a patient with a clinical suspicion of AIHA. Once the diagnosis is confirmed, the steroid therapy can be stopped. There is no role of IVIg in cases of PCH. Rituximab can be considered in refractory cases, though such situations are infrequent.

■ MIXED AUTOIMMUNE HEMOLYTIC ANEMIA

Mixed AIHA is the least common of all, accounting for <5% of all AIHA in children.[5] The DCT is typically positive for IgG and C3d but may be positive for only IgG or only C3d in the minority. The C3d titer may be <1:64. The antibodies involved are both IgG and IgM. Mixed AIHA has the serological characteristics of both warm AIHA as well as cold agglutinin syndrome. The hemolysis is primarily extravascular with an intravascular component.

A secondary cause of hemolysis may be present in 50% of patients, with SLE being an important cause. The treatment should be like warm AIHA, though the disease may become chronic in several patients. Steroid dependence or refractoriness to first-line therapy is often seen.[4] Immunosuppressive therapy and treatment of underlying etiology help in improving outcomes.

■ CONCLUSION

Autoimmune hemolytic anemia remains a rare but significant cause of hemolysis in children. Rapid advances have occurred in the understanding of the genetic mechanisms underlying AIHA and Evans syndrome. Immunological disorders form the majority of secondary AIHA. The first-line treatment option remains oral or parenteral steroids. Steroids should be tapered gradually to prevent a relapse, while monitoring for steroid toxicity and adverse effects. Although mortality rates have decreased, there is a significant morbidity associated with AIHA. Patients with cold agglutinin syndrome and PCH are significantly more likely to attain long-term remission as compared to those with warm AIHA.

■ KEY POINTS

- Secondary AIHA contributes to one-third to two-thirds of all cases with warm AIHA.
- Evaluation of the secondary causes of warm-AIHA is essential at diagnosis. Immunological diseases are the most common cause of secondary AIHA.

- Steroids are the front-line therapy of warm AIHA.
- Autoimmune lymphoproliferative syndrome is increasingly being recognized as a cause of warm AIHA; sirolimus is an effective second-line agent to treat these patients.
- Primary immunodeficiency associated AIHA may need hematopoietic stem cell transplantation (HSCT) for definitive treatment, rather than escalation of immunosuppressive agents.
- Autoimmune hemolytic anemia with IgG or IgG+C3d positive DCT has a significantly worse prognosis than other forms of AIHA.

■ REFERENCES

1. Aladjidi N, Jutand MA, Beaubois C, Fernandes H, Jeanpetit J, Coureau G, et al. Reliable assessment of the incidence of childhood autoimmune hemolytic anemia. Pediatr Blood Cancer. 2017;64(12).
2. Voulgaridou A, Kalfa TA. Autoimmune hemolytic anemia in the pediatric setting. J Clin Med. 2021;10(2):216.
3. Aladjidi N, Leverger G, Leblanc T, Picat MQ, Michel G, Bertrand Y, et al. New insights into childhood autoimmune hemolytic anemia: a French national observational study of 265 children. Haematologica. 2011;96(5):655-63.
4. Hill QA, Stamps R, Massey E, Grainger JD, Provan D, Hill A, et al. The diagnosis and management of primary autoimmune haemolytic anaemia. Br J Haematol. 2017;176(3):395-411.
5. Ladogana S, Maruzzi M, Samperi P, Perrotta S, Del Vecchio GC, Notarangelo LD, et al. Diagnosis and management of newly diagnosed childhood autoimmune haemolytic anaemia. Recommendations from the Red Cell Study Group of the Paediatric Haemato-Oncology Italian Association. Blood Transfus. 2017;15(3):259-67.
6. Sankaran J, Rodriguez V, Jacob EK, Kreuter JD, Go RS. Autoimmune Hemolytic Anemia in Children: Mayo Clinic Experience. J Pediatr Hematol Oncol. 2016;38(3):e120-4.
7. Naithani R, Agrawal N, Mahapatra M, Kumar R, Pati HP, Choudhry VP. Autoimmune hemolytic anemia in children. Pediatr Hematol Oncol. 2007;24(4):309-15.
8. Miano M. How I manage Evans Syndrome and AIHA cases in children. Br J Haematol. 2016;172(4):524-34.
9. Hadjadj J, Aladjidi N, Fernandes H, Leverger G, Magérus-Chatinet A, Mazerolles F, et al; members of the French Reference Center for Pediatric Autoimmune Cytopenia (CEREVANCE). Pediatric Evans syndrome is associated with a high frequency of potentially damaging variants in immune genes. Blood. 2019;134(1):9-21.
10. Heddle NM. Acute paroxysmal cold hemoglobinuria. Transfus Med Rev. 1989;3(3):219-29.

Oncology

CHAPTER 16

Tumor Markers

Julius Xavier Scott, Ajeitha Loganathan

■ INTRODUCTION

Tumor markers are produced either by the neoplastic tissue or the body in response to a neoplasm. Depending on the site of the underlying neoplasm, they may be detectable in blood, cerebrospinal fluid (CSF), serum, urine, pleural or ascitic fluid or in the tumor tissue.[1] These markers are normally expressed in the fetus during various stages of development, but approach reference ranges for specific age groups in the postnatal period. When present, they can assist in establishing a diagnosis, occasionally obviating the need for a histopathological diagnosis. In addition, depending on the underlying diagnosis, they may play a role in predicting the prognosis, assessing the response to therapy and detecting recurrence. However, caution is necessary in the interpretation of results, as the tumor markers may not be specific and may be elevated in various benign disorders.

The most common tumor markers used in children are the following:
- *Alpha-fetoprotein (AFP)* (seen in yolk sac tumors and hepatic tumors, especially hepatoblastoma)
- *Beta fraction of human chorionic gonadotropin (hCG)* (seen in germ cell tumors, especially choriocarcinoma)
- *Serum and urinary catecholamines* (e.g., neuroblastoma).

In this chapter, we review the tumor markers useful in the diagnosis and management of common pediatric malignancies.

■ WHAT IS AN IDEAL TUMOR MARKER?

An ideal tumor marker should demonstrate:
- High specificity to the tumor
- High sensitivity to detect all those who have the malignancy
- Ability to correlate with response to therapy or detect recurrence early.

In addition, the tumor marker levels should, ideally, correlate with the tumor burden and its half-life should be short to allow serial measurements. Not all tumor markers fulfill these criteria.[2]

■ TUMOR MARKERS AND THEIR BIOLOGICAL STRUCTURE

Tumor markers can be categorized based on their molecular make-up and functions as proteins, enzymes, hormones and carbohydrate antigens:[3]

- *Proteins produced by the neoplastic tissue:* They are normally produced in the fetus and decline after birth. They are known as oncofetal proteins, e.g., AFP and carcinoembryonic antigen (CEA).
- *Enzymes:* They are normally produced in the body and elevated in malignancies. Examples include lactate dehydrogenase (LDH), which is elevated in aggressive and rapidly proliferating hematological malignancies (e.g., acute leukemia) and high-grade lymphomas (e.g., Burkitt lymphoma) and neuron-specific enolase seen in neuroblastoma.
- *Hormones:* Examples include beta-hCG, catecholamines and triiodothyronine.
- *Carbohydrate antigens (CA).* These include CA125 and CA19.9.

■ ALPHA-FETOPROTEIN

Alpha-fetoprotein is one of the most clinically significant tumor markers. It is an oncofetal protein normally produced in the liver of the developing fetus and the embryonic yolk sac. It is not specific for tumors of hepatic origin or hepatic disorders and is elevated in yolk sac tumors as well. AFP levels in fetus peak at 14 weeks of gestation and declines gradually to approximately 30,000 ng/mL at term.[4] It remains elevated in infancy and gradually declines to the adult values of 10 ng/mL by 1 year of age. Hence AFP levels need to be interpreted using the age-based nomograms in infancy.[5]

Alpha-fetoprotein levels are sometimes reported to be falsely low due to a process called "hook effect". Hook effect occurs when the very high AFP level in the specimen overpowers the assay leading to low levels. Hence, it is necessary to do AFP assays with serial dilutions of serum when there is a strong suspicion of hepatic malignancy or germ cell tumors despite low AFP levels.[6]

Alpha-fetoprotein from hepatic tumors includes a sub-fraction which binds to lens culinaris hemagglutinin (LCH) detected by immunoassay, whereas AFP from benign hepatic disorders does not.[7] A greater fraction (>25%) of AFP that is nonreactive to concanavalin-A differentiates AFP from yolk sac tumors from hepatic tumors. These tests are, however, not available commercially and have limited use in clinical practice. AFP is elevated in pancreatic, lung and gastrointestinal malignancies in adults.[8] AFP is a negative acute phase reactant following liver dysfunction and toxic insult, and hence typically is not elevated in these conditions.[9]

Table 16.1 lists the common causes of elevated AFP in children.

TABLE 16.1: Causes of elevated AFP in children.[10]

Hepatic tumors	Benign liver disorders	Nonhepatic causes
Malignant: • Hepatoblastoma • Hepatocellular carcinoma • Hepatocellular malignant neoplasm - not otherwise specified (HC-NOS) *Benign*: • Mesenchymal hamartoma • Infantile hemangioma	• Cirrhosis • Drug-induced liver damage • Acute and chronic hepatitis • Biliary obstruction • Tyrosinemia • Citrullinemia	• Non-seminomatous germ cell tumors • Yolk sac tumors (gonadal and extragonadal) • Teratoma (rare) • Sertoli-Leydig cell tumors (rare) • Wilms tumor (very rare) • Colitis • Ataxia telangiectasia • Fanconi anemia

AFP and Hepatic Tumors

Elevated AFP is seen in both hepatoblastoma (HB) and hepatocellular carcinoma (HCC). AFP is elevated in 95–98% of children with HB and 50–70% of children with HCC.[11] HB occurs in infants whereas HCC usually occurs in older children, either de novo or more commonly with an underlying cholestatic or metabolic liver disease. However, AFP levels tend to be higher in HB than HCC (often in tens of thousands to lakhs, i.e., more than 100,000 ng/mL). A hepatic tumor detected in infants with imaging and high AFP levels consistent with HB obviates the need for a biopsy and histological diagnosis.

Alpha-fetoprotein may be normal or low in an unfavorable histological type of HB viz. small cell undifferentiated (SCU) type. SCU variants that fail to express integrase interactor-1 (INI-1) in immunohistochemistry may in fact represent an aggressive malignant rhabdoid tumor.[12] SCU variants being undifferentiated do not produce AFP and low AFP (less than 100 ng/mL) is designated as a poor prognostic factor in the new international stratification called Children's Hepatic tumors International Collaboration—Hepatoblastoma Stratification (CHIC-HS).[13] AFP greater than 1 million ng/mL has been recognized as a prognostic factor in some protocols.[14]

Alpha-fetoprotein is also elevated in "hepatocellular malignant neoplasm-not otherwise specified (HC-NOS)" and benign tumors such as mesenchymal hamartoma or infantile hemangioma.[15,16] These can be differentiated based on the age at presentation and imaging findings, and are finally confirmed with biopsy.

Alpha-fetoprotein levels decline steadily with treatment and may be used as a surrogate marker for response to treatment. However, caution should be made since AFP levels may rise initially during treatment despite contrary evidence of tumor shrinkage by imaging due to tumor lysis. AFP has a half-life of approximately 5.5 days, but it may be longer (about 10 days) in young infants.[17] AFP declines following chemotherapy or surgery and hence needs to be interpreted in this light. In children with unresectable HB, a decline of <2 logs in AFP levels may identify poor responders to chemotherapy who might benefit from a change in therapy protocol.[18] AFP can be used in the follow up of children with HB post-therapy and in remission to detect recurrence even prior to radiological recurrence.

Alpha-fetoprotein and Germ Cell Tumors

Malignant germ cell tumors (GCT) with a yolk sac component (teratoma) or pure endodermal sinus tumor (yolk sac tumor, YST) produce AFP. These tumors may be gonadal or extragonadal. The common locations of extragonadal tumors are sacrococcygeal, mediastinal and intracranial midline areas. Hence in any midline intracranial tumor, AFP and beta-hCG assays should be done to identify a secretory non-seminomatous GCT.[19] These assays can be done in both serum and CSF. Midline intracranial GCT presents with elevated intracranial pressure, nystagmus or isosexual precocious puberty. In patients where biopsy of deep midline brain lesions is deemed to be hazardous, elevated AFP and/or beta-hCG either in serum or CSF may assist in the diagnosis. AFP levels are also of prognostic importance in GCT. AFP is typically increased in YST, but also in embryonal carcinoma and immature teratoma.

The International Germ Cell Consensus Classification (IGCCC) stratifies GCTs based on tumor histology, metastasis, and AFP levels.[20] Based on AFP levels the tumors are classified as follows:
- AFP less than 1000 ng/mL – good prognosis
- AFP between 1000 and 10000 ng/mL – intermediate prognosis
- AFP more than 10000 ng/mL – poor prognosis

As in HB, serial AFP monitoring can be used to assess treatment response as well as for follow up post-therapy to detect recurrence.

Alpha-fetoprotein in Other Disorders

Elevated serum AFP has been rarely reported in children with *Wilms tumor* wherein it declines post-surgery.[21]

Some childhood diseases, e.g., *hereditary tyrosinemia*, are associated with elevated serum AFP. However, AFP levels are significantly lower than in children with HB or GCT.[22] Children with hereditary tyrosinemia type 1 are at great risk of developing HCC but the fact that AFP might be elevated already and might fluctuate hampers its use in early detection of HCC.

Alpha-fetoprotein is also elevated in children with *ataxia telangiectasia* and increases with age. The raised AFP in ataxia telangiectasia is from the liver and the postulated cause is the aberrant transcriptional control of the regulatory proteins necessary for hepatic maturation.[23]

Though serum AFP has been suggested as a rapid screening tool for *Fanconi anemia*, this fact has not been consistently proven in many reports; chromosome breakage studies and/or genetic studies remain the gold standard for Fanconi anemia. The cause of elevated AFP in Fanconi anemia is still elusive.[24]

BETA SUBUNIT OF HUMAN CHORIONIC GONADOTROPIN

Human chorionic gonadotropin (hCG) is a glycoprotein composed of alpha and beta peptide subunits. It is normally synthesized by the syncytiotrophoblasts of the placenta during pregnancy. The alpha subunit shares structural similarity with that of other peptide hormones such as luteinizing hormone (LH), follicle stimulating hormone (FSH) and thyroid stimulating hormone (TSH). It is the beta subunit which is unique and is used in assays. Small amounts of beta-hCG (less than 5 IU/mL) are normally detected in adults. The half-life of beta-hCG is 24–36 hours. Elevated beta-hCG in children with suspected GCT (gonadal or extragonadal) indicates the presence of syncytiotrophoblast as in choriocarcinoma or the syncytiotrophoblast giant cells as in germinoma. Gestational choriocarcinoma is a well-known entity in adults. In children, choriocarcinoma arises in the gonads, mediastinum, retroperitoneum, or brain.[25]

As discussed earlier, like AFP, beta-hCG assay needs to be done in all children with midline tumors. Beta-hCG can also be detected in serum or CSF in children with secretory intracranial GCT rendering biopsy unnecessary.[26] Beta-hCG assay can be used for assessing response to treatment and in follow up. One caveat of estimating beta-hCG is that rising levels of beta-hCG can be seen in iatrogenic hypogonadism either following surgery or medical orchiectomy/oophorectomy because of cross-reactivity with elevated LH.[27]

Another important condition which warrants mention is infantile choriocarcinoma. The affected newborn presents with severe anemia, hepatomegaly and hemorrhagic symptoms. Though this condition is rare, it mandates immediate detection as it constitutes a medical emergency and is potentially curable with chemotherapy. Elevated serum beta-hCG provides a rapid diagnosis for infantile choriocarcinoma.[28] Rarely, liver tumors such as HB produce beta-hCG in the serum leading to isosexual precocious puberty or virilization.[29]

Table 16.2 lists the common causes of elevation of beta-hCG in children and adults.

CLINICAL APPLICATIONS OF AFP AND BETA-hCG ASSAYS IN GCT

Germ cell tumors (GCT) arise from totipotent and pluripotent cells in children. They are histologically diverse and may be gonadal or extragonadal.

TABLE 16.2: Causes of elevated beta-human chorionic gonadotropin (hCG).	
Childhood malignancies	**Adults**
• Choriocarcinoma • Embryonal carcinoma • Dysgerminoma (low levels) • Infantile choriocarcinoma • Benign teratoma (rare)	• Pregnancy • Gestational trophoblastic disease • Choriocarcinoma • Dysgerminoma (low levels) • *Other malignancies*: Hepatic, neuroendocrine, breast, ovarian, pancreatic, cervical and gastric malignancies (rare)

They are broadly classified as seminomatous and non-seminomatous. The term germinoma encompasses "seminoma" and "dysgerminoma"—germinomas of testis and ovary, respectively. AFP and beta-hCG are negative in histologically "pure germinoma" but elevated in germinoma with other types of secretory GCT tissue intermixed. Hence pure germinomas are non-secretory GCTs.

Embryonal carcinoma comprising undifferentiated, totipotent embryonal cells, though rare in children, is a major component of the malignant GCT of the testis and mediastinum in adolescents. Elevated AFP levels are seen in approximately 70% of children with embryonal carcinoma.[30]

Teratoma is the most common GCT in children with sacrococcygeal site being the most common. Serum AFP levels may be high in teratoma with a yolk sac component. Children diagnosed with immature teratoma, and high AFP have a high risk of malignant recurrence.[31]

■ OTHER MARKERS FOR GERM CELL TUMORS

Carbohydrate Antigen 125

Carbohydrate antigen 125 (CA 125) is a glycoprotein expressed in celomic epithelium during embryogenesis. In adults, serum CA 125 is elevated in patients with epithelial ovarian cancers, carcinoma of the endometrium and benign conditions such as pelvic inflammatory disease and endometriosis. The clinical significance of CA 125 in children is limited. A majority of gonadal tumors in children are GCTs and epithelial origin tumors and account for about one-third of gonadal tumors in adolescents. CA 125 may be useful in this population.[32] Elevated serum CA 125 is also observed in children with yolk sac tumor and embryonal carcinoma and it can be used as a prognostic marker.[33]

■ OTHER MARKERS FOR HEPATIC TUMORS

The serum unsaturated vitamin B12-binding protein (transcobalamin I [TC1] or haptocorrin) is raised in the fibrolamellar variant of HCC (arising in the non-cirrhotic liver of older children). As AFP levels are not elevated in this variant of HCC, haptocorrin can be used as a surrogate marker for response to therapy.[34]

Neurotensin, a polypeptide hormone of the nervous system and gastrointestinal tract is also elevated in the fibrolamellar variant of HCC.[35]

ROLE OF CATECHOLAMINES AND THEIR METABOLITES IN NEUROBLASTOMA

Neuroblastoma is the most common intra-abdominal solid tumor of childhood. It is one of the embryonal "small round blue cell" tumors of childhood. Tumor markers in neuroblastoma are used to define disease activity and monitor the response to therapy. Catecholamines and their metabolites are confirmatory markers, whereas serum neuron-specific enolase (NSE) is useful in monitoring the disease activity. LDH and ferritin are used for prognostication.

Neuroblastoma arises from the neural crest cells of sympathetic nervous system. The neural crest cells mature into cells of adrenal medulla and extra-adrenal sympathetic nervous system. The neuronal tumors may be classified as neuroblastoma, ganglioneuroblastoma or ganglioneuroma based on the degree of differentiation.[36]

Neuroblasts differ from the functional neuronal cells in the following ways:
- Malignant transformation leads to defective storage of dopamine in the storage vesicles. On release, the catecholamines are degraded into vanillylmandelic acid (VMA) and homovanillic acid (HVA) which are excreted in urine.
- Lack of the enzyme phenylethanolamine-N-methyltransferase (PNMT) involved in the conversion of norepinephrine to epinephrine leads to the major urinary metabolite excreted as HVA, with some VMA.

Plasma and Urinary Catecholamines

Dopamine and norepinephrine and their metabolites in urine, such as HVA and VMA are used to diagnose and monitor children with neuroblastoma and other neuroendocrine tumors. The synthesis and catabolism of catecholamines is shown in **Figure 16.1**. Norepinephrine and epinephrine are primarily metabolized into VMA. Dopamine is primarily metabolized into HVA. Urinary catecholamine metabolites are elevated in 90–95% of patients with neuroblastoma as detected by high-performance liquid chromatography (HPLC) assays. Urinary VMA and HVA are commonly assayed and have a sensitivity of more than 90% in combination. Normetanephrine and dopamine are the other metabolites used. A combination of normetanephrine with HVA or VMA has up to 100% sensitivity and specificity for neuroblastoma. Serum VMA and HVA are less consistent than the urinary levels. High

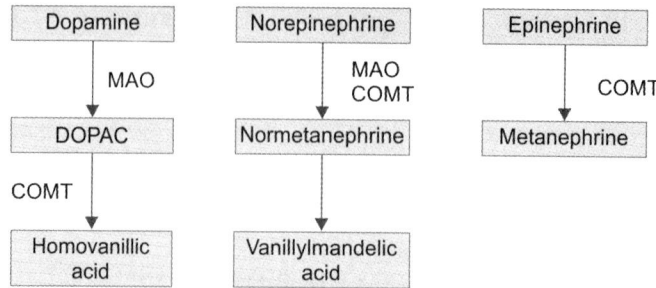

Fig.16.1: Catecholamine catabolism.
(MAO: Monoamine oxidase; COMT: Catechol-O-methyl transferase; DOPAC: Dihydroxyphenylacetic acid)

> **BOX 16.1:** Causes of elevated urine catecholamine metabolites.
> - Duchenne muscular dystrophy
> - Foods (such as fruits and nuts)
> - Drugs
>   - Paracetamol
>   - Theophylline
>   - L-dopa
>   - Chlorpromazine
>   - Sympathomimetics

VMA levels were associated with biologically favorable and high dopamine levels with biologically unfavorable neuroblastoma. For metastatic neuroblastoma of infancy, dopamine/VMA ratio is useful to discriminate between stage 4 and stage 4S.[37]

Mass screening for neuroblastoma of infants by estimation of urinary HVA and VMA with the aim of early detection and intervention, possibly leading to improved outcomes, were initially conducted in the 1980s. In 1985 the Japanese Welfare Ministry initiated a national screening program for neuroblastoma with urinary VMA and HVA. Children with high VMA/HVA levels were further assessed and referred to a regional center when neuroblastoma was detected. Majority of these tumors were biologically favorable and N-MYC non-amplified. N-MYC non-amplified tumors have better outcomes than N-MYC amplified tumors. The final conclusion was that the early identification did not necessarily lead to rapid identification of metastatic disease or disease progression.[38,39] Mass screening for neuroblastoma in infants is less likely to reduce mortality due to neuroblastoma.

Catecholamine metabolites can be elevated falsely in certain disorders and with intake of certain food substances and drugs which are listed in **Box 16.1**.

Traditionally 24-hr urine collections were used due to the diurnal variation of catecholamine metabolite secretion. This is cumbersome and difficult to collect especially in infants. Hence spot urinary measurements expressed as milligrams per gram of creatinine are increasingly being used. The catecholamine metabolites are less sensitive in detecting recurrence and are not used clinically for this purpose.

NEUROSECRETORY PROTEINS

Chromogranin A and neuropeptide-Y (NPY) are peptide markers of neuronal differentiation that have been identified in the serum of patients with neuroblastoma. These are helpful in characterizing differentiation status of neuronal tumors. Chromogranin A is an acidic protein stored and released along with catecholamines from the storage vesicles. In earlier studies, serum chromogranin A was reported as a useful marker with a sensitivity of 91% and specificity of 100% in the diagnosis of neuroblastoma. It was also a prognostic marker with increasing levels correlating with poor outcomes.

Neuropeptide-Y is a 33 amino acid peptide seen in the adrenal medulla and sympathetic nervous system. NPY is also produced by B-cell precursor lymphoblasts. Elevated plasma levels of NPY are seen in pheochromocytoma and ganglioneuroblastoma and appear to correlate with favorable outcomes.

NEURON-SPECIFIC ENOLASE

Enolase is a glycolytic enzyme present in several human tissues. The m-enolase subunit found in neural tissues or tumors is named neuron-specific enolase (NSE). NSE was first demonstrated by immunohistochemistry in tissue specimens and later, in serum of children with neuroblastoma. NSE is a sensitive tumor marker of embryonic tumors of neuroectodermal origin such as neuroblastoma, pheochromocytoma, medullary thyroid carcinoma, pancreatic islet cell carcinoma, and carcinoids.[40,41] Though NSE is sensitive, it is not specific and is also elevated in children with Ewing sarcoma, Wilms tumor and dysgerminoma. NSE can be used to monitor disease activity and treatment response but has not been widely used in clinical practice.

ROLE OF CATECHOLAMINE AND ITS METABOLITES IN CHROMAFFIN TUMORS

Pheochromocytoma and paraganglioma are chromaffin tumors, which arise from the neural crest cells of the adrenal medulla and extra-adrenal tissue respectively. These are catecholamine-secreting cells. Malignancy is seen in about 10% of cases and difficult to define histologically. Children present with features of catecholamine excess such as paroxysmal headaches, palpitations, sweating or persistent hypertension. Diagnosis is based on elevated urinary catecholamines, and their metabolites followed by identification of the tumor by imaging.[42,43] The pattern of metabolite excretion is different from neuroblastoma. Though the VMA may be elevated, the HVA and dopamine levels tend to be within normal limits. More recently, urinary metanephrines are used. Normetanephrine and metanephrine are methylated metabolites of noradrenaline and adrenaline respectively. In physiological state, the metabolites of norepinephrine and epinephrine are excreted as sulphate conjugates. In contrast, chromaffin tumors cannot proceed with sulphate conjugation and their catecholamine metabolites are excreted in the methylated unconjugated form [free normetadrenaline (fNMA) and free metadrenaline (fMA)]. Plasma free metadrenalines also known as free metanephrines are reported as the first choice for excluding or confirming with a high sensitivity of 99%.

■ CARCINOID TUMORS

Carcinoid tumors originate from enterochromaffin cells of the neural crest. These are rare tumors, may be either benign or malignant. The most common site is appendix and can mimic acute appendicitis.[44] Clinical symptoms of carcinoid syndrome such as flushing, diarrhea, and wheezing may not be found unless it has a large tumor mass or is metastatic. The tumor cells produce excess serotonin and histamine resulting in the symptoms of carcinoid syndrome. 5-hydroxyindolacetic acid (5-HIAA), the metabolite of serotonin can be measured in a 24-hour urinary sample for diagnosis of carcinoid.[45]

■ VASOACTIVE INTESTINAL POLYPEPTIDE IN NEUROGENIC TUMORS

Vasoactive intestinal polypeptide (VIP) secreted by some of the neuroblastic tumors cause the secretory symptoms of severe diarrhea, hypokalemia, dehydration and malnutrition. VIP is produced by the differentiated or differentiating cells of ganglioneuroma or ganglioneuroblastoma and, not by the undifferentiated neuroblastoma. In general, VIP-secreting neurogenic tumors have good prognosis.[46]

■ WILMS TUMOR

Wilms tumor is the most common renal tumor in children. The usual presentation is an asymptomatic abdominal mass. The plasma renin and prorenin levels are raised in children with Wilms tumor and result in hypertension.[47] Urinary hyaluronic acid is also elevated in children with Wilms tumor.[48] However, none of these markers are useful clinically.

■ BONE TUMORS

Many tumor markers have been studied in osteosarcoma. These include:
- *Major markers*: Markers of natural immunity, e.g., tumor-associated natural IgM antibodies.

- *Minor markers*: Thyroid hormone, e.g., triiodothyronine.
- *Additional markers*: Bone tumor angiogenesis markers, e.g., angiogenin and vascular endothelial growth factor (VEGF).

However, the lack of sensitivity and specificity is a major issue. Combinations of major, minor and additional markers are being studied as a "gold standard" for monitoring of children with osteosarcoma.[49] Other markers studied include free polyamines, insulin-like growth factor-1 (IGF-1), tumor necrosis factor-beta, bone alkaline phosphatase (ALP) and various chemokines and interleukins.

■ CARCINOEMBRYONIC ANTIGEN

Carcinoembryonic antigen (CEA) is an oncofetal glycoprotein normally expressed by mucosal cells in fetal intestine and liver. It is commonly elevated in adults with colorectal adenocarcinoma. Elevated serum CEA values are seen in children with malignancies such as Wilms tumor, hepatoblastoma and GCT.[50] It is neither sensitive nor specific for any pediatric tumor and its use is limited.

■ HORMONES AS TUMOR MARKERS

Endocrine tumors are rare in childhood. Levels of various hormones are elevated in these tumors because of their production by benign or malignant tumors or due to ectopic hormone production **(Table 16.3)**.[51] Many a times the hormonal production is a para-neoplastic manifestation of the tumor. The presence of endocrine tumors in childhood should alert the pediatrician for underlying genetic syndromes such as multiple endocrine neoplasia, *DICER1* syndrome (caused by mutation in *DICER1* gene which aids in the prevention of tumors), familial adenomatous polyposis, and Li-Fraumeni syndrome.[52,53]

■ OTHER NON-SPECIFIC TUMOR MARKERS

Lactate Dehydrogenase

Lactate dehydrogenase (LDH) is a widely distributed enzyme that converts pyruvate to lactate. LDH is elevated in many childhood malignancies including leukemia, lymphoma, Wilms tumor, hepatoblastoma and neuroblastoma.[54] There are five isoforms of LDH, and each isoenzyme is a tetramer made of two subunits, H and M. An increase in isoforms LDH2 and LDH3 is seen in neuroblastoma. Elevated LDH1 is seen in GCT including YST and germinoma. Though LDH is non-specific, the absolute levels of LDH are found to be prognostic in many tumors such as neuroblastoma and non-Hodgkin lymphomas.[55,56]

TABLE 16.3: Hormonal tumor markers.

Hormonal tumor marker	Tumor	Associated syndromes
Androgens	• Leydig cell tumor (testis) • Sertoli-Leydig cell (ovary) (rarely adrenal adenoma/carcinoma)	• Isosexual precocity in male • Virilization in female
Cortisol/Aldosterone	Adrenal adenoma/carcinoma	Cushing/Conn syndrome
Gastrin	Gastrinoma	Zollinger–Ellison syndrome
Glucagon	Glucagonoma/Carcinoid	Hyperglycemia
Insulin	Insulinoma/Carcinoid	Hypoglycemia
Estrogens	• Granulosa cell tumor (ovary) • Sertoli cell tumor (testis) • Rarely adrenal adenoma/carcinoma	• Isosexual precocity in female • Feminization in male
Parathyroid hormone (PTH)	Parathyroid hyperplasia/adenoma/carcinoma (rarely ectopic production from renal carcinoma/hepatoma)	MEN I and IIa
Prolactin/ACTH/Growth hormone/TSH/ LH/FSH	Secretory adenomas (rarely ectopic production from neuroblastoma, pheochromocytoma, hepatoblastoma)	• Galactorrhea • Cushing syndrome • Gigantism • Hyperthyroidism • Precocious puberty
Renin	Wilms tumor	Hypertension
T3/T4 (thyroxine)	Thyroid adenoma/carcinoma	Hyperthyroidism
Thyrocalcitonin	Medullary thyroid carcinoma (C-cell)	MEN IIa and IIb
Vasoactive intestinal peptide (VIP)	VIPoma	Watery diarrhea, hypokalemia

Ferritin

Ferritin is a protein for iron storage. It is an acute phase reactant and elevated in inflammation and infections. Ferritin is elevated in neuroblastoma and hematological malignancies.[57] Increased levels of ferritin seen in neuroblastoma normalize with disease remission. Ferritin is also used as a prognostic tumor marker in neuroblastoma with high levels correlating with poor disease outcomes.[55]

Creatinine Kinase

Creatinine kinase (CK) catalyzes the conversion of adenosine triphosphate to adenosine diphosphate. CK has three isoforms—CK-BB, CK-MB and

CK-MM. The CK-BB isozyme levels are elevated in neuroblastoma. CK-BB also has prognostic importance with levels greater than 15 ng/mL correlating with poor prognosis in a study.[58]

Alkaline Phosphatase

Alkaline phosphatase (ALP) is derived from the cell membrane of osteoblasts. It was evaluated as a marker of osteosarcoma. However, ALP may be elevated in children due to variations in age, healing fractures and liver disorders. Hence it has limited clinical use as a tumor marker. ALP was a prognostic marker in a meta-analysis of published data on osteosarcoma.[59]

■ CONCLUSION

Population-based screening of children for malignancy with tumor markers is not appropriate. Elevations in tumor markers need to be evaluated with the clinical context to distinguish malignancy from non-malignant conditions. Most used and clinically important tumor markers are AFP, beta-hCG and urinary catecholamines, useful in diagnosis and prognosis of certain pediatric malignancies such as GCT, hepatoblastoma and neuroblastoma. The progress toward early diagnosis, therapy, and favorable outcomes in children with malignancies depends on the precise diagnosis and targeted therapy, for which the tumor markers might be potentially useful.

■ KEY POINTS

- Tumor markers play an important role in the diagnosis, prognosis and follow up of malignancies in children.
- The most important clinically relevant tumor markers used in children are different from those used in adults. These important tumor markers in children include AFP, beta-hCG and urinary catecholamines.
- The other important tumor markers are hormones which are elevated in endocrine tumors or as a part of para-neoplastic manifestations of tumors.
- Tumor markers are not recommended as a population-based screening tool to diagnose malignancies in children.
- Many of the markers are not tumor-specific and can be elevated physiologically, in benign conditions or in other malignancies. Hence, interpretation of the reports of tumor markers warrants caution and detailed evaluation.

■ REFERENCES

1. Diamandis EP. Tumor Markers: Past, Present, and Future. In: Diamandis EP, Fritsche HA, Lilja H, Chan DW, Schwartz ML (Eds). Tumor Markers: Physiology, Pathobiology, Technology, and Clinical Applications. Washington DC: AACC Press; 2002. pp.1.
2. Sharma S. Tumor markers in clinical practice: general principles and guidelines. Indian J Med Paediatr Oncol. 2009;30(1):1-8.

3. Rustin GJ, van der Burg ME, Berek JS. Advanced ovarian cancer. Tumour markers. Ann Oncol. 1993;4 (Suppl):S71-7.
4. Lahdenne P, Kuusela P, Siimes MA, Rönnholm AK, Salmenperä L, Heikinheimo M. Biphasic reduction and concanavalin A binding properties of serum alpha-fetoprotein in preterm and term infants. J Pediatr. 1991;118(2):272-6.
5. Ferraro S, Panzeri A, Braga F, Panteghini M. Serum α-fetoprotein in pediatric oncology: not a children's tale. Clin Chem Lab Med. 2019;57(6):783-97.
6. Jassam N, Jones CM, Briscoe T, Horner JH. The hook effect: a need for constant vigilance. Ann Clin Biochem. 2006;43(Pt 4):314-7.
7. Johnson PJ, Poon TC, Hjelm NM, Ho CS, Blake C, Ho SK. Structures of disease-specific serum alpha-fetoprotein isoforms. Br J Cancer. 2000;83(10):1330-7.
8. Spear BT. Alpha-Fetoprotein. In: Maloy S, Hughes K (Eds.). Brenner's Encyclopedia of Genetics (Second edition). Gurugram, India: Elsevier; 2013. pp. 89-91.
9. Mizejewski GJ. Alpha-fetoprotein (AFP) and inflammation: Is AFP an acute and/or chronic phase reactant? J Hematol Thrombo Dis. 2015;3:1.
10. Van Houwelingen L, Sandoval JA. Alpha-fetoprotein in malignant pediatric conditions. In: Saxena SK (Ed). Proof and concepts in rapid diagnostic tests and technologies. New York: Intechopen; 2016.
11. Sergi CM. Carcinoma of the liver in children and adolescents. In: Sergi CM (Ed). Liver Cancer (internet). Brisbane: Exon Publications; 2021. pp. 1-38.
12. Trobaugh-Lotrario AD, Tomlinson GE, Finegold MJ, Gore L, Feusner JH. Small cell undifferentiated variant of hepatoblastoma: adverse clinical and molecular features similar to rhabdoid tumors. Pediatr Blood Cancer. 2009;52(3):328-34.
13. Meyers RL, Maibach R, Hiyama E, Häberle B, Krailo M, Rangaswami A, et al. Risk-stratified staging in paediatric hepatoblastoma: a unified analysis from the Children's Hepatic tumors International Collaboration. Lancet Oncol. 2017;18(1):122-31.
14. Fuchs J, Rydzynski J, Von Schweinitz D, Bode U, Hecker H, Weinel P, et al. Pretreatment prognostic factors and treatment results in children with hepatoblastoma: a report from the German Cooperative Pediatric Liver Tumor Study HB 94. Cancer. 2002;95(1):172-82.
15. Arrunategui AM, Caicedo LA, Thomas LS, Botero V, García O, Carrascal E, et al. Giant mesenchymal hamartoma in pediatric patients: A new indication for liver transplantation. J Pediatr Surg Case Rep. 2017;21:1-3.
16. Itinteang T, Chibnall AM, Marsh R, Dunne JC, de Jong S, Davis PF, et al. Elevated serum levels of alpha-fetoprotein in patients with infantile hemangioma are not derived from within the tumor. Front Surg. 2016;3:5.
17. Wu JT, Book L, Sudar K. Serum alpha fetoprotein (AFP) levels in normal infants. Pediatr Res. 1981;15(1):50-2.
18. Van Tornout JM, Buckley JD, Quinn JJ, Feusner JH, Krailo MD, King DR, et al. Timing and magnitude of decline in alpha-fetoprotein levels in treated children with unresectable or metastatic hepatoblastoma are predictors of outcome: a report from the Children's Cancer Group. J Clin Oncol. 1997;15(3):1190-7.
19. Dieckmann K-P, Simonsen-Richter H, Kulejewski M, Anheuser P, Zecha H, Isbarn H, et al. Serum tumour markers in testicular germ cell tumours:

frequencies of elevated levels and extents of marker elevation are significantly associated with clinical parameters and with response to treatment. BioMed Res Int. 2019:5030349.
20. Mead GM, Stenning SP, Cook P, Fossa SD, Horwich A, Kaye SB, et al. International Germ Cell Consensus classification: a prognostic factor-erased staging system for metastatic germ cell cancers. J Clin Oncol. 1997;15(2):594-603.
21. Dhungel S, Cheng LJ, Hai ZZ. Elevated serum alpha-fetoprotein in Wilms' tumor: a case report with review of literature. J Pediatr Surg Case Rep. 2014;2(3):153-5.
22. Chinsky JM, Singh R, Ficicioglu C, van Karnebeek CD, Grompe M, Mitchell G, et al. Diagnosis and treatment of tyrosinemia type I: a US and Canadian consensus group review and recommendations. Genet Med. 2017;19(12):101.
23. Ishiguro T, Taketa K, Gatti RA. Tissue of origin of elevated alpha-fetoprotein in ataxia-telangiectasia. Dis Mark. 1986;4(4):293-7.
24. Alter BP, Giri N. Serum alpha fetoprotein levels in Fanconi anaemia. Br J Haematol. 2019;184(6):1074-6.
25. Betz D, Fane K. Human Chorionic Gonadotropin. Florida: StatPearls [Internet]; 2020.
26. Hu M, Guan H, Lau CC, Terashima K, Jin Z, Cui L, et al. An update on the clinical diagnostic value of β-hCG and αFP for intracranial germ cell tumors. Eur J Med Res. 2016;21:10.
27. Porakishvili N, Jackson AM, de Souza JB, Chiesa MD, Roitt IM, Delves PJ, et al. Epitopes of human chorionic gonadotropin and their relationship to immunogenicity and cross-reactivity of β-chain mutants. Am J Reprod Immunol. 1998;40(3):210-4.
28. Alsharif S, Karsou A. Infantile choriocarcinoma of the liver: Case report and review of the literature. Oncol Cancer Case Rep. 2017;3(124):2.
29. Al-Jumaily U, Sammour I, Al-Muhaisen F, Ajlouni F, Sultan I. Precocious puberty in an infant with hepatoblastoma: a case report. J Med Case Rep. 2011;5(1):1-4.
30. Aldrink JH, Glick RD, Baertschiger RM, Kulaylat AN, Lautz TB, Christison-Lagay, et al. Update on pediatric testicular germ cell tumors. J Pediat Surg. 2021;S0022-3468(21)00295-5.
31. van Heurn LJ, Knipscheer MM, Derikx JP, van Heurn LW. Diagnostic accuracy of serum alpha-fetoprotein levels in diagnosing recurrent sacrococcygeal teratoma: A systematic review. J Pediatr Surg. 2020;55(9):1732-9.
32. Taskinen S, Fagerholm R, Lohi J, Taskinen M. Pediatric ovarian neoplastic tumors: incidence, age at presentation, tumor markers and outcome. Acta Obstet Gynecol Scand. 2015;94(4):425-9.
33. Kim JH, Park JY, Kim JH, Kim YM, Kim YT, Nam JH. The role of preoperative serum cancer antigen 125 in malignant ovarian germ cell tumors. Taiwan J Obstet Gynecol. 2018;57(2):236-40.
34. Lildballe DL, Nguyen KQ, Poulsen SS, Nielsen HO, Nexo E. Haptocorrin as marker of disease progression in fibrolamellar hepatocellular carcinoma. Eur J Surg Oncol. 2011;37(1):72-9.
35. Collier NA, Weinbren K, Bloom SR, Lee YC, Hodgson HJ, Blumgart LH. Neurotensin secretion by fibrolamellar carcinoma of the liver. Lancet. 1984;1(8376):538-40.
36. Sharma R, Mer J, Lion A, Vik TA. Clinical presentation, evaluation, and management of neuroblastoma. Pediatr Rev. 2018;39(4):194-203.

37. Strenger V, Kerbl R, Dornbusch HJ, Ladenstein R, Ambros PF, Ambros IM, et al. Diagnostic and prognostic impact of urinary catecholamines in neuroblastoma patients. Pediatr Blood Cancer. 2007;48(5):504-9.
38. Sawada T. Past and future of neuroblastoma screening in Japan. Am J Pediatr Hematol Oncol. 1992;14(4):320-6.
39. Hsiao RJ, Seeger RC, Yu AL, O'Connor DT. Chromogranin A in children with neuroblastoma. Serum concentration parallels disease stage and predicts survival. J Clin Invest. 1990;85(5):1555-9.
40. Galli S, Naranjo A, Van Ryn C, Tilan JU, Trinh E, Yang C, et al. Neuropeptide Y as a biomarker and therapeutic target for neuroblastoma. Am J Pathol. 2016;186(11):3040-53.
41. Isgrò MA, Bottoni P, Scatena R. Neuron-specific enolase as a biomarker: Biochemical and clinical aspects. Adv Exp Med Biol. 2015;867:125-43.
42. Bholah R, Bunchman TE. Review of pediatric pheochromocytoma and paraganglioma. Front Pediatr. 2017;5:155.
43. Lenders JW, Pacak K, Walther MM, Linehan WM, Mannelli M, Friberg P, et al. Biochemical diagnosis of pheochromocytoma: which test is best? JAMA. 2002;287(11):1427-34.
44. Spunt SL, Pratt CB, Rao BN, Pritchard M, Jenkins JJ, Hill DA, et al. Childhood carcinoid tumors: the St Jude Children's Research Hospital experience. J Pediatr Surg. 2000;35(9):1282-6.
45. Doede T, Foss HD, Waldschmidt J. Carcinoid tumors of the appendix in children-epidemiology, clinical aspects and procedure. Eur J Pediatr Surg. 2000;10(06):372-7.
46. Yeh PJ, Chen SH, Lai JY, Lai MW, Chiu CH, Chao HC, et al. Rare cases of pediatric vasoactive intestinal peptide secreting tumor with literature review: a challenging etiology of chronic diarrhea. Front Pediatr. 2020;8.430.
47. Maas MH, Cransberg K, van Grotel M, Pieters R, van den Heuvel-Eibrink MM. Renin-induced hypertension in Wilms tumor patients. Pediatr Blood Cancer. 2007;48(5):500-3.
48. Longaker MT, Adzick NS, Sadigh D, Hendin B, Stair SE, Duncan BW, et al. Hyaluronic acid-stimulating activity in the pathophysiology of Wilms' tumors. J Natl Cancer Inst. 1990;82(2):135-9.
49. Savitskaya YA, Rico-Martínez G, Linares-González LM, Delgado-Cedillo EA, Téllez-Gastelum R, Alfaro-Rodríguez AB, et al. Serum tumor markers in pediatric osteosarcoma: a summary review. Clin Sarcoma Res. 2012;2(1):1-9.
50. Mann JR, Lakin GE, Leonard JC, Rawlinson HA, Richardson SG, Corkery JJ, et al. Clinical applications of serum carcinoembryonic antigen and alpha-fetoprotein levels in children with solid tumours. Arch Dis Child. 1978;53(5):366-74.
51. Sun Q, Zhao Z. Peptide hormones as tumor markers in clinical practice. Enzymes. 2017;42:65-79.
52. Anik A, Abaci A. Endocrine cancer syndromes: an update. Minerva Pediatr. 2014;66(6):533-47.
53. Millar S, Bradley L, Donnelly DE, Carson D, Morrison PJ. Familial pediatric endocrine tumors. Oncologist. 2011;16(10):1388-96.

54. Al-Saadoon EA, Al-Naama LM, Hassan JK. Serum lactate dehydrogenase (LDH) activity in children with malignant diseases. Bahrain Med Bull. 2003;25(2):1-7.
55. Moroz V, Machin D, Hero B, Ladenstein R, Berthold F, Kao P, et al. The prognostic strength of serum LDH and serum ferritin in children with neuroblastoma: a report from the International Neuroblastoma Risk Group (INRG) project. Pediatr Blood Cancer. 2020;67(8):e28359.
56. Cairo M, Auperin A, Perkins SL, Pinkerton R, Harrison L, Goldman S, et al. Overall survival of children and adolescents with mature B cell non-Hodgkin lymphoma who had refractory or relapsed disease during or after treatment with FAB/LMB 96: a report from the FAB/LMB 96 study group. Br J Haematol. 2018;182(6):859-69.
57. Wang F, Lv H, Zhao B, Zhou L, Wang S, Luo J, et al. Iron and leukemia: new insights for future treatments. J Exp Clin Cancer Res. 2019;38(1):406.
58. Ishiguro Y, Kato K, Akatsuka H, Ito T. The diagnostic and prognostic value of pretreatment serum creatine kinase BB levels in patients with neuroblastoma. Cancer. 1990;65(9):2014-9.
59. Ren HY, Sun LL, Li HY, Ye ZM. Prognostic significance of serum alkaline phosphatase level in osteosarcoma: a meta-analysis of published data. BioMed Res Int. 2015;2015:160835.

Rheumatology

Biologicals and Other Targeted Therapies in Rheumatology

Jagatshreya Satapathy, Narendra Bagri

■ INTRODUCTION

Pediatric rheumatic disorders are characterized by periods of remissions and exacerbations and if unchecked, the inflammation leads to significant morbidity and mortality. Traditionally, conventional disease-modifying anti-rheumatic drugs (DMARDs) and steroids form the sheet anchor for managing these disorders. However, the limited efficacy of the conventional DMARDs and steroid toxicity are the commonly encountered challenges while caring for these patients. To overcome these limitations, during the last few decades, the therapeutic armamentarium for the management of pediatric rheumatic disorders has expanded with the addition of various biological agents. *Biologics* are proteinaceous molecules produced from biologic processes and include monoclonal antibodies, receptor antagonists and other agents engineered to target specific molecules on the cell surface or inflammatory pathways. As per the nomenclature system for these agents, the monoclonal antibodies end with "mab" (*source identifier:* u = human, e.g., adalim*u*mab; zu = humanized, e.g., tocili*zu*mab; and xi = chimeric e.g., ritu*xi*mab), while all receptors end in "cept" (e.g., etanercept and abatacept). **Table 17.1** summarizes the list of various biological agents that are commonly used in pediatric rheumatology practice.

With the availability of various biological agents, clinical remission is becoming a reality in an increasing number of rheumatic disorders. While being effective, these agents also pose a significant risk of infections, particularly tuberculosis in Indian settings and should be used judiciously. This chapter shall focus on the latest updates on various classes of biologics, their mechanism of action, prerequisites, monitoring, and adverse effects.

■ TUMOR NECROSIS FACTOR INHIBITORS

Tumor necrosis factor-alpha (TNF-α) is an inflammatory cytokine that is involved in the pathogenesis of juvenile idiopathic arthritis (JIA). It acts by binding to receptors on cell surface TNF receptors (TNFR), leading to downstream production of transcription factors such as activation protein-1

TABLE 17.1: Commonly used biologics in pediatric rheumatology.

Biologic	Route	Dose	Indications	Adverse effects	Laboratory monitoring
Etanercept	SC	0.8 mg/kg q wk or 0.4 mg/kg twice weekly	Polyarticular JIA, ERA, PsA	TB, other infections, demyelinating disease	CBC, ALT, AST q 2–3 months
Adalimumab	SC	15–30 kg: 20 mg q 2 wk > 30 kg: 40 mg q 2 wk	JIA, uveitis, Behçet's disease, PsA	TB, other infections, demyelinating disease	CBC, ALT, AST q 2–3 months
Infliximab	IV	6–10 mg/kg q 2 wk–2 mo Refractory KD: 5 mg/kg single infusion	JIA, KD, sarcoidosis, uveitis, PsA	Infusion reactions, TB, other infections, MS	CBC, ALT, AST q 2–3 months
Rituximab	IV	Polyarticular JIA: 375–500 mg/m² q 2 wk × 2 doses AAV: Induction: 375 mg/m²/wk × 4 wk, or 2 fixed doses 500 mg/m² (max 1 g) administered 2 weeks apart Maintenance: 500 mg 6-monthly (adult data)	Polyarticular JIA, AAV, SLE, JDM	Infusion reactions, hypogammaglobulinemia, PML	• CBC, AST, ALT q 2–3 months • B cell number at baseline and 1 month later • Ig levels at baseline, followed by every 6–12 months
Tocilizumab	IV	SJIA <30 kg: 12 mg/kg q 2 wk ≥30 kg: 8 mg/kg q 2 wk Polyarticular JIA <30 kg: 10 mg/kg q 2 wk >30 kg: 8 mg/kg q 2 wk	SJIA, polyarticular JIA	Infection, TB, malignancy, hypersensitivity, gastrointestinal perforation, anaphylaxis	• CBC (for neutropenia and thrombocytopenia), AST, ALT q 2–3 months • Lipid profile at 4–8 weeks, then every 6–12 weeks
	SC	162 mg ≥30 kg: once every 2 wk ≤30 kg: once every wk			
Abatacept	IV	10 mg/kg q 2 wk × 3 doses, then q 4 wk	JIA	Injection site reactions, infections	CBC, ALT, AST q 2–3 months

(AAV: ANCA-associated vasculitis; ALT: alanine aminotransferase; APLA: Anti-phospholipid antibody; AST: aspartate aminotransferase; BD: twice daily; CBC: complete blood count; ERA: enthesitis-related arthritis; IV: intravenous; JDM: juvenile dermatomyositis; JIA: Juvenile idiopathic arthritis; KD: Kawasaki disease; kg: kilogram; mg: milligram; mo: month; MS: multiple sclerosis; PML: progressive multifocal leukoencephalopathy; PsA: Psoriatic arthritis; SC: subcutaneous; SJIA: systemic JIA; SLE: systemic lupus erythematosus; SSc: Systemic sclerosis; TB: tuberculosis; wk: week)

(AP-1) and nuclear factor kappa B (NF-κB).[1] This causes inflammation in the joints by the recruitment and activation of monocytes, macrophages, and resident fibroblasts. To limit such harmful effects of TNF-α, its receptors are thrown off the cell surface into the plasma. This constitutes the fraction of soluble TNFRs that helps in the prevention of interaction between TNF-α and its receptors. Hence, the use of drugs that antagonize the actions of TNF-α, either by binding to circulating TNF-α molecules, or by binding to receptors on the cell membrane have proved to be useful in TNF-α-mediated diseases such as polyarticular JIA, inflammatory bowel disease, psoriasis, and seronegative spondyloarthropathy. TNF-α inhibitors approved for pediatric use include infliximab, adalimumab, golimumab, certolizumab, and etanercept.

TNF-α inhibitors are the most widely used biologics in pediatric population. Hence, being aware of their potential adverse effects is important. Patients have a significantly high risk of reactivation of latent tuberculosis while being on therapy with anti-TNF agents *(vide infra)*. There is also an increased risk of systemic infections (bacterial and viral), upper respiratory tract infections, and injection-site reactions (mostly mild) in these patients.[2] These children should be fully vaccinated as per the national schedule, including against varicella, prior to initiation of these drugs.

Etanercept

Etanercept is a completely human, dimeric protein consisting of the extracellular portion of the human TNFR and Fc region of IgG1 being fused together. Soluble TNF-α (sTNF-α), transmembrane TNF-α as well as lymphotoxin are inactivated by etanercept. Inactivation of predominantly sTNF-α and prevention of interaction between it and its receptor, are the reasons behind its effectiveness in chronic inflammatory disorders. Additionally, T-cell activation, dendritic cell functions, and neutrophil migration too are altered, thus influencing the attenuation of production of cytokines and chemokines. It is slowly absorbed and eliminated by the metabolism of the formed TNF-α-etanercept complexes.

It was one of the very first biologics to be approved by the Food and Drug Administration (FDA) for use in children with JIA. Etanercept may be used in children above 2 years of age with polyarticular JIA, enthesitis-related arthritis, and psoriatic arthritis who demonstrate inadequate response to a 12-week trial of NSAIDs and methotrexate.[3] However, it is not indicated in uveitis associated with JIA. Its half-life is around 4 days.

In pediatric patients, the clearance of etanercept is influenced by the body surface area and its volume of distribution is governed by the patient's body weight, unlike in adults. It is administered subcutaneous (SC) at a dose of 0.4 mg/kg twice a week or 0.8 mg/kg once a week (maximum dose 50 mg).

Clinical response to etanercept is usually observed after three to four doses. Methotrexate is usually administered concomitantly with etanercept in order to improve and sustain its efficacy by preventing the development of antibodies against etanercept (human antichimeric antibodies, HACAs). Hemogram and liver function tests (LFT) should be monitored every 3-4 months while on anti-TNF agents.

Various cases of patients developing antinuclear antibodies (ANA), anticardiolipin antibodies (aCL) and anti-dsDNA antibodies after initiation of etanercept have been published.[3] However, only a few of these patients developed overt systemic lupus erythematosus (SLE) or SLE-like illness. Discontinuation of the drug usually leads to subsidence of the symptoms. Occasionally, treatment with steroids may be necessary. Current guidelines do not mention any need of documenting a patient's baseline antibodies prior to and during treatment with etanercept.[3]

Infliximab

Infliximab is a chimeric anti-TNF-α antibody made by amalgamation of the mouse Fab' fragment with the constant region of human IgG1. It is administered as an intravenous (IV) infusion and is recommended for use in polyarticular JIA, refractory Kawasaki disease (KD) and granulomatous disorders such as sarcoidosis.[4]

The usual starting dose for JIA is 6 mg/kg/infusion over 2 hours on weeks 0, 2, and 6. The subsequent doses are administered every 4-8 weekly and the dose may be escalated up to 10 mg/kg depending on clinical response.[5] To prevent the development of anti-infliximab antibodies, methotrexate is usually given with infliximab. It is administered intravenously (IV) at a dose of 5 mg/kg over 2 hours for refractory KD. In a study on the use of infliximab in the primary treatment of KD, it was concluded that it decreased the duration of fever, erythrocyte sedimentation rate (ESR), and coronary artery Z-scores, though the development of treatment resistance was unaltered.[6]

Like etanercept, infections are the most important concern with use of infliximab. Reactivation of latent tuberculosis is more likely with infliximab than with etanercept.[7] Infusion reactions can range from mild allergic reactions to severe, life-threatening events such as hypotension and shock. To reduce the occurrence of such infusion reactions, the infusion is started at a slow rate and doubled every 15-30 minutes, if tolerated. Premedication with an antihistaminic and paracetamol is advocated before infusion. Infliximab should be discontinued in case of allergic reactions. Response may be expected after third or fourth infusion. Complete blood counts, LFT, and serum albumin need to be monitored every 3-4 months in children undergoing infliximab therapy.

Adalimumab

Adalimumab is a human monoclonal antibody against TNF-α. It neutralizes both cell surface-bound and soluble TNF-α. The major use of adalimumab is in polyarticular JIA, enthesitis-related arthritis, and noninfectious uveitis in JIA and Behçet's disease.[8]

It is administered subcutaneously (SC) at a fixed dose of 10 mg every 2 weeks for children weighing 10–15 kg, 20 mg every 2 weeks in children between 15 and 30 kg and 40 mg every 2 weeks in children weighing ≥30 kg. Coadministration of methotrexate reduces the formation of antiadalimumab antibodies (which may reduce the trough levels of the drug) and thus, should be considered while using adalimumab. At the authors' center, conventional DMARDs are usually coadministered with biological agents.[9,10] Adverse effects consist of mild injection site reactions and a heightened risk of infections. Monitoring includes hemogram and LFT, including serum albumin every 3–4 months.

Golimumab

Golimumab is an IgG antibody against TNF-α produced by recombinant DNA technology. It is used at a dose of 30 mg/m^2 SC once a month, maximum dose being 50 mg.

Certolizumab Pegol

It is the Fab segment of a monoclonal antibody against TNF-α. Pegylation increases its half-life. The doses are 50 mg for patients between 10 and 20 kg, 100 mg for 20–40 kg, and 200 mg for children weighing >40 kg to be administered SC every fortnight. It is usually very well tolerated; upper respiratory tract infections and infections of urinary tract are amongst the most frequent infections with certolizumab therapy.

Considerations with use of TNF-α Inhibitors

Anti-TNF Therapy and Tuberculosis

As TNF-α is involved in the initial and long-term control of tuberculosis, its blockade makes the patient vulnerable to development of tuberculosis, mostly due to reactivation of latent tuberculosis. Therefore, a thorough evaluation to rule out active or latent tuberculosis must be undertaken prior to the initiation of TNF-α inhibitors. A baseline chest radiograph and tuberculin skin test (TST) and/or interferon gamma release assay (IGRA), such as QuantiFERON TB Gold (QFT) or T.SPOT TB test are used to rule out latent tuberculosis.[11] Unlike IGRA, the TST results have been shown to be negatively influenced by immunosuppressive medications and Bacillus Calmette–Guérin (BCG) vaccination.[12] With the availability of commercial tests for IGRA, we suggest using IGRA alone or in combination with TST for diagnosis of latent tuberculosis wherever feasible. To rationalize the cost constraints and availability of IGRA, TST may be performed as the first test and IGRA may be ordered for a negative TST. In this context, it is important to note that initiation of anti-TNF therapy based on a negative TST

Flowchart 17.1: Algorithm showing screening of latent tuberculosis while initiating anti-TNF therapy.

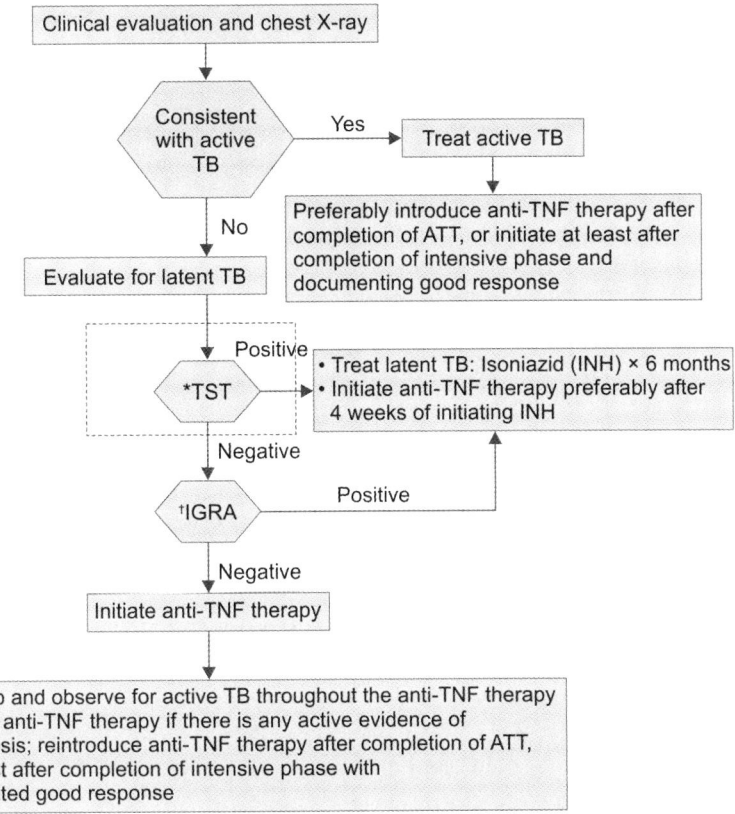

(ATT: antituberculous therapy; IGRA: interferon gamma release assay; TB: tuberculosis; TNF: tumor necrosis factor; TST: tuberculin skin test)
*TST: TST is considered positive in presence of >10 mm induration within 48–72 hours of intradermal administration of 0.1 mL (5 TU).
†IGRA: Interferon-gamma release assay (IGRA) is less influenced by previous BCG status and immunosuppressive drugs and hence is a better screening test for latent tuberculosis.
Inset (dashed box) represents skipping TST and considering IGRA upfront, wherever feasible. However, as IGRA tests are cost prohibitive, we suggest stepwise use of TST and IGRA. Negative TST and normal chest X-ray along with a close follow-up may also be an acceptable approach in resource-poor settings.

and normal chest X-ray along with a close follow-up, may also be an acceptable approach in resource-poor settings. The positivity of either test should be considered as an indicator of latent tuberculosis and warrants prophylaxis with isoniazid **(Flowchart 17.1)**. In such cases, anti-TNF agents should be preferably initiated after 4 weeks of isoniazid prophylaxis. Nevertheless, some clinicians begin simultaneous etanercept and isoniazid therapy too.[11]

All patients on anti-TNF agents should also be carefully monitored for the development of active tuberculosis during therapy. The development of active tuberculosis warrants discontinuation of anti-TNF and initiation of antituberculous therapy (ATT). Anti-TNF therapy may be restarted after 2 months of intensive ATT after documenting good therapeutic response.[11]

TNF-α Inhibitor and Malignancies

Patients with inflammatory conditions such as JIA, SLE, and psoriatic arthritis are inherently predisposed to a higher risk of malignancies due to the presence of an inflammatory milieu. While in the past, concerns had been raised about the possibility of such malignancies arising due to the use of TNF-α inhibitors *per se,* recent evidence suggests that such patients have no increased risk of development of malignancies such as lymphoma with long-term exposure to these agents. But patients with a history of malignancies did carry an increased risk of a future new or recurring malignancy.[13]

TNF-α Inhibitor and Demyelination

Iatrogenic demyelination is being reported more often with an increase in the ambit of use of TNF-α inhibitors. A possible explanation of this phenomenon is due to the blockade of TNF-type 2 receptor (TNFR2), which is abundantly expressed in central nervous system (CNS) and has a role in promoting myelination and cell survival and decreasing inflammation. Almost one-third of demyelination progresses to full-blown cases of multiple sclerosis. Fortunately, a complete or partial response is seen in most of these patients with discontinuation of the offending agent and use of steroids or other immunomodulators.[14] In children with previously diagnosed history or family history of demyelinating disorders or multiple sclerosis, it is advisable to avoid the use of anti-TNFs.[14] A baseline magnetic resonance imaging (MRI) would be helpful in identifying hitherto undiagnosed, silent demyelination in those with a history of familial occurrence of multiple sclerosis or demyelinating disorders.[14]

■ INTERLEUKIN-6 INHIBITORS

In autoinflammatory diseases such as systemic-onset JIA (SJIA), activation of inflammatory cells such as phagocytes leads to formation of inflammatory cytokines such as interleukin-6 (IL-6). Serum levels of IL-6 correlate with fever spikes, thrombocytosis, and arthritis in SJIA. Inhibition of IL-6-mediated inflammatory pathway through IL-6 inhibitors such as tocilizumab offers therapeutic benefits in many rheumatic disorders such as SJIA.

Tocilizumab

Tocilizumab is a humanized monoclonal antibody against soluble fraction of IL-6 receptors, which is produced by attaching the complementarity-determining region of mouse anti-human IL-6 receptor antibody to human IgG1. It can attach to soluble as well as cell membrane-bound IL-6 receptor.

Dosages vary according to weight and disease. For children with polyarticular JIA, it is given at a dose of 10 mg/kg and 8 mg/kg for patients weighing less than and above 30 kg, respectively. In SJIA, the dosage for patients <30 kg is 12 mg/kg, while the dose remains at 8 mg/kg for children above 30 kg.

Tocilizumab has been found to be highly effective in inducing remission in patients with refractory SJIA.[15,16] It has also shown its efficacy in inducing and maintaining long-term remission with a good safety profile in methotrexate-resistant polyarticular JIA. Additionally, tocilizumab rapidly improves ocular parameters in children with uveitis associated with JIA, which was resistant to conventional immunosuppressants and other biologics.[17]

Though large-scale, randomized studies on its use in Takayasu arteritis are lacking, small case series do suggest that tocilizumab may be effective in those who fail to demonstrate adequate improvement with initial immunosuppressive agents.[18] Desirable effects of tocilizumab used off label in other rheumatological conditions in children such as SLE, juvenile dermatomyositis (JDM), KD, scleroderma, and TNF receptor associated periodic syndrome (TRAPS) have been reported in small case series and reports, thus highlighting the untapped potential it carries and scope of future research.[19]

Despite the initial enthusiasm of its benefits in suppressing the hyperinflammatory state in COVID-19, due to the lack of benefits demonstrated in randomized controlled trials in adults and long-lasting immunosuppressive effect of tocilizumab, the American College of Rheumatology (ACR) does not favor the use of tocilizumab in hyperinflammatory syndrome secondary to COVID-19.[20]

Neutropenia, transaminitis, and increased risk of infections are the commonly observed adverse effects. Serious adverse events warranting cessation of therapy include anaphylactic reactions. Gastrointestinal hemorrhage has also been occasionally reported and it should be used cautiously in patients with history of diverticulitis or intestinal ulceration.

Recently, in 2018, the SC formulation of tocilizumab was approved by the FDA for polyarticular JIA and SJIA in patients between 2 and 17 years. Pharmacokinetics and pharmacodynamics of this route are comparable to the IV route in efficacy and adverse effects. The only new adverse effect noted was injection site reactions, consistent with SC route of administration, while the infection rates and formation of anti-tocilizumab antibodies remained the same.[21]

Clazakizumab and sarilumab are few of other anti-IL-6 monoclonal antibodies that are under study for potential use in children suffering from JIA.

■ INTERLEUKIN-1 INHIBITORS

The proinflammatory cytokine, IL-1, has been well documented in the causation of SJIA and many other autoinflammatory entities. In the inflammatory milieu of these disorders, high levels of ILs-1, 6, 18, and S-100 proteins are found, thus providing us an exciting target in the treatment of diseases and monitoring of therapeutic efficacy of these drugs.[22] IL-1 also leads to joint destruction by stimulating chondrocytes and synovial cells to produce other inflammatory molecules such as prostaglandins and matrix metalloproteinases (MMP).

Anakinra

Anakinra is a recombinant human IL-1 antagonist which acts by competitively blocking the attachment of IL-1 to its receptor, interleukin-1 type-1 receptor (IL1R1). Due to a short half-life of 4–6 hours, anakinra is injected daily via the SC route, usually at 1–2 mg/kg (maximum dose 100 mg).

Treatment of SJIA with anakinra has been found to reverse the gene expression patterns in peripheral blood cells.[22] Its use is recommended in poorly controlled SJIA with steroid dependence. Anakinra reduces the need of steroids and their accompanying side effects. SJIA patients with shorter duration of disease, lesser joint involvement, pronounced systemic symptoms, and higher serum ferritin levels are more likely to respond to IL-1 inhibitors, while others may demonstrate partial response. Anakinra has also been used successfully in macrophage activation syndrome (MAS)—one of the most dreaded complications of rheumatic disorders such as SJIA, SLE, and KD. Cytokine-specific therapy using anakinra is increasingly being used in the treatment of MAS in SJIA, the usual starting dose being 1–2 mg/kg, which may be increased up to 10–15 mg/kg/day (especially in KD associated MAS).[23] In this regard, it may be given IV as well, which is advantageous in patients with shock, thrombocytopenia, disseminated intravascular coagulation, or very young age.[24,25]

IL-1β also drives the pathogenesis of familial Mediterranean fever (FMF), an autosomal recessive autoinflammatory disorder. The use of anakinra leads to remission in addition to normalization of serum amyloid A levels in FMF refractory or intolerant to colchicine.[26] In addition, anakinra holds its position in the management of various other autoinflammatory disorders with IL-1 pathway dysregulation such as mevalonate kinase deficiency, TRAPS, deficiency of interleukin 1 receptor antagonist (DIRA), and cryopyrin-associated periodic syndrome (CAPS).[23] The role of anakinra has also been elucidated in other disorders including refractory KD and Behçet's syndrome.[27-30]

Recently, anakinra has been used in multisystem inflammatory syndrome in children (MIS-C) temporally related to coronavirus disease 2019 (COVID-19) pandemic. Clinical guidance by the ACR suggests the use of high-dose anakinra (>4 mg/kg/day) for MIS-C refractory to steroids or where steroids are contraindicated.[20]

Adverse effects of anakinra mostly consist of local injection site reactions such as erythema, rash, and pruritus which can be well managed with simple measures such as application of ice packs. Anakinra also confers increased risk of serious bacterial infections. However, its use in Indian settings is precluded by the lack of availability and high cost.

Rilonacept and Canakinumab

Rilonacept and canakinumab are two other IL-1 inhibitors that have been found useful in the treatment of CAPS and colchicine-resistant or intolerant FMF.[31-33] Canakinumab in addition has been seen to induce rapid and sustained clinical and biochemical responses in SJIA.[34] In Indian scenario, the widespread use of both these agents in the near future seems unlikely due to lack of availability and cost issues.

■ ANTI-B CELL ANTIBODY

Rituximab

Rituximab (RTX) is a chimeric mouse anti-CD20 monoclonal antibody. CD20 molecule is present on pre-B and mature B cells. Rituximab removes B cells from circulation by apoptosis, antibody-dependent cellular cytotoxicity and complement-dependent cellular cytotoxicity. In this manner, antigen presentation by B cells, cytokine production, tissue infiltration by B cells, and antibody production by memory B cells are hampered, even though plasma cells continue to produce antibodies.

Its use in anti-neutrophil cytoplasmic antibody (ANCA)-associated vasculitis (AAV) was established in the seminal rituximab (RTX) in AAV (RAVE) trial, which demonstrated its non-inferiority in a dose of 375 mg/m^2/week for 4 weeks to daily cyclophosphamide (2 mg/kg/day) in induction of remission.[35] It is also superior to azathioprine (2 mg/kg/day) in maintenance of remission in AAV, when given at a fixed dose of 500 mg at 0 and 2 weeks, followed by three doses 6-monthly, without any concomitant rise in adverse events, as concluded in the MAINRITSAN trial.[36] However, both these trials were conducted in adults. RTX also improves the disease activity and modified Rodnan score in scleroderma. Beneficial effects are also exerted on lung involvement in systemic sclerosis. In juvenile dermatomyositis (JDM), autoantibodies and B-cell activation are implicated in the pathogenesis of myositis and other manifestations and the use of RTX is advocated by the European Alliance of Associations for Rheumatology (EULAR) for refractory or severe JDM.[37]

Despite no evidence of superiority of adding RTX in both non-renal and renal lupus in two adult trials, the EXPLORER and LUNAR trials respectively, RTX is used in clinical settings for disease control in SLE including severe lupus nephritis and severe non-renal manifestations of SLE such as autoimmune hemolytic anemia, immune thrombocytopenia, and antiphospholipid antibody syndrome (APLA).[38]

RTX is given IV at 375 mg/m^2 weekly for 4 weeks or more conveniently at 500 mg/m^2 in two doses separated by a fortnight.[39] Premedication with steroids should be instituted prior to infusion. Infection with HIV, hepatitis B and C viruses, and latent tuberculosis should be ruled out prior to initiation of RTX. Rarely, reactivation of John Cunningham (JC) virus or human polyomavirus-2 may lead to progressive multifocal leukoencephalopathy in patients with autoimmune diseases. As it knocks off B cells, hypogammaglobulinemia is a known phenomenon in patients treated with RTX. Children may be more susceptible to RTX-induced hypogammaglobulinemia.[40] Documentation of immunoglobulin levels at baseline and subsequently every 6–12 months till at least a year after cessation of therapy is advisable to detect RTX-induced hypogammaglobulinemia. Hypogammaglobulinemia accompanied with severe or recurrent infections warrants replacement with IV immunoglobulin (IVIG) at 0.4 mg/kg/month. Subsequent IVIG doses may be adapted to the clinical response, trough IgG levels and presence of infections.[41]

Belimumab

Belimumab is a human IgG1 monoclonal antibody directed against B-lymphocyte stimulating factor [also known as B-lymphocyte stimulator (BLyS)]. By blocking the interaction between BLyS and its receptor, it decreases the survival of autoreactive B cells. It is given IV at a recommended dose of 10 mg/kg q2 weekly for the first three doses, followed by every 4 weeks. Two randomized control trials (RCTs) conducted in adult population—BLISS-52 and BLISS-76 (excluding severe active lupus and CNS lupus) showed better disease control, reduction in the number of disease flares, and improved quality of life in patients in the belimumab arm.[42] It was well-tolerated and resulted in good outcome scores in children with SLE in the PLUTO trial, which matched with the results obtained in adult studies.[43,44] It was approved by the FDA in 2019 for use in childhood SLE between 5 years and 17 years of age. A trial on subcutaneous belimumab in childhood SLE (cSLE) is currently underway (ClinicalTrials.gov Identifier: NCT04179032).

■ INHIBITION OF COSTIMULATORY PATHWAY

Abatacept

Abatacept is the fusion product of cytotoxic T lymphocyte–associated antigen-4 (CTLA-4) and IgG1. For activation of resting T cells, in addition to antigen presentation in appropriate major histocompatibility complex (MHC) by antigen presenting cells (APC), costimulation signal too is essential by binding of CD 28 (on T cells) with CD 80/86 (on APC). CTLA-4 prevents this costimulation by binding to CD 80/86 with a greater affinity than CD 28. Administered IV, it is approved for use in children above 6 years of age for polyarticular JIA. Response may be seen after three or four doses but may be delayed by as much as 6 months. Recently, subcutaneous route has also been found to be well-tolerated in a phase III open-labeled study and led to remission of symptoms in polyarticular JIA.[45] It is also used sparingly in refractory cases of JIA-associated uveitis. Major adverse effects include increased risk of infections.

■ INTERLEUKIN-23 INHIBITORS
Ustekinumab and Guselkumab

Ustekinumab is a monoclonal antibody against the common p40 subunit of two cytokines, IL-23 and IL-12. By preventing the interaction between these cytokines and their receptors, it inhibits IL-17 secreting T helper 17 (Th17) cells.

■ INTERLEUKIN-17 INHIBITORS
Secukinumab and Ixekizumab

These are monoclonal antibodies against IL-17, which have not yet been approved for pediatric use. Secukinumab is undergoing trials for its efficacy in pediatric psoriatic arthritis and enthesitis-related arthritis (ClinicalTrials.gov Identifier: NCT03031782).

■ JANUS KINASE-SIGNAL TRANSDUCTION AND ACTIVATION OF TRANSCRIPTION INHIBITORS

The Janus kinase-signal transduction and activation of transcription (JAK-STAT) is an intracellular cytokine-signaling pathway that is involved in various rheumatic disorders. It transduces the downstream effects of multiple inflammatory cytokines, interferons, and hormones. After a cytokine binds to its receptor on the cell surface, the associated tyrosine kinase is activated and phosphorylates STAT protein. Upon being phosphorylated, monomers of STAT polymerize to form homo- or heterodimers. They enter the cell nucleus and act as transcription factors for expression of various genes involved in the pathogenesis of diseases.

The blockade of single cytokine such as TNF-α with the use of biologics may not lead to complete clinical remission owing to activation of alternative pathways via other cytokines. Unlike biological agents, the Janus kinase inhibitors (Jakinibs) offer the potential advantage of blocking the final signal transduction pathway of multiple inflammatory cytokines by a single drug. Also, unlike biologics, hypersensitivity reactions are seldom seen with their use.[46] Nonetheless, the risk of serious infections, especially viral [herpes zoster, JC virus, BK virus (a polyoma virus)] and opportunistic infections, are the same as with use of biologics.[47]

Jakinibs may be *nonspecific* JAK inhibitors like tofacitinib or *selective* JAK inhibitors, such as filgotinib and upadacitinib (Jak-1 inhibitors). The selective Jakinibs offer an increased precision and efficacy of therapy and better safety profile owing to decreased suppression of other cytokine pathways.

Tofacitinib

Tofacitinib is an orally administered nonspecific Jakinib which inhibits the downstream signaling of multiple proinflammatory cytokines including ILs-2, 4, 7, 9, 15, and 21 through blockade of Jak 3 and IL-6, 10, 11, IFN-α/β and IFN-γ via Jak1 inhibition. A phase III clinical trial of the safety and efficacy of tofacitinib in children with polyarticular JIA has been completed and awaits publication (A3921104; ClinicalTrials.gov: NCT02592434). A long-term, phase-III, open-label study on the safety of tofacitinib in previously enrolled participants of other JIA is still ongoing (A3921145; ClinicalTrials.gov: NCT01500551). A case report mentions it to be effective in management of arthritis, serositis, and other systemic symptoms in a case of recalcitrant SJIA.[48] Tofacitinib is also useful in the management of rash and improving the muscle strength in patients with refractory JDM. It also benefits those with interferonopathies such as stimulators of interferon genes (STING)-associated vasculopathy with onset in infancy (SAVI).[49]

Serious adverse effects include various infections including tubercular, bacterial, viral, and fungal. Hence, a careful watch on reactivation of latent tuberculosis, absolute neutrophil count, liver enzymes, and complete blood counts is important during therapy.

Baricitinib

Baricitinib is a Jak-1/Jak-2 inhibitor that has been approved by the FDA for use in rheumatoid arthritis. Oral baricitinib has shown some promise in treatment of rare, monogenic autoinflammatory diseases with increased expression of interferons such as chronic atypical neutrophilic dermatosis with lipodystrophy and elevated temperature (CANDLE) syndrome and SAVI, though without complete normalization in disease scores in SAVI patients.[49] There are anecdotal reports of its use in COPA syndrome; caused by mutation in *coatomer protein complex subunit alpha* (*COPA*) gene.[50]

Ruxolitinib

Ruxolitinib inhibits Jak-1/2 and its downstream signaling of cytokines. It has been used successfully in a few cases of refractory hemophagocytic lymphohistiocytosis (HLH) and interferonopathies.[49,51,52] These patients stayed in remission even till 1 year of therapy, thus giving rise to hopes of steroid-free HLH treatment regimen.

■ PHOSPHODIESTERASE INHIBITORS

Phosphodiesterase-4 (PDE-4) is responsible for production and degradation of various pro- and anti-inflammatory cytokines via cyclic adenosine monophosphate (cAMP). PDE-4 blockade leads to accumulation of c-AMP, which in turn leads to production of anti-inflammatory cytokines via activation of protein kinase A (PKA).

Apremilast
It is an orally administered PDE-4 antagonist that has demonstrated efficacy in decreasing the number and pain of oral ulcers and improving the disease activity scores in Behçet's disease, primarily in adults.

■ BIOSIMILARS

A biosimilar is a biotherapeutic drug that is highly similar, but not identical to an already licensed drug with respect to its safety, potency, and quality but may be different from the originally approved drug in clinically inactive components. They have minor variations in structure (like glycosylation or amino acid sequences) due to the manufacturing processes. To be adjudicated as a biosimilar for clinical use, the molecule must demonstrate structural and functional similarities with comparable pharmacokinetic (PK) and pharmacodynamic (PD) properties to the reference product in appropriately designed clinical trials. The comparatively low cost of biosimilars may overcome the affordability issue of original molecules for most of the patients, if not all.

■ KEY ISSUES FOR IMMUNIZATION PRACTICES DURING BIOLOGICAL THERAPY

The use of immunosuppressive agents is associated with various adverse effects including increased risk of infections. Hence, it is imperative to properly document the immunization status of patients and advise the needful vaccines during use of biological agents. The following key points should be considered while administering vaccines to children with underlying rheumatic disorders.[53,54]

- The following doses are immunosuppressive:
    - *Glucocorticoids* ≥ 2 weeks in dosages equivalent to prednisolone 20 mg/day or 2 mg/kg/body weight
    - *Methotrexate* at ≥ 0.4 mg/kg/week or *azathioprine* ≥ 3.0 mg/kg/day
    - Use of any biological DMARD
- Ideally the patient should be vaccinated during the quiescent state of the disease and live vaccines should be administered *at least 4 weeks prior to initiation* of immunosuppressive therapy, particularly anti-B cell therapy

- In case prior vaccination is not possible, it should be carried out *at least 6 months after and 4 weeks before* the administration of next dose of B cell-depleting therapy
- Nonlive vaccines can be administered while on treatment with steroids and DMARDs.
- A child should be vaccinated against *varicella* prior to immunosuppression if prior infection with varicella is absent.
- *Pneumococcal vaccination* should be advised for most patients with rheumatic diseases. For those with unknown or no history of pneumococcal immunization, i.e., a PCV-13 prime-PPSV23 boost strategy, with an interval of at least 8 weeks between the two vaccines, is recommended by the Center for Disease Control and Prevention (CDC), USA.
- Annual *influenza vaccination* is also advisable for most patients with rheumatic disorders.
- Girls with SLE must be advised bivalent or quadrivalent *human papillomavirus (HPV) vaccine* during adolescence.

■ CONCLUSION

With the expanding knowledge of the pathogenesis of pediatric rheumatic disorders, newer biologic drugs are being developed every year. Judicious use of biological agents under close surveillance makes a huge difference in the lives of children with wide spectrum of rheumatic disorders. Albeit effective in controlling the disease, they are not devoid of adverse effects particularly the risk of infection and hence children on biologicals should be kept under close follow-up.

■ KEY POINTS

- Biologics are produced from biologic processes and include monoclonal antibodies, antagonists of receptors, and specific cellular inflammatory pathways.
- TNF-α inhibitors are the most widely used biological agents in pediatric population for various disorders including JIA (polyarticular, enthesitis-related, and psoriatic), Behçet's disease, KD, and sarcoidosis.
- Latent tuberculosis should be ruled out before initiation of biologics (particularly TNF-α inhibitors) and these patients should be monitored closely for symptoms of tuberculosis during treatment with these agents.
- Tocilizumab is an IL-6 inhibitor that is available both in IV and SC formulations and may be used for systemic JIA, polyarticular JIA, and uveitis associated with JIA.
- IL-1 inhibitors such as anakinra are used in diseases with involvement of innate immunity such as SJIA, autoinflammatory syndromes, MIS-C temporally associated with COVID-19, and macrophage activation syndrome.
- Rituximab is an anti-CD20 monoclonal antibody used in therapy of SLE, ANCA-associated vasculitis, and JDM in children.

- Rituximab use carries a risk of developing rituximab-induced hypogammaglobulinemia, and hence immunoglobulin levels should be monitored at baseline and 6- and 12-monthly.
- JAK-STAT inhibitors block multiple cytokines by blocking the final common pathway of cell signaling and are being studied in a wide spectrum of pediatric rheumatic disorders.
- All children under treatment with biologicals and other targeted therapies are inherently predisposed to infections, making immunization with recommended vaccines a matter of paramount importance.

■ REFERENCES

1. Baugh JA, Bucala R. Mechanisms for modulating TNF alpha in immune and inflammatory disease. Curr Opin Drug Discov Devel. 2001;4(5):635-50.
2. Lovell DJ, Giannini EH, Reiff A, Cawkwell GD, Silverman ED, Nocton JJ, et al. Etanercept in children with polyarticular juvenile rheumatoid arthritis. Pediatric Rheumatology Collaborative Study Group. N Eng J Med. 2000:342(11):763-9.
3. Kerensky TA, Gottlieb AB, Yaniv S, Au SC. Etanercept: efficacy and safety for approved indications. Expert Opin Drug Saf. 2012;11(1):121-39.
4. Tynjälä P, Vähäsalo P, Tarkiainen M, Kröger L, Aalto K, Malin M, et al. Aggressive combination drug therapy in very early polyarticular juvenile idiopathic arthritis (ACUTE-JIA): A multicentre randomised open-label clinical trial. Ann Rheum Dis. 2011;70(9):1605-12.
5. Tambralli A, Beukelman T, Weiser P, Atkinson TP, Cron RQ, Stoll ML. High doses of infliximab in the management of juvenile idiopathic arthritis. J Rheumatol. 2013;40(10):1749-55.
6. Tremoulet AH, Jain S, Jaggi P, Jimenez-fernandez S, Pancheri JM, Sun X, et al. Infliximab for intensification of primary therapy for Kawasaki disease : a phase 3 randomised, double-blind, placebo-controlled trial. Lancet. 2014;383(9930):1731-8.
7. Wolfe F, Michaud K, Anderson J, Urbansky K. Tuberculosis infection in patients with rheumatoid arthritis and the effect of infliximab therapy. Arthritis Rheum. 2004;50(2):372-9.
8. Ho M, Chen LJ, Sin HPY, Iu LPL, Brelen M, Ho ACH, et al. Experience of using adalimumab in treating sight- threatening paediatric or adolescent Behçet's disease-related uveitis. J Ophthal Inflamm Infect. 2019-9:14.
9. Klein A, Becker I, Minden K, Foeldvari I, Haas JP, Horneff G. Adalimumab versus adalimumab and methotrexate for the treatment of juvenile idiopathic arthritis : Long-term data from the German BIKER registry. Scand J Rheumatol. 2019;48(2):95-104.
10. Weinblatt ME, Keystone EC, Furst DE, Moreland LW, Weisman MH, Birbara CA, et al. Adalimumab, a fully human anti-tumor necrosis factor alpha monoclonal antibody, for the treatment of rheumatoid arthritis in patients taking concomitant methotrexate: the ARMADA trial. Arthritis Rheum. 2003;48(1):35-45. Erratum in: Arthritis Rheum. 2003 Mar;48(3):855.
11. Shim TS. Diagnosis and treatment of latent tuberculosis infection due to initiation of anti-TNF therapy. Tuberc Respir Dis (Seoul). 2014;76(6):261-8.

12. Starke JR; Committee on Infectious diseases. Interferon-γ release assays for diagnosis of tuberculosis infection and disease in children. Pediatrics. 2014;134(6).e1763-73.
13. Mariette X, Matucci-Cerinic M, Pavelka K, Taylor P, van Vollenhoven R, Heatley R, et al. Malignancies associated with tumour necrosis factor inhibitors in registries and prospective observational studies: a systematic review and meta-analysis. Ann Rheum Dis. 2011;70(11):1895-904.
14. Kemanetzoglou E, Andreadou E. CNS demyelination with TNF-α blockers. Curr Neurol Neurosci Rep. 2017;17(4):36.
15. De Benedetti F, Brunner HI, Ruperto N, Kenwright A, Wright S, Calvo I, et al; PRINTO; PRCSG. Randomized trial of tocilizumab in systemic juvenile idiopathic arthritis. N Engl J Med. 2012;367(25):2385-95.
16. Yokota S, Itoh Y, Morio T, Origaza H, Sumitomo N, Tomobe M, et al. Tocilizumab in systemic juvenile idiopathic arthritis in a real-world clinical setting: results from 1 year of postmarketing surveillance follow-up of 417 patients in Japan. Ann Rheum Dis. 2016;75(9):1654-60.
17. Calvo-Río V, Santos-Gómez M, Calvo I, González-Fernández MI, López-Montesinos B, Mesquida M, et al. Anti-interleukin-6 receptor tocilizumab for severe juvenile idiopathic arthritis-associated uveitis refractory to anti-tumor necrosis factor therapy: A multicenter study of twenty-five patients. Arthritis Rheumatol. 2017;69(3):668-75.
18. Batu ED, Sönmez HE, Hazırolan T, Özaltın F, Bilginer Y, Özen S. Tocilizumab treatment in childhood Takayasu arteritis: Case series of four patients and systematic review of the literature. Semin Arthritis Rheum. 2017;46(4):529-35.
19. Jung JY, Kim MY, Suh CH, Kim HA. Off-label use of tocilizumab to treat nonjuvenile idiopathic arthritis in pediatric rheumatic patients: a literature review. Pediatr Rheumatol Online J. 2018;16(1):79.
20. Henderson LA, Canna SW, Friedman KG, Gorelik M, Lapidus SK, Bassiri H, et al. American College of Rheumatology clinical guidance for pediatric patients with multisystem inflammatory syndrome in children associated with SARS-CoV-2 and hyperinflammation in COVID-19. Version 2. Arthritis Rheumatol. 2021;73(4):e13-e29.
21. Ruperto I, Brunner HI, Ramanan AV, Horneff G, Cuttica R, Henrickson M, et al. Pediatric Rheumatology INternational Trials Organisation (PRINTO) and the Pediatric Rheumatology Collaborative Study Group (PRCSG), Subcutaneous dosing regimens of tocilizumab in children with systemic or polyarticular juvenile idiopathic arthritis. Rheumatology (Oxford). 2021;60(10): 4568-80.
22. Pascual V, Allantaz F, Arce E, Punaro M, Banchereau J. Role of interleukin-1 (IL-1) in the pathogenesis of systemic onset juvenile idiopathic arthritis and clinical response to IL-1 blockade. J Exp Med. 2005;201(9):1479-86.
23. Maniscalco V, Abu-Rumeileh S, Mastrolia MV, Marrani E, Maccora I, Pagnini I, et al. The off-label use of anakinra in pediatric systemic autoinflammatory diseases. Ther Adv Musculoskelet Dis. 2020 Oct 16;12:1759720X20959575.
24. Bagri NK, Gupta L, Sen ES, Ramanan AV. Macrophage activation syndrome in children: Diagnosis and management. Indian Pediatr. 2021:S097475591600308.
25. Phadke O, Rouster-Stevens K, Giannopoulos H, Chandrakasan S, Prahalad S. Intravenous administration of anakinra in children with macrophage activation syndrome. Pediatr Rheumatol Online J. 2021;19(1):98

26. Cetin P, Sari I, Sozeri B, Cam O, Birlik M, Akkoc N, et al. Efficacy of interleukin-1 targeting treatments in patients with familial mediterranean fever. Inflammation. 2015;38(1):27-31.
27. Cohen S, Tacke CE, Straver B, Meijer N, Kuipers IM, Kuijpers TW. A child with severe relapsing Kawasaki disease rescued by IL-1 receptor blockade and extracorporeal membrane oxygenation. Ann Rheum Dis. 2012;71(12):2059-61.
28. Sánchez-Manubens J, Gelman A, Franch N, Teodoro S, Palacios JR, Rudi N, et al. A child with resistant Kawasaki disease successfully treated with anakinra: a case report. BMC Pediatr. 2017;17(1):102.
29. Kone-Paut I, Cimaz R, Herberg J, Bates O, Carbasse A, Saulnier JP, et al. The use of interleukin 1 receptor antagonist (anakinra) in Kawasaki disease: A retrospective cases series. Autoimmun Rev. 2018;17(8):768-74.
30. Cantarini L, Vitale A, Scalini P, Dinarello CA, Rigante D, Franceschini R, et al. Anakinra treatment in drug-resistant Behçet's disease: a case series. Clin Rheumatol. 2015;34(7):1293-301.
31. Hoffman HM, Throne ML, Amar NJ, Sebai M, Kivitz AJ, Kavanaugh A, et al. Efficacy and safety of rilonacept (interleukin-1 Trap) in patients with cryopyrin-associated periodic syndromes: results from two sequential placebo-controlled studies. Arthritis Rheum. 2008;58(8):2443-52.
32. Hashkes PJ, Spalding SJ, Giannini EH, Huang B, Johnson A, Park G, et al. Rilonacept for colchicine-resistant or -intolerant familial Mediterranean fever: a randomized trial. Ann Intern Med. 2012;157(8):533-41.
33. Gülez N, Makay B, Sözeri B. Long-term effectiveness and safety of canakinumab in pediatric familial Mediterranean fever patients. Mod Rheumatol. 2020;30(1):166-171.
34. Ruperto N, Brunner HI, Quartier P, Constantin T, Wulffraat N, Horneff G, et al; PRINTO; PRCSG. Two randomized trials of canakinumab in systemic juvenile idiopathic arthritis. N Engl J Med. 2012;367(25):2396-406.
35. Stone JH, Merkel PA, Spiera R, Seo P, Langford CA, Hoffman GS, et al; RAVE-ITN Research Group. Rituximab versus cyclophosphamide for ANCA-associated vasculitis. N Engl J Med. 2010;363(3):221-32.
36. Guillevin L, Pagnoux C, Karras A, Khouatra C, Aumaître O, Cohen P, et al; French Vasculitis Study Group. Rituximab versus azathioprine for maintenance in ANCA-associated vasculitis. N Engl J Med. 2014;371(19):1771-80.
37. Bellutti Enders F, Bader-Meunier B, Baildam E, Constantin T, Dolezalova P, Feldman BM, et al. Consensus-based recommendations for the management of juvenile dermatomyositis. Ann Rheum Dis. 2017;76(2):329-340.
38. Fanouriakis A, Kostopoulou M, Alunno A, Aringer M, Bajema I, Boletis JN, et al. 2019 update of the EULAR recommendations for the management of systemic lupus erythematosus. Ann Rheum Dis. 2019;78(6):736-45.
39. Cassidy J, Petty R, Laxer R, Lindlsey C. Pharmacology: Biologics. Textbook of Pediatric Rheumatology, 6th edition. Netherlands: Elsevier;2010. pp. 161-75.
40. Khojah AM, Miller ML, Klein-Gitelman MS, Curran ML, Hans V, Pachman LM, et al. Rituximab-associated Hypogammaglobinemia in pediatric patients with autoimmune diseases. Pediatr Rheumatol Online J. 2019;17(1):61.
41. Wijetilleka S, Jayne DR, Mukhtyar C, Ala A, Bright PD, Chinoy H, et al. Recommendations for the management of secondary hypogammaglobulinaemia due to B cell targeted therapies in autoimmune rheumatic diseases. Rheumatology (Oxford). 2019;58(5):889-96.

42. Furie R, Rovin BH, Houssiau F, Malvar A, Teng YKO, Contreras G, et al. Two-year, randomized, controlled trial of belimumab in lupus nephritis. N Engl J Med. 2020;383(12):1117-28.
43. Brunner HI, Abud-Mendoza C, Viola DO, Penades IC, Levy D, Anton J, et al; Paediatric Rheumatology International Trials Organisation (PRINTO) and the Pediatric Rheumatology Collaborative Study Group (PRCSG). Safety and efficacy of intravenous belimumab in children with systemic lupus erythematosus: results from a randomised, placebo-controlled trial. Ann Rheum Dis. 2020;79(10):1340-48.
44. Bass DL, Okily M, Hammer A, JI B, Roth D, Quasny H. Efficacy of intravenous belimumab in children with systemic lupus erythematosus with markers of high disease activity: across-trial comparison with adult belimumab studies. Lupus Science & Medicine. 2020;7.
45. Brunner HI, Tzaribachev N, Vega-Cornejo G, Louw I, Berman A, Penadés IC, et al; Paediatric Rheumatology International Trials Organisation (PRINTO) and the Pediatric Rheumatology Collaborative Study Group (PRCSG). Subcutaneous abatacept in patients with polyarticular-course juvenile idiopathic arthritis: Results from a phase iii open-label study. Arthritis Rheumatol. 2018;70(7): 1144-54.
46. Kotyla PJ. Are janus kinase inhibitors superior over classic biologic agents in RA patients? Biomed Res Int. 2018;2018:7492904.
47. Schwartz DM, Kanno Y, Villarino A, Ward M, Gadina M, O'Shea JJ. JAK inhibition as a therapeutic strategy for immune and inflammatory diseases. Nat Rev Drug Discov. 2017;16(12):843-62.
48. Huang Z, Lee PY, Yao X, Zheng S, Li T. Tofacitinib treatment of refractory systemic juvenile idiopathic arthritis. Pediatrics. 2019;143(5):e20182845.
49. Kerrigan SA, McInnes IB. JAK Inhibitors in rheumatology: Implications for paediatric syndromes? Curr Rheumatol Rep. 2018;20(12):83.
50. Krutzke S, Rietschel C, Horneff G. Baricitinib in therapy of COPA syndrome in a 15-year-old girl. Eur J Rheumatol. 2019;7(Suppl 1):1-4.
51. Broglie L, Pommert L, Rao S, Thakar M, Phelan R, Margolis D, et al. Ruxolitinib for treatment of refractory hemophagocytic lymphohistiocytosis. Blood Adv. 2017;1(19):1533-6.
52. Jianguo L, Zhixuan Z, Rong L, Xiaodong S. Ruxolitinib in alleviating the cytokine storm of hemophagocytic lymphohistiocytosis. Pediatrics. 2020;146(2): e20191301.
53. Heijstek MW, Ott de Bruin LM, Bijl M, Borrow R, van der Klis F, Koné-Paut I, et al. EULAR recommendations for vaccination in paediatric patients with rheumatic diseases. Ann Rheum Dis. 2011;70(10):1704-12.
54. Groot N, Heijstek MW, Wulffraat NM. Vaccinations in paediatric rheumatology: an update on current developments. Curr Rheumatol Rep. 2015;17(7):46.

Genetics

CHAPTER 18

Recent Advances in the Diagnosis and Treatment of Genetic Disorders

Alec Reginald Errol Correa, Madhulika Kabra

■ INTRODUCTION

Although individually rare, collectively genetic disorders account for a significant proportion of diseases in children. Broadly, genetic disorders can be divided into chromosomal, monogenic, and multifactorial disorders. *Chromosomal disorders* are due to numerical or structural abnormalities in the chromosomes. These abnormalities result in an alteration in the normal number of many genes present on the affected chromosome leading to disease. Numerical abnormalities may be due to a gain (trisomy; e.g., trisomy 13, 18, or 21) or a loss of a chromosome (monosomy; e.g., monosomy X). Structural abnormalities include deletions, duplications, translocations, and inversions. *Monogenic disorders* are due to an alteration in a single gene. These mutations are due to nucleotide substitutions, deletions, or insertions resulting in decreased amount of protein formation or the formation of a protein with altered function. Genetic disorders can be classified based in the pattern of inheritance **(Box 18.1)**. *Multifactorial disorders* are complex diseases caused by the interaction of multiple genetic loci with environmental factors.

Advances in technology have not only enabled the discovery of a genetic etiology for an ever-increasing number of diseases but have paved way for newer therapies. This chapter will focus on the recent advances in the diagnosis and treatment of genetic disorders.

■ INVESTIGATIONS

Chromosomal Disorders

Conventional methods to detect chromosomal abnormalities include karyotyping and fluorescence in situ hybridization (FISH). Karyotyping involves the staining of cultured cells arrested in the metaphase of mitosis to detect chromosome abnormalities based on specific banding patterns of each chromosome. Conventional karyotyping has several limitations:
- It cannot detect abnormalities smaller than 5 megabases
- It requires living cells for culture
- It is labor-intensive and requires skilled manpower for interpretation.

BOX 18.1: Patterns of inheritance.

Autosomal dominant:
- Manifest in the heterozygous state
- Disease present across multiple generations
- Affects both males and females
- 50% chance of transmission to offspring

E.g., Marfan syndrome, neurofibromatosis

Autosomal recessive:
- Manifest in homozygous or compound heterozygous state
- Disease present in the same generation (affects siblings)
- Affects both males and females
- 25% chance of transmission to offspring, if both parents are carriers

E.g., Gaucher disease, beta-thalassemia, cystic fibrosis

X-linked recessive:
- Manifests in males (hemizygous), most females are heterozygous carriers
- Female carriers have 50% chance of an affected male offspring and 50% chance of carrier female offspring
- Affected males cannot transmit disease to male offspring, 100% chance of carrier female offspring

E.g., Duchene muscular dystrophy, hemophilia A and B

X-linked dominant:
- Manifests both in heterozygous females and hemizygous males
- More severe disease or lethal in males
- Affected females can transmit disease to 50% of offspring; affected males can transmit disease to 100% of female offspring

E.g., Incontinentia pigmenti, X-linked hypophosphatemic rickets

Mitochondrial inheritance:
- Due to mutations in the mitochondrial DNA
- Inherited exclusively from the mother, males do not transmit to offspring
- Transmitted from a female to both male and female offspring
- Heteroplasmy—presence of mitochondria with and without the mutation in a cell
- Threshold effect—disease manifests only if a certain percentage of mitochondria carry the mutation

E.g., MELAS (mitochondrial encephalopathy, lactic acidosis, stroke-like episodes)

Triplet repeat disorders:
- Due to expansion in the number of trinucleotide repeats
- Cause disease beyond a certain threshold level
- Dynamic mutations—the number may change on transmission to offspring
- Anticipation—subsequent generations may have earlier onset of disease due to expansion of repeat size

E.g., Fragile X syndrome, myotonic dystrophy

Imprinting disorders:
- Due to abnormalities in imprinted genes
- Genetic imprinting is the silencing of certain genes based on parent of origin

E.g., Prader–Willi syndrome, Angelman syndrome, Russell–Silver syndrome

Uniparental disomy:
- Inheritance of both copies of a chromosome or part of a chromosome from a single parent.

E.g., Prader-Willi syndrome, Beckwith-Wiedemann syndrome

(DNA: deoxyribonucleic acid)

However, karyotyping can detect-balanced rearrangements such as inversions and balanced translocations that cannot be picked up by a chromosomal microarray (CMA). FISH is a technique that utilizes a fluorescent-labeled probe, designed for specific genetic loci. These probes hybridize with deoxyribonucleic acid (DNA) in either interphase or metaphase cells and the resultant fluorescent signals are used to detect chromosomal abnormalities. Other molecular techniques used to detect chromosomal disorders include quantitative fluorescence polymerase chain reaction (PCR) and multiplex ligation-dependent probe amplification.[1]

Chromosomal Microarray

Chromosomal microarray is a molecular cytogenetic technology used to detect copy number variants (CNV; deletions and duplications) in the genome. There are two types of techniques used, namely array-based comparative genomic hybridization (aCGH) and single nucleotide polymorphism (SNP) arrays. SNP arrays are commonly used in the evaluation of chromosomal disorders. In aCGH, the patient's DNA is compared to that of a control sample by staining the two samples after enzymatic degradation and subsequent hybridization to oligonucleotide probes on an array. Any imbalance in the amount of DNA between the two samples will be detected by changes in the intensity of the florescence at specific probes **(Fig. 18.1)**. SNP arrays use probes designed to identify SNPs spread across the genome. The intensity of the fluorescence is measured to determine the copy number state and genotype. In contrast to aCGH, a control sample is not used during the test as the platform software compares the patient's data to reference data **(Fig. 18.2)**. **Table 18.1** describes the differences between the different aCGH and SNP arrays and compares them to conventional karyotyping.

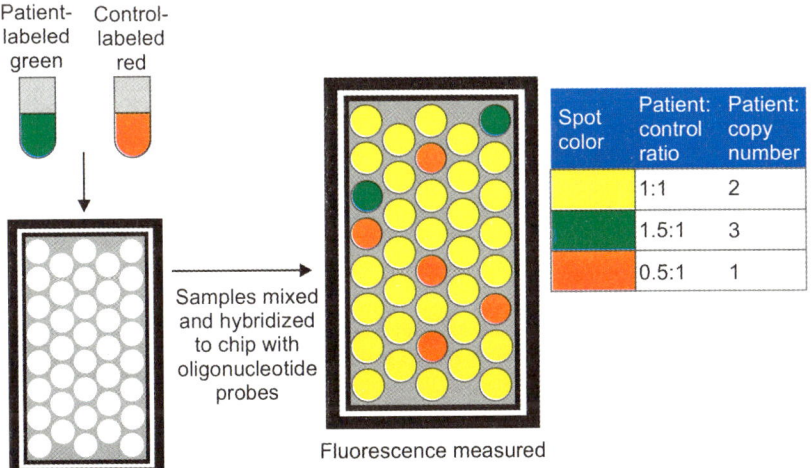

Fig. 18.1: Array-based comparative genomic hybridization (aCGH).

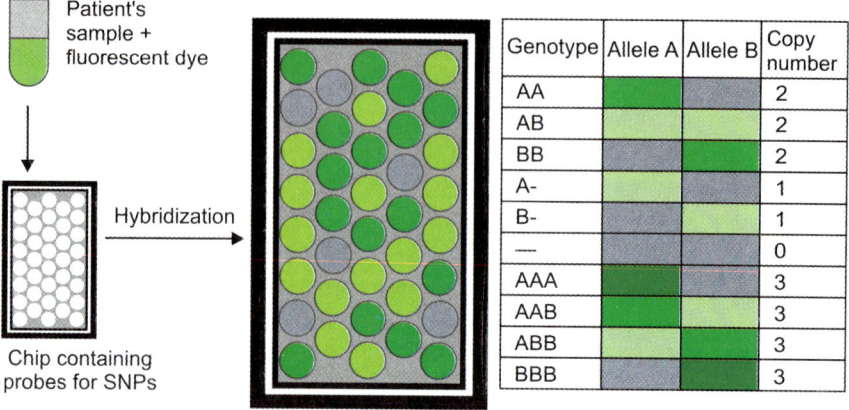

Fig. 18.2: Single nucleotide polymorphism (SNP) chromosomal microarray.

Technique	Aneuploidy	CNV	Unbalanced translocation	Balanced translocation and inversion	Triploidy	LOH/UPD
Conventional karyotyping	+	+ >5 mb	+	+	+	–
CGH array	+	+	+	–	–	–
SNP array	+	+	+	–	+	+

TABLE 18.1: Comparison between conventional karyotyping, array CGH, and SNP array.

(CGH: comparative genomic hybridization; CNV: copy number variations; LOH: loss of heterozygosity; SNP: single nucleotide polymorphism; UPD: uniparental disomy)

Figure 18.3 shows the CMA report of a patient with an 8 megabase deletion. In addition to CNVs, SNP arrays can also detect uniparental disomy (UPD) and regions of loss of heterozygosity (LOH).[2,3]

Chromosomal microarray is currently indicated as a first line test in the evaluation of patients with unexplained intellectual disability (ID), autism spectrum disorders (ASD), and multiple congenital anomalies (MCA).[2,4] CMA is used for a variety of prenatal and postnatal disorders. Prenatal indications include structural abnormality of the fetus on ultrasound, abnormal antenatal screening, recurrent miscarriages (on product of conception), and a previous child with a chromosomal abnormality or a parent with a chromosomal rearrangement. Postnatal indications include MCA, developmental disorders, abnormal growth parameters, ambiguous genitalia, and delineation and confirmation of a previously-detected cytogenetic abnormality.[1] CMA offers a significantly higher resolution than conventional karyotyping (10–50 kilobases vs. 5 megabases), resulting in a significantly higher diagnostic yield of between 15 and 20%, as compared to 3% for conventional

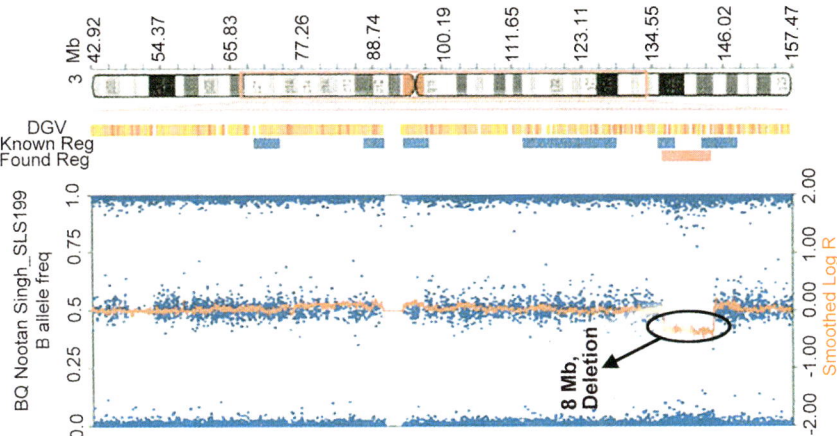

Fig. 18.3: Chromosomal microarray report showing 8 Mb deletion.

karyotyping in the evaluation of patients with unexplained ID, ASD, or MCA.[2] Advantages of CMA include the following:
- The ability to detect cryptic abnormalities
- Better characterization of breakpoints
- Objective data and results
- It can be performed on DNA from a variety of sources (unlike karyotyping that requires living cells)
- It can detect regions of copy neutral loss of heterozygosity

Limitations of CMA include:
- The inability to identify-balanced rearrangement
- It cannot detect low levels of mosaicism
- It cannot detect abnormalities below a certain level depending on probe coverage.

Furthermore, CMA does not provide information about the physical position and mechanism of the abnormality, which may be important for counseling regarding recurrence.[5]

Monogenic Disorders

Mutations causing a monogenic disorder were traditionally identified using PCR-based methods or by Sanger sequencing. Sanger sequencing, developed in the 1970s, is still considered the gold standard sequencing technology. It utilizes fluorescence-labeled chain-terminating dideoxynucleotides to sequence a specific region of DNA. Only short sequences of DNA (500–1000 bases) can be sequenced at a time. Furthermore, these techniques require prior knowledge of the mutations or genes causing the disease which limit their utility in diseases caused by mutations in several genes or in conditions with nonspecific phenotypic features such as ID. These limitations have been overcome by next generation sequencing technologies.

Next Generation Sequencing

Next generation sequencing (NGS) includes massively parallel sequencing technologies that are capable of sequencing millions of fragments of DNA simultaneously. NGS offers very high throughput allowing the sequencing of entire genomes and multiple samples simultaneously, thus revolutionizing the field of genetic testing by bringing down the time and cost of sequencing the genome tremendously. The basic steps of NGS include the fragmentation of genomic DNA into many short sequences that are subsequently sequenced in parallel. Bioinformatic software is then used to align the sequence of these fragments to a reference genome sequence to detect variants.[6,7]

Exome Sequencing

Whole exome sequencing (WES) is the process of sequencing the exomes of all the genes in the genome. This enables detection of variants in the exons which account for over 85% of disease-causing variants although the exome accounts for just 1–2% of the genome.[6,7] Often regions of the introns flanking the exons are also sequenced, allowing the detection of splice junction variants. Alternately, instead of sequencing the entire exome, another approach is to sequence the exons of specific genes called a gene panel. Commercially available gene panels may range from fewer than 10 genes to thousands of genes. "Clinical exome sequencing" commonly available in India covers the exons of a panel of approximately 5,000–6,000 genes that are known to be associated with disease **(Fig. 18.4)**.

Genome Sequencing

Whole genome sequencing (WGS) involves the sequencing of the entire genome, including exons, introns, and intergenic regions. This enables the detection of variants in most regions of the genome. Current platforms cover nearly 90% of the genome only, excluding difficult to sequence areas such as GC-rich (guanine-cytosine-rich) repetitive regions, centromeres, and telomeres. Additionally, copy number variants and chromosomal rearrangements can also be detected. Genome sequencing generates significantly more data than exome sequencing requiring more data handling and processing resources.[7] Additionally, the interpretation of intronic variants is difficult. Currently, genome sequencing is used to a limited extent in clinical practice due to the complexity of interpretation and higher cost involved. The diagnostic yield of genome sequencing and exome sequencing has been calculated to be 43% and 34%, respectively.[8] The differences between whole exome and genome sequencing are mentioned in **Table 18.2**.

Recent Advances in the Diagnosis and Treatment of Genetic Disorders

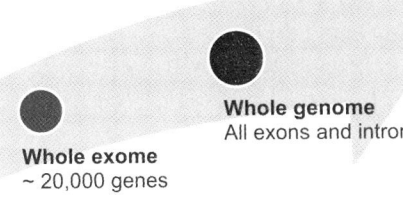

Whole genome
All exons and introns

Whole exome
~ 20,000 genes

Clinical exome
~5,000 to 6,000 disease-associated genes

Targeted gene panel
IEM, LSD, neuromuscular, immune deficiency, and epilepsy

Fig. 18.4: Tests using next generation sequencing.
(IEM: inborn errors of metabolism; LSD: lysosomal storage disorders)

TABLE 18.2: Differences between whole exome sequencing and whole genome sequencing.

	Whole exome sequencing	**Whole genome sequencing**
Coverage	<2% of genome ~20,000 gene	Covers all the genes, introns, and intergenic regions
Cost	Low	High
Data	4–5 Gb	90 Gb
Advantages	• Detects majority of disease-causing variants • Allows for higher sequencing depth and less data storage infrastructure required • Easier data analysis and interpretation	• Able to detect deep intronic and intergenic variants • Can identify structural variants • No exon capture required • Uniform coverage across the genome
Disadvantages	• Limited utility in detecting CNVs • Cannot detect deep intronic and intergenic variants	• Generates large amounts of data • Difficulty in interpreting noncoding variants
Uses	Monogenic disorders	Monogenic disorders, chromosomal disorders, and genotyping for complex disorders

(CNVs: copy number variants)

Indications for Exome or Genome Sequencing

Recently published American College of Medical Genetics guidelines recommend exome or genome sequencing as the first or second line test for patients with congenital anomalies and ID or developmental delay.[8]

Exome sequencing should be used for clinical diagnosis in individuals with a suspected genetic disorder in the following situations:[9]
- Targeted testing is not available
- The disorder is genetically heterogeneous
- Targeted testing has not detected any variants
- The cost of NGS would be less than that of sequencing individual candidate genes sequentially.

Exome sequencing is currently being extensively used in the diagnosis of monogenic disorders, prenatal diagnosis, and carrier screening.

■ MANAGEMENT

Most genetic disorders have no definitive treatment options and are managed with symptomatic and supporting care. However, advances in knowledge and technology have unleashed a flood of new therapeutic options for several genetic diseases. Presently, treatment is available for approximately 5% of genetic disorders.

Enzyme Replacement Therapy

The principle of enzyme replacement therapy (ERT) is to supplement the body with the deficient enzyme to promote normal physiological functioning of the cell and prevent the accumulation of harmful substrates in the cells. Ever since the first ERT with alglucerase, developed for the treatment of Gaucher disease, was approved for use in 1991, there has been sustained development of new ERTs. Currently ERT is available for several lysosomal storage disorders (LSD) including mucopolysaccharidosis (MPS, types I, II, IV, and VI), Pompe disease, and Fabry disease. Additionally, apart from lysosomal storage disorders, ERT has been developed for hypophosphatasia and adenosine deaminase (ADA) deficiency, and late infantile form of ceroid lipofuscinosis 2 (CLN2). **Table 18.3** gives information on currently available ERTs.

The enzymes are produced by recombinant DNA technology in human, plant, or animal cell lines. These enzymes, designed to mimic the natural enzyme in structure and function, are chemically modified with mannose-6-phosphate residues to direct them into the lysosomes. Most ERTs are administered as a weekly or two-weekly intravenous infusion. Although clinical trials have demonstrated clear therapeutic efficacy, real world benefits depend on several factors such as disease severity and complications, organ systems involved, and the age at initiation of treatment. To date, patients

TABLE 18.3: Commercially available enzyme replacement therapy.

Disease	Enzyme replacement therapy	Brand name
Gaucher disease	• Imiglucerase • Taliglucerase alpha • Velaglucerase alpha	• Cerezyme® • Elelyso® • VPRIV®
Pompe disease	Alglucosidase alpha	Myozyme® Lumizyme®
MPS I	Laronidase	Aldurazyme®
MPS II	• Idursulfase alpha • Idursulfase beta	Elaprase® Hunterase®
MPS IVA	Elosulfase	Vimizim®
MPS VI	Galsulfase	Naglazyme®
MPS VII	Vestronidase	Mepsevii®
Fabry disease	• Agalsidase alpha • Agalsidase beta	Replagal® Fabrazyme®
Lysosomal acid lipase deficiency	Sebelipase alpha	Kanuma®
Late infantile neuronal ceroid lipofuscinosis type 2 (CLN2)	Cerliponase alpha	Brineura®
Hypophosphatasia	Asfotase alpha	Strensiq®

(MPS: mucopolysaccharidosis)

with Gaucher disease have shown the best response to therapy. Although ERTs are safe drugs with acceptable side effect profiles, rare instances of hypersensitivity reactions have been reported.

Enzyme replacement therapies collectively share several common drawbacks. As presently available ERTs are unable to cross the blood brain barrier, ERTs have no effect on serious neurological manifestations of disease, resulting in limited utility in patients with severe cognitive impairment or neurological deficits. Efforts to overcome this impediment by direct infusion of ERT into the central nervous system (CNS) by means of lumbar puncture, intrathecal infusion catheters, and intraventricular infusion through reservoir devices are being investigated. Additionally, ERTs have been seen to have poor penetration into certain tissues (e.g., bone and cartilage) and are unable to repair already damaged tissues. Administration of ERTs requires considerable compliance from patients and their caregivers, as it involves frequent intravenous infusions in a day care setting that may result in significant time and monetary expenditure. Furthermore, the prohibitive cost of most commercially available ERT precludes its wider use in resource-limited countries such as India. Patients may develop immune reactions to the ERT. Antibodies against the exogenous ERT may reduce effectiveness of the medication; this phenomenon has been most striking on Pompe disease, and current treatment guidelines incorporate immunosuppressive medication to mitigate this problem.[10-12]

Gene Therapy

Gene therapy is the process of altering the genetic material in a cell to bring about a therapeutic change. It involves the transfer of a transgene, i.e., an artificially designed DNA molecule into the cells. The genetic modification of somatic cells is termed *somatic gene therapy*. The genetic modifications are limited to the individual being treated and cannot be transmitted to future offspring. Currently gene therapy research is directed toward somatic therapy. On the other hand, modifications to the DNA of gametes or the zygote are termed as *germline gene therapy*. This entails serious ethical issues regarding the transmission to future generations and long-term adverse effects of treatment. Human germline gene therapy is currently banned in most countries.

Broadly, gene therapy follows one of the two strategies to treat diseases—modification of disease cells and killing disease cells **(Flowchart 18.1)**. The former is used to treat monogenic disorders while the latter is used to treat cancers.

An important aspect of gene therapy is the transfer of the genetic material into the cell. This depends on several factors such as target cell type, location, and whether the cells are dividing or nondividing. The transfer can be achieved using viral (transduction) or nonviral vectors (transfection). Viral vectors include retroviruses, lentiviruses, adeno-associated viruses, and adenoviruses. They are highly efficacious and result in high levels of gene expression. Additionally, therapies can be targeted to a specific cell line by choosing viruses that can infect the target cells. Immunogenic reactions are important adverse effects of the viral vector, as the host mounts an immune response against the

Flowchart 18.1: Gene therapy strategies.

```
                    Gene therapy
                   /            \
    Modifying disease cells      Killing disease cells
    • Gene augmentation:         • Direct killing:
      – A copy of the deficient    – Transfer of a suicide gene to the cell
        gene is transferred to       resulting in cell death
        the cell to produce      • Indirect killing:
        the desired protein        – Genes transferred to immune cells
      – Useful for loss of           into enhance immune responses
        function mutations           against cancer cells
    • Gene silencing:
      – Production of a toxic
        gene product is inhibited
      – Useful for gain of
        function mutations
    • Gene repair:
      – Defective gene is edited
        using the correct sequence
```

virus. These can be severe reactions and result in death. Immunosuppressant therapy may be required to prevent immunological reactions.

Another important adverse effect that is seen with the use of integrating vectors such as retroviruses is that the DNA material integrates nonspecifically into the host genome. This may result in the activation of an oncogene resulting in cancer. This was a common adverse effect of the initial gene therapies designed to treat severe combined immunodeficiency. However, the use of lentivirus vectors which are less likely to integrate near oncogenes has reduced the risk of cancer. Nonviral transfer methods include lipid delivery systems, cationic lipid vesicles, and DNA nanoparticles. Although they are safer than viral vectors, their use is not as common as viral vectors, and they are less efficacious.

Depending on whether the therapeutic gene is given directly to the patient or not, gene therapy may be divided into *in vivo* and *ex vivo*. In *in vivo* therapy, the patient is directly given the genetic material carried in the appropriate vector either by injection directly into the target organ or intravenously. The vectors enter the cells resulting in the transfer of the genetic material into the target cells. In contrast, in *ex vivo* gene therapy, the patient's cells are extracted and cultured outside the body. The gene therapy is applied in vitro to these cultured cells. The cells with the desired modification are then selected and further cultured. This final product is then transplanted back into the patient. *Ex vivo* therapy can be used in situations where the target tissue is easily accessible such as blood.[13] **Table 18.4** lists the gene therapies currently approved for use in patients.

Gene editing is the process by which alterations are made to the normal DNA sequence at specific predetermined regions of the genome. It can be carried out *in vitro* or *in vivo*. The basic principle involves the creation of breaks in the DNA using programmable nucleases followed by the repair of these breaks by normal DNA repair mechanisms. The targetable nucleases, zinc-finger nuclease, transcription activator-like effector nuclease (TALEN), and CRISPR/Cas9 systems are designed to bind to specific sequences of DNA where the desired alteration is required. Gene editing can be used to inactivate a gene, upregulate a gene or correct a gene by supplying a normal DNA sequence simultaneously. Clinical trials for the development of therapies to treat several diseases including monogenic disorders (beta-thalassemia, sickle cell disease, hemophilia B, neurofibromatosis type 1, Leber congenital amaurosis, etc.), cancers, and infectious diseases such as human immunodeficiency virus (HIV) infection are currently underway. Furthermore, gene editing technologies are extensively used in the research setting in order to study the molecular basis of monogenic, cancer, and multifactorial disease through the development of disease specific cell lines, model organisms, and the production of induced pluripotent stem cells.[13,14]

TABLE 18.4: Examples of approved gene therapies for monogenic disorders.

Name	Vector	Disease	Comments
In vivo:			
Onasemnogene abeparvovec (ZOLGENSMA)	AAV9	Spinal muscular atrophy	• FDA approval 2019 • *Dose*—single dose of 1.1×10^{14} vector genomes/kg intravenous infusion • Systemic immunosuppression with corticosteroids for 30 days • *Adverse effects*—elevated aminotransferases and thrombocytopenia
Voretigene neparvovec (LUXTURNA)	AAV	RPE65-associated retinal dystrophy	• FDA approval 2017 • *Dose*—1.5×10^{11} vector genomes (vg) administered by subretinal injection per eye • Systemic oral corticosteroids (prednisolone 1 mg/kg/day) for a total of 7 days (starting 3 days before administration)
Alipogene tiparvovec (Glybera)	AAV1	Lipoprotein lipase deficiency	• EMA approval in 2012 • Currently withdrawn from market
Ex vivo:			
Strimvelis	γ-retrovirus	Adenosine deaminase deficiency (ADA-SCID)	• EMA approval 2016 • Autologous CD34+ enriched cell transduced with retroviral vector encoding for the human adenosine deaminase (ADA) cDNA • *Dose* - 2 and 20 million CD34+ cells/kg by intravenous infusion • Pre-treatment conditioning with Busulfan
Betibeglogene autotemcel (Zynteglo)	Lentivirus	β-thalassemia Sickle cell anemia	• Conditional authorization by EMA autologous CD34+ cell containing hematopoietic stem cells (HSC) transduced with lentiviral vector (LVV) encoding the βA-T87Q-globin gene • *Indication*—transfusion-dependent β-thalassemia (TDT) who do not have a β^0/β^0 genotype • *Dose*—minimum 5.0×10^6 CD34+ cells/kg • Full myeloablative conditioning required • Use suspended in 2021 as three patients in sickle cell trial developed myelodysplastic syndrome and acute myeloid leukemia

(EMA: European Medicines Agency; FDA: United States Food and Drug Administration)

Ribonucleic Acid Therapeutics

Ribonucleic acids (RNAs) play an important role in cellular pathways. In eukaryotic cells, RNA not only acts as an intermediary molecule in the transmission of genetic information between DNA and proteins, but also have enzymatic and regulatory functions. RNA therapeutics use RNA-based drugs to modulate diverse biological pathways to treat diseases. In recent years, several RNA-based therapies have been approved for clinical use. Additionally, clinical trials for numerous drugs for both genetic and complex disorders are currently being undertaken. The scope of RNA therapeutics is enormous as these drugs are easy to design and manufacture. Based on their composition and mechanism of action, RNA therapeutics can be divided into the following categories.

Antisense Oligonucleotides

Antisense oligonucleotides (ASO) are short single stranded RNA molecules that have sequences which are complementary to their target DNA/RNA sequences. Most common targets of these drugs are messenger RNAs (mRNAs). They bind to their complementary targets such as mRNA and act by altering the normal splicing of mRNA or degrading the mRNA through cellular pathways or preventing the translation of the mRNA. These molecules have chemical modification to the nucleotide base and sugars to increase stability, affinity, and reduce side effects.

Nusinersen is a drug developed to treat spinal muscular atrophy (SMA). It acts by binding to the survival of motor neuron 2 (SMN2) pre-mRNA and altering its splicing. Normally, exon 7 is not spiced into the SMN2 mRNA. Nusinersen prevents the exclusion of exon 7 from the SMN2 mRNA resulting in the production of a full-length protein like that produced by the *SMN1* gene (**Fig. 18.5**). Conversely, ASOs such as eteplirsen and goldodirsen result in skipping of exon 51 and 53 in Duchenne muscular dystrophy (DMD) mRNA. This helps to correct errors in the reading frame caused by deletions ending at these exons. By converting an out of frame deletion into an in-frame deletion, these treatments result in the production of a functional albeit shorter protein (**Fig. 18.6**).

Small Interfering Ribonucleic Acids

Small interfering RNAs (siRNAs) are short double stranded RNAs that act through the RNA interference (RNAi) cellular pathway. RNAi is a normal cellular pathway used to regulate gene expression by degrading RNA molecules in a process also called RNA silencing.

Ribonucleic Acid Aptamers

These are short single stranded RNA molecules that are designed to bind to specific targets such as proteins or peptides and inhibit their function. These drugs have high affinity and specificity for their targets.

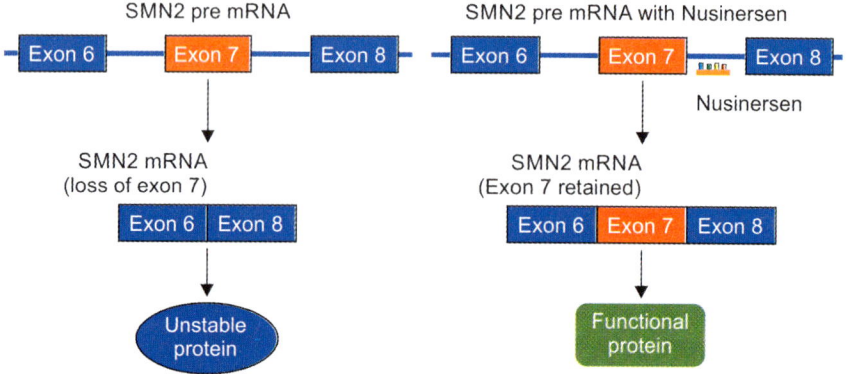

Fig. 18.5: Mechanism of action of Nusinersen.
(mRNA: messenger ribonucleic acid; SMN2: survival of motor neuron 2)

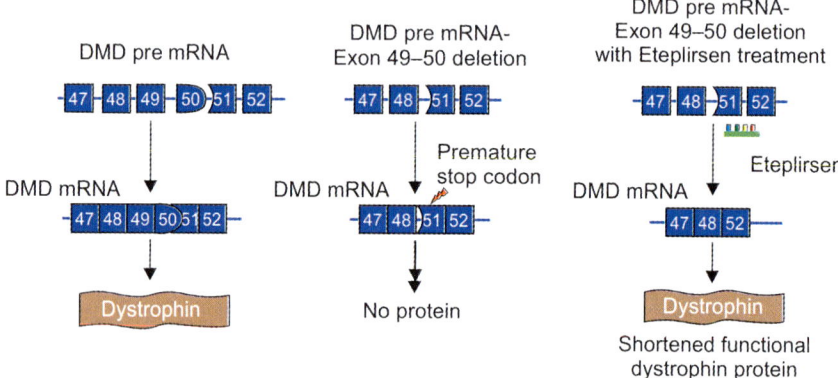

Fig. 18.6: Mechanism of action of eteplirsen.
(DMD: Duchenne muscular dystrophy; mRNA: messenger ribonucleic acid)

Messenger Ribonucleic Acid

Drugs based on mRNA use externally-produced mRNA molecules to produce proteins *in vivo*. These RNAs are designed to be similar to naturally occurring mRNA, and consist of a 5' cap, coding sequence, and 3' poly A tail. They enter the cytoplasm and are translated into proteins. They are rapidly eliminated from the cytoplasm by normal degradative pathways. The mRNA drugs can be used for:
- Replacement of deficient or defective protein
- Vaccines
- Cell therapy—mRNA is used to modify cells, cultured ex vivo, that are subsequently transfused into patients.[15-17]

The RNA therapeutic agents currently commercially available for use in patients are listed in **Table 18.5**.

TABLE 18.5: Currently approved RNA therapies.

	Name	Disease	Mechanism of action	Date of approval
Antisense oligonucleotides	Mipomersen	Familial hypercholesterolemia	Binds to mRNA and induces degradation	2013
	Nusinersen	Spinal muscular atrophy	Alternative splicing of SMN2 to include exon 7, resulting in increased functional SMN protein	2016
	Eteplirsen	Duchenne muscular dystrophy	Skipping of exon 51 during splicing	2016
	Inotersen	Hereditary transthyretin amyloidosis	Binds to mRNA and induces degradation	2018
	Golodirsen	Duchenne muscular dystrophy	Skipping of exon 53 during splicing	2019
	Volanesorsen	Familial chylomicronemia syndrome	Binds to apoC-III mRNA, leading to its degradation, preventing translation of apoC-III protein	2019
	Casimersen	Duchenne muscular dystrophy	Skipping of exon 45 during splicing	2021
Small Interfering RNA	Patisiran	Hereditary transthyretin amyloidosis	Reduces protein production through RNAi	2018
	Givosiran	Acute hepatic porphyria	Reduces protein production through RNAi	2019
	Inclisiran	Hypercholesterolemia	Reduces protein production through RNAi	2020
RNA aptamer	Pegaptanib	Age-related macular degeneration	Binds to VEGF and blocks its action	2004
mRNA	BTN162b2	COVID-19	Antigen production	2020
	Mrna-1273	COVID-19	Antigen production	2020

(mRNA: messenger ribonucleic acid; RNAi: RNA interference; SMN2: survival of motor neuron 2; VEGF: vascular endothelial growth factor)

Small Molecule Therapy

Substrate Reduction Therapy

Substrate reduction therapy (SRT) refers to a class of drugs that work on the principle of reducing the synthesis of compounds that accumulate in the cell in lysosomal storage disorders; these compounds are normally degraded (i.e., the substrate for the enzymes) by the specific enzyme that is deficient in that disorder. These drugs offer theoretical advantages over ERT—they are available in oral forms, can cross the blood brain barrier, and do not elicit immunological responses. Additionally, a single drug may be effective in several disorders. SRTs currently commercially available are miglustat, for the treatment of Gaucher disease and Niemann-Pick type C, and eliglustat tartrate for Gaucher disease.[18,19]

Stop Codon Read through Therapy

Nonsense mutations lead to the formation of premature stop codons, resulting in truncated proteins that are degraded. These therapies prevent translation of the premature stop codon without affecting translation termination at the normal stop codon site, allowing the formation of a functional protein. Two classes of drugs currently available are aminoglycosides (e.g., gentamycin) and nonaminoglycosides (e.g., ataluren). Ataluren is currently approved in the European Union and the UK for the treatment of Duchenne muscular dystrophy caused by nonsense mutations. Approximately 10–15% of DMD is caused by nonsense mutations and is amenable to treatment with ataluren. However, the medication did not show significant benefits for the primary endpoints in a phase 3 trial. Additionally, trials in patients with cystic fibrosis also failed to show benefit.[20]

Risdiplam

It is a small molecule therapy for SMA. It modifies the splicing of SMN2 pre mRNA leading to the production of a full-length protein. It is given via the oral route. It has been shown to be efficacious in trial with patients with SMA type 1, type 2, and type 3.[21]

Chaperone Therapy

Chaperone therapy is a therapeutic strategy to treat diseases caused by misfolded proteins. These drugs act either by binding to the misfolded proteins themselves or by inducing endogenous protein chaperones to correct misfolding. Thus, they prevent premature degradation of the protein and result in normal function of the protein. Presently, many drugs are being tested for the treatment of numerous genetic disorders. Migalastat and Tafamidis are chaperone therapies approved for Fabry disease and transthyretin amyloidosis, respectively.

CONCLUSION

Recent advances in diagnostics and therapeutics have revolutionized the field of clinical genetics. Genetic testing is increasingly being used in the diagnosis and management of patients across all pediatric subspecialties. Hence, an up-to-date knowledge about the utility and limitations of genetic testing and treatment options is essential for all pediatricians.

KEY POINTS

- Chromosomal microarray offers higher resolution compared to traditional tests for chromosomal abnormalities.
- Next generation sequencing technologies have reduced cost and turnaround time of sequencing and have permitted the sequencing of the whole exome or genome.
- Exome or genome sequencing is recommended as first line tests for the evaluation of congenital anomalies, intellectual disability or developmental delay.
- Enzyme replacement therapy is the first line treatment for a number of lysosomal storage disorders.
- Recently approved gene therapies offer treatment options for SMA, RPE65-associated retinal dystrophy, ADA deficiency, β-thalassemia, and sickle cell anemia.
- RNA therapeutics show promising therapeutic benefits for several disorders.

REFERENCES

1. Silva M, de Leeuw N, Mann K, Schuring-Blom H, Morgan S, Giardino D, et al. European guidelines for constitutional cytogenomic analysis. Eur J Hum Genet. 2019;27(1):1-16.
2. Miller DT, Adam MP, Aradhya S, Biesecker LG, Brothman AR, Carter NP, et al. Consensus statement: chromosomal microarray is a first-tier clinical diagnostic test for individuals with developmental disabilities or congenital anomalies. Am J Hum Genet. 2010;86(5):749-64.
3. Karampetsou E, Morrogh D, Chitty L. Microarray technology for the diagnosis of fetal chromosomal aberrations: Which platform should we use? J Clin Med. 2014;3(2):663-78.
4. Manning M, Hudgins L; Professional Practice and Guidelines Committee. Array-based technology and recommendations for utilization in medical genetics practice for detection of chromosomal abnormalities. Genet Med. 2010;12(11):742-5.
5. South ST, Lee C, Lamb AN, Higgins AW, Kearney HM; Working Group for the American College of Medical Genetics and Genomics Laboratory Quality Assurance Committee. ACMG Standards and guidelines for constitutional cytogenomic microarray analysis, including postnatal and prenatal applications: revision 2013. Genet Med. 2013;15(11):901-9.
6. Rehm HL, Bale SJ, Bayrak-Toydemir P, Berg JS, Brown KK, Deignan JL, et al. ACMG clinical laboratory standards for next-generation sequencing. Genet Med. 2013;15(9):733-47.
7. Rehder C, Bean LJH, Bick D, Chao E, Chung W, Das S, et al. Next-generation sequencing for constitutional variants in the clinical laboratory, 2021 revision:

A technical standard of the American College of Medical Genetics and Genomics (ACMG). Genet Med. 2021;23(8):1399-415.
8. Manickam K, McClain MR, Demmer LA, Biswas S, Kearney HM, Malinowski J, et al. Exome and genome sequencing for pediatric patients with congenital anomalies or intellectual disability: an evidence-based clinical guideline of the American College of Medical Genetics and Genomics (ACMG). Genet Med. 2021.
9. ACMG Board of Directors. Points to consider in the clinical application of genomic sequencing. Genet Med. 2012;14(8):759-61.
10. Desnick RJ, Schuchman EH. Enzyme replacement therapy for lysosomal diseases: Lessons from 20 years of experience and remaining challenges. Annu Rev Genomics Hum Genet. 2012;13(1):307-35.
11. Parini R, Deodato F. Intravenous enzyme replacement therapy in mucopolysaccharidoses: Clinical effectiveness and limitations. Int J Mol Sci. 2020;21(8):2975.
12. Li M. Enzyme Replacement Therapy: A review and its role in treating lysosomal storage diseases. Pediatr Ann. 2018;47(5):e191-7.
13. Strachan T, Read AP. Human Molecular Genetics, 5th edition. Garland Science; 2018. p. 784.
14. Li H, Yang Y, Hong W, Huang M, Wu M, Zhao X. Applications of genome editing technology in the targeted therapy of human diseases: mechanisms, advances and prospects. Signal Transduct Target Ther. 2020;5(1):1.
15. Damase TR, Sukhovershin R, Boada C, Taraballi F, Pettigrew RI, Cooke JP. The Limitless Future of RNA Therapeutics, Volume 9, Frontiers in Bioengineering and Biotechnology. 2021. p. 161.
16. Kim Y-K. RNA Therapy: Current Status and future potential. Chonnam Med J. 2020;56(2):87-93.
17. Wang F, Zuroske T, Watts JK. RNA therapeutics on the rise, Volume 19, Nature reviews. Drug discovery. England; 2020. pp. 441-2.
18. Yue WW, Mackinnon S, Bezerra GA. Substrate reduction therapy for inborn errors of metabolism. Emerg Top Life Sci. 2019;3(1):63-73.
19. Coutinho MF, Santos JI, Alves S. Less is more: Substrate reduction therapy for lysosomal storage disorders. Int J Mol Sci. 2016;17(7):1065.
20. Keeling KM, Xue X, Gunn G, Bedwell DM. Therapeutics based on stop codon read through. Annu Rev Genomics Hum Genet. 2014;15:371-94.
21. Dhillon S. Risdiplam: First approval. Drugs. 2020;80(17):1853-8.

Otorhinolaryngology

Obstructive Sleep Apnea

Siddharth Mahesh, Mahesh Babu Ramamurthy

■ INTRODUCTION

As humans, we spend up to a third of our lifetime sleeping! The importance of sleep to the health and well-being cannot be overemphasized. Sleep plays a crucial role in brain development, enhances learning and memory, regulates emotion and appetite as well as maintains the integrity of immune system. It is not just the quantity of sleep, but the quality of sleep that is paramount. One of the most common disorders that impair quality of sleep is "sleep disordered breathing (SDB)". This chapter mainly addresses obstructive sleep apnea (OSA) syndrome, a form of SDB with significant effects on the human body.

■ EPIDEMIOLOGY

Sleep disordered breathing, particularly OSA, is seen across all age groups in children from neonates to adolescents. Snoring is a primary symptom that parents recognize and is widely prevalent in children globally. Various studies have reported a prevalence of 21–68% of snoring in children. A large study from UK reported that 59.7% of children aged between 1 and 4 years had snoring at some time in the past 12 months.[1] Children who snore for more than three nights a week on a regular basis are called "habitual snorers" and the prevalence of habitual snoring in children has been reported as 3–12%.[2-4] Children with habitual snoring who have no apnea, hypopnea, or hypoxic events are called "primary snorers (PS)". Only a small percentage of about 2–3% of children who snore have OSA according to global studies.[4,5] The prevalence of OSA varies with the mode of diagnosis. A prevalence of 9.6% has been reported in 5–10 years old children from India in studies using questionnaires.[6] However, based on overnight sleep studies, this number is likely to be smaller.

■ ETIOPATHOGENESIS

Obstructive sleep apnea is typically characterized by multiple episodes of either complete or partial cessation of oronasal airflow due to repeated upper airway obstruction. The upper airway in humans is quite a complex

TABLE 19.1: The different causes contributing to development of obstructive sleep apnea (OSA) in children and examples of pathologies.

Categories of causes contributing to development of pediatric OSA	Examples of pathologies
Structural causes	• Craniofacial anomalies—maxillary and mandibular hypoplasia and retrognathia • Nasal obstruction—choanal stenosis and nasal polyps • Adenotonsillar hypertrophy • Large tongue
Neuromuscular causes	• Congenital or acquired hypotonia due to any neuronal or muscular cause • Central hypoventilation syndromes • Cerebral palsy
Genetic associations	Syndromic associations such as trisomy 21, mucopolysaccharidosis, and Prader–Willi syndrome
Obesity	
Systemic inflammation	Rhinosinusitis

structure and is involved in three critical processes—swallowing, breathing, and speech. The walls of upper airway are supported mainly by a multitude of small muscles of the pharyngeal wall and some soft tissue structures such as the tonsils, soft palate, and the tongue. The only bony structures lending stability are the mandible and the floating hyoid. The site of obstruction in OSA is different in adults (retropalatal and retroglossal areas) and in children (adenoids, soft palate, and tonsils).

From a therapeutic standpoint, OSA can be due to various processes, either in isolation or combination: (1) anatomical (structural) narrowing of upper airway, (2) inflammatory swelling of the lymphoid tissue, and (3) obesity.

Causes for OSA can be varied in children **(Table 19.1)**. Upper airway stability and patency depend on two discrete factors—structural and neuromuscular. Since the upper airway wall is mainly formed by musculature, it is not difficult to imagine that the lumen will tend to collapse when there is hypotonia of the muscles, as observed in myopathies. The other major factor is the structure of the airway. Anything that reduces the luminal diameter will cause upper airway resistance and collapse. Interplay between these two factors is important and helps to understand why two children with similar sized adenoids and tonsils have different clinical pictures. One with good muscle tone might be normal while the other with decreased muscle tone will present with OSA. Obesity is a new age pandemic, which causes OSA by more than one mechanism,

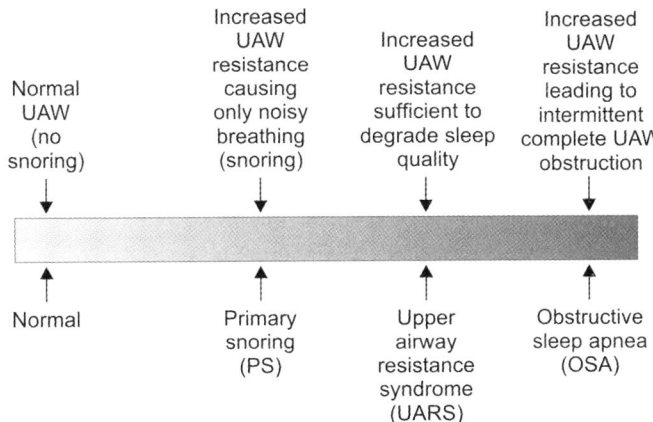

Fig. 19.1: Spectrum of obstructed sleep disordered breathing. (UAW: upper airway)

with structural narrowing of airway and airway inflammation being significant factors. The upper airway obstruction that occurs in OSA results in frequent arousals and intermittent short hypoxia events. These two pathophysiological processes underlie most of the sequelae that occurs in OSA.

CLINICAL FEATURES AND CLASSIFICATION

Obstructive SDB is not a single clinical entity but a spectrum with varied clinical manifestations and implications. Snoring is a common thread across the spectrum and patients can be categorized clinically based on signs and symptoms **(Fig. 19.1)**.

Primary Snorers

These are children with habitual snoring who do not have any apnea/hypopnea, gas abnormalities or who do not experience any arousals during sleep. These patients were initially thought to have a benign condition, but today we know that these children not only have a higher incidence of behavioral, attentional (such as hyperactivity and inattention), and social problems but also have a higher mean diastolic blood pressure.[7,8]

Upper Airway Resistance Syndrome

These are children with habitual snoring who have increased work of breathing, nasal airflow limitation, and increased arousals during sleep without associated respiratory events (apnea/hypopnea) or gas abnormalities. Children with upper airway resistance syndrome (UARS) complain of daytime tiredness and fatigue. They also tend to experience somatized symptoms.[9]

Obstructive Sleep Apnea

This is the extreme form of SDB with recurrent partial or complete obstruction of upper airway leading to abnormalities in saturation, carbon dioxide clearance, and sleep architecture.

■ HISTORY AND EXAMINATION

A detailed history is the first step in assessing a child for SDB. *Snoring* is the primary symptom that needs to be asked about first. Snoring is present in most children with OSA, but snoring is not specific to OSA. Once a history of snoring is obtained, it is then important to establish other features sequentially including the loudness of snoring, regularity of snoring, and witnessed apnea. Many parents will provide a history of snoring only when the child is tired or during upper respiratory tract infections, with no snoring in between. These children need to be monitored.

Daytime symptoms in pediatric OSA differ from adults **(Table 19.2)**. While most adults with OSA tend to have increased daytime somnolence, most children with OSA tend to be hyperactive and restless during daytime. However, a subgroup of children with significant obesity with OSA tends to follow adult behavior and sleep more during the day.[10]

Though most children with OSA may not have any specific findings on clinical examination, it is good to systematically look for physical signs. Some children will either have telltale signs of contributing factors or sequelae of OSA. *Adenotonsillar hypertrophy* is a common finding, though not an indispensable feature. Children with chronic adenoid hypertrophy often have characteristic adenoid facies, mouth breathing, long and elongated facial features, short upper lips, thin nostrils, high arched palate, and dull looking facies. Whether these features are a cause or effect of OSA still remains unknown.[11] Craniofacial features must be particularly looked for. These include maxillary hypoplasia, retrognathia, or micrognathia. A quick look at the lateral profile of the face is also important to pick up mandibular abnormalities.

TABLE 19.2: Nocturnal and daytime symptoms in a child with suspected OSA.

History-taking in a child with obstructive sleep apnea (OSA)

Nocturnal symptoms	Daytime symptoms
Snoring	Difficulty in waking up
Witnessed apnea	Morning headaches
Labored breathing/ paradoxical breathing	Dry mouth
Restlessness	Daytime somnolence
Enuresis	Hyperactivity/poor attention
Neck hyperextension	Poor school performance
Parasomnias	Poor growth

In children with longstanding OSA, clinical features of sequelae may be increasingly prevalent. There is an increased prevalence of behavioral dysregulation (hyperactivity, attention deficits, and impulsivity), impaired memory and learning, impaired executive functioning (planning and carrying out problem solving skills), and impaired verbal reasoning and general intelligence in children with longstanding OSA.[12] Cardiovascular complications of OSA include systemic hypertension, pulmonary hypertension (evidenced by loud P2 in longstanding OSA) and left ventricular remodeling on echocardiography. OSA has been implicated in failure to thrive, with better growth patterns seen in children after adenotonsillectomy.[13]

DIAGNOSIS

While snoring is relatively common in children, diagnosis of OSA in children has proven to be a challenge. As with most medical conditions, a good history and clinical examination are the first steps in the diagnosis. However, even a good history has its limitations, and it is difficult to diagnose primary snoring from OSA and to grade the severity of OSA. Whilst the overnight polysomnogram/polysomnography (PSG) is considered the gold standard in diagnosis of OSA, its limited availability and high cost globally have limited its use. As a result, there have been many attempts over the years to create diagnostic tools to diagnose and grade OSA. These are reviewed below.

Sleep Questionnaires

There have been several sleep questionnaires that have been developed for screening and diagnosing OSA.[14] An initial score by Brouillette based on observed apnea, dyspnea, and snoring had a high sensitivity but low specificity. OSA-18 is an 18 item-based questionnaire that is frequently used. Though it had good reports initially, later analysis revealed a sensitivity of only 40%. Another commonly used pediatric OSA questionnaire is the sleep-related breathing disorder scale (SBD scale). This was shown to have a sensitivity of 85% and specificity of 81% in diagnosing OSA. Children's sleep habits questionnaire (CSHQ) with a subsection on OSA has also been used. The general limitations of these questionnaires are the low specificity and the time taken to complete these questionnaires in a busy clinic. Researchers are still looking at a shortened item list which can be validated. So, at this point, though a good history can be used as a screening tool, it cannot be used to diagnose OSA with confidence.

Home Audio and Video Recording

This is a relatively low hanging fruit in diagnostics. With the wide use of smartphones in most countries, it is easy for parents to record events at home. In fact, many parents bring recordings of their children's sleep to the clinics. The onus is then on the pediatrician to make the diagnosis. Unfortunately, this form of diagnosis is not evidence-based at present. In the 1990's, Goldstein et al. tried correlating audio recordings with PSG scores. Though the audio recordings had a sensitivity of 92%, the specificity was only 29%. Furthermore, while the negative predictive value was 83%, the positive predictive value was only 50%.[15] Hence, these recordings could potentially be used only as screening tools. Sivan et al. analyzed parent-initiated video recordings of their child's sleep with PSG. When compared to PSG, the video recordings had a sensitivity of 94% but a specificity of only 68% and hence these cannot be used for definitive diagnosis.[16] However, with improving technology, these diagnostic modalities still have a lot of potential for the future.

Pulse Oximetry

Intermittent transient hypoxia is the hallmark of OSA. Therefore, measuring hypoxia with pulse oximetry overnight during sleep has been used as an investigative tool for OSA. However, since SDB is not a single entity but a spectrum, measuring overnight saturations will only help diagnose children with extreme conditions such as OSA, and conditions such as primary snoring, UARS, and obstructive hypoventilation (which do not have hypoxia) are bound to be missed.

Transient hypoxia in OSA is not defined as a drop in oxygen below a specific saturation (such as 92% for example), but is instead defined as a drop in saturation of ≥3% from baseline (i.e., a drop to 95% from 98% is recorded as a desaturation event). These events are very transient lasting for just a few seconds. Hence, the oximetry device must have the appropriate sensitivity to pick these transient desaturations. Most oximetry instruments used in hospitals and intensive care units display an output that is averaged over a long period of time (12–16 seconds). Therefore, we need equipment with shorter averaging times of 2–6 seconds for overnight pulse oximetry.

The main advantage of pulse oximetry is the fact that it can be done at home, in the natural environment for the child. A minimum of 6 hours of recording in the night is recommended. Conducting studies across multiple nights is preferred, although some studies have shown that one night is sufficient.[17] If the pulse oximetry is positive for recurrent hypoxia, then it is confirmatory of an existent problem. However, if the result is negative or inconclusive, then a PSG is indicated. Most modern pulse oximeters come with a recording software capable of beat-to-beat recording. It is then possible to download this data with a trend of saturations with time and other useful information. Many scoring systems have been developed to analyze overnight pulse oximetry studies. One of the commonly used scoring algorithms is McGill score.[18] **Table 19.3** shows the approach this scoring system uses.

TABLE 19.3: Different types of study results for the diagnosis of OSA as defined by the McGill score.[18]

Description	Definition
A "desaturation"	≥4% fall in saturation
A "cluster"	≥5 desaturations within a 30-minute period
A "positive" study	≥3 clusters with ≥3 desaturations to <90%
An "inconclusive" study	Not a positive study (i.e., <3 clusters or <desaturations below 90%)

TABLE 19.4: Management of OSA based on oximetry scores.[19]

| Oximetry score | Comment | Criteria | | | Recommendation |
		Number of drops in $SaO_2 < 90\%$	Number of drops in $SaO_2 < 85\%$	Number of drops in $SaO_2 < 80\%$	
1	Normal study/inconclusive for OSA	<3	0	0	Additional evaluation of breathing during sleep required
2	OSA, mild	≥3	≤3	0	Required T&A on waiting list
3	OSA, moderate	≥3	>3	≤3	
4	OSA, severe	≥3	>3	>3	Recommend urgent surgery

(SaO_2: oxygen saturations by pulse oximetry; T&A: adenotonsillectomy)

For use in resource-crunched centers, a modified approach has been used to predict management of pediatric OSA based on pulse oximetry **(Table 19.4)**.[19]

However, pulse oximetry also comes with its limitations. As noted earlier, a negative study does not rule out OSA. Children with cold and vasoconstricted peripheries are not ideal candidates. There are bound to be motion artifacts in the study, though some of the newer software do have the ability to cancel them. Since different types of hemoglobins have varied adsorption spectrum, hence children with abnormal hemoglobin types are not candidates for this study either.

In summary, pulse oximetry is an affordable, reliable, and reproducible test that can be used for diagnosing OSA. Children with negative tests will still need PSG to rule out OSA and investigate further.

Polysomnography

Polysomnography is considered the gold standard for diagnosis of OSA in children. As the name suggests, it literally means recording many channels during sleep. PSG is an overnight recording and a minimum of 6 hours of

TABLE 19.5: A list of the most used channels in PSG.

Channels	Purpose	Sensors
EEG, EOG, Chin EMG	Staging of sleep	Electrodes on scalp, chin and face
Airflow	Recognizing apnea and hypopnea	Thermistor and nasal pressure transducer
Respiratory effort	Recognizing respiratory effort	Chest and abdominal belts (either RIP or piezoelectric)
Peripheral oxygen saturation	Recognizing desaturations	Pulse oximeter
Carbon dioxide (CO_2)	Recognizing hypoventilation	Either transcutaneous or endotracheal CO_2
ECG	Measuring heart rate	Thoracic electrodes
Audio	Recognizing snoring	Microphone over neck
Video	Recognizing awake state, body position and abnormal movements	Infrared camera in the room

(EEG: electroencephalogram; EOG: electrooculogram; EMG: electromyogram; ECG: electrocardiogram; CO_2: carbon dioxide monitoring, RIP: respiratory inductance plethysmography)

sleep recording is required, although 8 hours are preferred. Most pediatric PSGs are hospital-based and technician-monitored. A child-friendly sleep lab and technician are preferred, especially in young children who tend to remove the leads frequently. While home PSG is accepted in adults, it is not yet part of guidelines in children. There are many studies now, with advancing technology, to show that home polygraphy [limited channels without electroencephalogram (EEG)] is acceptable to make a diagnosis of OSA in the majority of children.[20,21] However, one needs to be careful in validating the data and interpreting it. The channels used in PSG commonly are shown in **Table 19.5**.

In a pediatric PSG, a limited number of EEG channels are recorded using a 10–20 system of electrode placement. Generally, pairs of frontal, central, and occipital leads are used. Additionally, two channels are used to record oronasal airflow; the thermistor (a temperature sensor which recognizes the warm expiratory breath and can hence measure the presence/absence of airflow) and the pressure transducer (device measuring subtle airflow resistance and inspiratory flow). The thermistors are useful in detecting complete cessation of breath (apnea), while the nasal pressure transducers are useful in detecting drop in airflow (hypopnea) and UARS.[22] The abdominal and the respiratory belts not only aid in detecting respiratory movements, but also the asynchrony between abdominal and thoracic movements which suggests upper airway resistance/obstruction.

TABLE 19.6: Description of some of the respiratory events recorded by a polysomnogram (PSG).[23]

Events	Description
Central apnea	>90% drop in airflow signal associated with absence of inspiratory effort that lasts for 20 seconds (without associated criteria) or lasts for a duration of two normal breaths and is associated with any of the following: • Drop of ≥3% saturations or • Cortical arousal or • Associated with drop in the heart rate to <50/min for at least 5 seconds
Obstructive apnea	>90% drop in airflow signal that lasts for duration of at least two normal breaths associated with continued or increased inspiratory effort during the entire period
Mixed apnea	>90% drop in airflow signal that lasts for a duration of at least two normal breaths associated with absent respiratory effort during one portion of the event and presence of inspiratory effort in another portion, regardless of which portion comes first
Hypopnea	≥30% decrease in airflow signal lasting for duration of at least 2 normal breaths associated with either • Cortical arousal or • ≥3% drop in saturation
Respiratory effort-related arousal (RERA)	Respiratory event (increased respiratory effort, flattening of the inspiratory portion of the nasal pressure waveform, snoring or an elevation in end tidal CO_2 ($ETCO_2$) that leads to arousal and does not qualify as an apnea or hypopnea
Sleep-related hypoventilation	End tidal or transcutaneous CO_2 >50 mm Hg for >25% of the total sleep time

Polysomnography in modern times is a digital recording. The monitor screen is calibrated to show a set duration of sleep called an "epoch". Traditionally, 30-second epochs are used while looking at an EEG and staging sleep whilst two-minute epochs are used while scoring the respiratory leads. Reading and scoring sleep studies are often challenging and time-consuming. Conventionally, interpreters normally start by staging sleep (staged as awake, non-REM sleep stages 1, 2, and 3, and REM sleep) followed by scoring arousals in EEG, suggesting interruption of sleep. This is then followed by scoring of respiratory events. Some of the respiratory events that are scored are listed below **(Table 19.6)**.[23]

Based on the respiratory events, the obstructive apnea-hypopnea index (OAHI) is calculated to grade OSA. This is calculated by dividing the sum of all obstructive apneas and hypopneas by the total sleep time in hours. A normal score is an OAHI of less than one. **Table 19.7** shows the grading of OSA in children as per the OAHI score.

TABLE 19.7: Grading of OSA in children according to the obstructive apnea-hypopnea index (OAHI) score.

OAHI	Grading of OSA in children
1–4.9	Mild OSA
5–9.9	Moderate OSA
>10	Severe OSA

Though a PSG should ideally be performed for all children with suspected OSA, it is impractical considering the costs and availability. If a child in the typical age group (2–10 years) presents with symptoms of OSA associated with unequivocal enlarged tonsils/adenoids, then there is no need for PSG in such a child, particularly in resource-crunched areas. Indications for pediatric PSG in the context of OSA can be listed as:
- In children with comorbidities such as obesity, craniofacial syndromes, trisomy 21, and neuromuscular disorders.
- If there is discrepancy between history and clinical findings.
- Recurrence/persistence of symptoms after adenotonsillectomy.
- Titration of positive airway pressure (PAP)—continuous positive airway pressure or bilevel positive airway pressure (CPAP and BiPAP) for OSA.

There are certainly limitations with PSG as well. The cost and the availability of pediatric PSG beds are globally limited. As it is organized in a hospital environment, it certainly is affected by the "first night effect" with children sleeping for longer in the supine position and having less rapid eye movement (REM) and stage 3 sleep. However, these factors affect the sleep parameters but not the respiratory parameters. PSG is currently mainly used to score OAHI and does not look at the end organ morbidity.

Drug-induced Sleep Endoscopy

While a nasal endoscopy is often done to estimate the size of adenoids before a surgery, it is not required for diagnosis. Drug-induced sleep endoscopy (DISE) is a variation where upper airway dynamics are studied in simulated sleep.

It is now becoming clear that adenotonsillectomy is not curative in many children with OSA. A significant number will have residual OSA and while a repeat PSG will show the presence of residual OSA, it will not show the site of obstruction. In these scenarios, an upper airway endoscopy in children with drug-induced sleep will demonstrate the level of obstruction. It is performed with sedation under strict protocols. The medications commonly used are propofol and midazolam. The usual sites of obstruction cited in literature include lingual tonsil, residual/regrowth of adenoids, tongue base prolapse, and laryngomalacia. DISE-directed surgery is a practical possibility.[24]

While there are many smart watch and smart phone apps which are proposed to look at sleep in children, these are not useful for OSA at present. They are not evidence-based. There is a lot of promise of alternative source of diagnosis, and this is an exciting space to look out for.

■ MANAGEMENT

There is no controversy that children with moderate-to-severe OSA need definitive management. However, there is variability in the management of mild OSA. There is literature to show that watchful waiting results in improvement in a sizable population of patients with mild OSA. This, however, might not hold for children with moderate-to-severe OSA.[25] While it is important to know the PSG results when available, the management of a child with OSA should be guided by a sum of clinical presentation, presence of risk factors, and the associated comorbidities.

Adenotonsillectomy

Adenotonsillectomy is the first line of treatment for OSA in otherwise normal children. This however, is not a recent advance.[26] Adenotonsillectomy has been documented to improve symptoms and OAHI scores in children with OSA. In fact, there have been good studies to show that there is significant improvement of cognition after surgery as well. Adenotonsillectomy is a relatively safe surgery today. However, one needs to look for complications such as respiratory compromise, secondary hemorrhage, and postoperative pulmonary edema in children with severe OSA.

Since the beginning of the millennium, there have been quite a few papers demonstrating residual OSA in children after adenotonsillectomy. This is particularly more prevalent in children with other risk factors including obesity, severe OSA presurgery, older age (>7 years), craniofacial anomalies, trisomy 21, and children with neuromuscular diseases. In fact, there is now evidence that even those who normalize their OAHI scores after surgery within the first 6 months start having recurrence of symptoms within the first few years postoperatively.[27] Hence, it is imperative that the physicians follow-up all children who undergo adenotonsillectomy for recurrence.

Other Surgical Options

Rapid maxillary expansion (RME), a procedure that gradually helps to increase the transverse breadth of hard palate over time has been found to be useful, particularly in children with high arched narrow palate and retrusive bites.[28] Similarly mandibular distraction surgery is known to help children with significant retrognathia.[29]

Positive Airway Pressure Therapy

Unlike adults, PAP therapy is not the first line in an otherwise normal child with OSA. It is, however, should be considered in children with:
- Significant obesity
- Craniofacial anomalies and structural defects
- Residual moderate/severe OSA after adenotonsillectomy
- Contraindications for surgery (adenotonsillectomy)
- Neuromuscular diseases.

While CPAP is usually the mode of PAP chosen, children with neuromuscular diseases and nocturnal hypoventilation will benefit from BiPAP.

One of the greatest hurdles with PAP therapy, apart from cost, is adherence, which is extremely poor. It is important to have a conversation with the parents and the child (if appropriate) at the beginning. Once PAP has been initiated, the family is encouraged to use the device with minimal pressure for a couple of weeks before a titration PSG is organized. During this period, PSG is done with the child using the PAP device and the PAP pressures are individually titrated to suit the child. These children should then be followed up closely as outpatients and it helps to see them at regular intervals. The new PAP machines come with a memory card. It is extremely beneficial to have patients bring the past few months of recording from their memory card. This helps to estimate the adherence and the pressure requirements.

There are a few side effects which need to be monitored for, which include nasal bridge pressure marks secondary to mask use, discomfort due to air leaks, oral dryness, and abdominal distention. It is also important to note that children requiring long-term PAP (and for extended hours) tend to develop skeletal changes (flattening of mid face) due to pressure of masks.

Medical Therapy

Tonsils removed from children with OSA are known to express increased levels of leukotriene receptors.[30] Similarly, the lymphoid tissues from adenoids and tonsils in children with OSA have been shown to secrete cytokines IL-6, IL-8, and TNF-α. Therefore, antileukotrienes such as montelukast and anti-inflammatory inhaled nasal steroids (INS) have been trialed in management of OSA. At present they are considered in children with residual OSA after adenotonsillectomy and in children who are being managed conservatively. If considered, they have to be given a 4-week trial. INS showed a moderate decrease in OAHI in children with OSA and can be given alone.[31] If there is improvement, then the duration of medication can be prolonged. Though montelukast has also showed some response, its use is limited by the possibility of neuropsychiatric symptoms as side effects.[32]

Other Modalities of Noninvasive Management

In the recent past, there has been an increased interest in myofunctional therapy. Having known that muscle tone actively contributes to OSA in children, myofunctional therapy aims to teach children oropharyngeal exercises and improve tongue posture. While some studies have shown benefit, the main challenges are sustaining adherence and practicing proper technique.

Weight loss is another measure which has been shown to help, especially children with obesity.[33] Considering the difficulties associated with achieving weight loss, it is preferable to treat children with obesity associated with significant OSA using CPAP while concurrently encouraging weight loss.

■ FUTURE DIRECTIONS

While a lot has been achieved in the past two to three decades in pediatric sleep, there is still a long way to go. PSG is useful in providing us with an OAHI score, but it does not give us information of end organ morbidity of OSA on the individual child. Whilst there have been studies looking at biomarkers (urine, blood, and breath), these have not been consistent. This is probably the way to move forward to try and individualize approach and move towards precision therapy.

■ KEY POINTS

- Snoring is quite prevalent in children of all ages.
- Prevalence of OSA is about 2–3% in children.
- Adenotonsillar hypertrophy is the most common cause of OSA in an otherwise normal child.
- Overnight PSG is currently considered gold standard for diagnosis, however, overnight saturation study can be used in picking up children with OSA.
- Adenotonsillectomy is the first line of treatment for children with OSA.
- Continuous positive airway pressure is useful in managing children with structural issues and children with residual OSA after adenotonsillectomy.

■ REFERENCES

1. Kuehni CE, Strippoli MPF, Chauliac ES, Silverman M. Snoring in preschool children: Prevalence, severity and risk factors. Eur Respir J. 2008;31(2):326-3.
2. Brockmann PE, Bertrand P, Pardo T, Cerda J, Reyes B, Holmgren NL. Prevalence of habitual snoring and associated neurocognitive consequences among Chilean school aged children. Int J Pediatr Otorhinolaryngol. 2012;76(9):1327-31.
3. Hornero R, Kheirandish-Gozal L, Gutiérrez-Tobal GC, Philby MF, Alonzo-Álvarez ML, Álvarez D, et al. Nocturnal oximetry-based evaluation of habitually snoring children. Am J Respir Crit Care Med. 2017;196(12):1591-8.
4. Kaditis AG, Finder J, Alexopoulos EI, Starantzis K, Tanou K, Gampeta S, et al. Sleep-disordered breathing in 3,680 Greek children. Pediatr Pulmonol. 2004;27(6):499-509.

5. Lumeng JC, Chervin RD. Epidemiology of pediatric obstructive sleep apnea. Proc Am Thorac Soc. 2008;5(2):242-52.
6. Goyal A, Pakhare AP, Bhatt GC, Choudhary B, Patil R. Association of pediatric obstructive sleep apnea with poor academic performance: A school-based study from India. Lung India. 2018;35(2):132-6.
7. Hagström K, Saarenpää-Heikkilä O, Himanen S-L, Lampinlampi AM, Rantanen K. Neurobehavioral outcomes in school-aged children with primary snoring. Arch Clin Neuropsychol. 2020;35(4):401-12.
8. Li AM, Au CT, Ho C, Fok TF, Wing YK. Blood pressure is elevated in children with primary snoring. J Pediatr. 2009:115(3):362-8.
9. Guilleminault C, Kirisoglu C, Poyares D, Palombini L, Leger D, Farid-Moayer M, et al. Upper airway resistance syndrome: A long-term outcome study. J Psych Res. 2006:40(3):273-9.
10. Dayyat E, Kheirandish-Gozal L, Gozal D. Childhood Obstructive Sleep Apnea: One or Two Distinct Disease Entities? Sleep Med Clin. 2007;2(3):433-44.
11. Eber E, Midulla F. ERS Handbook of Paediatric Respiratory Medicine. United Kingdom: European Respiratory Society Publication; 2021.
12. O'Brien LM, Mervis CB, Holbrook CR, Bruner JL, Klaus CJ, Rutherford J, et al. Neurobehavioral implications of habitual snoring in children. Pediatrics. 2004;114(1):44-9.
13. Katz ES, Moore RH, Rosen CL, Mitchell RB, Amin R, Arens R, et al. Growth after adenotonsillectomy for obstructive sleep apnea: An RCT. Pediatrics. 2014;134(2):282-9.
14. Kadmon G, Shapiro CM, Chung SA, Gozal D. Validation of a pediatric obstructive sleep apnea screening tool. Int J Pediatr Otorhinolaryngol. 2013;77(9):1461-4.
15. Goldstein NA, Sculerati N, Walsleben JA, Bhatia N, Friedman DM, Rapoport DM, et al. Clinical diagnosis of pediatric obstructive sleep apnea validated by polysomnography. Otolaryngol Head Neck Surg. 1994;111(5):611-7.
16. Sivan Y, Kornecki A, Schonfeld T. Screening obstructive sleep apnoea syndrome by home videotape recording in children. Eur Respir J. 1996;9(10):2127-31.
17. Pavone M, Cutrera R, Verrillo E, Salerno T, Soldini S, Brouillette RT. Night-to-night consistency of at-home nocturnal pulse oximetry testing for obstructive sleep apnea in children. Pediatr Pulmonol. 2013;48(8):754-60.
18. Brouillette RT, Morielli A, Leimanis A, Waters KA, Luciano R, Ducharme FM. Nocturnal pulse oximetry as an abbreviated testing modality for pediatric obstructive sleep apnea. Pediatrics. 2000;105(2)405-12.
19. Nixon GM, Kermack AS, Davis GM, Manoukian JJ, Brown KA, Brouillette RT, et al. Planning adenotonsillectomy in children with obstructive sleep apnea: the role of overnight oximetry. Pediatrics. 2004;113(1):19-25.
20. Kingshott RN, Gahleitner F, Elphick HE, Gringras P, Farquhar M, Pickering RM, et al. Cardiorespiratory sleep studies at home: Experience in research and clinical cohorts. Arch Dis Child. 2019;104(5):476-81.
21. Chiner E, Cánovas C, Molina V, Sancho-Chust JN, Vañes S, Pastor E, et al. Clinical Medicine Home Respiratory Polygraphy is Useful in the Diagnosis of Childhood Obstructive Sleep Apnea Syndrome. J Clin Med. 2020;9(7):2067.
22. Medscape. (2020). Polysomnography: Overview, Parameters Monitored, Staging of Sleep. [online] Available from https://emedicine.medscape.com/article/1188764-overview#showall [Last accessed December, 2021].

23. Grigg-damberger AM. (2019). Overview of polysomnography in infants and children. [online] Available from https://www.uptodate.com/contents/overview-of-polysomnography-in-infants-and-children?topicRef=6357&source=related_link [Last accessed December, 2021].
24. He S, Peddireddy NS, Smith DF, Duggins AL, Heubi C, Shott SR, et al. Outcomes of drug-induced sleep endoscopy-directed surgery for pediatric obstructive sleep apnea. Orig Res Otolaryngol Otolaryngol Neck Surg. 2018;158(3):559-65.
25. Marcus CL, Moore RH, Rosen CL, Giordani B, Garetz SL, Taylor HG, et al. A randomized trial of adenotonsillectomy for childhood sleep apnea. N Engl J Med. 2013;368(25):2366-76.
26. Hill W. On some causes of backwardness and stupidity in children: and the relife of these symptoms in some instances by naso-pharyngeal scarifications. Br Med J. 1889;2(1500):711-2.
27. Huang YS, Guilleminault C, Lee LA, Lin CH, Hwang FM. Treatment outcomes of adenotonsillectomy for children with obstructive sleep apnea: a prospective longitudinal study. Sleep. 2014;37(1):71-7.
28. Villa MP, Rizzoli A, Rabasco J, Vitelli O, Pietropaoli N, Cecili M, et al. Rapid maxillary expansion outcomes in treatment of obstructive sleep apnea in children. Sleep Med. 2015;16(6):709-16.
29. Noller MW, Guilleminault C, Gouveia CJ, Mack D, Neighbors CL, Zaghi S, et al. Mandibular advancement for pediatric obstructive sleep apnea: A systematic review and meta-analysis. J Craniomaxillofac Surg. 2018;46(8):1296-1302
30. Kheirandish L. Intranasal steroids and oral leukotriene modifier therapy in residual sleep-disordered breathing after tonsillectomy and adenoidectomy in children. Pediatrics. 2006;117(1):e61-6.
31. Brouillette RT, Manoukian JJ, Ducharme FM, Oudjhane K, Earle LG, Ladan S, et al. Efficacy of fluticasone nasal spray for pediatric obstructive sleep apnea. J Pediatr. 2001;138(6):838-44.
32. Goldbart AD, Goldman JL, Veling MC, Gozal D. Leukotriene modifier therapy for mild sleep-disordered breathing in children. Am J Respir Crit Care Med. 2005;172(3):364-70.
33. Gillberg Andersen I, Holm J-C, Homøe P. Impact of weight-loss management on children and adolescents with obesity and obstructive sleep apnea. Int J Pediatr Otorhinolaryngol. 2019;123:57-62.

Developmental Pediatrics

CHAPTER 20

Nurturing Care for Early Childhood Development

Nandita Chattopadhyay

■ INTRODUCTION

Growth and development are unique for children. Development is a process whereby children learn gradually to gain control over themselves and their environment, through phases of maturation in different domains. This process continues seamlessly from conception to adulthood. Early childhood development (ECD) alludes to the initial few years when development occurs at a peak velocity. Though the World Health Organization (WHO) refers to the first 8 years of life as the period of early development, in common parlance ECD refers to the **first three years**, as this is the period when the most rapid brain development transpires.

■ NEUROBIOLOGY OF DEVELOPMENT

Neurobiology explains how the brain develops in the first few years and indicates the importance of this period. By the age of 1 year, the total brain volume reaches 72% of the adult size; thereafter it increases by an additional 15% over the second year.[1] In the first year of life, the neurons form new connections at a tremendous rate of 700–1,000 per second.[2] The prolific neuronal growth results in approximately 100 billion neurons, each with an average of 15,000 synapses by 3 years of age.

Eventually, there is systematic trimming of this "overgrowth" by a process of pruning of the synapses. This pruning pattern depends on the experiences gained by the brain. Synapses in the "often-used" pathways are preserved, whereas the "less-used" ones atrophy. This unique characteristic, referred to as *neuroplasticity* is most marked in the early years but continues into adolescence, though at a slower pace. During this later phase of life we observe remarkable development of the prefrontal cortex, which is concerned with planning, decision-making and emotional control. This gradual shaping of the brain and its neural connections are largely driven by the child's environment.

Significant changes are noted in the anatomical and physiologic characteristics of the brain in preschool children. Total cortical area is seen to increase while cortical thickness is diminished. In the gray and white matter of the brain, cellular properties of neuronal tissues such as diffusion in the cerebral fiber tracts change drastically leading to an increase in metabolic demands of the brain.

As the brain structure evolves, the child learns new functions. These skills or functions build from "bottom up".[3] A child first learns simple skills; based on them more complex and finer skills are acquired. If there is a learning gap at the initial stage, difficulties may ensue at a later age in learning finer skills. For example, early fine motor skills like fingering, grasping and manipulating small toys form the basis for good pencil grip and early writing skills.[1] Not only motor skills but cognitive and behavioral development will also falter if the functional connectivity of the neurons is disrupted, thereby sometimes leading to psychiatric and developmental disorders. Functional magnetic resonance imaging (fMRI) studies have demonstrated such disruptions.

A child's physical and mental health, cognitive development, social skills as well as the lifelong capacity to learn, adapt to change, and develop psychological resilience are dependent largely on the environmental stimulation available to the developing brain.[3] Thus, the early years provide a window of opportunity to influence brain development through adequate environmental stimulation to bring out the best in the child. Now, let us examine what comprises this optimum stimulating environment and what are the determinants for early development.

■ DETERMINANTS OF EARLY CHILDHOOD DEVELOPMENT

Numerous factors influence the development of the fetus in-utero and the baby in the first few years, both as risk factors and protective factors (**Flowchart 20.1**). The risk factors may be biological as well as social or environmental.[4,5] The biological risk factors include neonatal risk factors, genetic disorders, malnutrition and illnesses whereas the social or environmental factors include lack of stimulation, poor parenting, child neglect/abuse, poverty, etc. The protective factors on the other hand are breastfeeding, family support and resilience along with peer interaction.

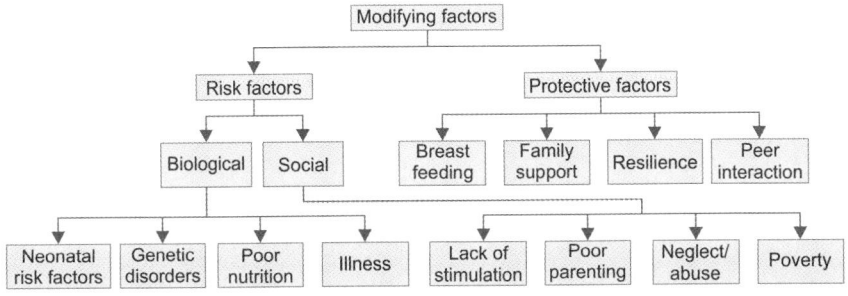

Flowchart 20.1: Determinants of early childhood development.

Biological Factors

Various biological factors may influence brain development.[4] They range from genetic constitution, in utero exposure to teratogens, perinatal insult to the developing brain as a result of prematurity, low birth-weight (LBW), birth asphyxia and other postnatal illnesses such as hypoglycemia, sepsis, and meningitis. Exposure to hazardous substances (e.g., lead and mercury), inborn errors of metabolism and various other systemic illnesses can also affect development, both directly and indirectly. The indirect effects of systemic illness include poor nutrition, lack of parental attention, and poor engagement with peers. A child's temperament and behavior may also be influenced by maternal prenatal and perinatal stress and anxiety, possibly through the effect of stress hormones.[5]

Environmental Factors

Environment plays a major role in shaping the structure and function of the young brain, thereby determining the level of early development of a child.[5] Genes provide the blueprint for brain development on which the environment works to give final shape to the brain.[6] The richer the psychomotor stimulation, the better will be a child's brain development. The young child develops a cause-and-effect logic of her/his own, based on the response she/he receives to the cues she/he provides and vice-versa. Every time a cue given by the baby is responded to promptly, it sends a signal to the tiny brain that this cue is effective, so now the child gives a counter-response. Thus, the to-and-fro interaction continues, stimulating the growing brain. This mechanism has been termed as the "serve and return" principle of learning, based on the analogy from the game of tennis.[7] The more effective and consistent our responses are, the better is the learning process. In many situations caregivers are unaware about normal child development and the necessity to augment brain development through simple interventions and fail to provide necessary environmental stimulation, which eventually hampers adequate development in a child.

Research has shown that the greatest threats to ECD are inadequate psychomotor stimulation, extreme poverty, poor parenting, neglect, abuse, insecurity, gender inequities, violence, environmental toxins, and poor maternal mental health.[8,9] These threats are not rare events. Presently it is estimated that 250 million children are living in countries affected by armed conflict, while 160 million are likely to suffer from famine and food insecurity.[10]

Life Cycle Approach to Developmental Risk Factors[11]

Though the target age for stimulating early childhood development is from conception to 3 years, interventions at all ages directly or indirectly affects the

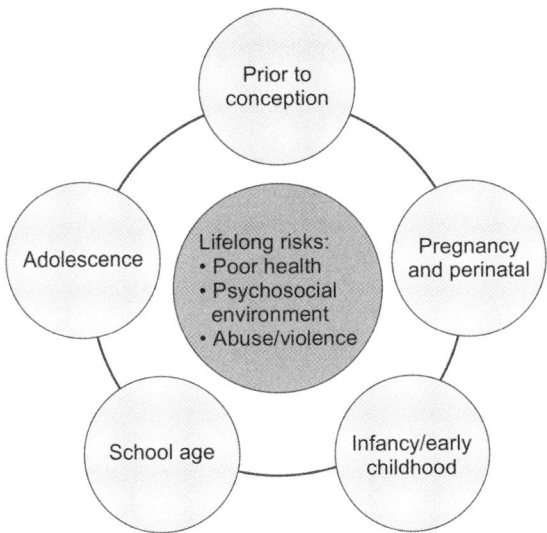

Fig. 20.1: Life cycle approach to developmental risk factors.

Source: Adapted from Chattopadhyay N. Early childhood development: the buzz word in child health today. J Community Med Public Health Care. 2019;6:061.

wellbeing of the little ones **(Fig. 20.1)**. Care of a pregnant mother directly helps in the growth and development of the growing fetus. Her nutrition, physical and mental health, understanding about childcare and the preparedness for child rearing are all essential elements. The father also needs to be primed and sensitized toward a wholesome parenthood. Young women, adolescent girls and boys need proper diet, healthy habits, and health education to prepare the ground for a healthy family life. Measures to prevent early marriage and adolescent pregnancy are effective in this age group.

Going further back, young children should be provided adequate health care, nutrition, and education, so that they grow up into healthy, stable parents. A stunted, malnourished little girl will grow into a stunted, anemic woman, who is more prone to deliver a low birthweight (LBW) or preterm baby. Moreover, if this girl enters family life early and has an early pregnancy in her adolescent years, the problems multiply few folds, leading to poor early childhood development in the baby. Parental care and attitude remain inadequate among parents with poor education. So, we see that positive intervention at every age will augment early childhood development; hence the importance of a life cycle approach is paramount.

■ WHY IS EARLY CHILDHOOD DEVELOPMENT IMPORTANT?

Early childhood forms the basis of future adult life. A child who gets appropriate stimulation from her/his environment to promote early learning and who gets adequate attention, love and care grows up into a well-adjusted, sociable adult, who performs well in life and makes a good citizen. The foundations for lifelong health, social and emotional wellbeing and productivity are predominantly built in the first 3 years. For example, social and emotional skills gained through secure, emotionally stable relationships with parents help generate empathy and self-control in later life, which inhibit criminal tendencies and violence.[8,12] So, it is evident that today's focus on ECD will lay the foundation for tomorrow's healthy and prosperous society.

Good learning opportunity in the early years enhances later educational achievement, which leads to better economic productivity. An increased adult income in the new generation helps to break the intergenerational cycle of poverty and raises the human capital in a community.[9] These educated youngsters will also become successful parents in future. Conversely, it has been estimated that adults who were exposed to adversity in the early years, earn nearly one-third less than their peers and are often more prone to anti-social behavior and crimes with poor emotional adjustment.[13]

The WHO endorses the adage that "enabling young children to achieve their full developmental potential is a human right and a critical requisite for sustainable development". Though all babies are born with a birthright to growth and development to the best of their potential, unfortunately, due to extreme social, economic, and cultural variations, the basic requirements for early development are not always met. The Lancet series (2017), "Advancing early childhood development: from science to scale" highlight the profound benefits of investing in ECD.[9,14] For any country, such investment promotes economic growth and helps in building peaceful and sustainable societies by reducing poverty and inequality.[15-17] Moreover, promotion of ECD helps to uphold the right of every child to survive and thrive.[18]

Today, on account of better healthcare facilities, we are witnessing significant reduction in perinatal, infant and under-5 mortality. Global data shows a 53% drop in childhood mortality between 1990 and 2015.[19] Illness and morbidity in children have also decreased drastically. In contrast, the load of developmental challenges is still alarmingly high. Many of the very sick children, who are surviving, are not reaching their developmental potential. In the developing world, even today, 250 million children (43% of child population) are at risk of not achieving their cognitive developmental potential in first 5 years of life and they all need adequate support to promote ECD.[13,14] Missing out in this investment early in life can turn out to be very costly to the family, society, and the nation at large.

For healthy brain development, children need a safe, secure, and nurturing environment, with proper nutrition, responsive care and early learning activities provided by their parents or other caregivers.[20]

NURTURING CARE FRAMEWORK

Evolution of the Nurturing Care Framework

Considering the gravity of the situation, experts across the world are today focusing on promotion of ECD to ensure optimum brain development of every single child. The WHO, the United Nations Children's Fund (UNICEF), the World Bank Group, the United Nations Educational, Scientific, Cultural Organization (UNESCO), and other global institutions have given priority to ECD in their action plans. ECD has been prominently featured in the *Sustainable Development Goals (SDG)* laid down by the United Nations (UN). It is accepted today that the key to the transformation that the world intends to achieve by 2030 lies in optimum development of young children.[21] The UN Secretary-General's Global Strategy for Women's, Children's, and Adolescents' Health 2016–2030 conceptualized a new vision, where the goal is to *"Survive, Thrive and Transform"*.[22] This involves 17 SDG targets, many of which involve promotion of ECD. The Lancet series on ECD in 2007, 2011 and 2017 have provided a plethora of scientific evidence to support the importance of ECD and the *Nurturing Care Framework (NCF)* has evolved as a roadmap to channelize this science to action, with a vision to build a world in which every child is able to develop to his/her full potential and no child is left behind.[23] NCF highlights on five SDG targets: Goal 1, target 1.2, Goal 2, target 2.2, Goal 3, target 3.2, Goal 4, target 4.2, Goal 16, target 16.2.

SDG Targets in NCF

1.2. By 2030, reduce at least by half the proportion of men, women and children of all ages living in poverty in all its dimensions according to national definitions.

2.2. By 2030, end all forms of malnutrition, including achieving, by 2025, the internationally agreed targets on stunting and wasting in children under 5 years of age, and address the nutritional needs of adolescent girls, pregnant and lactating women and older persons.

3.2. By 2030, end preventable deaths of newborns and children under 5 years of age, with all countries aiming to reduce neonatal mortality to at least as low as 12 per 1,000 live births and under-5 mortality to at least as low as 25 per 1,000 live births.

4.2. By 2030, ensure that all girls and boys have access to quality early childhood development, care and pre-primary education so that they are ready for primary education.

16.2. End abuse, exploitation, trafficking and all forms of violence against and torture of children.

What is Nurturing Care Framework?

Keeping in mind that adequate child development is dependent on adequate healthcare and nutrition for the mother and child, protection from threats,

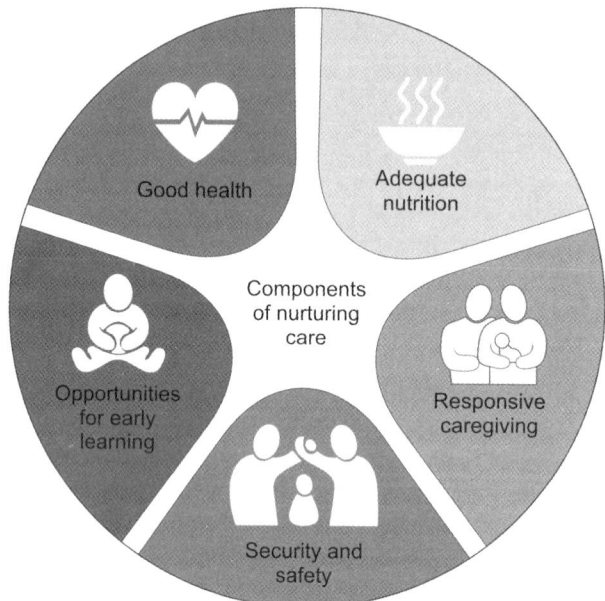

Fig. 20.2: Domains of nurturing care.

provision of learning opportunities through stimulating interactions by the caregivers and responsive, and emotionally supportive care, an optimum environment surrounding a child has been conceptualized in the WHO's NCF for ECD, which was presented at the World Health Assembly in May 2018.[2] This framework comprises five closely linked components—(1) good health, (2) nutrition, (3) safety and security, (4) early learning opportunity and (5) responsive caregiving **(Fig. 20.2)**.

Guiding Principles

The guiding principles for NCF are as follows:[8]
- The child's right to survive and thrive
- Leave no child behind
- Family-centered care
- "Whole-of-government" action, with multisectoral involvement involving health, nutrition, education, labor, finance, water-sanitation, and child protection[8]
- A "whole-of-society" approach, involving all sections of society.[8]

To effectively provide all these services to every child in an integrated manner, various organizations, governments and individuals must work together in a concerted manner. Hence the NCF addresses a wide range of stakeholders, including policymakers and program managers at both national and local level, nonprofit organizations, professional and academic bodies, and funding agencies, both global and national. Different sectors such as health, nutrition, education, child protection and social protection are involved in rolling out the NCF. Eventually, at the ground level, the parents and caregivers who attend to children on an everyday basis are reached through these various stakeholder channels with an aim to empower them to deliver proper nurturing care to their children.

Many countries are already addressing the first two components of NCF, namely (1) "good health" and (2) "adequate nutrition". The newer aspects of NCF are "responsive caregiving", "early learning opportunity" and "safety-security", which were not taken into much consideration hitherto. Responsive caregiving and early learning opportunity are integral components of good-quality care for young children. The NCF demonstrates how various existing programs can be brought together to provide comprehensive childcare, taking into account all the needs of young children. NCF promotes the use of locally available assets, utilized in a locally acceptable manner through promotion of ownership at community level. Emphasis is also laid on protection of young children from the worst effects of adversity. This leads to lifelong and intergenerational benefits for health, productivity, and social cohesion.

Components of Nurturing Care

Good Health

This includes health and wellbeing of children as well as their caregivers, as compromised physical and mental health of mothers can negatively influence their ability to take care of their children.

Good health does not just mean freedom from illness; provision of good health is not synonymous to care in illness and immunization. It goes further to include personal hygiene, prevention of infection, proper sleep and physical activity and protection from potential danger. Caregivers need to respond affectionately to the daily needs children. Parents are encouraged to utilize all available health services, both promotive and preventive so that the child receives proper treatment for all illnesses. Regular monitoring of their physical and emotional status is also of great importance.

Healthcare of the pregnant mother is equally important. Care should be taken of the mother's regular check-up with special reference to prevention/treatment of infections and immunization, support for mental health care, and avoiding domestic violence, substance use (such as alcohol and tobacco) and environmental toxins. Family life counseling for parents is essential to address issues like infertility, child spacing, and violence.

Suggested interventions for promotion of good health include essential newborn care, immunization of mother and child, prevention and treatment of childhood illness, growth monitoring, care for children with developmental difficulties or disabilities, promotion of health and wellbeing including health care seeking behavior, care for maternal physical and mental health problems, family planning, testing for human immunodeficiency virus (HIV) and prevention of mother-to-child HIV transmission.

Adequate Nutrition

Attention needs to be paid to both the child's and the mother's nutrition. From birth to the age of 6 months babies must get exclusive breastfeeding. After 6 months complementary foods need to be introduced, based on local availability. This should provide the necessary nutrients, (macro- and micro-) to support their rapidly growing bodies and brains. The diversity of food and frequency of feeds will increase with age. Breastfeeding needs to be continued till at least 2 years of age. Parents are expected to help the little child during meals, respond to her/his feeding needs. This is termed as responsive feeding. Parents can help them make the transition to eating nutritious family foods by 1 year of age. Micronutrient supplements, such as vitamin A or zinc may be considered when needed. The mother's nutrition is of paramount importance all through. Nutrition of the pregnant mother affects the growth of the fetus. For proper breastfeeding the lactating mother must get good food. To provide proper childcare the mother must be healthy and well nourished.

Suggested interventions include the following early initiation and exclusive breastfeeding for 6 months, introduction of appropriate complementary feeding along with breastfeeding from 6 months, responsive feeding practices, micronutrient supplementation for mother and child, and management of undernutrition as well as overweight and obesity.

Prior to conceptualization of the NCF, we were accustomed to considering mostly health care and nutrition to ensure wellbeing of the child. Now we need to delve deeper into the other three components (i.e., security and safety, opportunities for learning and responsive caregiving) and see how they impact child development.

Safety and Security

Safe and secure environments for children and their families are essential. Physical dangers as well as emotional stress, environmental risks, and access to proper food and water need to be addressed. To feel secure and safe, young children need the following:
- Access to nutritious food, clean water and sanitation
- Clean indoor and outdoor air, free of pollution
- Good hygiene
- Safe spaces to play and home environment free of health hazards

- Protection from physical punishment, mental or emotional abuse, domestic violence and neglect
- Protection from sexual abuse and child trafficking.

Major risks to children in the developing countries are extreme poverty and lack of basic living amenities, financial hardship and child labor, air pollution and exposure to toxic chemicals, unsafe play environments, harsh punishment, and violence. Availability of social and child protection services is also critical for obtaining financial and other support for the vulnerable families. The suggested interventions include the following:

- Birth registration
- Social care services including cash transfer to the most vulnerable families
- Child-proofing at home for safe environment
- Promotion of positive parenting
- Protection from natural and political calamities like war, famine etc.
- Care for vulnerable population (refugees, under-privileges communities, etc.).

Opportunities for Early Learning

This refers to the scope provided to the young child to interact with his/her immediate environment through which he/she learns new skills. The child's environment comprises persons, objects, and the surroundings. Every interaction with the child, whether positive, negative, or absent, contributes to the development of the child's brain and lays the foundations for later learning.

Learning begins right after conception, and as soon as babies are born, they begin to acquire various skills through their interactions with other people—smiling and eye contact, talking and singing, modeling and imitation, and simple games like "wave bye-bye" are common examples. Acquisition of these skills is promoted by interactive stimuli provided by caregivers. Children constantly give cues to evoke responses from the surroundings, based on which they learn to understand their environment and manipulate it too. The baby also learns to follow the cues provided by the parent or caregiver. Hence, a prompt, clear and consistent response from the parent makes learning easier for the child.

To support early learning, the caregivers need to undertake the following:
- Talk, play, and interact with children during all routine activities throughout the day
- Encourage them to move their bodies, use their five senses, listen, use language for communication, and explore the surroundings
- Smile, imitate/copy gestures, and play simple games (e.g., peek a boo)
- Engage actively in age-appropriate play with the child with household objects. Involve other family members and peers.
- Tell stories and explore storybooks together.

Responsive Caregiving

This refers to the parents' ability to take cognizance of the cues given by the child and respond to them appropriately and consistently. This is the fundamental component, because this responsive attitude enables caregivers to be better at providing the other four components.

Responsive care giving includes attentive observation of all the movements, sounds, gestures and verbal requests the child makes. Various outcomes of responsive caregiving are enumerated as follows:
- Protecting children against any imminent trauma
- Preventing the negative effects of adversity by picking up early signs of danger
- Recognizing and responding to illness or deprivation at the earliest
- Proper mindful interaction with the child
- Enriched learning through enjoyable interactions
- Building a strong bondage with the child, based on trust and dependence.

Responsive care giving starts before birth, when the mother should start fondly responding to the baby's movements in utero.[24] Hearing develops in a fetus by 24 weeks and it has been studied that the mother's voice can have a stimulating and comforting effect on the growing fetus. From birth, the baby can recognize the mother's voice and face distinctive from others.[24]

Even before young children begin to speak, they engage with their caregivers through cuddling, eye contact, smiles, vocalizations, and gestures; early bonding is facilitated when parents actively engage in the above modes of communication from early life. These mutually enjoyable interactions create close bonding, which augments emotional development and builds a level of confidence in the surrounding environment in the developing young child. Bonding with parents builds the foundation for social bonding and good communication skills in later life. Responsive caregiving interacts with all the other components of NCF and is essential for achieving good health, adequate nutrition, security and safety, and early learning. It includes responsive feeding, which is especially important for low-weight or ill infants. Feeding is a process of bonding with the child actively, not just a mechanical process of pushing food into the child's mouth.

To promote responsive care giving, parents/caregivers need to be sensitized to the following:
- Making eye contact, smile, cuddle, praise the child at every opportunity
- Being attentive to their child and taking note of the cues she/he provides
- Responding appropriately to the child with sensitivity, promptness and consistency
- Identifying early signs of hunger, satiety, illness, emotional distress, interest to play, and pleasure

- Looking for opportunities in everyday life to interact and play with their child
- Most importantly, enjoying the company of the child.

All this takes active vigilance on the part of the parents with deep mental involvement.

■ SUPPORT LEVELS FOR NURTURING CARE

The level of nurturing care support required by a family depends on their requirements and vulnerability. Accordingly, three levels of support have been identified as universal support, targeted support, and indicated support.

Universal Support

This is to be provided for all families of young children, through the available services, rendering health promotion and primary prevention. Through universal support nurturing care will reach every single child.

Targeted Support

This focuses on families at-risk. The various risk factors include poverty, malnutrition, adolescent pregnancy, HIV, violence, and other humanitarian emergencies. Timely and adequate intervention in this group will help reduce the damaging effects of severe stress and deprivation and provide support in developing proper coping mechanism.[20]

Examples of targeted support include home visit programs, group activity in the community ensuring participation by the marginalized families and provision of day-care centers.[8]

Indicated Support

This is aimed at families with greater needs where extra services need to be provided. This group includes:
- Premature and LBW babies
- Young children without caregivers
- Mothers working in informal sectors deprived of child-care facilities
- Children living with depressed mothers
- Children living in violent homes, exposed to domestic conflict
- Children with disabilities or developmental difficulties
- Children with severe malnutrition
- Children exposed to various emergency situations such as a disease outbreak, large-scale food contamination, chemical or radioactive spills, and natural disasters.

Premature and LBW babies are vulnerable to illness, poor health, stunted growth, brain damage and developmental challenges. Moreover, they are often neglected in the family due to their frailty. Consequently, they remain at a greater risk of developmental delay.

Mothers from lower income settings are prone to depression, anxiety, and adjustment disorders due to exposure to socioeconomic stresses, domestic violence, unplanned and early pregnancy, and lack of support. Poor maternal mental health predisposes to inadequate childcare. These children are seen to suffer more from acute illnesses, malnutrition, incomplete immunization, and socioemotional difficulties.

Violence against children is often caused by parents and other primary caregivers involving physical, sexual, and emotional abuse and neglect. Global data from various sources have revealed that physical abuse affects about 23% of children, emotional abuse reported in 36% and neglect in 16%. Sexual abuse has been reported in an estimated 18% of girls and 8% of boys.[9,25]

Special "indicated support" for these vulnerable groups include the following:
- Treatment and help with perinatal depression and other mental problems
- Good-quality care for preterm and LBW
- Early detection, early interventions and rehabilitation with a family-centered approach and adequate community support for developmental challenges and disability
- Risks for neglect and abuse need to be addressed and protective measures taken at four levels: individual, relationship, community, and society.[20]

■ IMPLEMENTATION STRATEGIES FOR NCF-ECD

It is evident that NCF has an ambitious goal to provide every child on this planet with optimum childcare facilities. To make this a reality, certain strategies need to be adopted.

As this is a global issue, all countries need to be involved and country-wise customized programs must evolve. As wellbeing of the child involves numerous issues including health, food, security, education, etc., coordination of multiple stakeholders is imperative. There needs to be a shared understanding of context, and activity across sectors. Accelerated action on nurturing care requires "whole-of-government" action. Stakeholders must come together to formulate a work plan. Implementation by different sectors and at different levels will also require a vigilant, comprehensive monitoring. Effective coordination and accountability are essential. All the relevant stakeholders involved in creating environments for nurturing care include:
- Policymakers and program managers in ministries of health, nutrition, education, child protection, social protection, finance

- Local government representatives
- Civil-society groups and private-sector organizations
- Professional associations
- Academic institutions, such as training institutes, colleges, and universities
- Funding initiatives, both global and national
- Local media
- Local law enforcement
- Parents and caregivers: the pivotal persons.

A unique "whole-of-society" approach is being adopted by NCF, which involves the coalition of parents, caregivers, local community, and society at large.

Though stakeholders are many, the delivery point remains single. Through this terminal delivery point the package needs to be delivered to the focal persons in charge of the child: the parents/primary caregivers. Policies, programs, and services must be designed to enable and empower them.

■ GLOBAL GUIDELINES
WHO Guidelines on ECD

World Health Organization has come up with definite guidelines for caregivers and health workers, who are at the forefront of providing nurturing care, as they need to be supported through policies and services in order to have knowledge, skills, time and material resources for appropriate child care.[26] To improve early childhood development, WHO has endorsed the NCF and has come up with the following recommendations:

1. *Responsive caregiving*: All infants and children should receive responsive care during the first 3 years of life; parents and other caregivers should be supported to provide responsive care.
2. *Promote early learning*: All infants and children should have early learning activities with their parents and other caregivers during the first 3 years of life; parents and other caregivers should be supported to engage in early learning with their infants and children.
3. *Integrate caregiving and nutrition interventions*: Support for responsive care and early learning should be included as part of interventions for optimal nutrition of infants and young children.
4. *Support maternal mental health*: Psychosocial interventions to support maternal mental health should be integrated into early childhood health and development services.

Country-wise Strategic Plans

Nurturing Care Framework, as we see, is an all-encompassing concept for ECD, but global implementation across all barriers is a very ambitious goal and the path is fraught with numerous hurdles. Keeping these issues in mind, the universal recommendations laid down by global bodies such as WHO, UNICEF and the World Bank require some need-based country-wise and community-wise customization, as the threats to ECD vary and the workforce and implementation mechanisms vary. Today most countries have responded to this global movement towards "ECD for all", through nurturing care, and have devised their own unique ECD programs tailor-made to their needs. Let us take a brief bird's eye view of how some of the countries are approaching ECD through NCF.

Brazil is running the world's biggest ECD program, "Criança Feliz" since 2016, through home-visits, to promote comprehensive development of children in their early years.[27]

Jamaica has focused on a strong legal framework.[28] Their "Early Childhood Commission (ECC)" serves as an institutional anchor coordinating across sectors. Their core ECD policy goals are: (1) establishing an enabling environment, (2) wide implementation and (3) monitoring and quality assurance.

Peru has been successful in reaching out to 32% of their rural population across the country by 2016, with locally trained personnel and community participation (*Cuna Mas*) by adopting the Early Childhood Workforce Initiative (ECWI), a global, multisectoral effort.[29] They have laid major emphasis on generous funding and proper remuneration for field workers. The recommendations laid down to make this program successful and scalable are as follows:

- Supervision in the field is critical
- Develop indigenous educational material
- Address communication issues for remote areas
- Proper incentive and remuneration.

Challenges faced in **Mexico** include lack of equity and cultural differences. Moreover, the transition from a disease-based model to a development-based model is difficult. There is also a tendency to emphasize on physical development and neglect social, emotional, and cognitive development.[30]

The successful 'Side-by-side' campaign in **South Africa**[31] has been created by the health department, supported by civil societies, academics, multi-lateral agencies, and private foundations.[31] They are also keen on involving other government departments besides health education. This campaign is centered on their 'Road to Health booklet (RtHB)', popularizing the five pillars of NCF.

Ethiopia has also developed a multi-sectoral approach to the nurturing care agenda.[32]

The Government of the Republic of **Zambia** with support from UNICEF and the LEGO Foundation has launched a national campaign 'I play, I learn, I thrive', highlighting the benefits of play for Zambian children.[33]

Country-wise information, as available from the Nurturing Care website (https://nurturing-care.org) has provided information about many other countries too, as mentioned below:

Ghana has called upon other government agencies, donors, non-governmental actors, and the media to increase their investments, and attention to ECD, focusing on 0–3 years.

Vietnam has come up with a holistic parenting model through parenting clubs at commune and village levels.

In western **Kenya**, the Governor is leading the scale-up of policies, programs, and services in support of nurturing care.

Mozambique has leveraged funding from the Global Financing Facility and World Bank to integrate early learning and responsive caregiving into the national nutrition package.

The Government of **Bulgaria**, in partnership with UNICEF, has established a universal home visiting programme for all families.

In **Greece**, Refugee Trauma Initiative (2016) set up an Early Childhood Care and Development (ECCD) program for refugee children aged 0–6 years.

Kazakhstan has refined their home visiting program to ensure families receive coordinated support from health professionals and social workers.

USA introduced the 'Global Child Thrive Act' in U.S. Senate, which directs the US administration to advance policies for advancement of ECD internationally (https://nurturing-care.org/global-child-thrive-act).

Thus, we see, different nations are trying in their unique ways to ultimately reach a common goal.

■ ECD EFFORTS IN INDIA

The ECD promotion concept is not new in India. We can boast of the oldest and largest national program on child development, the Integrated Child Development Services (ICDS) launched in 1976. We presently have a wide network of ICDS centres strewn across the country, delivering comprehensive healthcare, nutrition, and pre-school education to children 0–6 years.

Many national policies have evolved with a multi-sectoral and multi-dimensional perspective, which include the following: The National Policy for Children (1974); the National Policy for Education (1986); the National Nutrition Policy (1993), the National Plan of Action for Children (2005); the National Early Childhood Care and Education (ECCE) Policy (2013); the National Health Policy (2017) to name a few. The Universal Salt Iodization program is an intervention with definite implication for child development, which has made significant progress. Presently the Centre has about 38 programs that can be linked to and categorized in the NCF.

Services are delivered at the grass-root level by our field level workers (FLW) from both health and education sectors (e.g., ASHA, ANM, and AWWs) who by now have been well-primed in home-based newborn care, integrated healthcare of young children, nutrition, immunization, and hygiene through programs like Home based newborn care, IMNCI, POSHAN, WASH etc. All these activities work towards child health and wellbeing. Follow up clinics for high-risk newborns for early detection and early intervention for incipient developmental delay is being emphasized at the facilities, to prevent neuro-developmental disorders.

In 2018, the *Rashtriya Bal Surakhsha Karyakram (RBSK)* program was launched to identify and treat all common illnesses in children up to 18 years, laying a major emphasis on developmental delays and congenital defects. The concept of 'District early intervention center (DEIC)' would provide early intervention for all detected developmental delays at a district level. So, we may rightly conclude that our government has harnessed multiple initiatives to augment ECD in India. Yet, we have a long way to go to reach the countdown to the 2030 SDG target. The major reason is the magnitude of our child population at risk. Our 0–6 age group comprise 13.2% of population and the estimated total 0–6 child population is 158,789,287, of which the rural child population is 117,585,514 (**74%**). A majority of these are under-privileged and marginalized, hence difficult to reach.

Though we have good schemes in vogue, implementation and monitoring are often inadequate. There exists a lack of coordination between the different sectors involved. Many NGOs are active, but they mostly work in small pockets with inadequate scaling up. ECD is still not fully in focus and a poor awareness is visible at various levels.

The Way Forward in India

To make NCF for ECD an effective program in India we need to urgently focus on the following:
- Generate awareness at all levels
- Advocacy for prioritization of ECD
- Formulate a robust strategic plan along "Nurturing Care" model to fit our national delivery system
- Technical skill development among caregivers and field level workers—presently they are deficient in the knowledge and skill on child development promotion
- Convergence of various stakeholders, such as health and education sectors, government and nongovernment bodies, implementing organizations and academic bodies, national and global bodies—all need to join hands for a common cause
- Involvement of professional and academic bodies and systematic documentation and research.

We must ensure that the following are made available to all beneficiaries:
- *Parent education and family support* for early intervention
- *Primary health care and nutrition* for mother and child
- *Prevent substance exposure* (lead, mercury)
- *Stimulating home environment:* Language exposure, social interaction, and early literacy
- *Attend to behavioral and emotional needs* of child and mother
- *Prevent toxic stress:* Maternal depression, abuse and neglect, extreme poverty, family violence.

India has already started her journey toward the 2030 SDG goal. If we can sincerely take up these issues and try to fill our lacunae, we will succeed in helping our children achieve the best of their potential.

The *NCF* focuses on reaching out to all children, leaving none behind, and enabling them to survive and thrive. Through this endeavor alone the health and human potential of people across all boundaries may be transformed.

CONCLUSION

Brain development occurs at a prolific rate in the early years of life; influence of various biological and environmental factors prompting the optimum brain development at this stage determines the ultimate holistic development of the individual as an adult and his/her success in life. Hence it is of paramount importance to address the factors influencing child development, which have been compiled under five major headings namely good health, adequate nutrition, safety and security, early learning opportunity and responsive care giving. Together, this comprises the *"Nurturing Care Framework"*, as conceptualized by the WHO.

KEY POINTS

- Holistic development of a child from conception to 3–5 years of age is of paramount importance from a medical, social, cultural, and financial point of view.
- Simultaneous attention needs to be paid to a child's good health, adequate nutrition, stimulating environment for early learning opportunity, responsive care giving and assured safety and security to promote a child's optimum development.
- These five aspects comprise the five components of the nurturing care framework.
- All stakeholders, beginning from parents to policy makers need to prioritize on ECD and focus on the nurturing care framework.
- ECD–NCF is a highlighted issue globally; the international bodies such as WHO, UNICEF, and World Bank are actively working on this and most countries across the globe have taken up ECD–NCF with great seriousness and urgency. India is a forerunner in this drive.

REFERENCES

1. Feigelman S. Assessment of fetal growth and development. In: Kliegman RM, Stanton BF, Schor NF, St Geme III JW, Behrman RE (Eds). Nelson Textbook of Pediatrics, 20th edition. Philadelphia: Elsevier; 2016. pp. 60-1.
2. Nelson CA. The neurobiological bases of early intervention. In: Shonkoff JP, Meisels SJ, (Eds). Handbook of Early Childhood Intervention, 2nd edition. Cambridge, MA: Cambridge University Press; 2000. pp. 204-27.
3. Building Better Brains. New Frontiers in Early Childhood Development. [online] Available from: https://www.childrenandaids.org/sites/default/files/2017-04/Building%20Better%20Brains.pdf. [Last Accessed January, 2022].
4. World Health Organization. Developmental Difficulties in Early Childhood. Available from: http://apps.who.int/iris/bitstream/handle/10665/97942/9789241503549_eng.pdf;jsessionid=79575F44E19458AE669DE36928F0E32B?sequence=1. [Last Accessed January, 2022].
5. Gopnik A. Cognitive development domains and theories. In: Kliegman RM, Stanton BF, Schor NF, St Geme III JW, Behrman RE (Eds). Nelson Textbook of Pediatrics, 20th edition. Philadelphia: Elsevier; 2016. pp. 54-9.
6. Britto PR, Singh M, Dua T, Kaur R, Yousuafzai AK. What implementation evidence matters: scaling-up nurturing interventions that promote early childhood. Ann NY Acad Sci. 2018:1419(1):5-16.
7. Shonkoff JP. The science of early childhood development. January 2007 National Scientific Council on the Developing Child. Second Printing—November 2007. Cambridge: Harvard University; 2021.
8. Nurturing Care for Early Childhood Development. A Framework for Helping Children Survive and Thrive to Transform Health and Human Potential. [online] Available from: https://apps.who.int/iris/bitstream/handle/10665/272603/9789241514064-eng.pdf [Last Accessed January, 2022].
9. Black MM, Walker SP, Fernald LCH, Andersen CT, DiGirolamo A, Lu C, et al. Early childhood development coming of age: science through the life course. Lancet. 2017;389(10064):77-90.
10. Bouchane K, Yoshikawa H, Murphy KM, Lombardi J. Early childhood programs for refugees. Paris: UNESCO; 2018.
11. Chattopadhyay N. In Early Childhood Development: The Buzz Word In Child Health Today. J Community Med Public Health Care. 2019;6:61.
12. Nofziger S, Rosen NL. Building self-control to prevent crime. In: Teasdale B, Bradley M, (Eds). Preventing crime and violence. Basel, Switzerland: Springer International Publishing; 2017. pp. 43-56.
13. Gertler P, Heckman J, Pinto R, Zanolini A, Vermeerch C, Walker S, et al. Labor market returns to an early childhood stimulation intervention in Jamaica. Science. 2014;344(6187):998-1001.
14. Lu C, Black MM, Richter LM. Risk of poor development in young children in low-income and middle-income countries: an estimation and analysis at the global, regional, and country level. Lancet Glob Health. 2016;4(12):e916-22
15. World Health Organization. Executive summary: Nurturing Care Framework for early childhood development: A framework for helping children survive and thrive to transform health and human potential. Geneva: WHO; 2018.
16. Heckman JJ. Skill formation and the economics of investing in disadvantaged children. Science. 2006;312(5782):1900-2.

17. Shonkoff JP. Leveraging the biology of adversity to address the roots of disparities in health and development. Proc Natl Acad Sci USA. 2012;109 (Suppl 2):17302-7.
18. UNICEF. (1989). The United Nations Convention of the Rights of the Child. New York: United Nations; 1989.
19. Chattopadhyay N. Early Childhood Development: The Buzz Word in Child Health Today. J Community Med Public Health Care. 2019;6:61.
20. Nurturing Care Handbook. [online] Available from: https://nurturing-care.org/handbook-start-here. [Last Accessed January, 2022].
21. Transforming our World: The 2030 Agenda for Sustainable Development. New York: United Nations; 2015.
22. Survive, Thrive, Transform: The Global Strategy for Women's, Children's and Adolescents' Health (2016–2030). New York: United Nations; 2015.
23. Britto PR, Lye SJ, Proulx K, Yousafzai AK, Matthews SG, Vaivada T, et al. Nurturing care: promoting early childhood development. Lancet. 2017;389(10064):91-102.
24. Murray L, Andrews E. The Social Baby: Understanding Babies' Communication from Birth. Richmond, UK: The Children's Project; 2002.
25. Stoltenborgh M, Bakermans-Kranenburg MJ, van Ijzendoorn MH. The neglect of child neglect: a meta-analytic review of the prevalence of neglect. Soc Psychiatry Psychiatr Epidemiol. 2013;48(3):345-55.
26. WHO. Improving Early Childhood Development: WHO Guidelines https://www.who.int/publications-detail-redirect/97892400020986. [Last Accessed January, 2022].
27. Buccini G, Venancio SI, Pérez-Escamilla R. Scaling up of Brazil's Criança Feliz early childhood development program: an implementation science analysis. Ann N Y Acad Sci. 2021;1497(1):57-73.
28. UNICEF. SABER Country Report 2013, Jamaica. An analysis of early childhood development (ECD) programs and policies affecting children in Jamaica. [online] Available from: https://www.unicef.org/jamaica/reports/saber-country-report-jamaica. [Last Accessed January, 2022].
29. Repositorio. Supporting Early Childhood Workforce at Scale: The Cuna Mas Home Visiting Program at Peru. Washington DC: Results for Development; 2017.
30. Myers RG. Desarrollo infantil temprano en México: avances y retos [Early child development in Mexico: advances and challenges]. Bol Med Hosp Infant Mex. 2015;72(6):359-61.
31. Nurturing-Care. South Africa, Campaigning side-by-side. [online] Available from: https://nurturing-care.org/resources/south-africa/. [Last Accessed January, 2022].
32. Advancing Nutrition. Nurturing Care to Improve Early Childhood Development: Ethiopia Country Profile. [online] Available at https://www.advancingnutrition.org/sites/default/files/2021-10/ecd_landscape_brief_ethiopia.pdf. [Last Accessed January, 2022].
33. UNICEF. "I play, I learn, I thrive" playful parenting campaign. [online] Available from: https://www.unicef.org/zambia/press-releases/coinciding-fathers-day-government-republic-zambia-unicef-and-lego-foundation-launch. [Last Accessed January, 2022].

Adolescent Pediatrics

CHAPTER 21: Media Use

Nidhi Bedi, Piyush Gupta

■ INTRODUCTION

Screen time has ever been increasing in the last half of the century but with the 2020 COVID-19 pandemic an unprecedented rise was recorded. India declared its national lockdown on 24 March 2020, and since then children have been spending most of their time indoors.[1] Schools had been shut down and outdoor games got restricted. Most of the cities continued to be partially locked out with limited relaxations. Markets and malls has become a risky place to venture. Recreational and sporting activities had almost come to a halt. In such a situation, media had become the only source of leisure and entertainment, in terms of education and recreational activities besides connecting to people. Thereby, screen time increased multiple folds leading to significant side effects. All categories of people including parents, and physicians started seeking answers for multiple questions such as what is screen time, what are the ill effects of excessive screen time, what content is permissible to watch, how much a child or an adolescent should be allowed to watch per day etc. Hence, it becomes essential for us to understand more about screen time and its judicious use.

■ SCREEN TIME AND TYPES OF MEDIA

Screen time also known as digital engagement time, is the total time spent in watching screens such as televisions, computers, laptops, tablets, smartphones, and video games in a day.[2,3] Often digital media is a word used synonymously with screen time, but they are not the same. Media refers to the different modes of mass communication. These include print, broadcast, and internet media. Print and broadcast media are the traditional media, which were the main means of mass communication before the launch of digital media. While newspapers and magazines are examples of the print media, television and radio are the broadcast media. Digital media or internet media or newer media is defined as a group of internet-based applications that are built on the ideological and technological foundations of Web 2.0 and allow the creation and exchange of user-generated content.[4] Thus it includes any content that is transmitted over the internet or computer networks on all devices such as smartphones, laptops, desktops, tablets, etc. Digital media is more interactive, engaging, and provides personalized communication. Again, digital media can be available as audio such as digital radio stations and podcast or as video. Video digital media can be on different platforms. These include streaming platforms such as Netflix, Amazon Prime, and YouTube channels, social media platforms such as Facebook, Twitter, WhatsApp, and Instagram, multiplayer games platforms such as PUBG and Candy Crush, news and literature platforms, and lastly the advertisements which are often seen as part of programs or uploaded individually and remain the major source of financial gains.

■ EXTENT OF THE PROBLEM
Global Outlook
The prevalence of excess screen time in under-five children has varied from 10 to 93.7% in the high-income countries, and 21 to 98% in the middle-income countries.[5] There is some nonhomogeneity due to the difference in criteria used to define excess screen time. Some studies classified it as more than 1 hour/day and others as >2 hours/day. The overall screen time in under-five children has varied between 0.1 and 5 hours/day. In a systematic review of 130 studies conducted since the year 2000 in children and adolescents, 52.3% of the participants had a screen time exceeding >2 hours/day.[6] The average screen time recorded was 3.6 hours/day, varying from 1.3 to 7.9 hours/day.

As per the American Academy of Pediatrics (AAP), three-fourths of teenagers use at least one social media site, mainly Facebook, Twitter, and Instagram, and nearly 80% households own a device used to play videogames.[7]

Indian Scene
Exposure to screens in Indian children has also been reported from all age groups starting as early as 2 months though the median age of first exposure was found to be 10 months. In a study by Meena et al., published in 2020, it was found that almost all (99.7%, n = 370) children were exposed to screen-based media by 18 months of age. Screen time of > 1 hour/day was noted in 88.7% and > 2 hours/day in 56.5% of toddlers. Smartphone use was noted more commonly (96%) than television viewing (89%).[8] Many studies have reported television watching while having dinner; the above study reporting it in more than 50% of the families. This behavior has been found to have significant correlation with increased screen time. In a study by Dubey et al. in 2018 on adolescent population,[9] it was found that nearly three-fourths (76.4%) of the adolescents were viewing television during mealtime and only one-fifth (22.9%) had any family rules for watching television. Smartphone addiction among adolescents, ranged from 39 to 44% (p < 0.0001). Among those going

to school, screen time was more during vacation than school days [3.9 (±2.8) and 3.2 (±2.8) hours/day, respectively]. The most used device was television followed by mobile phone (96.5 vs. 56.7%, respectively). This was unlike the findings seen in preschoolers in the other study by Meena et al. where smartphones were the most used devices, primarily for games and videos.[8,9]

Many studies have found smartphones to be the most common screen used, especially among late adolescents and college students. In a study by Gupta et al. in 2018, of adolescents and young adults in undergraduate colleges, most common computing devices owned by the students were smartphones (95.8%), followed by laptop (64.0%), desktop (26.8%), and tablets (15.53%).[10] Some other studies have shown that a lot of adolescent children are very active on social media sites making them the major reason to spend time on screen.[11] In a school-based survey of adolescents from Manipur in 2019, a total of 38.6, 36.2, and 15.6% children had account on Facebook, WhatsApp, and Instagram, respectively. About 28.7% of the participants used their laptop/smartphones till late at night.[12]

■ FACTORS ASSOCIATED WITH INCREASED SCREEN TIME

Various factors have been associated with increased screen time. These can be divided into three—(1) child-related, (2) parent-related, and (3) environment-related.

Child-related Factors

- *Daily sleep duration*: Lesser sleep duration is associated with more screen time.[13]
- *Sedentary preferences:* Higher the sedentary activities, more is the screen time recorded across multiple studies.[13]
- *Gender:* Boys were found to have higher screen time than girls though not noted in all studies.[13]
- *Age:* Age has been an inconsistent factor with some studies reporting an increase in screen time with age and others reporting vice versa. Introduction of screen time at an early age has also been associated with increased propensity of exaggerated use with increase in age, though not in all studies.[14,15]
- *Mealtime:* Practice of having meals while having television leads to higher screen time.[16] In one of the Indian studies, almost 80% greater odds of higher screen time exposure were found in those watching television while having meals. Such habits were more commonly noted in urban population.[17]

■ PARENT-RELATED FACTORS

Parents are the role models for children and their behavior has a big impact on children. Parental screen time also has significant impact on screen time in their children.[18]

- *Screen time of parents:* More the parental screen time, higher the screen time in children. Cell phone use by mothers was shown to cause a twofold increase in the odds of high screen time of children.[16,17]
- *Maternal stress:* Maternal stress and higher working hours are associated with higher screen time in children in various studies.[19]
- *Parity:* Children of first-time mothers had higher screen time. This was attributable to a lack of knowledge, less time for mothers to manage household works, and no sibling available to play.[19]
- *Maternal education:* Some studies reported higher maternal education (intermediate/equivalent and above) to be associated with decreased screen time, though not noted in all studies. This difference may be due to increased awareness among educated mothers.[15,16]
- *Socioeconomic status:* Parents from lower socioeconomic class often consider screen as learning tool and have rather promoted its use.[20]
- *Parental knowledge, attitudes, and beliefs:* These have been found to impact the screen time in children.[21,22]

Environmental-related Factors

- *Access*: Easier access to digital media, high background television time, and mealtime television viewing are factors found to be directly affecting screen time.[19,21]
- *Number of devices available*: Higher number of screen devices at home promotes higher screen viewing in children (60% odds of increased screen time recorded in families with two or less devices versus those with three and more). Besides, presence of television in bedroom has been associated with increased screen time in multiple studies.[17,23]
- *Place of care*: Increased screen time is seen in children receiving home-based care compared to those in day care centers.[24]
- *Device availability*: Previously, watching TV was preferred over other digital media but last decade has seen maximum increase in mobile phone screen time followed by laptop.

■ EFFECTS OF INCREASED SCREEN TIME

In today's time when COVID-19 pandemic has completely taken over, electronic media has become the most important source of learning and interaction. Studies show exponential increase in screen time during this period. The risk-benefit ratio in such a situation needs to be weighed closely. To count on the benefits, it helps in better connectivity, improved spatial skills in younger children, easier ways to gain knowledge, improved academic development, more job opportunities, and health promotion by promoting behavioral change such as encouraging exercises, maintaining healthy diet and preventing substance abuse, and experiencing positive emotions and moral values.[25-30] But all these benefits come with a long list of ill effects. The negative effects associated with increased screen time are discussed below.

Sleep

Decreased sleep duration, poor quality of sleep, and prolonged sleep latency are noted. Sleep deprivation leads to obesity, reduced immunity, growth retardation, and mental health issues. Significant worsening of sleep score leads to excessive daytime sleepiness and poor academic performance.[31]

Obesity

There are various theories proposed for the mechanism of screen exposure and obesity, the most prominent of which are decreased physical activity, increased intake of high calorie, low energy food, and decreased sleep.[32] Increased screen time also leads to poor sleep quality. This further promotes obesity by changes in ghrelin and leptin causing increased hunger and decreased satiety, increased snacking beyond normal mealtimes, especially at night and consumption of more unhealthy calories during increased snacking time.[32] Multiple studies have shown a dose response relationship of television viewing and body mass index (BMI).[33] In one of the US based studies, it was seen that the odds of being overweight were 4.6 times higher in children watching television for >5 hours/day as compared to 0-2 hours/day in 10-15 years of age group.[34]

Altered Recognition and Comprehension

Cognitive development depends on quantity and quality of program and social content of media viewed. In children < 3 years of age, each hour of television viewing was associated with significant deleterious effect on reading, recognition, and comprehension. Exposure to adult-directed television in early life, and high background television exposure was found to have a negative correlation with the child's executive functioning and cognitive development.[35,36] In children > 6 years of age, watching media that is directed to adults has been associated with antisocial aggressive behavior, fights, and poor school performance. Frequent exposure to violent media may increase the child's baseline arousal level. After some time, children get habituated and desensitized, and their baseline arousal decreases. Such kind of mental state can lead to attention deficit hyperactivity disorder (ADHD)-related behavior.[37,38]

Eating Disorders

Adolescent children have poor body image perception and eating disorder. Social media exposure of 1-1.5 hours/day has been associated with significant calorie reduction and strong emotional reaction.[39]

Psychological Disorders

Unrealistic image of female beauty causes dissatisfaction and psychological effects including low self-esteem. It was seen that people who were extroverts further became more active but those with low self-esteem showed features of depression in due course of time. Exposure to smoking in movies is identified as a risk factor for smoking uptake among children. Similarly, alcohol consumption, which is casually depicted in movies and videos, may promote early addiction to these substances.[40] Viewing alcohol advertisements is found to increase immediate alcohol consumption when compared with viewing nonalcohol advertisements.[41]

Physical Effects

Many people with excessive screen time develop physical side effects such as wear and tear of cervical spine, leading to posture-related disorders.[42]

Eye Problems

Refractive errors have also been commonly associated with screen time. Viewing > 3 hours of television has been found to cause significant visual impairment including myopia, heterophoria, astigmatism, refractive errors, dryness of eyes, blurring, itching, and irritation. Even 1 hour of smart phone or tablet use is found to be associated with eyestrain, discomfort, reduced blink rate, and headache.[43]

■ INTERVENTIONS

The initial interventions started way back in 1980s in western world when the ill effects of prolonged screen time started becoming visible, but the peak work was done from 2000 to 2020. Interventions were made at various levels such as community, school, home/family-based, clinic, or multicentric. Similarly, mode of intervention varied from knowledge-providing interventions, behavioral interventions, environmental interventions, regulatory interventions, or a combination of these.

Behavioral change theories (BCTs) have been used most successfully, of which social cognitive theory (SCT) is the most used intervention. BCTs attempt to explain why behavioral changes occur. Each BCT focuses on a different factor to explain behavioral change. SCT takes environmental, personal, and behavioral characteristics into account. In SCT individual acquires and maintains a behavior along with the social environment in which the person performs the behavior. Various components of SCT include reciprocal determinism, behavioral capability, observational learning, reinforcements, expectations, self-efficacy, and self-control. It also has certain limitations like the assumption that the change in environment will automatically change the person.[5]

In a review article by Schmidt et al. in 2011, 47 studies with children <12 years of age were included.[44] Almost all had home/family interventions with many having more than one setting. Nearly 75% of them were randomized controlled trials (74%). Most of the interventions lasted for <1 year (68%). The major interventions made were educational sessions, physical activity, resources/curricula for teachers, resource kit/newsletter for parents, electronic TV time monitors, incentives, open or close loop contingent system, and community advertising. They found that 29/47 (62%) studies showed significant reduction in screen time. Behavioral change theory and knowledge transfer were the most common interventions. The most effective interventions noted were electronic monitoring device, contingent open and close feedback system, clinic-based counseling, and high parental involvement.

Maniccia et al.[45] in same year conducted another review of 29 randomized controlled trials including 5–11 years (20/29). The most common intervention noted was again behavioral theory (social cognitive), most common place of intervention being school (13/29) followed by home (8/29). Interventions included information provision component to change behavior, 9/29 facilitating behavior change by controlling the environment using a television-control device. Other common methods for behavioral change included setting goals, television-viewing budget or plan, behavioral contract where children agreed that they will spend a predeceded time in front of a screen, increasing awareness amongst children by making them monitor themselves and record their own screen time, identifying alternative activities for the child, providing opportunities for physical activity, and environmental modification by restricting access to the television or computer with the help of a television-control device. They noted that during intervention period effect was large and statistically significant, whereas after intervention most studies showed small favorable effect. By 2016, more studies were published using SCT and knowledge transfer as interventions. Newer methods of screen control like TV/computer control device to budget time spent, TV turn off period and goal setting within the intervention were used.[46]

Downing et al.[47] in a meta-analysis of 17 studies in 2017 found that those with longer duration (>6 months) of intervention, those conducted in a community-based or preschool/childcare setting and studies with greater parental involvement were most effective.

In one of the latest meta-analyses by Nguyen et al., in 2020, effective interventions included education sessions on healthy lifestyle, newsletters, health promotion materials, strategies for self-monitoring, reinforcement behavior, motivational counseling, and goal setting.[48]

■ EXISTING GUIDELINES

International Guidelines

The American Academy of Pediatrics (AAP) released the first ever screen time guidelines for pediatricians and other healthcare professionals in

2001.[49] They conveyed that parent should know how much and what types of media their children are watching. They should serve as good role models for children by using television appropriately. The guidelines stated that total entertainment media time for children should be not more than 1–2 hours of quality programming per day. They advised not to have television in children's bedrooms. Parents were guided to discourage television viewing for children younger than 2 years and encourage more interactive activities for them to promote proper brain development. The content of the programs was suggested to be monitored to ensure they are informational, educational, and nonviolent. The same could be done by parents by watching the program along with children and discuss the content. Parents were encouraged to find alternative entertainment for children, including reading, athletics, hobbies, and creative play. Pediatricians were urged to not only educate parents but also initiate policies at school levels, hospitals, community, school education department, and media groups.

In 2013, these guidelines were revised to focus on young adolescents along with children.[50] The new guidelines recommended that youth should not have access to the Internet or TV in their bedrooms, and reinforced parents to monitor media use for their children. They also asked local chapters to make socially responsible decisions on marketing products to youth. They advised local bodies to educate schools about the ill effects of using unlimited and unsupervised media and to teach school authorities more about violence prevention, sex education, and drug use prevention program. They suggested maximizing prosocial content in media and minimizing harmful effects.

Further in 2016, the guidelines became more elaborate to cover all aspects of healthy living, which guided parents and pediatricians to promote children of all age groups to daily physical activity recommended for their age along adequate sleep varying from 8–12 hours (as per the age). They advised that children should not have any devices in their bedrooms while sleeping, not to watch screen at least an hour before sleep, avoid entertainment media during homework, to have media-free times in the day. This time should also be utilized as the time spent together with family, to have media-free places in homes, promote activities that will promote development and health, like talking, and playing together and last but very importantly to communicate guidelines to other caregivers so that media rules are followed consistently. Parents should have regular conversation with children about online safety. They should be aware about how to treat others, avoiding cyber bullying and sexting, and avoiding communications that can compromise personal privacy and safety.[7,25]

In 2020, American Academy of Child and Adolescent Psychiatry made some changes to the above guidelines.[51] The new changes permitted screen time for <18 months for video chatting in supervision of an adult. For children

18–24 months screen watch was limited to educational viewing along with an adult, though the permitted duration has not been mentioned. For children more than 2 years and till 5 years of age, entertainment screen time was permitted to 1 hour per day on weekdays and up to 3 hours on the weekend days. For >5 years, children were motivated for healthy habits and limit activities that include screens. For all age groups, parents were encouraged to turn off all screens during family meals, outings, and 30–60 minutes before bedtime. They were advised not to use screens as pacifiers, babysitters, or stop tantrums.

Like the United States, many other countries released their recommendations, especially in last 5 years. The Canadian Society for Exercise Physiology involving representatives of national organizations, research experts, methodologists, stakeholders, and end-users came together in 2017 to create the Canadian 24-Hour Movement Guidelines for the Early Years (0–4 years) and in older children. The guidelines recommended that children under 2 years should not have any screen time, 2–5 years should have not >1 hour a day and those over five should have not >2 hours a day of screen time.[52]

Australia too had similar guidelines along with parenting tips for younger kids and teens. The main features were to install parental controls, use age-appropriate sites with high learning potential, bookmark favorite sites so that children only go to the sites they are interested in, parents to sit with kids to check what they are seeing, time limit the sessions and avoid just-before-bed computer time and setting up good family guidelines and be the role models.[53]

In 2019, World Health Organization once again recommended no screen time for infants and no >1 hour for 2–4-year-old, with as less time possible to be preferred.[54]

Indian Guidelines

Indian Psychiatry Society 2020 Guidelines

The year 2020–21 saw the release of three guidelines from India. The first one was from Indian Psychiatry Society in 2020 where they advocated screen time for children in 2 subgroups.[55] They recommended no screen time for children 2 years of age and younger. For those between 2 and 5 years of age, screen time may be introduced but only under parent supervision. Further, for this age group, viewing was advised to be limited to educational media, not longer than 30 minutes per session, with a maximum of two sessions per day. Adult interaction with the child during media use has been stressed upon. It should be ensured that media watching should not turn into addiction. Screen watching affects the brain structurally and functionally, which becomes difficult to regulate in later ages and adolescents. Parents have been cautioned against fast-paced programs, those with violent content or having distracting elements. Such programs lead to concentration difficulties and behavioral problems later. They again stressed on not using screen time as a pacifier or to keep the child engaged. Screen-free areas and times like bedroom, mealtimes, and parent-child playtimes should be available. No screens one hour before bedtime and no screens in bedrooms have been advocated. Parents should be good role models.

For children between 5 and 18 years of age, besides following the above recommendations, they should also be taught "digital literacy". They should be explained on how to use technology in healthy and safe way. There should be some rules and time monitored plans for screen time, but they should be realistic. Media use should be strongly discouraged during mealtimes and doing homework. Preferably all screen watching should be done in common areas or with parents rather than in secluded separate room or place. Software such as parental control software, control filters, PIN passwords, or safe search may be used for healthy browsing. Content of social media platforms should be discussed by parents patiently to help children build trust and feel comfortable to communicate with their parents. Children should have a daily physical activity for at least 1 hour, and adequate sleep of 8–12 hours, as per age. They should be engaged in other activities such as reading, talking, and playing together which facilitate development and health. Children should not sleep with devices with them or around them. Children should be encouraged to discuss any new platform with parents before they join. Parents should guide children on how to avoid themselves getting exploited online and what to do if they come across any disturbing or inappropriate content. Parents should be patient and good listeners and should carry an empathetic attitude. It should be ensured that the family rules for media watching are explained to all members at home so that everyone in family understands and follows media rules.

PRAGYATA Guidelines

The next guidelines were from Ministry of Information and Broadcasting in association with National Council for Education, Research and Training (NCERT), named as PRAGYATA guidelines for online teaching in view of ongoing COVID-19 pandemic.[56] They suggested that screens should be limited to not more than 30 minutes for preprimary children while children of classes first till eighth to limit online classes to two sessions (30–45 min duration each). For classes from ninth to twelfth, it was permitted up to four sessions (30–45 min duration each).

Indian Academy of Pediatrics 2021 Guidelines

Further in 2021, Indian Academy of Pediatrics (IAP) released its parental guidelines for screen time, which, in accordance with AAP guidelines, does not permit screen time for children <2 years of age except video calls with relatives under adult supervision.[57] For those between the age of 2 and 5 years, screen time was limited to not >1 hour, with a word of caution that lesser the better. For children above 5 years, the academy advises to learn balancing screen time with other activities. These include all those activities needed for a complete overall development such as physical activity for at least an hour, adequate duration for sleep (as per age), homework completion, meal, and family timings, and extracurricular activities especially growing hidden talents and hobbies, etc. Screen should be used only over and above the time for these activities and should not be a restriction for the complete personality development of the child.

They have also suggested on the benefits and risks of digital media, how to ensure healthy use and the right age for use of various platforms of social media. Various steps to ensure digital hygiene were included such as to have a supportive and secure environment in family, to avoid using screen as pacifier, and to ensure that the child is getting adequate time to complete activities needed for overall growth as mentioned above. There should be no screen exposure at least an hour before sleeping. It has been reemphasized to have correct posture while sitting in front of the television, laptop, and mobile phones and to follow 20-20-20 rule to reduce eye strain and dryness **(Box 21.1)**. All digital devices should be switched off while watching television, and multitasking should be avoided. Parents should monitor the online content and interactions made and read by children. Programs and games with violent content should be avoided. Safe search engines and all safety and privacy measures should be followed. Digital free zones and free times should be maintained, and parents should be the role models for children.

■ CONCLUSION

In the present time, when digital media has become the major means of communication, following digital hygiene and online manners can help young children to live a more healthy and happy life. As pediatricians, we should educate parents and children about judicious use of media. We should educate them on how to maximize benefits and minimize the side effects. Simple take home measures like limiting screen time as per the age, parental

---

BOX 21.1: Steps to maintain correct posture and healthy eyes while watching screen.

1. Sit on a table and chair
2. The top of the screen to be at eye level
3. Shoulders should be relaxed
4. Legs should be bent at 90–100 degree angle
5. Feet should be flat on the floor
6. Chair should completely support the thighs and have a backrest for lower back
7. Forearm should be parallel to the floor
8. Device should be looked at by lowering the eyes rather than bending the neck
9. Every 20 minutes take a break for 20 seconds to look at an object 20 feet away

involvement, avoiding screen before sleep and in bedrooms, following 20-20-20 rule and to maintain screen free time and zones can help us to overcome these unprecedented difficult times during the current pandemic.

■ KEY POINTS

- Some of the key factors affecting screen time include higher sedentary activities, mealtime screen exposure, parental screen time, and accessibility to devices.
- Most common consequences of increased screen time are obesity, poor sleep pattern, poor cognition in young, psychological disorders, and visual problems.
- Behavioral change theories, using social cognitive approach, have been found to be the most successful intervention.
- American Academy of Pediatrics does not recommend screen time for less than 2 years and not more than 1–2 hours of quality programming per day beyond 2 years.
- Indian Academy of Pediatrics parental guidelines recommend for zero screen time, other than video calling, in children <2 years. Further for 2–5 years, not >1 hour is advised. Above 5 years, IAP suggests to learn balancing screen time with other activities.
- Avoiding screen an hour before sleep, no screen in bed rooms, screen-free family times, increased physical activities, parental monitoring, child friendly atmosphere, and parents as role model have been suggested in most guidelines.

■ REFERENCES

1. Anitha GFS, Narasimhan U. Coronavirus disease 2019 and the inevitable increase in screen time among Indian children: Is going digital the way forward? Ind Psychiatry J. 2020;29(1):171-5.
2. Dickson K, Richardson M, Kwan I. Screen-based activities and children and young people's mental health: A systematic map of reviews, London: EPPI-Centre, Social Science Research Unit, UCL Institute of Education, University College London; 2018.
3. Viner R, Davie M, Firth A. (2019). The health impacts of screen time: a guide for clinicians and parents. [online] Available from: https://www.rcpch.ac.uk/sites/default/files/2018-12/rcpch_screen_time_guide_-_final.pdf [Last accessed December, 2021].
4. Chassiakos YLR, Radesky J, Christakis D, Moreno MA, Cross C; Council on Communications and Media. Children and adolescents and digital Media. Pediatrics. 2016;138(5):e20162593.
5. Kaur N, Gupta M, Malhi P, Grover S. Screen time in under-five children. Indian Pediatr. 2019;56:773-88.
6. Thomas G, Bennie JA, De Cocker K, Castro O, Biddle SJH. A Descriptive epidemiology of screen-based devices by children and adolescents: a scoping review of 130 surveillance studies since 2000. Child Indicators Res. 2020;13:935-50.
7. AAP Council on Communications and Media. Media use in school-aged children and adolescents. Pediatrics. 2016;138:e20162592.
8. Meena P, Gupta P, Shah D. Screen time in Indian children by 15-18 months of age. Indian Pediatr. 2020;57:1033-6.

9. Dube M, Nongkynrih B, Gupta SK, Kalaivani M, Goswami AK, Salve HR. Screen-based media use and screen time assessment among adolescents residing in an urban resettlement colony in New Delhi, India. J Med Prim Care. 2018;7:1236-42.
10. Gupta A, Khan A, Rajoura O, Srivastava S. Internet addiction and its mental health correlates among undergraduate college students of a university in North India. J Fam Med Prim Care. 2018;7:721-7.
11. Yu L, Luo T. Social networking addiction among Hong Kong university students: Its health consequences and relationships with parenting behaviors. Front Public Health. 2021;8:555990.
12. Lyngdoh M, Akoijam BS, Agui R, Singh KS. Diet, physical activity, and screen time among school students in Manipur. Indian J Community Med. 2019;44:134-7.
13. Christakis DA, Garrison MM. Preschool-aged children's television viewing in child care settings. Pediatrics. 2009;124:1627-32.
14. Carson V, Janssen I. Associations between factors within the home setting and screen time among children aged 0–5 years: A cross-sectional study. BMC Public Health. 2012;12:539.
15. Barber SE, Kelly B, Collings PJ, Nagy L, Bywater T, Wright J. Prevalence, trajectories, and determinants of television viewing time in an ethnically diverse sample of young children from the UK. Int J Behav Nutr Phys Act. 2017;14:88.
16. Kourlaba G, Kondaki K, Liarigkovinos T, Manios Y. Factors associated with television viewing time in toddlers and preschoolers in Greece: the GENESIS study. J Public Health (Oxf). 2009;31:222-30.
17. Shah R, Fahey N, Soni A, Phatak A, Nimbalkar S. Screen time usage among preschoolers aged 2-6 in rural Western India: A cross-sectional study. J Fam Med Prim Care. 2019;8:1999-2002.
18. Duch H, Fisher EM, Ensari I, Harrington A. Screen time use in children under 3 years old: a systematic review of correlates. Int J Behav Nutr Phys Act. 2013;10:102.
19. LeBlanc AG, Katzmarzyk PT, Barreira TV, Broyles ST, Chaput JP, Church TS, et al. Correlates of total sedentary time and screen time in 9-11 year-old children around the world: The international study of childhood obesity, lifestyle and the environment. PLoS One. 2015;10(6):e0129622.
20. Paudel S, Jancey J, Subedi N, Leavy J. Correlates of mobile screen media use among children aged 0-8: A systematic review. BMJ Open. 2017;7:e014585.
21. Ravikiran SR, Baliga BS, Jain A, Kotian MS. Factors influencing the television viewing practices of Indian children. Indian J Pediatr. 2014;81:114-9.
22. Faltýnková A, Blinka L, Ševčíková A, Husarova D. The Associations between family-related factors and excessive Internet use in adolescents. Int J Environ Res Public Health. 2020;17(5):1754.
23. Chang HY, Park EJ, Yoo HJ, Lee JW, Shin Y. Electronic media exposure and use among toddlers. Psychiatry Investig. 2018;15:568-73.
24. Griffith SF, Hagan MB, Heymann P, Heflin BH, Bagner DM. Apps as learning tools: A systematic review. Pediatrics. 2020;145(1):e20191579.
25. Council on Communications and Media. Media and Young Minds. Pediatrics. 2016;138(5):e20162591.
26. Lenhart A, Duggan M, Perrin A. (2015). Teens, social media & technology overview 2015. [online] Available from: https://www.pewresearch.org/wp-content/uploads/sites/9/2015/10/pi_2015-10-01_teens-technology-romance_final.pdf [Last accessed December, 2016].

27. McClurg PA, Chaillé C. Computer games: Environments for developing spatial cognition? J Educ Comput Res. 1987;3:95-111.
28. Evans WD. Social marketing campaigns and children's media use. Future Child. 2008;18:181-203.
29. Bhanderi DJ, Pandya YP, Sharma DB. Smartphone use and its addiction among adolescents in the age group of 16-19 years. Indian J Community Med. 2021;46:88-92.
30. Li C, Cheng G, Sha T, Cheng W, Yan Y. The relationships between screen use and health indicators among infants, toddlers, and preschoolers: A meta-analysis and systematic review. Int J Environ Res Public Health. 2020;17(19).7324
31. Robinson TN, Banda JA, Hale L, Lu AS, Fleming-Milici F, Calvert SL, et al. Screen media exposure and obesity in children and adolescents. Pediatrics. 2017;140 (Suppl 2):S97-S101.
32. Braithwaite I, Stewart AW, Hancox RJ, Beasley R, Murphy R, Mitchell EA, et al. The worldwide association between television viewing and obesity in children and adolescents: Cross sectional study. PLoS One. 2013;8(9):e74263.
33. Gortmaker SL, Must A, Sobol AM, Peterson K, Colditz GA, Dietz WH. Television viewing as a cause of increasing obesity among children in the United States, 1986-1990. Arch Pediatr Adolesc Med. 1996;150:356-62.
34. Barr R, Lauricella AR, Zack E, Calvert SL. Infant and early childhood exposure to adult-directed and child-directed television programming. Merrill-Palmer Quarterly. 2010;56:21-48.
35. Schmidt ME, Pempek TA, Kirkorian HL, Lund AF, Anderson DR. The effects of background television on the toy play behavior of very young children. Child Dev. 2008;79:1137-51.
36. Murray JP. Media Violence: The effects are both real and strong. Am Behav Scientist. 2008;51:1212-30.
37. Gentile DA, Lynch PJ, Linder JR, Walsh DA. The effects of violent video game habits on adolescent hostility, aggressive behaviours, and school performance. J Adolesc. 2004;27:5-22.
38. Jett S, Laporte DJ, Wanchisn J. Impact of exposure to pro-eating disorder websites on eating behaviour in college women. Eur Eat Disord Rev. 2010;18:410-6.
39. Nigg JT. What causes ADHD?: Understanding what goes wrong and why. United States: Guilford Press; 2006. pp. 433 p.
40. Dalton MA, Beach ML, Adachi-Mejia AM, Longacre MR, Matzkin AL, Sargent JD, et al. Early exposure to movie smoking predicts established smoking by older teens and young adults. Pediatrics. 2009;123(4):e551-8.
41. McComb SE, Mills JS. A systematic review on the effects of media disclaimers on young women's body image and mood. Body Image. 2020;32:34-52.
42. Hansraj KK. Assessment of stresses in the cervical spine caused by posture and position of the head. Surg Technol Int. 2014;25:277-9.
43. Saxena R, Vashist P, Tandon R, Pandey RM, Bhardawaj A, Gupta V, et al. Incidence and progression of myopia and associated factors in urban school children in Delhi: The North India Myopia Study (NIM Study). PloS One. 2017;12(12):e0189774.
44. Schmidt ME, Haines J, O'Brien A, McDonald J, Price S, Sherry B, et al. Systematic review of effective strategies for reducing screen time among young children. Obesity (Silver Spring). 2012;20:1338-54.

45. Maniccia DM, Davison KK, Marshall SJ, Manganello JA, Dennison BA. A meta-analysis of interventions that target children's screen time for reduction. Pediatrics 2011;128:e193-210.
46. Altenburg TM, Holthe JK, Chinapaw MJM. Effectiveness of intervention strategies exclusively targeting reductions in children's sedentary time: a systematic review of the literature. Int J Behav Nutr Phys Act. 2016;13:65.
47. Downing KL, Hnatiuk JA, Hinkley T, Salmon J, Hesketh KD. Interventions to reduce sedentary behaviour in 0–5-year-olds: a systematic review and meta-analysis of randomised controlled trials. Br J Sports Med. 2018;52:314-21.
48. Nguyen P, Le LK-D, Nguyen D, Gao L, Dunstan DW, Moodie M. The effectiveness of sedentary behaviour interventions on sitting time and screen time in children and adults: an umbrella review of systematic reviews. Int J Behav Nutr Phys Act. 2020;17:117.
49. American Academy of Pediatrics. Children, adolescents, and television. Pediatrics. 2001;107:423-6.
50. Council on Communications and Media. Children, adolescents, and the media. Pediatrics. 2013;132:958-61.
51. AACAP. (2020). Screen time and children. [online] Available from: https://www.aacap.org/AACAP/Families_and_Youth/Facts_for_Families/FFF-Guide/Children-and-Watching-TV-054.aspx#contentstart [Last accessed December, 2020].
52. Canadian Society for Exercise Physiology. (2017). Canadian 24-Hour Movement Guidelines for the Early Years (0–4 Years): An Integration of Physical Activity, Sedentary Behaviour, and Sleep. [online] Available from: https://www.participaction.com/sites/default/files/downloads/PAR7972_24h_Guidelines_EY_En.pdf [Last accessed December, 2021].
53. Australian Department of Health. (2019). Australia Physical activity and sedentary Behaviour guidelines and the Australian 24 Hour movement guidelines. Australian Department of Health 2019. [online] Available from: http://www.health.gov.au/internet/main/publishing.nsf/content/health-pubhlth-strateg-phys-act-guidelines#npa05 [Last accessed December, 2021].
54. World Health Organization. (2019). Guidelines on physical activity, sedentary behaviour and sleep for children under 5 years of age. [online] Available from: https://apps.who.int/iris/handle/10665/311664 [Last accessed December, 2021].
55. Indian Psychiatric Society. (2020). Recommendations for screen use. [online] Available from: https://indianpsychiatricsociety.org/wp-content/uploads/2020/06/E-Booklet-RECOMMENDATIONS-FOR-SCREEN-USE.pdf [Last accessed December, 2021].
56. PRAGYATA: Guidelines for digital education. (2021). Department of School Education & Literacy Ministry of Human Resource Development Government of India. [online] Available from: https://www.education.gov.in/sites/upload_files/mhrd/files/pragyata-guidelines_0.pdf [Last accessed December, 2021].
57. Indian Academy of Pediatrics. (2021). Screen time guidelines for parents. [online] Available from: https://iapindia.org/pdf/Screentime-Guidelines-for-Parents-Ch-005.pdf [Last accessed December, 2021].

Environmental Medicine

Noise-induced Hearing Loss

Alok Gupta

Don't make noise!
Loud sounds in a classroom or in a library meant a disturbance or an irritant to students and the teacher. Well, this still holds true.

■ INTRODUCTION
What is "Sound"?
Vibrations from any source make the particles in that medium to quiver "to and fro", moving the particles around them, without getting displaced themselves, causing a "wave effect". This pressure wave moves outward in a direction, which is dependent on the source as well as the medium. When we clap in air or drop a stone in a pond with still water, air or the water particles are pressed and then decompresses by pressure, which gets transmitted ahead causing a "ripple effect". These pressure changes are felt by other objects in the vicinity. The mammalian ears including those of humans perceive this as "sound". This sound is described and measured in various ways.[1]

■ ASSESSMENT OF SOUND
Volume or loudness of sound depends on the quantum of pressure changes particles are subjected to or the distance moved by them. When these pressure changes are plotted on a graph, the height of graph is proportionate to the "amplitude" or the "loudness" of the sound.

Decibel (dB) is the relative measure of loudness, volume, or intensity of sound. In air, a 10 dB sound is the softest that human beings can hear whereas 130 dB becomes painful. The term "dB(A)" is A-weighted measurement, which is believed to correlate better with the relative risk of noise-induced hearing loss (NIHL) and used when dB is used in relation to sound's effect on hearing.

Pitch of sound is the frequency of vibrations of particles per second.

Wavelength is the gap between two vibrations or waves. The wavelength of the sound is indirectly proportional to the pitch or frequency of sound. High-pitched sounds have shorter wavelengths. Humpback whales making low-pitched sounds have up to 100 metres between the peaks of their sound waves.

Frequency: The number of sound waves passing in a fixed period is frequency of that sound. Hertz (Hz) is a measure of frequency. Hertz is the vibrations made by sound originator per second. At a fixed point, if 20 waves pass in 1 second it would mean that the sound is of 20 Hz. Normal human beings can hear sounds between the ranges of 20 and 20,000 Hz. 1,000 Hz is equal to 1 kHz and normal human beings can hear sounds up to 20 kHz only. The density of air and water is different, water being denser. A comparison factor of 61.5 dB needs to be added to measure sound in water. 343 m/s sound speed in air equals to 1,484 m/s when in water. Increase in amplitude relates to volume whereas the frequency change is the "pitch" of the sound.[1]

■ ORGANS OF HEARING

The principal organ of hearing in human beings is the ear **(Fig. 22.1)**, which collects the sounds mostly outside the body and transmits it to the brain, which deciphers the sound. Human ear is made of three parts:

1. *Outer ear*: Outer ear consists of the "pinna", a passage known as the "ear canal" and the eardrum or the "tympanic membrane". Tympanic membrane transmits the mechanical sound waves to the middle ear.[2,3]
2. *Middle ear*: Middle ear extends from the tympanic membrane laterally to the "oval window" medially. This small air-filled chamber is connected to the nasopharynx through the Eustachian tube. Middle ear contains three of the tiniest bones or ossicles in the human body, namely hammer or the malleus (most lateral), anvil or the incus and the stirrup or the stapes, the most medially placed. These three ossicles transmit the sound

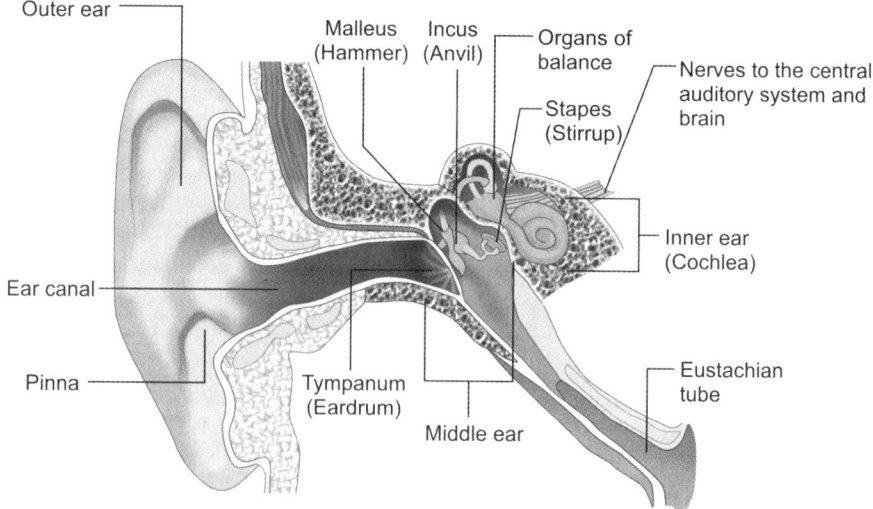

Fig. 22.1: Organs of hearing in human beings.

wave vibrations or pulses from the tympanic membrane to the inner ear. The muscles attached to these three ossicles regulate the intensity of sound transmitted to inner ear and thus present the sound safely and appropriately to be forwarded inside through stapes attached to the oval window. The round window is the other membrane window that transmits mechanical sound waves to the inner ear filled with fluid.[2,3]

3. *Inner ear:* Inner ear contains the cochlea, a fluid filled spiral tube, which is divided lengthwise by the organ of Corti. Organ of Corti converts the mechanical signals of varied intensity into neuronal signals of corresponding action potentials. Organ of Corti consists of very sensitive and specialized hair cells and basilar membranes bathed in endolymph. It also transmits these neuronal signals to the auditory nerve and the central nervous system (CNS).[2,3] The number of outer and inner hair cells of cochlea is fixed at birth. In mammalian spices including human beings, regeneration of these sensory cells does not occur once they have been damaged.

■ SOUND FREQUENCIES

Sound is produced in varying frequencies ranging from 0 Hz and more. Human beings with normal hearing can hear the frequencies that range from 20 to 20,000 Hz. This range of frequency (audible range) is known as the *audio frequency (AF)*. Sounds below 20 Hz are infrasonic and the sounds above 20,000 Hz are ultrasonic sounds. Animals, other than human beings, can perceive sounds of ultrasonic as well as infrasonic frequencies as per their natural requirement.

Average sound levels with their safe limits at common places we inhabit are given in **Table 22.1**. We should remember that these are averages and

TABLE 22.1: Sound levels and safe duration at common places (approximate).

Common places	Decibel (dB)	Safe duration
Spacecraft/rocket launching time	220	Nil
Airplane taking off (from 25 m distance)	140	Nil
Night club	110–120	1 hour
Construction activity	100	4 hours
Medium road traffic	80–90	4–8 hours
Busy office	80	8 hours
Normal talk	60	16 hours
Study room	30–40	16 hours
Sleeping areas	20–30	16 hours
Outer space	0	–

hearing loss can occur at lower sound levels as well at lesser duration in an individual.[4]

■ NOISE

When does "Sound" become a "Noise"?

Sound is referred to as "noise" subjectively. Any undesirable sound can be called noise. Technically, sounds which are not pure or rhythmic are known as noise.

Sound wave making a sine-shape graph is called a "pure note". Vibrating tuning fork of a particular frequency produces a smooth wave-line and thus a pure sound of one note. Harmonics are created by combining a number of pure notes in various combinations that form the basis of musical instruments.

Impure notes are not pleasant to ears and are referred to as noise. The graph of "noise" if plotted is random and not smooth. These unpleasant sounds are screened out by our ears to a varying extent and are very subjective. Sounds under the water to humans are messed up or jumbled sounds with unclear pure-tones or patterns.

A sound, source of which may be visible or invisible but is intense, inappropriate, causes irritation or disturbance, or leads to harm or diminishes or disrupts one's quality of life, which may be temporary or permanent is known as *noise*.[5,6] When this sound occurs in the environment for a time or intensity causing reversible temporary or irreversible permanent adverse effect on animals or humans, it comes to be called *noise pollution*.[7,8] Now we have evidence that loud sound and its associated vibrations cause damage to the monuments, architecture, buildings, and other similar nonliving things. Evidence that plants too are disturbed by noise is a matter of concern. Noise adds to the hearing damage caused by other factors and vice versa. The resultant loss of hearing, partial or complete becomes a handicap for comfortable living.

■ HEARING LOSS

As per the estimates of the World Health Organization (WHO), 1.5 billion people (nearly 20%) out of 7.9 billion global population experience some hearing loss in their life, of whom at least 430 million (6%) will require care.[9] The consequences of hearing loss if unidentified or unaddressed early are grave. Hearing loss affects the development of language and speech, cognitive development, listening, communication, education, psychosocial health, earning, employment, mental health, relationships, identity issues, stigma and quality of life and could lead to loss of nearly 1 trillion dollars every year.[9]

Loud music for long time puts nearly 1.1 billion young people of age 12–23 years at the risk of hearing loss, which is permanent but totally preventable as the public in general does not know the risk of exposure to loud music. Increasing public awareness is essential to prevent this noise-induced hearing loss (NIHL).[1,9]

Worldwide, children constitute about 40 million of the 430 million people having hearing loss that is disabling. WHO estimates that 60% of the hearing loss occurring in childhood is preventable.[9] National Health and Nutrition Examination Survey (NHNES), USA (1994-2006) data shows that hearing loss in teenagers increased from 3.5 to 5.3%. Use of personal audio device (PAD) music increased by 75% between 1990 and 2005, mostly with the risky behavior of using them for 16-18 hours every day at high volumes. Nearly 50% of people aged 12-35 years use PAD with high volumes. Excessive sound at workplaces causes NIHL in 16% adults.[9] Noise affects other systems of the body but these too are totally preventable.

Hearing loss (HL) occurs when a person cannot perceive the sounds within the audible range clearly. This can occur naturally with aging (presbycusis) or due to some event disrupting the hearing apparatus (outer, middle or inner ear), auditory nerve or specified areas in the brain. The hearing loss may be minor where hearing of only some frequencies are lost or major when it is spread across a wide range of frequencies. Tinnitus and hallucinations can occur due to a complex mechanism affecting the hearing system.

■ CLASSIFICATION OF HEARING LOSS

The classification of HL is done based on the etiology or type or degree of hearing loss as shown in **Box 22.1**.[1,9-11]

BOX 22.1: Classification of hearing loss.

- **Based on etiology of hearing loss**
  - Hereditary
  - Congenital
  - Aging/presbycusis
  - Acquired
- **Based on the types of hearing loss**
  - *Conductive*: Involvement of outer and middle ear
  - *Sensorineural (SNHL)*: Involvement of Inner ear, auditory nerve or brain
  - *Mixed*: Conductive and sensorineural
- **Based on the degree** [in decibel HL (dBHL)] **of hearing loss**[9]
  - Slight (16–25 dBHL)
  - Mild (26–34 dBHL)
  - Moderate (35–49 dBHL)
  - Moderately severe (50–64 dBHL)
  - Severe (65–80 dBHL)
  - Profound (81–94 dBHL)
  - Total or complete (95 and above)
  - Unilateral (< 20 dB in the better ear, 35 dB or greater in the worse ear)

■ AREAS OF NOISE POLLUTION

The most common areas of noise pollution in a community are:
- *Public transport hubs*: Bus stands, airports, railway stations, shipyards, highways and parking lots
- Industries, mining, and commercial zones
- Residential, educational, institutional and office areas
- Entertainment, social, religious, and public places
- *Other areas*: Noisy workplaces, heavy construction work belts, tunneling, combat training and war zones, health care areas such as hospitals, sport centers such as stadiums, pet zones, and recreational habitats like gymnasium.

■ SOURCES OF NOISE

The common sources of noise leading to pollution and hearing loss include:
- *Motorized vehicles:* Motorcycles, autos, cars, emergency vehicles, buses, trucks, large trailers, trains, airplanes, helicopters, jets, combat aircrafts, cargo vehicles, maintenance vehicles, etc.
- *Large machines:* Drills, land-movers and diggers, and machines used in construction and maintenance of buildings, etc.
- *Mechanical equipment:* Mixers, grinders, hammers, mowers, air cooling systems as well as kitchen, home, educational and office appliances.
- *Leisure:* Noisy toys, play stations, radio, television (TV), bands, music systems, loudspeakers, movie halls, concerts, rock bands, processions, discotheques, PADs such as earphones, ear buds, headphones, and other Bluetooth audio devices.
- *Communications:* Public address systems, headphones, and handheld phones, etc.

■ HEALTH HAZARDS OF ENVIRONMENTAL NOISE POLLUTION

Only in the recent past, noise and noise pollution have been identified to have adverse effects on hearing. This effect is across all spectrums of ages. Environmental noise pollution (ENP) causes two main effects on hearing—(1) auditory and (2) nonauditory **(Table 22.2)**.

TABLE 22.2: Health hazards of environmental noise pollution (ENP).

Auditory	Nonauditory
Tinnitus	Noise annoyance and noise sensitivity
Hidden hearing loss (HHL)	Insomnia and sleep disturbances
Noise-induced hearing loss (NIHL)	Cognitive impairment
	Cardiovascular manifestations

Auditory Hazards

Tinnitus

Hissing, buzzing, ringing, whistling, grinding or similar abnormal sounds are often heard by many in one or both ears. They seem to arise closeby in the surroundings just like sounds of crickets. When these sounds occur frequently or become continuous, they are known as tinnitus. Tinnitus can be very annoying and distracting often hampering normal activities such as study, meditation, prayer, work and sleep. Origin of tinnitus has been found to be sensorineural with the two most important causes being noise pollution and aging.

Hidden Hearing Loss (HHL)

In hidden hearing loss (HHL) hyperacusis, difficulty in hearing and tinnitus occur though undetectable on pure tone audiometry. Normal hearing is present in 250–8,000 Hz range. Cochlear synaptopathy occurs before hair cell destruction, which then finally progresses to permanent hearing loss.[9]

Noise-induced Hearing Loss

Nearly 5% population in the world is suffering from NIHL. NIHL accounts for about 50% acquired hearing loss in human beings. As per WHO estimates, 50% of the children and adults between ages of 12 and 35 years using PAD remain at risk of loss of hearing and more so when the use is prolonged, or the level of the sound is high.[9] Very loud sound that is sudden may lead to perforation of eardrums or acute tympanitis due to sudden strong force of the sound waves. Gradual loss of hearing due to prolonged exposure of noise is sensorineural hearing loss (SNHL). This is due to irreversible damage to the hearing organs of the inner ear, the auditory nerves and/or the nervous tissues in the CNS.[12] NIHL may be temporary or permanent.

Temporary NIHL: A brief but very loud sound like an exploding firecracker, or an explosive, a jet-plane landing or take off may lead to temporary or reversible loss in hearing. A few hours of exposure to moderately loud sound like in a discotheque or a rock-concert may also lead to temporary hearing loss. Wide range of frequencies are affected in such losses and fortunately near full recovery usually ensues within hours to weeks depending on the intensity of exposure and damage to the hearing organs.

Permanent NIHL: Irreversible hearing loss occurs due to constant exposure to sound frequencies of 80 dB(A) or a single sudden exposure above 120 dB(A). The hearing loss occurs over a small or wide range of frequencies, which are difficult to predetermine.

US Environment Protection Agency (USEPA) has labeled 70 dB(A) of sound as the safe upper cut-off range. Sounds above this level have decreasing safe duration. Sounds at or above 85 dB have a safe limit of eight hours per 24 hours only while sound of 100 dB has a safe limit of only 15 min. Correspondingly a brief sound above 120 dB will be permanently damaging to the human hearing organs.[6]

Cochlear damage by loud sounds happens by two mechanisms:

1. *Mechanical*: The rigidity and effective functioning of sensory hair cells is lost by regular exposure to loud sounds gradually over a period till they are permanently destroyed and become non-functional.
2. *Cellular level intense metabolic activity*: Intense exposure to loud sounds requires high energy levels to protect themselves. The high oxygen consumption leads to increased levels of free-radical generation in the cochlea. Antioxidant defense system of the ear fails to neutralize the free radicals generated and permanent cell death results.

Personal Audio Devices

Personal audio devices are now a proven cause for NIHL. The output regulations for PADs vary from country to country and are not followed strictly. The commonly used PADs have an output, which ranges from 75 to 136 dB. The volume set by users of these devices commonly ranges from 75–105 dB.[9,13-17] 50% of the young children and adults including adolescents use PADs constantly or at high volumes. When this habit of routine daily use of PADs persists for some years, high frequency hearing (4 kHz) starts getting affected. With time the higher and lower frequencies start getting affected leading to permanent irreversible SNHL.[9] This NIHL gets worse with aging and other causes of hearing loss pitch in. In a US study, 12.5% of the children between 6 and 19 years of age had a varying degree of permanent hearing loss due to increasing noise pollution.[6,18]

Hazards of unsafe use of personal audio devices
The hazards of unsafe use of PADS include:
- Low quality ear buds do not block ambient noise out
- Music by tiny speakers is directed right into the ear canal
- Bass transmission is poor by ear buds
- The user keeps increasing the volume for better sound effect
- Better space buffering between the ear canal and music is provided by outside-the-canal headphones but they too do not transmit bass effectively, being of poor quality
- Compromised road safety, reduced social communication, cognitive overload and impaired performance
- Air-block, ear numbness, wax accumulation, otitis, tinnitus and NIHL.

Non-auditory Hazards

Environmental noise pollution (ENP) is any sound occurring in the habitat for a time or intensity causing temporary (reversible) or permanent (irreversible) adverse effect on animals or humans. All animals are affected by sound. Unpleasant sound causes them to move away from the source, become irritable, aggressive or show some abnormal behavior. They may lose concentration and get hurt or resort to become quieter or louder themselves.[19]

Noise has varied effects on human beings. Mental as well as physical health has been proved to be adversely affected. Psychomotor effects of noise pollution are well established. Noise affects the human beings in the following ways:[6,9,20,21]

- Noise annoyance and noise sensitivity
- Sleep disturbance and insomnia
- Cognitive impairment
- Cardiovascular disorders.

Noise Annoyance and Noise Sensitivity

Anyone and everyone get annoyed by a wrong sound at a wrong time, at a wrong place of a wrong intensity. A sound of an airplane taking off or landing is expected at an airport, a train at train station, large trucks on the highway, loud music in a discotheque or a concert, roaring cars and motorbikes on the racetrack, machine sounds in a factory but not in a home, classroom, or a quiet workplace. If it happens, it will be annoying leading to negative responses such as loss of concentration, communication difficulties, inadvertent raising of voice to be heard properly, mood and behavior disturbances, withdrawal, depression, distraction, dissatisfaction, disappointment, irritability, change in body language, anger, unsocial behavior, etc. When these noises occur with increasing frequencies or regularities the effects will correspondingly increase. These effects in turn will start affecting the normal physiology of individuals ranging from newborn, infants, children, adolescents, adults, pregnant women, and elderly.[12,22] Effects on the pregnant women will affect the developing fetus. Hence the entire range of the population will be affected including the entire animal kingdom and possibly the plants and heritage structures. Noise-annoyance causes loss of more than 0.5 million disability-adjusted life years (DALYs) among the urban population in European Region countries alone (WHO). The effect is more established and pronounced in those with noise sensitivity and other personality traits like neuroticism.[21]

Sleep Disturbance and Insomnia

The effect of noise during sleep is dependent on the stage of sleep and occurrence of awakening. Chronic effects of "nocturnal environmental noise (NEN)" on health lead to suppression of hypothalamic-pituitary-adrenal (HPA) axis and sympathetic nervous system. Disturbances of sleep and arousal also affect the release of anabolic growth hormones. Insomnia and sleep deprivation also affect the immune system, appetite, and carbohydrate metabolism. Hormonal imbalances between ghrelin, insulin and leptin occur leading to adiposity, increased body mass index (BMI) and risk of type 2 diabetes.[21]

Cognitive Impairment

Sleep deprivation and annoyance lead to cognitive impairment of varying proportions.

Cardiovascular Disorders

Blood pressure, heart rate and cardiovascular events are similarly affected depending on personality traits. Systemic inflammation is increased as reflected by increase in C-reactive protein (CRP), tumor necrosis factor-α (TNF-α) and interleukin-6 (IL-6) levels that are causes of increased morbidity and mortality.

■ HAZARD RECOGNITION

Recommendations for newborn hearing tests soon after birth are well in place. This detects the hearing disability in a newborn for the congenital and hereditary causes. It is not a common pediatric practice to perform hearing tests in childhood unless a hearing loss is suspected by a parent or a teacher because of child's lack of attention, poor school performance or delayed development. Older children and adolescents may directly or indirectly indicate hearing issues by selective use of a better ear, using louder sound volumes or hearing difficulties in them as well as in their siblings and peers. Unfortunately, by this time as it is with vision, the hearing loss has become permanent which can only increase with time. The effects of moderate sounds are cumulative in nature as well as the other factors damaging the cochlear structures including aging process, which adds to gradual loss of hearing.

Noise pollution though omnipresent, unfortunately, till recent past, happens to be an area that has been neglected totally. It is only now that noise pollution has been identified as a hazard to health and has found an established place as a distinct entity in the policies for environmental pollution.[9,23] "Silent Zone" and "No Horn Zone" in India are still signs that can be seen placed in schools, hospitals, and VIP areas. Loud music and use of loudspeakers are banned during the night hours but only in bigger cities and local authorities take action only when the affected people lodge a complaint. Surprisingly all the noisy and heavy vehicles can run during these night hours.

Fortunately, the learned people including the children have started to recognize the "value of silence" during the resting hours and concerns are being raised. The "last Wednesday of April" every year is now observed as "International Noise Awareness Day" and "No Horn Day" by the concentrated efforts of the Center of Hearing and Communication (CHC) since the year 1996. Concerned public and professional bodies discuss deafness,

NIHL, and related issues on this day to increase the public awareness about the hazards of noise and it being a totally avoidable source of pollution.[24]

■ NOISE POLLUTION: GUIDELINES AND RULES

The Situation in India

The Central Pollution Control Board (CPCB), Ministry of Environment, Forest and Climate Change, Government of India enacted "The Noise Pollution (Regulation and Control) Rules, 2000" (Updated June 12, 2020).[25]

Guiding Principles

The major guiding principles are summarized here:
- Whereas the increasing ambient noise levels in public places from various sources, inter-alia, industrial activity, construction activity, generator sets, loudspeakers, public address systems, music systems, vehicular horns and other mechanical devices have deleterious effects on human health and the psychological well-being of the people; it is considered necessary to regulate and control noise producing and generating sources with the objective of maintaining the ambient air quality standards in respect of noise.
- An area comprising not less than 100 meters around hospitals, educational institutions and courts may be declared as silence area/zone for the purpose of these rules.
- "Area/Zone" means all areas which fall in either of the four categories categorized by the State Government, viz., industrial, commercial, residential or silence areas/zones for the purpose of implementation of noise standards for different areas.
- "Educational institution" means a school, seminary, college, university, professional academies, training institutes or other educational establishment, not necessarily a chartered institution and includes not only buildings, but also all grounds necessary for the accomplishment of the full scope of educational instruction, including those things essential to mental, moral, and physical development.
- "Hospital" means an institution for the reception and care of sick, wounded, infirm or aged persons, and includes government or private hospitals, nursing homes and clinics.
- The Act describes in detail, the responsibilities of the local administration in control of ENP under the following headings and the maximum permissible levels of sound **(Table 22.3)**.
- Responsibility as to enforcement of noise pollution control measures.
- Restrictions on the use of loudspeakers/public address system.
- Consequences of any violation in silence zone/area.
- Complaints to be made to the authority.
- Power to prohibit, etc., continuance of music sound or noise.

TABLE 22.3: Ambient air quality standards in respect of noise as specified by CPCB.

SCHEDULE
(see rule 3(1) and 4(1))
Ambient Air Quality Standards in respect of Noise

Area code	Category of area / zone	Limits in dB(A) Leq*	
		Day time	Night time
(A)	Industrial area	75	70
(B)	Commercial area	65	55
(C)	Residential area	55	45
(D)	Silence zone	50	40

Note:
1. Day time shall mean from 6.00 a.m. to 10.00 p.m.
2. Night time shall mean from 10.00 p.m. to 6.00 a.m.
3. Silence zone is an area comprising not less than 100 metres around hospitals, educational institutions, courts, religious places or any other area which is declared as such by the competent authority
4. Mixed categories of areas may be declared as one of the four above mentioned categories by the competent authority.

* dB(A) Leq denotes the time weighted average of the level of sound in decibels on scale A which is relatable to human hearing.

A "decibel" is a unit in which noise is measured.

"A", in dB(A) Leq, denotes the frequency weighting in the measurement of noise and corresponds to frequency response characteristics of the human ear.

Leq: It is an energy mean of the noise level over a specified period.

TABLE 22.4: Recommendation for upper limits of most common sources of noise.

Areas of noise	Average daily exposure (dB)	Night exposure (dB)	Strength of evidence
Road traffic	53	45	Strong
Railway noise	54	44	Strong
Aircraft	45	40	Strong
Wind turbine	45	–	Conditional
Leisure noise	70 (yearly)	–	Conditional

European Region

WHO European Region Guidelines (2018): Guiding Principles: Reduce, Promote, Coordinate and Involve

- Reduce exposure to noise, while conserving quiet areas
- Promote interventions to reduce exposure to noise and improve health

- Coordinate approaches to control noise sources and other environmental health risks
- Inform and involve communities potentially affected by a change in noise exposure.[21]

The recommendations, source by source, are shown in **Table 22.4**. Though these WHO recommendations have been issued for European Region but global data has been taken into account and thus can be used for policy making by any country in the world.

NOISE-INDUCED HEARING LOSS
Diagnosis of Noise-induced Hearing Loss[1,4,9]

- Tinnitus or difficulty in hearing in one or both the ears is the presenting complaint. Onset may be sudden or gradually increasing difficulty in hearing conversation in a party, meeting, noisy workplace or crowd.
- Thorough examination of the ear, tuning fork tests and audiometry will be needed to confirm hearing loss and its extent.
- Appropriate audiometry tests are chosen taking age and other possible factors into consideration. The tests used may be pure tone audiometry, otoacoustic emissions (OAE), auditory brainstem responses (ABR), brainstem auditory evoked response (BAER) or behavior audiometry evaluation (BAE).

Treatment of Noise-induced Hearing Loss[4,9,26,27]

Reversal or treatment of NIHL by medical or surgical intervention is not possible, as of now. Research in future may help. Stem cell and gene therapy, neurotropins and pharmacological agents may come to rescue and improve quality of life in future.

Acute NIHL

- Person should be shifted into a quiet room immediately.
- Antioxidants and hyperbaric oxygen can help in limiting the damage.
- Exposure to loud sounds in future has to be avoided to protect cochlear structures.
- Ear buds and ear muffs to be used for protection of hearing in noisy places. When used singly and together 15–30 dB and 25-45 dB sound reduction is achieved, respectively.

Chronic NIHL

- Hearing protection and exposure to loud sounds have to be avoided strictly to prevent further HL.
- Hearing aids, cochlear implants, bone conduction and middle ear implants, sign language, speech reading and other rehabilitative technology can be helpful as per individual requirements.

■ PREVENTION OF HARMFUL EFFECTS OF NOISE

Individuals[9]
- Keep sound volume low
  - Use good quality PADs with lowest possible volume and for least possible time (at 60% of maximum volume for less than 1 hour in a day)
  - Use speaker phone whenever possible
- Minimizing time spent in noisy places
  - If possible, avoid residence near bus stands, railway stations, airports, highways, etc.
  - Avoid loud sounds, music events and noisy areas
- Protect ears and hearing in noisy places
  - Use ear buds and ear muffs.
- Monitor personal sound exposure and hearing
  - Maximum total sound exposure be kept below 80 dB for 40 hours/week
  - Check hearing regularly by smart phone apps such as 'hearWHO' app and by ENT doctors.

Community[9]
- Administrative controls and sound engineering for the reduction of noise levels and exposure
  - The CPCB of India Act will be a definite deterrent.
  - Loudspeakers, motor vehicle horns, pressure horns, sirens, etc., be made punishable except in emergency situations.
  - Noisy vehicles and machinery be prohibited in residential, hospital and quiet areas and sound barriers are installed around noisy areas.
  - Noise inside hospitals and quiet areas needs to be addressed.
  - Music programs should be held in closed areas or away from quite areas with a clear warning of harmful effects of noise unless hearing protection in place.
  - Public transport hubs such as railway stations, bus stands, airports, etc., should be moved away from residential areas.
  - Electric vehicles, optimum speed limits, good smooth roads, and smooth flowing traffic can bring down traffic noise considerably.
- Noise monitoring
  - Strict compliance of local noise pollution guidelines be enforced 24 × 7 by noise monitoring.
- Use of hearing protectors
  - Hearing protectors such as ear buds, headphones, and ear muffs should be used and made available at all places of loud noise.
- Public education
  - The CPCB should choose a few focus areas of concern like loudspeakers in public places and traffic noise to start with. Campaigns for public awareness will educate the public about the repercussions of

these noises and the need to avoid them. Public is usually not aware that such laws exist and therefore bear them as inevitable.
- Roadside hoardings, road signs, etc., will be helpful in educating the people of their rights about noise pollution. Complaints can be lodged under Section 16 (f) of the Air (Prevention and Control of Pollution) Act, 1981.[25]
- Hearing surveillance
  - Hearing surveillance at birth, school, elderly and at-risk population is the key to early identification and rehabilitation. A smartphone app, *hearWHOpro* can be used as screening tool by the healthcare workers.

■ CONCLUSION

Environmental noise pollution (ENP) is a serious health issue, which is now drawing increased attention. It is the leading cause of temporary as well as permanent loss of hearing in all age groups starting from intrauterine life. Nonauditory effects of ENP are alarming. Sleep disturbance is the major effect of nocturnal environmental noise (NEN), which in turn leads to metabolic, endocrine, cardiac and psychiatric disorders, developmental delay and antisocial behavior in children as well as adults. Biological effects akin to endogenous sleep disorders result in altered sleep patterns, sleep quality and stress. These consequences trigger daytime sleepiness, mood changes, annoyance, irritability, nervousness and tiredness leading to impaired decision taking normally as well as in emergency situations, diminished cognitive performance, and decreased well-being the following day. These effects occurring daily can be disastrous to individuals as well as public at large depending on the occupation of the individual. Awareness, public health measures and counseling can prevent and treat these concerns. Normal hearing and adequate sleep are essential for normal functioning. ENP as well as NEN need to be addressed and adequate measures must be taken to prevent adverse effects caused by them.

■ KEY POINTS

- An intense and inappropriate sound that causes irritation or disturbance, or leads to harm, or diminishes or disrupts one's quality of life, whether temporary or permanent is defined as 'noise'.
- When the sound occurs in the environment for a time or intensity causing reversible temporary or irreversible permanent adverse effect on humans, it is called environmental noise pollution.
- Gradual loss of hearing due to prolonged exposure of noise is sensorineural hearing loss (SNHL).
- Unwanted, undesired sound of low or high intensity becomes noise, which has adverse auditory hazards and effects on other systems of the body.
- Auditory health hazards of noise pollution include tinnitus, hidden hearing loss and noise-induced hearing loss.

- Persistent daily long-term use of personal audio devices (PADs) leads initially to high frequency hearing (4 kHz) followed by permanent irreversible SNHL of both higher and lower frequencies.
- Nonauditory health hazards of noise pollution are noise annoyance and noise sensitivity, insomnia and sleep disturbances, cognitive impairment and cardiovascular manifestations.
- Noise-induced hearing loss (NIHL) is very common but is entirely preventable.
- Avoid noise and use hearing protection when unavoidable.
- NIHL is irreversible and permanent. Nearly 5% population in the world is suffering from NIHL. NIHL accounts for about 50% acquired hearing loss in human beings.
- Public awareness is very important to protect hearing.

■ DISCLAIMER

No funding or conflict of interest.

■ REFERENCES

1. CDC. (2018). Audiometry Procedures Manual. NHANES. [online] Available from: https://wwwn.cdc.gov/nchs/data/nhanes/2017-2018/manuals/2018-Audiometry-Procedures-Manual-508.pdf. [Last Accessed January, 2022].
2. WHO. The anatomy and physiology of the ear and hearing. [online] Available from: www.who.int/occupational_health/publications/noise2.pdf. [Last Accessed January, 2022].
3. Healy AF, Proctor RW. Handbook of Psychology: Experimental Psychology. New Jersey: John Wiley and Sons; 2003.
4. Gupta A, Gupta A, Jain K, Gupta S. Noise pollution and impact on children health. Indian J Pediatr. 2018:85(4):300-6.
5. Goines L, Hagler L. Noise pollution: a modern plague. South Med J. 2007;100(3); 287-94.
6. United States Environment Protection Agency. Clean Air Act Title 4. [online] Available from: https://www.epa.gov/clean-air-act-overview/clean-air-act-title-iv-noise-pollution. [Last Accessed January, 2022].
7. EPA. Noise Pollution and Abatement Act of 1972. Senate Public Works Committee. S. Rep. No. 1160, 92nd Cong. 2nd session. Washington, D.C.: United States Environment Protection Agency; 1976.
8. Hogan CM, Latshaw GL. The relationship between highway planning and urban noise. Proceedings of the ASCE, Urban Transportation by American Society of Civil Engineers. Chicago, Illinois: Urban Transportation Division; 1973.
9. WHO. World Report on Hearing. [online] Available from: https://www.who.int/publications/i/item/world-report-on-hearing. [Last Accessed January, 2022].
10. Martini A, Mazzoli M, Kimberling W. An introduction to the genetics of normal and defective hearing. Ann N Y Acad Sci. 1997;830:361-74.
11. Clark JG. Uses and abuses of hearing loss classification. ASHA. 1981;23(7):493-500.
12. Thakur N, Batra P, Gupta P. Noise as a health hazard for children, time to make a noise about it. Indian Pediatr. 2016;53(2):111-4.
13. Mazlan R, Saim L, Thomas A, Said R, Liyab B. Ear infection and hearing loss amongst headphone users. Malays J Med Sci. 2002;9(2):17-22.

14. Huh A, Choi Y, Moon KW. The effects of earphone use and environmental lead exposure on hearing loss in the Korean population. Korean National Health and Nutrition Examination Survey. PLoS One. 2016:15-24.
15. Kiran N, Sunil P. High frequency hearing loss in students used to earphone music: a randomized trial of 1000 students. Indian J Otol. 2014;20(1):29-32.
16. Krug E, Cieza MA, Chadha S, Sminkey L, Morata T, Swanepoel D, et al. Hearing loss due to recreational exposure to loud sound, 1st edition. Geneva: World Health Organization; 2015.
17. Khaiwal R, Singh T, Tripathy JP, Mor S, Munjal S, Patro B, et al. Assessment of noise pollution in and around a sensitive zone in North India and its non-auditory impacts. Sci Total Environ. 2016;566-67:981-7.
18. Martin WH, Sobel J, Griest SE, Howarth L, Yongbing S. Noise induced hearing loss in children; preventing the silent epidemic. J Otol. 2006;1(1):11-21.
19. Buxton RT, McKenna MF, Mennitt D, Fristrup K, Crooks K, Angeloni L, et al. Noise pollution is pervasive in U.S. protected areas. Science. 2017;356 (6337);531-3.
20. Rosen S, Olin P. Hearing loss and coronary heart disease. Arch Otolaryngol. 1965;82:236-43.
21. World Health Organization. (2018). Environmental Noise Guidelines for the European Region. [online] Available from: https://www.euro.who.int/en/health-topics/environment-and-health/noise/publications/2018/environmental-noise-guidelines-for-the-european-region-2018. [Last Accessed January, 2022].
22. Monazzam MR, Karimi E, Abbaspour M, Nassiri P, Taghavi L. Spatial traffic noise pollution assessment - a case study. Int J Occup Med Environ Health. 2015;28(3):625.
23. Andersen ZJ, Sram RJ, Ščasný M, Gurzau ES, Fucic A, Gribaldo L, et al. Newborns health in the Danube Region: Environment, biomonitoring, interventions and economic benefits in a large prospective birth cohort study. Environ Int. 2016;88:112-22.
24. Pluhar ZF, Piko BF, Kovacs S, Uzzoli A. "Air pollution is bad for my health": Hungarian children's knowledge of the role of environment in health and disease. Health Place. 2009;15(1):239-46.
25. CPCB. (2000). The Noise Pollution (Regulation and Control) Rules, 2000 [online]. Available from: http://cpcbenvis.nic.in/noisepollution/noise_rules_2000.pdf. [Last Accessed January, 2022].
26. Oishi N, Schacht. Emerging treatments for noise-induced hearing loss. Expert Opin Emerg Drugs. 2011;16(2):235-45.
27. American Hearing Research Foundation. Noise Induced Hearing Loss. Hearing and Balance. [online] Available from: http://american-hearing.org/disorders/noise-induced-hearing-loss. [Last Accessed January, 2022].

Critical Care

CHAPTER 23: Management of Burns

K Ravikumar, Bala Ramachandran

■ INTRODUCTION

Burns are a leading cause of morbidity and mortality in children. Burns in children account for 17–25% of total admissions due to burns in our country.[1] Most burns in children are due to household accidents. Scald burns are common in younger children, whereas flame burns are more common in older children. Children are different compared to adults when it comes to management of burns. The body surface area (BSA) to body mass ratio is higher in children. Younger children have thin skin and less subcutaneous fat. These factors predispose to more loss of heat and water in children with burns. Therefore, children with burns have more complications due to fluid loss and hypothermia compared to adults. Assessment of the depth of burns is difficult in children due to their thin skin.

■ INITIAL ASSESSMENT AND STABILIZATION IN THE EMERGENCY ROOM

The initial assessment and stabilization of a child with burns is similar to a child with polytrauma. Systematic assessment with primary survey followed by secondary survey should be done in all children with major burns.[2]

Primary survey includes the following steps—airway management, breathing with ventilation, circulation and cardiovascular stabilization, disability and neurological examination, and exposure.

Airway management is crucial in children with thermal burns involving the face and head or in children with inhalational injury and these children may require intubation and mechanical ventilation for airway edema. Breathing and ventilation may be affected in children with full thickness circumferential burns involving the chest or in acute lung injury secondary to burns or sepsis.

The hemodynamic status of the patient may be affected due to excess fluid loss combined with a lack of adequate fluid intake or resuscitation prior to arrival in emergency room (ER). Fluid boluses are required only if there are features of shock. Fluid management will be based on the body surface area involved.

Disability management includes assessment of mental status using the Glasgow Coma Scale in children with suspected inhalational injury or hypoxia.

Exposure includes removal of clothes to assess the degree of burns involvement and prevent the effects of heat/chemicals in thermal and chemical burns respectively.

Secondary survey includes assessment of the percentage of surface area and depth of burns, in addition to looking for any nonburn injuries.[2] Assessment of the percentage of surface area of burns in children should be done using the Lund-Browder chart **(Fig. 23.1; Table 23.1)** as it considers the disproportionate body surface area of head and extremities, rather than the "Rule of Nines".[2,3] Assessment of depth of burns is difficult as depth may change due to fluid resuscitation and wound infection.

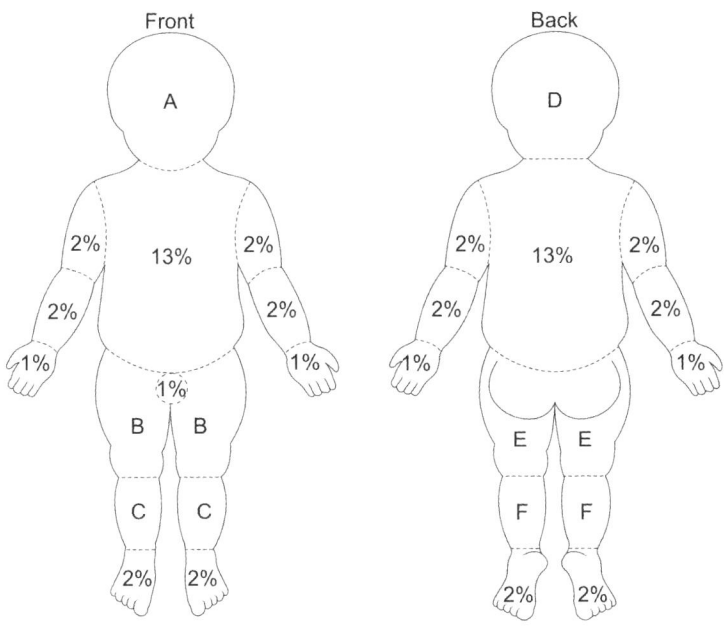

Fig. 23.1: Burns surface area calculation.

TABLE 23.1: Lund-Browder Chart used to assess surface area of burns in children.[3]					
Relative percentage of body surface area (% BSA) at different ages					
	Age				
Body Part	0 year	1 year	5 years	10 years	15 years
A/D = ½ of head	9 ½	8 ½	6 ½	5 ½	4 ½
B/E = ½ of 1 thigh	2 ¾	3 ¼	4	4 ¼	4 ½
C/F = ½ of 1 lower leg	2 ½	2 ½	2 ¾	3	3 ¼

TABLE 23.2: Hospital admission criteria for children with burns.[1,2]

S. No.	Criteria
1.	Burns involving face, hands, genitalia, perineum, or major joints
2.	Partial thickness burns involving more than 10% total body surface area (TBSA) and any partial thickness burns in infants
3.	All third-degree burns
4.	High voltage electrical burns and chemical burns
5.	Circumferential burns involving extremities/chest/abdomen
6.	Inhalational injury
7.	Burns in children with other co-morbidities or concomitant trauma
8.	Suspected child abuse

Once initial assessment is completed, children with smaller area of burns with good mental status and stable hemodynamics can be sent home on simple management remedies (e.g., paracetamol for pain relief) after initial first aid and dressing. Children requiring admission should be stabilized and shifted to the 'Burns ward' or the pediatric intensive care unit (PICU) based on the clinical condition. **Table 23.2** lists the criteria for admission to the hospital.[1,2]

TYPES OF BURN INJURIES

Electrical Burns

Electrical burns are rare in children but cause significant underlying tissue damage. Electrical injuries can cause direct and indirect damage.[4] Direct damage is tissue or organ damage directly from the current. Indirect damage can be due to trauma secondary to a fall following electric shock or problems caused by forceful muscle contractions. Electrical injuries are classified as low or high voltage injury. Low voltage injuries generally result from sources with voltage less than 1,000 V and have less morbidity. Children with low voltage injuries can be managed as outpatient cases, if the electrocardiograph (ECG) is normal and mental status is good. High voltage injuries result from source with voltage more than 1,000 V and can be fatal.[5] Children with high voltage electrical injuries will need hospital admission for monitoring. Deep tissue and organ involvement is common with electrical injuries and complications such as arrhythmias, muscle damage, compartment syndrome, rhabdomyolysis, or renal failure may ensue. Fluid requirements may be higher in electrical burns. In children with renal failure, fluid requirements will be variable and early renal replacement therapy should be started.

Chemical Burns

Chemicals cause protein denaturation and tissue destruction. Tissue damage is directly proportional to the duration of exposure, concentration of chemical and tissue solubility.[1] Tissue damage is more with alkalis as compared to acid burns. Chemical burns are most likely due to accidental ingestion of colored liquids by children and cause more of gastrointestinal, upper and lower airway and facial injuries. The most important first aid is to clean the affected area with copious amounts of running water and remove any contaminated clothing to prevent further damage due to the chemicals. Neutralizing solutions are neither available nor useful in most of the chemical burns.

Inhalational Injury

Inhalational injury refers to airway or pulmonary damage secondary to direct thermal or chemical injury.[2] Cyanide or carbon monoxide toxicity due to inhalation of gases generated during combustion of plastics and other substances are also included under inhalational injury. Hoarseness of voice, history of burns happening within an enclosed space, burns above the clavicle, singed nasal hairs, respiratory distress with lung parenchymal involvement and carbonaceous sputum are clues suggestive of probable inhalational injury.[1,2]

In children with inhalational injury without respiratory distress or stridor, careful clinical monitoring for worsening of respiratory symptoms is a safe option.[1] These children may get better with supportive care in most of the situations. The other alternative is to visualize the airway under general anesthesia using laryngoscopy or bronchoscopy to assess the extent of airway involvement. Children with inhalational injury having respiratory distress or upper airway obstruction symptoms will most likely need some form of respiratory support (noninvasive or invasive ventilation) and airway evaluation. These children will require aggressive physiotherapy, early identification, and treatment of pneumonia. Nebulized heparin, epinephrine, mucolytics and systemic steroids have not shown consistent benefits.[6,7] Systemic steroids may increase the risk of new-onset infection and should be used with caution.

■ FLUID MANAGEMENT

Burns involving more than 15–20% of total body surface area (TBSA) commonly result in increased capillary permeability secondary to inflammation and increased hydrostatic pressure. Both under- and over-resuscitation are detrimental. Under-resuscitation leads to hypoperfusion, organ dysfunction and further worsening of inflammation. Over-resuscitation, also called as fluid-creep, leads to increase in burn wound depth due to tissue edema, compartment syndrome, acute lung injury and multiorgan dysfunction.[2,8,9]

The timing of starting resuscitation is extremely important since delay is associated with worse outcomes. In a retrospective study of 133 children with burns involving > 50% TBSA, the mortality when resuscitation was started within 2 hours of injury, between 2–4 hours and 4–12 hours was 14%, 61% and 91%, respectively. Early start of resuscitation was associated with less sepsis, acute kidney injury and cardiac arrest.[10]

In children, burns involving more than 10% of TBSA will require fluid resuscitation for fluid losses from skin damage.[8] Resuscitation fluid does not include the maintenance fluids. Fluid resuscitation in burns has evolved over time starting from the 17th century to the most recent Parkland/revised Brooke formulae used in adults **(Table 23.3)**. The calculated resuscitation fluids are administered over the first 24 hours, with 50% of the resuscitation fluids given over the first 8 hours and the remaining 50% given over the next 16 hours.[2,8]

Initial adult resuscitation formulae used a mixture of colloids and crystalloids and two-figure formulae (resuscitation and maintenance fluid containing dextrose separately). Newer resuscitation formulae do not have separate maintenance fluids preparations. Over time, the amount of fluids used for resuscitation has decreased and colloids have been removed from resuscitation formulae.[8]

Pediatric fluid resuscitation has been modified from adult formulae. The major problem with modification was the proportionally higher body surface area in children compared to adults. Fluid requirements are higher in children. Children also have less glycogen stores and will need dextrose-containing maintenance fluids along with resuscitation fluids.[1,2,8]

In children without venous access, oral or nasogastric (NG) route can be tried. During emergency, venous access (central/peripheral) can be inserted through burns affected skin and later changed to other sites. Children with up to 25–30% TBSA burns, who are alert and not in shock, can be started on oral/NG fluid resuscitation using oral rehydration solution (ORS) or salt/sugar or rice (*conjee*) water or vegetable soups with salt in a peripheral set up and then moved to a higher-level center. Oral/NG route can be used to give 15–20% of calculated resuscitation fluids.[2,11]

Endpoints of Resuscitation

The resuscitation formulae shown above are only a rough guide to administer IV fluids. Fluids must be adjusted based on endpoints in the patient to prevent under/over-resuscitation. The most used end point for resuscitation in burns is the urine output. Urine output > 0.5 mL/kg/h in children > 30 kg and urine output 0.5–1 mL/kg/h in children < 30 kg is a sign of adequate fluid resuscitation.[2,8] Urine output may be affected by inappropriate antidiuretic hormone (ADH) secretion secondary to pain and stress. The other end points of resuscitation are clinical parameters such as heart rate, pulse

TABLE 23.3: Newer fluid resuscitation formulae for burns in children.[2,8]

Formula	Age group	Crystalloid volume	Colloid volume	Maintenance dextrose fluids	Administration instructions
Parkland	Adult	4 mL/kg/% TBSA burns as RL	No	No	Half over first 8 hours, half over next 16 hours
Revised Brooke	Adult	3 mL/kg/% TBSA burns as RL	No	No	Half over first 8 hours, half over next 16 hours
Cincinnati	Younger children	4 mL/kg/% TBSA burn + 1500 mL/m² total BSA as RL	12.5 g of 25% albumin per liter of crystalloid in the last 8 hours of the first 24 hours	5% dextrose as needed to maintain glucose	• Half over first 8 hours, half over next 16 hours. Composition of fluid changes every 8 hours • First 8 hours—50 mEq/L of NaHCO$_3$ added to RL • Second 8 hours—RL alone • Third 8 hours—25% albumin mixed with RL
Cincinnati	Older children	4 mL/kg/% TBSA burn + 1,500 mL/m² total BSA as RL	No	5% dextrose as needed to maintain glucose	Half over first 8 hours, half over next 16 hours
Galveston	All children	5000 mL/m² TBSA burn + 2000 mL/m² TBSA as RL	12.5 g of 25% albumin per liter of crystalloid	5% dextrose as needed to maintain glucose	Half over first 8 hours, half over next 16 hours

(% TBSA: percent total body surface area; BSA: body surface area: RL: Ringer's Lactate; NAHCO$_3$: sodium bicarbonate) volume, peripheral perfusion, mental status, and laboratory markers such as base excess and lactate. Using these clinical and lab endpoints, initial fluid administration rates can be changed (decreased or increased) to avoid over/under-resuscitation.

■ ADMISSION TO PEDIATRIC INTENSIVE CARE UNIT

Children needing airway monitoring, respiratory support, and hemodynamic support should be monitored in the pediatric intensive care unit (PICU) **(Table 23.4)**. Infants with large area of burns also need to be admitted to the PICU for better hemodynamic monitoring.[1] In the PICU, resuscitation fluids initiated in the emergency room (ER), analgesia, wound care measures and other supportive measures should be continued. Organ dysfunction parameters should be monitored.

■ ROUTINE CARE OF THE BURNS PATIENT

Routine care involves, in addition to appropriate surgical management, careful assessment of the fluid balance to ensure that neither too much nor too little fluid is given, providing proper and adequate nutrition, preventing infection, detecting and treating established infection early, and maintaining metabolic homeostasis. Several advancements have occurred in the management of burns over the past few decades. These are related to early resuscitation, advances in airway management, nutrition, infection control, surgical management, transfusion therapy, management of hypermetabolism and the availability of various types of artificial skin covers.

■ WOUND MANAGEMENT

Wound care aims to maintain a moist environment, prevent burn wound infection, promote burn wound healing, and minimize discomfort for the patient.[12,13] Wound care begins with cleaning, gentle debridement, and dressing the wound with antimicrobial agents. Cleaning should ideally be done with running tap water rather than stored water in home-based settings or peripheral centers. Sterile water or saline can be used to clean in higher centers.

TABLE 23.4: Criteria for transfer to pediatric intensive care unit (PICU).

S. No.	Criteria
1	Children with burns involving face or neck
2	Inhalational injury
3	Children requiring mechanical ventilation for airway/lung involvement
4	Children with hemodynamic instability or multiorgan dysfunction
5	Children with burns involving more than 15% total body surface area (TBSA)
6	Children with burns and secondary sepsis

Clean uninfected wounds can be covered with biological dressings or skin substitutes. Biological dressings promote epithelialization, decrease pain and fluid losses from burnt skin and are preferred in children. Gauze or fine mesh gauze dressing with antimicrobials are preferred in infected wounds. Antimicrobial ointments are not required for superficial burn wounds. In heavily colonized wounds, antibiotic, and antifungal ointments along with wound excision are used to decrease the incidence of systemic infections. There is no role for prophylactic systemic antibiotics in the first week of burn injury. Systemic antibiotics are used only for suspected or proven burn wound infection.

Advances in Burn Wound Care

One of the most important advances in the care of burns is the concept of early wound excision and grafting. The burn wound has lost its protective skin cover and serves as a portal for entry of microorganisms. In addition, the wound potentiates the inflammatory process contributing to the hypermetabolism seen in burns patients. Burn wounds were initially covered with temporary dressings and subsequently subjected to split thickness skin grafting or allowed to heal by secondary intention. However, the currently preferred therapy is to excise the wound so that necrotic tissue is removed up to a depth where viable tissue is available. This is done by repeated tangential excision—when done within 48-72 hours of injury, it is called *"early excision"*. The excised wound must be covered by either the patient's own skin (autograft), or with other materials including allografts (cadaveric or donated human skin), or artificial skin. Early wound excision and wound cover is now the mainstay of burns therapy across the world and has been shown to be associated with less blood loss, shorter hospital length of stay, reduced morbidity, and mortality, when compared with delayed excision and grafting.[14]

Advances in Burn Wound Assessment

Accurate assessment of burn wound depth is challenging, even for experienced surgeons. Of late, laser technology is used to assess burn wound depth by measuring microvascular dermal perfusion. These techniques, called laser Doppler imaging (LDI), or laser Doppler Line scanning, are more accurate than regular visual assessment. A recent study showed that LDI done 48 hours to 5 days after injury had accuracy between 90 and 97%, compared with 53-71% by clinical assessment.[15]

Advances in Burn Wound Cover

Due to the limited availability of autografts from the patient and allografts, various alternatives have been tried to cover the burn wound after excision. Biological dressings include amniotic membrane and processed bovine collagen (Kollagen®). Amniotic membrane has been used for centuries and is even now quite popular in several parts of the world for treating partial-thickness burns. Collagen membrane is used extensively in India for both partial and full thickness burns.[16]

Several biosynthetic materials are available for use as temporary wound cover and include the following:
1. *Biobrane®*: Collagen chemically bound to nylon and encased in silicone film
2. *AWBAT®*: Like Biobrane®, but much more porous
3. *Suprathel®*: A synthetic copolymer film

In addition to these, several dermal analogs are available. The most widely used analog is Integra®—a tissue engineered composite skin substitute useful for deep burns.

Cultured epithelial autografts (CEA) are important advances in burn management. Full thickness samples of unburned skin are taken from the victim at admission and then subjected to a tissue culture process. The patient's wounds are excised and covered temporarily with allografts or other material. After 3 weeks, sheets of keratinocytes are available for use on the patient. This technique has been reported to give good results in patients with extensive (>75% TBSA) burns.[17]

In addition to these, other composite skin substitutes containing live fibroblasts are available (Orcel®, Apligraft®)—these are not widely used because they have a limited shelf life. ReCell® is a spray-on preparation consisting of live fibroblasts, melanocytes, Langerhans cells and keratinocytes that is useful to treat the donor area wound. Finally, active research is ongoing in the field of gene therapy and the use of growth factors to improve burn wound healing.[18]

■ PAIN MANAGEMENT

Pain management in an important cornerstone of burns management. Pain management starts with appropriate pain monitoring. Various validated pain-scoring systems are available. The burns specific pain anxiety scale (BSPAS) monitors pain as well as anxiety in patients with acute burns. It is based on a questionnaire that is scored by the patient and therefore cannot be used in young children. Critical care pain observation tool (CPOT) can be used when patients are not able to communicate or interact for pain assessment. It is an objective measurement using behavioral variables only.[19,20] The Comfort B scale is an objective measurement of pain and sedation in children using eight parameters including behavioral and physiological (heart rate, blood pressure and respiration) variables.[21] Comfort B scale is the preferred scoring system for pain and sedation assessment in children. Nurses should be trained in the use of appropriate pain monitoring tools.

Pharmacological therapies remain the mainstay, but nonpharmacological therapies should be tried in children with chronic burns to avoid drug dependence. Paracetamol or nonsteroidal anti-inflammatory drugs (NSAIDs) can be used for pain management, alone or in combination with opioids. Opioid analgesics (morphine/fentanyl/tramadol) are needed in major burns and in admitted patients.

Ketamine is an alternative to opioid for burn wound dressing procedures, as it gives good skin analgesia. Dexmedetomidine and clonidine are reasonable alternative to opioids but less effective. Gabapentin or pregabalin can be used in patients with neuropathic pain. Effective pain management is important for rehabilitation and long-term outcomes.[19]

■ NUTRITION

In patients with burns, the catabolic/hypermetabolic state is prolonged and can continue for months. Protein degradation and requirements are higher in patient with burns. Caloric requirements are higher and if not met appropriately, the catabolic state by itself leads to poor wound healing and higher risk of infection. Nutritional support is especially important in any child with burns. *Early enteral nutrition* is the best way to provide calories without increasing the risk of infection. Nasogastric tube feeding is a very good alternative to direct oral feeding and will help in reaching the target calorie and protein intake faster and in a consistent manner. Multiple studies have shown that initiation of enteral feeds early, within 24 hours, is associated with shorter ICU length of stay, fewer wound infections and lower mortality.[22]

Indirect calorimetry (IC) is the ideal method to calculate calorie requirements in any child with burns due to high and variable requirements. Unfortunately, IC is cumbersome and not freely available. Nutritional support is guided by formulae in the majority of centers. There are different formulae available to calculate calorie requirements in children with burns.[2] Few commonly used formulae are the Galveston Shriners Burn Center formula **(Table 23.5)** or Curreri Junior formula **(Table 23.6)**.[1,2,8] Again, these formulae are only rough guides for management. Besides these formulae, daily or frequent weight monitoring, clinical examination to look for edema and fluid overload, laboratory parameters such as urinary urea nitrogen, acute phase reactants such as serum albumin and C-reactive protein can be used to adjust the nutritional support.

TABLE 23.5: Galveston Shriners Burn Center formula for nutritional support.[1,8]

Age group	Daily calorie requirement
Infants (0–12 months)	2,100 kcal/m^2 + 1,000 kcal/m^2 burn
Children (1–11 years)	1,800 kcal/m^2 + 1,300 kcal/m^2 burn
Children (12 years and older)	1,500 kcal/m^2 + 1,500 kcal/m^2 burn

TABLE 23.6: Curreri Junior formula for nutritional support in children with burns.[1,2]

Age group	Daily calorie requirement
0–1 year	Basal RDA in kcal + 15 kcal per % burn
1–3 years	Basal RDA in kcal + 25 kcal per % burn
4–15 years	Basal RDA in kcal + 40 kcal per % burn

RDA: recommended dietary allowances, Basal RDA (kcal) varies with age

■ TRANSFUSION IN BURNS

Traditionally, hemoglobin in critically ill patients with burns has been maintained at a level higher than 10 g/dL. Proponents of this practice argue that this threshold is required to improve oxygen carrying capacity and improve wound healing. However, of late this strategy has been questioned. Blood transfusions are associated with many adverse effects, including transfusion-associated circulatory overload (TACO), transfusion-associated acute lung injury (TRALI), immunosuppression and transmission of infections. A study in patients with burns had shown that blood transfusion by itself is associated with 11% increase in the incidence of bloodstream infections for each unit transfused.[23] Subsequently, a randomized trial in adults with burns showed that a restrictive transfusion strategy (transfusion of packed cells only when Hb < 7 g/dL) was equivalent to a liberal policy of transfusion to maintain a hemoglobin > 10 g/dL. There were no differences in any outcome parameter, including incidence of bloodstream infections, ventilator days, time to wound healing, length of stay or 30-days mortality. The restrictive transfusion group received 50% less blood transfusions. Another single center study also confirmed that a restrictive transfusion strategy in children with burns is safe. Therefore, current recommendations are that blood transfusion should be given to patients with burns only for hemoglobin < 7 g/dL.[24]

■ HYPERMETABOLISM IN BURNS

Burn injury leads to a severe hypermetabolic state that is mediated by the exaggerated release of proinflammatory mediators, including tumor necrosis factor (TNF) and interleukins (IL-6 and IL-8). There are increased levels of catecholamines, glucagon and cortisol, and lower levels of growth hormone (GH) and testosterone. The net result is a catabolic state that causes profound metabolic derangement. There is glycolysis, gluconeogenesis, lipolysis, proteolysis, insulin resistance, hepatic dysfunction and loss of lean and total body mass.[25-27] The hypermetabolic state occurs in two distinct phases—the ebb and the flow phase. The ebb phase happens early, within 48 hours of injury and is associated with reduced cardiac output, oxygen consumption, and metabolic rate, along with impaired glucose tolerance and hyperglycemia. The flow phase starts as a gradual increase in metabolic rate, leading to hyperdynamic circulation, fever, tachycardia, insulin resistance and marked hyperglycemia. The flow phase can last for up to 12 months after injury, and the altered glucose homeostasis can persist for as long as 3 years.[27] There is net negative protein balance, immune dysfunction, decreased wound healing, and an inability to use lipids as an energy source.

Management of the Hypermetabolic Phase after Burns

Early wound excision and grafting reduces the magnitude of the hypermetabolic response. In addition, several agents can be used to attenuate this hypermetabolic phase—anabolic steroids, propranolol, metformin, and insulin.

Oxandrolone, a testosterone analog with less virilization, has been used successfully at a dose of 0.1 mg/kg (maximum 10 mg) orally twice daily. It improves nitrogen loss, reduces weight loss, and improves donor site wound healing. It can be used for up to 1 year following burns. Liver enzymes should be monitored, and female recipients checked for virilization. Oxandrolone has been associated with significantly decreased length of hospitalization and improved lean body mass.[27] Even though lean body mass increases, strength can be improved only with concomitant exercise.

Propranolol has been shown to oppose the effects of increased catecholamines, resulting in decreased metabolism, heart rate, resting energy expenditure and reduced muscle wasting. There is also some evidence to show that propranolol use reduces the incidence of hospital-acquired infection and sepsis in children and adults with burns.[28]

Glycemic Control

Hyperglycemia occurs during the hypermetabolic phase and has been associated with increased morbidity and mortality.[27] Hyperglycemia can be managed with either insulin or metformin. The exact glucose target is unknown. Insulin is associated with anabolic and anti-inflammatory responses and when used in the acute phase of burns has been shown to improve donor-site healing, and reduce infection rates and mortality. The use of insulin must be balanced with the risk of hypoglycemia. Metformin has been shown to reduce blood glucose equally well as insulin, with less hypoglycemia.[27]

■ GROWTH HORMONE

Children with burns have significant growth delay. Treatment with recombinant human growth hormone (rhGH) has been shown to have a significant improvement in height velocity.[27] However, rhGH should be used only in the chronic phase after burns, and only in the absence of active infection.

■ CONCLUSION

Recent advances in the management of burns in children include early excision with grafting, administering less fluids, fewer blood transfusions, avoiding prophylactic antibiotics, and the use of newer wound cover materials.

The management of burns in children is challenging and best results can be achieved through a multidisciplinary effort involving the burns surgeon, the pediatric intensivist, infectious disease specialist, pulmonologist, microbiologist, clinical pharmacologist, endocrinologist, nutritionist, anesthesiologist and physiotherapist. With careful attention to detail, it is possible to save even children with exceptionally large burns, involving > 70% TBSA.

■ KEY POINTS

- Up to 25% of the total admissions due to burns in India are reported in children.
- Most pediatric burns are accidental and preventable.
- Burn surface area in children should be determined by using the Lund-Browder chart, and not by the "Rule of Nines".
- Early adequate fluid resuscitation is extremely important—fluids should be titrated to achieve a urine output of 0.5–1 mL/kg/h.
- Prophylactic systemic antibiotics are not required during the initial phase of management of burns.
- Pain should be assessed with a clinical scoring system and treated adequately.
- Early enteral nutrition is the best policy for nutritional support.
- Packed RBC should be transfused only if hemoglobin is <7 g/dL.
- Propranolol is effective in treating the hypermetabolism after burns.

■ REFERENCES

1. Sharma RK, Parashar A. Special considerations in paediatric burn patients. Indian J Plast Surg. 2010;43(Suppl 1):S43-50.
2. ISBI Practice Guidelines Committee, Steering Committee, Advisory Committee; Ahuja RB, Gibran N, Greenhalgh D, Jeng J, Mackie D, Moghazy A, et al. ISBI Practice Guidelines for Burn Care. Burns. 2016;42(5):953-1021.
3. Broadis E, Chokotho T, Borgstein E. Paediatric burn and scald management in a low resource setting: A reference guide and review. Afr J Emerg Med. 2017;7(Suppl):S27-31.
4. Koumbourlis A. Electrical injuries. Crit Care Med. 2002;30(11 Suppl):S424-30.
5. Arnoldo B, Klein M, Gibran NS. Practice guidelines for the management of electrical injuries. J Burn Care Res. 2006;27(4):439-47.
6. Levine BA, Petroff PA, Slade CL, Pruitt BA Jr. Prospective trials of dexamethasone and aerosolized gentamicin in the treatment if inhalation injury in the burned patient. J Trauma. 1978;18(3):188-93.
7. Miller AC, Rivero A, Ziad S, Smith DJ, Elamin EM. Influence of nebulized unfractionated heparin and N-acetylcysteine in acute lung injury after smoke inhalation injury. J Burn Care Res. 2009;30(2):249-56.
8. Romanowski KS, Palmieri TL. Pediatric burn resuscitation: past, present, and future. Burns Trauma. 2017;5(1):1-9.
9. Duran C, Sheridan RL. Current concepts in the medical management of the pediatric burn patient. Curr Trauma Rep. 2016;2(4):202-9.
10. Barrow RE, Jeschke MG, Herndon DN. Early fluid resuscitation improves outcomes in severely burned children. Resuscitation. 2000;45(2):91-6.
11. Pham TN, Cancio LC, Gibran NS; American Burn Association. American Burn Association practice guidelines burn shock resuscitation. J Burn Care Res. 2008;29(1):257-66.

12. Norman G, Christie J, Liu Z, Westby MJ, Jefferies JM, Hudson T, et al. Antiseptics for burns. Cochrane Database Syst Rev. 2017;7(7):CD011821.
13. Yoshino Y, Ohtsuka M, Kawaguchi M, Sakai K, Hashimoto A, Hayashi M, et al; Would/Burn Guidelines Committee. The wound/burn guidelines – 6: Guidelines for the management of burns. J Dermatol. 2016;43(9):989-1010.
14. Lang TC, Zhao R, Kim A, Wijewardena A, Vandervord J, Xue M, et al. A Critical Update of the Assessment and Acute Management of Patients with Severe Burns. Adv Wound Care (New Rochelle). 2019;8(12):607-33.
15. Zuo KJ, Medina A, Tredget EE. Important developments in burn care. Plast Reconstr Surg. 2017;139(1):120e-138e.
16. Oliveira A, Simões S, Ascenso A, Reis CP. Therapeutic advances in wound healing. J Dermatolog Treat. 2020;1-21.
17. Jeschke MG, Shahrokhi S, Finnerty CC, Branski LK, Dibildox M. Wound coverage technologies in burn care: established techniques. J Burn Care Res. 2018;39(3):313-8.
18. Jeschke MG, Finnerty CC, Shahrokhi S, Branski LK, Dibildox M; ABA Organization and Delivery of Burn Care Committee. Wound coverage technologies in burn care: novel technologies. J Burn Care Res. 2013;34(6):612-20.
19. ISBI Practice Guidelines Committee; Advisory Subcommittee; Steering Subcommittee; Allorto N, Atieh B, Bolgiani A, Chatterjee P, Cioffi W, Dziewulski P, et al. ISBI Practice Guidelines for Burn Care, Part 2. Burns. 2018;44(7):1617-706.
20. Romanowski KS, Carson J, Pape K, Bernal E, Sharar S, Wiechman S, et al. American Burn Association Guidelines on the Management of Acute Pain in the Adult Burn Patient: A Review of the Literature, a Compilation of Expert Opinion and Next Steps. J Burn Care Res. 2020;41(6):1129-151.
21. Ista E, Van Dijk M, Tibboel D, De Hoog M. Assessment of sedation levels in pediatric intensive care patients can be improved by using the COMFORT "behavior" scale. Pediatr Crit Care Med. 2005;6(1):58-63.
22. Endorf FW, Ahrenholz D. Burn management. Curr Opin Crit Care. 2011;17(6):601-5.
23. Palmieri TL, Caruso DM, Foster KN, Cairns BA, Peck MD, Gamelli RL, et al; American Burn Association Burn Multicenter Trials Group. Effect of blood transfusion on outcome after major burn injury: a multicenter study. Crit Care Med. 2006;34(6):1602-7.
24. Palmieri TL. Burn injury and blood transfusion. Curr Opin Anaesthesiol. 2019;32(2):247-51.
25. Gauglitz GG, Williams FN, Herndon DN, Jeschke MG. Burns: where are we standing with propranolol, oxandrolone, recombinant human growth hormone, and the new incretin analogs? Curr Opin Clin Nutr Metab Care. 2011;14(2):176-81.
26. Gus EI, Shahrokhi S, Jeschke MG. Anabolic and anticatabolic agents used in burn care: What is known and what is yet to be learned. Burns. 2020;46(1):19-32.
27. UpToDate. (2018). Hypermetabolic response to moderate to severe burn injury and management. [online] Available from: https://www.uptodate.com/contents/hypermetabolic-response-to-moderate-to-severe-burn-injury-and-management/contributors. [Last Accessed January, 2022].
28. Jeschke MG, Norbury WB, Finnerty CC, Branski LK, Herndon DN. Propranolol does not increase inflammation, sepsis, or infectious episodes in severely burned children. J Trauma. 2007;62(3):676-81.

Critical Care

CHAPTER 24: Refractory Status Epilepticus

Soonu Udani, Suhani Shah

■ LEARNING OBJECTIVES
- To understand the various terms and timelines associated with the management of status epilepticus (SE) and focus on refractory status epilepticus (RSE).
- To understand the recent advances in the management of RSE.
- To be able to follow or devise an institutional algorithm for the management of SE.

Prehospital and domiciliary management will not be discussed.

■ INTRODUCTION

Epilepsy has been known since prehistoric times and there are references in cave paintings, in records of old South American civilizations and even in the Bible. Ancient Indian medical texts had prescribed cures for epilepsy and even today many of our patients seek alternative medicinal cures as adjuncts to what we prescribe. Shakespeare referred to it as the "falling sickness" for Julius Caesar. It was only in the 18th and 19th century, that epilepsy was emancipated from superstition to a disorder of the brain. Herbs and chemical substances such as potassium bromide were commonly used in the ancient times. Due to the anticonvulsant and sedative traits, potassium bromide became a choice of treatment for patients with epileptic seizures and nervous disorders until the discovery of phenobarbital in 1912.[1]

Convulsive, generalized status epilepticus (SE) is one of the most common emergencies both in office and in intensive care situations. Prompt management is usually effective in terminating seizures in addition to stabilizing vital signs and preventing secondary organ and brain damage. Most episodes will terminate spontaneously, but the acute care of continued seizure activity, despite routine treatment, poses a major challenge. Refractory status epilepticus (RSE) and super-RSE (SRSE) have poor overall long-term outcome. Recent advances in the management include immunotherapy and rarely, emergency surgery.

■ EPIDEMIOLOGY

The World Health Organization (WHO) estimates the global burden of epilepsy at 50 million with 4–10 per 1,000 being on active treatment. Nearly 80% of people with epilepsy live in low- and middle-income countries. It is estimated that up to 70% of people living with epilepsy could live seizure-free if accurately diagnosed and treated. The risk of premature death in people with epilepsy is up to three times higher than that for the general population.[2]

The overall prevalence (3.0–11.9 per 1,000 population) and incidence (0.2–0.6 per 1,000 population per year) of epilepsy in India are comparable to those of high-income countries despite significant variations in population and treatment characteristics.[3]

In a retrospective review of 154 children who had SE, 39% had RSE.[4] Mortality was 21% and survivors with RSE developed more new neurological deficits ($p < 0.001$) and more epilepsy ($p < 0.004$) than children with SE. Aggressive treatment had a better outcome ($p = 0.03$). The predictors of poor outcome were seizures of long duration ($p < 0.001$), acute symptomatic etiology ($p = 0.04$), nonconvulsive status epilepticus (NCSE) ($p = 0.01$), and age < 5 years ($p = 0.05$), thus emphasizing the need for quick resolution of even electrical seizures. In India, the outcome of SE and RSE may differ depending on the inconsistency and variations in prevailing healthcare delivery systems. In studies from three public hospitals, an overall mortality of 30–38% was reported. Sadik et al. found a higher correlation with central nervous system (CNS) infections.[5,6] Santhanam's emergency room (ER) data showed a low mortality of 4.6% in the short-term, based on the discharge from the ER.[7] Mortality correlated with shock and the need for ventilation. However, the cohort studied was mixed and included febrile status.

Good outcome goes beyond the measure of mortality or hospital discharge. Disability and severe epilepsy are common sequelae. In a meta-analysis that included pediatric studies, 20–40% of survivors had epilepsy, motor deficits, and cognitive issues.[8]

■ PATHOPHYSIOLOGY

Glutamate is the major amino acid excitatory neurotransmitter in the brain. Some affected individuals have prolonged seizures thought to be caused by excessive activation of excitatory amino acid receptors **(Fig. 24.1)**. Other excitatory neurotransmitters that contribute to SE include aspartate and acetylcholine. There are possibly many mechanisms involved, both in initiation and termination of seizures. When the normal mechanisms that limit the spread of seizures become ineffective, SE ensues. Gamma-aminobutyric acid (GABA) is the main inhibitory neurotransmitter in the brain, and antagonists to it may contribute to SE.[9] Many drugs used in the management of SE are GABA agonists. Antiepileptic drugs are also tailored

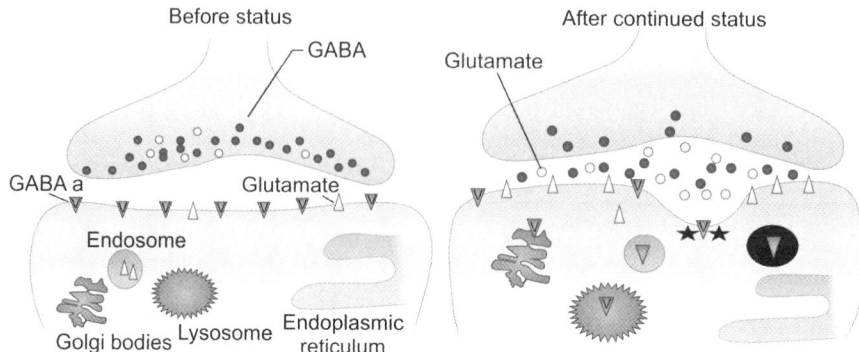

Fig. 24.1: Internalization of gamma-aminobutyric acid (GABA) receptors.[10]

Note: The panel "before status" on the left shows GABA receptors lined up to receive GABA. The panel "after continued status" on the right shows GABA getting released. The receptors are fewer and some are in the cell, so the excitation continues.

(*Source*: RESUS.co.au open access Internet available).

toward the blockage of several other receptors such as the N-methyl-D-aspartate (NMDA). The internalization of GABA receptors early in status and the up-regulation of glutamate receptors later in SE may help to explain the better response to first-line therapy with benzodiazepines (BZDs) early on within the first half-hour and the decline in effect later **(Fig. 24.1)**. Probably this may be one reason to consider NMDA receptor antagonists early in the management of RSE.

The principles of treatment of RSE would therefore be to use drug combinations that would target different receptors and work in tandem to suppress the excitatory activity that causes RSE.

■ DEFINITIONS AND TIMELINE

In 2015, The International League Against Epilepsy (ILAE) Task Force put forward an operational definition for time periods of SE for treatment ('t1' period) as 5 minutes for generalized tonic-clonic seizures, 10 minutes for focal seizures, and 10–15 minutes for absence seizures.[11] With growing recognition for urgency of treatment, the standard definition of SE as "a 30-minute seizure with no recovery of consciousness" has been abandoned in order to emphasize urgency ('t2' period for long-term consequences). When the seizure either fails to naturally terminate or cannot be medically terminated, *urgent upscaling of treatment should be initiated.* While this breaks it up into two timelines, there are definitions for the various phases that could be helpful in guiding therapy.

Definitions

Table 24.1 provides the definitions and correlations with a timeline.

TABLE 24.1: Definitions and correlation with timeline.

Epilepsy	Definition	Correlation with timeline
SE (Also called impending SE)	Any seizure lasting longer than 5 minutes, without a return to normal consciousness, or recurrent seizures without a return to normal consciousness between seizures	Stabilization phase 0–5 minutes
Established SE	Seizure/s that continue/s following first-line medications (benzodiazepines)	Initial treatment phase 5–30 minutes
RSE	Seizures that do not resolve following benzodiazepines plus one or two anticonvulsants	Second therapy phase 30–60 minutes
SRSE	Drug-resistant status that persists or recurs despite continuous intravenous coma induction for more than 24 hours	Third therapy phase >60 min (Ill defined)

(SE: status epilepticus; RSE: refractory status epilepticus; SRSE: super-refractory status epilepticus)

In treatment, 5 minutes and 30 minutes are important landmarks.[12] Most seizures last <5 minutes. Those that do not terminate, rarely stop spontaneously. A seizure lasting >30 minutes is associated with up to 19% mortality, and those with RSE have mortality as high as 60%. The 30-minute landmark, where neuronal damage is believed to occur and pharmacoresistance develops, is controversial and it is now believed that these changes may occur much earlier.

■ ETIOLOGY

Febrile SE remains the most common cause of SE. This often terminates with the first-line medication. Nevertheless, fever is a common association with many conditions that cause SE. Most children are normal prior to the onset of SE unless they have a premorbid neurological condition showing the first manifestation of epilepsy. Epilepsy due to any cause may have its first presentation with SE/RSE.

For the intensivist, SE in children can be classified broadly into categories based on etiology as shown in **Box 24.1**.

■ SYSTEMIC EFFECTS DURING RSE AND CORRESPONDING CLINICAL FEATURES

Initially, there is a rush of catecholamines, leading to tachycardia, and elevated blood pressure.[13] The danger of hypoxia from respiratory depression or choking should be recognized at every stage. Blood glucose is often elevated unless hypoglycemia is the cause. Hypotension, bradycardia,

> **BOX 24.1:** Classification of SE based on etiology.
>
> - *Symptomatic: Acute/remote/progressive*
>   - *Acute symptomatic SE* (acute symptom of a medical or neurologic disease)
>   - Central nervous system infections (meningitis and encephalitis)
>   - Acute hypoxic ischemic insult (cardiopulmonary resuscitation, drowning, and hypotension)
>   - Metabolic disease (hypoglycemia, inborn error of metabolism)
>   - Electrolyte imbalances (hyponatremia)
>   - Traumatic brain injury
>   - Drugs, intoxication, and poisoning
>   - Cerebrovascular event (infarcts, bleeds)
>   - *Remote symptomatic epilepsy/seizures* → caused by an insult early in life:
>   - Perinatal hypoxic-ischemic injury
>   - Trauma
>   - Infection
>   - Congenital brain malformation
>   - *Progressive* → brain tumors
>   - Progressive myoclonic epilepsy
>   - Syndromic epilepsies
>   - Inherited disorders
> - *Unknown or cryptogenic*—no known or identifiable cause

and hypoxemia with hypercarbia, will further complicate the picture as time elapses. Initial hyperemia with increased cerebral perfusion reduces as RSE continues and cerebral perfusion falls. Occasionally, intracranial pressure is also known to rise (especially in RSE/SRSE). Hypoxia and muscle activity increase the lactate levels and in extreme situations, rhabdomyolysis may also occur. Hence the emphasis of management should not be only on drugs but also on good supportive care in an intensive care setting.

■ MANAGEMENT

Out of Hospital Treatment

Since seizures beget seizures and if not terminated within 5 minutes, tend to last longer; hence rapid termination is the aim of management. Delay in treatment has been found to have poor treatment response. Details will not be discussed here as the discussion is on RSE and SRSE.

Initial Assessment and Management

At the first contact simultaneous efforts should be made to terminate the seizures along with assessment and stabilization. If you are alone, it is best to call an extra hand early. **Box 24.2** lists the various steps in initial management. **Box 24.3** lists the laboratory tests to be performed during the emergency management.

The American Epilepsy Society (AES) has recently published guidelines (2016) for adults and children which break up the management into four

> **BOX 24.2:** Initial management.
>
> - Brief physical examination is done to assess respiratory and circulatory status
> - Establish an adequate airway immediately if there is respiratory compromise
> - Place an intravenous (IV) catheter for sampling of blood and administration of medications
> - Supportive therapy (e.g., oxygen, mechanical ventilation) instituted as needed
> - Initiate ongoing monitoring of vital signs
> - Rapid neurologic examination
> - Preliminary classification of the type of status epilepticus (SE)
> - History obtained from a witness may help to determine the cause and semiology of the seizures

> **BOX 24.3:** Laboratory studies.
>
> - Blood glucose by fingerprick
> - Serum electrolytes, calcium, and magnesium levels
> - Arterial blood gases
> - Complete blood counts
> - Urine and blood toxicology (if toxin ingestion suspected)
> - Serum anticonvulsant drug levels (*subtherapeutic levels are found in almost one-third of children presenting in SE and dosing can be rationalized once the levels are known*) in those already on treatment
> - *Other investigations*: Imaging, metabolic screen, etc. as per clinical profile for suspected metabolic, genetic, or structural disorders

phases.[14] A timeline-based protocol for management of SE and RSE is provided in **Table 24.2** and discussed in detail below.

First Line

Initial Therapy Phase (5–20 minutes of Seizure Activity)

Benzodiazepines remain the first-line treatment for SE because they can rapidly control seizures **(Table 24.3)**. An additional drug is usually added to prevent further seizures pending the decision for long-term therapy. This could be phenytoin, phenobarbitone (not currently recommended) or more commonly now, levetiracetam as well as valproate.[15] *In the initial RSE two or more primary drugs have failed and in practical terms, close to an hour would have elapsed.*

Second Therapy Phase (30–40 minutes)

When this initial therapy phase fails to control seizures, additional second and third line therapy adds only marginal benefit (2.3-5%). The drugs added in this stage are additional doses of phenytoin, phenobarbitone, levetiracetam, or IV valproate. If seizures continue, these additional steps waste precious time with limited benefit and a switch to an *"accelerated protocol"* is now the

TABLE 24.2: Suggested protocol for management of SE and RSE based on stage and proposed timeline.

Stage	Management

Impending SE, 0–5 minutes
AES stabilization stage
	• No IV access/casualty:
	  – Consider buccal midazolam or rectal diazepam
	• Benzodiazepines:
	  – Lorazepam, 0.1 mg/kg IV (maximum, 5 mg) over 1 min
	  – Allow 5 minutes to determine whether seizure terminates
	• Supportive measures:
	  – All supportive care as needed—metabolic and hemodynamic
	• *Monitoring*:
	  – Begin EEG monitoring

Established SE, 5–10 minutes
AES initial therapy stage
	• *Antiepileptics*:
	  – Repeat benzodiazepine administration
	  – Administer fosphenytoin PE 30 mg/kg IV at 2–3 mg/kg/min (maximum 150 mg/min)
	  – If patient's age is <2 years, consider pyridoxine 100 mg IV push.
	• *Testing*:
	  – Bedside glucose, CBC, cultures, electrolytes, Ca, Mg, P, and LFT
	  – Toxicology screen if indicated (serum and urine; preserve till further clarity)
	  – AED levels, PT, PTT
	• *Urgent neuroimaging*:
	  – If treatable cause is suspected. MRI is preferred
	• *Supportive measures*:
	  – Support airway, respiration, and hemodynamics as needed
	  – Consult neurology service

Initial refractory SE
AES secondary therapy stage
	• *Anticonvulsants*:
	  – If seizure continues 10 minutes after fosphenytoin infusion, repeat 10 mg/kg dose of fosphenytoin
	  – Wait 10 minutes
	  – Administer levetiracetam 60 mg/kg IV at 5 mg/kg/min (maximum, 3 g)
	  – If contraindication to levetiracetam and no specific concern regarding liver/metabolic/mitochondrial disease, then administer valproate 40 mg/kg at 5 mg/kg/min (in 8–10 minutes)
	• *Consider "accelerated protocol"*:
	  – Midazolam infusion—directly

Contd...

Contd...

Stage	Management

Established RSE	• *Anticonvulsants*:
	  – If seizure continues 5 minutes after levetiracetam or valproate, administer phenobarbital 20–30 mg/kg IV at 2 mg/kg/min (maximum rate 60 mg/min).
	• *Admit to PICU and go to "Accelerated Protocol"*:
	  – Midazolam infusion—directly
	• *Supportive measures*:
	  – Prepare to secure airway, mechanically ventilate, and obtain central venous access and continuous hemodynamic monitoring through arterial line
	• *Monitoring*:
	  – After clinical seizure terminates, will likely need EEG monitoring to assess for subclinical seizures

Coma induction
AES third therapy stage
SRSE
	• *Coma induction*:
	  – If seizure continues 10 minutes after completion of phenobarbital infusion, then initiate coma with midazolam 0.2 mg/kg bolus (maximum, 10 mg) over 2 minutes, and then initiate infusion at 0.1 mg/kg/h
	  – If clinical seizures persist 5 minutes after initial midazolam bolus, then administer additional midazolam bolus of 0.2 mg/kg bolus
	  – Continue infusion
	  – Repeat and escalate midazolam
	• *Supportive measures*:
	  – Intubate, and secure ABP and CVP lines
	  – Prepare inotrope on standby
	• *Start*: Thiopental
	  – Dose 4–5 mg/kg load and 1–2 mg/kg/h
	  – Increase only on advice of consultant and under EEG for burst suppression according to neurology service
	• *Consider high dose phenobarbital therapy and Immunotherapy*

Coma phase	• *Continue pharmacologic coma* for 24 hours after last seizure, with EEG goal of burst suppression
	  – Continue EEG monitoring with at least 8-hourly reviews
	  – Continue initial medications (phenytoin goal level in blood, 20–30 µg/mL; phenobarbital goal level, 40–50 µg/mL)
	  – (Daily) phenobarbital and free phenytoin levels
	  – Continue levetiracetam at 40–80 mg/kg IV, divided every 6 hours (maximum, 3 g)
	• *Consider high dose phenobarbitone therapy instead of thiopental*
	  – Ketogenic diet if not already on

Contd...

Contd...

Stage	Management
Weaning phase If no electrical/clinical seizures for > 48 h	• Reduce midazolam by 0.05 mg/kg/h every 3 hours, with frequent EEG review • If no clinical or electrographic seizures, then wean until off • Continue EEG for at least 24 hours after end of infusion, to evaluate for recurrent electrographic seizures
Repeat coma phase	• If clinical or subclinical seizures occur, reinstitute coma with midazolam for 24 hours • Similarly for thiopental • *NB*: Midazolam does not cause burst suppression, the end point is loss of seizure activity
Repeat weaning phase	• Reduce midazolam by 0.06 mg/kg/h every 6 hours • If seizures persist, then manage as guided by neurology consultation for advanced therapies

(AES: American Epilepsy Society; SE: status epilepticus; RSE: refractory status epilepticus; SRSE: super-refractory status epilepticus; CBC: complete blood count; LFT: liver function tests; AED: antiepileptic drug; Ca: calcium; Mg: magnesium; P: phosphorus; PT: prothrombin time; PTT: partial thromboplastin time; MRI: magnetic resonance imaging; PICU: pediatric intensive care unit; EEG: electroencephalogram; ABP: arterial blood pressure; CVP: central venous pressure)

usual practice. In this, the *second therapy phase* (described above) can be bypassed and coma induction with midazolam, pentobarbital, or propofol (preferably with continuous EEG monitoring) is advocated. Thus, the patient directly enters the *third therapy phase* saving at least 15–25 precious minutes of time. The application of such treatment must be balanced with available expertise and intensive care infrastructure. Many children need transfer from primary care to a tertiary care center at this stage.

Third Therapy Phase

Prior to initiating this stage, it may be worthwhile, especially in known epileptics, to maximize existing anticonvulsants by rechecking levels if possible and reloading existing drugs. Midazolam is most often used for coma induction. After the loading dose, the increments should be at 10–15 minutes or when repetitive clinical or electrographic seizures are seen. *A common error here is to plan increments at fixed intervals of several hours, which leads to delay in aborting the seizures.* The end point is unclear. Further escalation of doses beyond 0.6–0.8 mg/kg/h may not have any added benefit if the GABA receptors are saturated or internalized. When midazolam was used as the initial agent for RSE, the rate of clinical seizure control was 76%, which was achieved on an average at 41 minutes after starting the infusion. When midazolam was used in conjunction with

TABLE 24.3: Drugs used in the management of SE and RSE.

Drugs	Loading dose	Maintenance dose	Side effects
Midazolam	0.2 mg/kg	0.2–1 mg/kg/h	• Hypotension • Respiratory depression • Tolerance
Propofol	2 mg/kg	1–5 mg/kg/h	• Hypotension • Respiratory depression • Propofol infusion syndrome (PRIS)—acute refractory bradycardia leading to asystole evidenced by rhabdomyolysis, shock, and metabolic acidosis • Increased risk with ketogenic diet • Monitor lactate, triglycerides (>400 mg/dL), CPK and potassium • Avoid in Infants
Thiopental	2–4 mg/kg	1–5 mg/kg/h	• Hypotension • Respiratory depression • Tolerance
High dose phenobarbital	30 mg/kg	Repeat 10–20 mg/kg/day over 4–5 days	• Hypotension • Respiratory depression • Avoid in NCSE and epilepsia partialis continua

(CPK: creatinine phosphokinase; NCSE: nonconvulsive status epilepticus)

continuous electroencephalography (EEG), the time to seizure control was much longer and the mean dose required for seizure control was 10.7 µg/kg/min compared with a lower dose (2.8 µg/kg/min) in the studies not using this form of monitoring, suggesting that continuous EEG provided additional targets for treatment escalation and suboptimal treatment may be given when EEG monitoring is not done.[16]

Thiopental and pentobarbital: These act by enhancing the action of the GABA receptors and may have the additional advantage of being neuroprotective **(Table 24.3)**. They exhibit zero order kinetics and *due to rapid redistribution* have a profound tendency to accumulation leading to an extended half-life in anesthesia and long recovery time.[17] This is especially important when high dose phenobarbital therapy, which is gaining ground, is employed.

Hemodynamics should be supported so that hypotension itself is not a reason to discontinue therapy unless it is refractory to support or poses a threat to organ or cerebral perfusion.

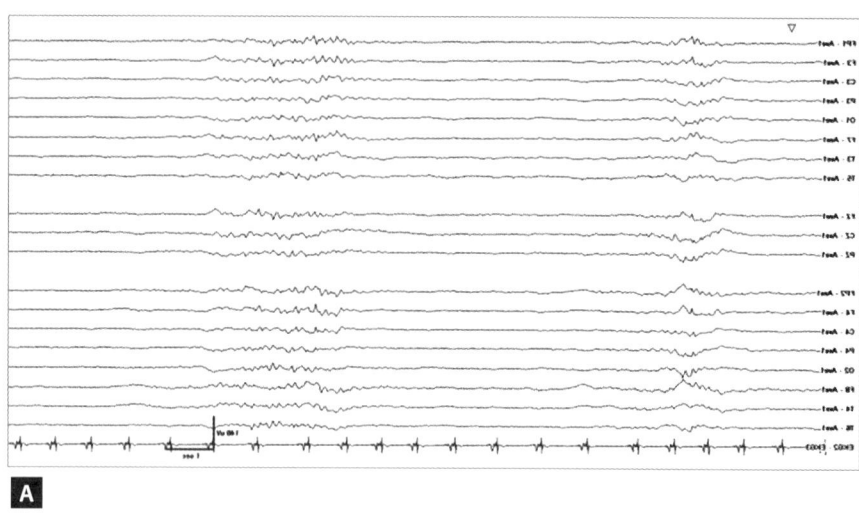

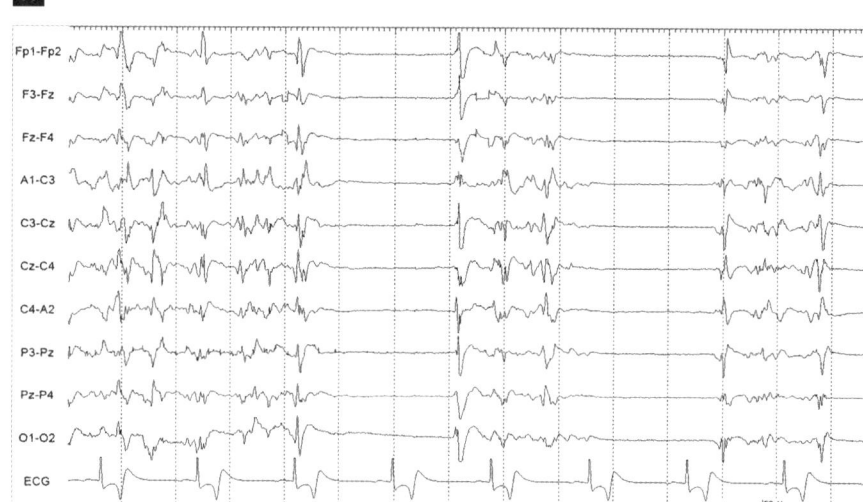

Figs. 24.2A and B: Continuous EEG monitoring. (A) Oversuppressed with very low amplitude; (B) Adequately suppressed with short suppression.

Profound suppression of brain activity may have a protective effect and "break the cycle" of seizures, making it easier to taper medications without recurrence. Among patients failing midazolam, barbiturate infusion was effective in 65%.[18]

Current recommendations suggest that early institution of continuous EEG monitoring helps in guiding therapy **(Figs. 24.2A and B)**. Debate continues regarding the recommended length of the periods of EEG suppression (the interburst interval) and how long the burst suppression pattern should be maintained. While data regarding the benefit of depth of EEG suppression versus only control with electrographic and clinical seizures is unclear. In a meta-analysis, patients treated with the goal of EEG background suppression with pentothal infusion had a 4% likelihood of breakthrough seizures compared with 53% for patients treated to control clinical and electrographic seizures only. Hence most units will aim for EEG suppression.[19]

Results for general anesthetics such as isoflurane and desflurane are usually limited as the number of children studied is very few. The action is by potentiation of postsynaptic GABAergic currents and thalamocortical pathways. Isoflurane 1.5–2.5% is employed with an honest gas scavenging system. Anesthesia often needs to be maintained for a mean (range) of 11 (2–26) days, which is challenging. The skill of the team and monitoring must be stepped up considerably for this step.

Weaning should be longer with intravenous anesthesia (pentobarbital) than volatile anesthetics, and it is reasonable to wean over 24 hours (but could also be for much longer with pentobarbital). A 24-hr electrographic seizure-free period is preferable but sometimes weaning needs to be done without that if toxicity risks outweigh medication benefits.

High-dose phenobarbitone: Very high-dose phenobarbital (VHDPB) has been used with increasing frequency in intensive care units.[20] The high levels are achieved over days to avoid the complications of severe CNS depression and reach a fatal dose.

The loading dose is 20–30 mg/kg. The dose is increased if seizures persist and it is recommended to add in increments of 5–10 mg/kg per dose once or twice a day. Dosage can go up to accumulated daily doses of up to 80–100 mg/kg/day. When this increment is used over several days, there are none of the side effects anticipated with the phenobarbital toxicity seen in an accidental overdose. The resulting serum level is immaterial, and >1,000 µmol/L has been reported with good tolerance.

It is highly effective in achieving seizure control, with milder adverse effects compared with thiopental or even high-dose midazolam infusions. Here too, the end point is burst suppression.

Ketamine: It is an NMDA receptor antagonist, with a rapid onset and is metabolized by cytochrome p450. It causes a dissociative state normally. GABA receptors exert an inhibitory influence on excitation. As the seizure continues, the GABA receptors get internalized by endocytosis, resulting in a lack of inhibitory control. This makes GABAergic agents ineffective. By this time, the number of excitatory NMDA receptors has increased and their stimulation by glutamate could be responsible for propagating seizures. Antagonistic action from ketamine may prevent this.

Variations from 30 to 60% were seen in different studies.[21] However, early use of ketamine may result in a greater efficacy.[22,23] Recommended dosage is 2–3 mg/kg bolus of ketamine every 5 minutes for a total of two administrations, followed by maintenance at a rate of 10–60 µg/kg/min) for several days. There are ongoing trials that include ketamine as a second-line drug after benzodiazepines in the early treatment of seizures. Other therapies in combination need to be applied at this stage.

Ketogenic Diet

This induces controlled ketosis. Mechanism of action is by altering brain energy metabolism, increasing synthesis of GABA, and reducing synthesis of reactive oxygen species. This can be started in the very initial phase by removing all glucose containing solutions from the management, including syrups, and reducing fluids to 60-70% of requirements. It is then started with tube feeds at 3: 1 or 4: 1 fat: nonfat ratio, with fats consisting of animal fat, vegetable oils, or medium chain triglycerides. Supplements with vitamins, calcium, phosphorus, magnesium, bicarbonate, and laxatives are sometimes needed. Short- and long-term complications include diarrhea, feed intolerance, constipation (12-50%), growth failure, hypoglycemia, acidosis, and renal stones (3-7%). This is started along with other adjuvant drugs that may help in controlling the SE and usually before going on to general anesthesia. Earlier introduction of ketogenic diet may be more efficacious; as after pentothal, gastric emptying time increases and may result in failure or intolerance to the diet.[24,25]

During this critical period of coma to induce burst suppression, there may be uncoupling of EEG and clinical seizures. Thus, many seizures designated as refractory status epilepticus may occur during weaning and may be only electrographic.

■ NEW-ONSET REFRACTORY STATUS EPILEPTICUS AND FEBRILE INFECTION-RELATED EPILEPSY SYNDROME

"New-onset refractory status epilepticus (NORSE)" is SE without a past history of epilepsy and without a clear cause. "Febrile infection-related epilepsy syndrome (FIRES)" has a history of fever either at onset or within the past few weeks. FIRES is more common in children whereas NORSE can be seen at any age. Both remain the quintessential paradigm for RSE and SRSE. The suggested pathway for treatment, already detailed earlier, applies to this condition. The last section on immunotherapy would apply to suspected or known immune-mediated SE and not to known epileptics with breakthrough SE.

Recommended Diagnostics and Therapeutics

These are discussed under various timelines below.[26]

Suspect Diagnosis

New onset acute repetitive seizures and intermittent SE in a previously healthy, normal developing child older than 2 years of age; preceding febrile illness within 2 weeks of seizure onset—*consider using an accelerated protocol early.*

First 24 hours

Perform lumbar puncture and rule out infective etiology by cerebrospinal fluid (CSF) polymerase chain reaction (PCR) and culture studies. Rule out a structural etiology by brain MRI. Continuous EEG monitoring is needed. Save serum and CSF for autoimmune panel [anti-NMDA, antivoltage-gated potassium channels (VGKC) and high IgG levels may be nonspecific]. If there is a positive panel for any of the antibodies and often even empirically, immune modulation is given **(Box 24.4)**.

Management as in Second and Third Therapy Phases

This is already outlined above.

Day 2-6: Establish FIRES determination—SRSE; strongly consider FIRES by day 6. Start ketogenic diet. Tolerate brief breakthrough seizures; try lift; or avoid barbiturate induced burst suppression. Competent PICU care and a multidisciplinary approach are essential **(Box 24.5)**.

ADJUNCTIVE DRUGS

Because of the pathophysiological changes in SE, there is a tolerance to the first and second line as well as the coma-inducing drugs as described earlier. The reasons are outlined in the **Box 24.6**.

Lacosamide

Lacosamide acts by low inactivation of voltage-gated sodium channels (VGNC), stabilization of hyperexcitable neuronal membranes, and inhibition of neuronal firing with decrease of long-term channel availability without affecting physiologic function. Only six case reports and series are published,

---

BOX 24.4: Management for positive CSF antibodies in the autoimmune panel: Immunotherapy.

- Consider methylprednisolone (30 mg/kg daily, max 1 g, for 3–5 days); IV immunoglobulin (IVIG, 2 g/kg divided over 2–3 days)
- If no response, try plasmapheresis, rituximab, or cyclophosphamide
- Send serum, and CSF, if available, for cytokine assays (specifically IL-1B, IL-6 and neopterin)
- Consider IL-1 RA Anakinra (subcutaneous injection 2–8 mg/kg). Consider other antiepileptic drugs (AEDs) including cannabidiol (CBD oil)[27,28]
- This may take up to 4 weeks and after that consider other immunomodulation such as tocilizumab (subcutaneous or intravenous injection 8–12 mg/kg) or canakinumab (subcutaneous injection 2–3 mg/kg)
- *Day 7–21*: Avoid prolonged burst suppression coma with barbiturates, ketamine, lidocaine, or propofol infusion. Extended trial of Anakinra (3–4 weeks) may be necessary before response is seen. Continue immunomodulatory therapy if positive response noted.

Note: Anakinra, canakinumab, and cannabidiol are not easily available but can be imported under special license.

> **BOX 24.5:** PICU care.
> - 1:1 nursing care with multimodal monitoring
> - Mechanical ventilation
> - Inotropes
> - Continuous EEG monitoring
> - Temperature
> - Arterial line for BP monitoring and maintenance
> - Central line as many drugs cannot be given for long periods peripherally
> - Indwelling urinary catheter for good output monitoring
> - Attention to downstream markers of tissue perfusion—lactate, bicarbonate, mixed venous oxygen saturation, etc.
> - Dietician for Ketogenic diet
> - Neurologist to guide therapy

> **BOX 24.6:** Causes for the development of tolerance.
> - Loss of GABA-mediated inhibition
> - Downregulation of GABA-A receptors
> - Upregulation of NMDA and glutamate receptors
> - Alterations of ion channels
> - Altered neuropeptide expression (substance P and neuropeptide Y)
> - DNA methylation, micro-RNA regulation, and altered gene expression
>
> (GABA: gamma-aminobutyric acid; NMDA: N-methyl-D-aspartate)

all of which employed a retrospective design. Overall, data from 36 pediatric SE patients are available with success rates in terminating SE of 45–78%.[29]

Topiramate

Topiramate also acts through VGNCs and high voltage-activated calcium channels. It may alter the activity of its targets by modifying their phosphorylation instead of by a direct action.[30] A dosage of 10 mg/Kg for 1–2 days followed by 5 mg/kg/day is often what is followed as the urgency of the situation does not allow for gradual increase.[30]

Novel Therapies

Electrical, Deep Brain, and Vagal Nerve Stimulation[31] and Magnetic Stimulation Therapy

It is postulated that these can alter the synchronization of epileptic discharges, increase the refractory period of neuronal discharge, or alter membrane or neurotransmitter function.[31]

Hypothermia

It reduces the cerebral metabolic rate, oxygen utilization, ATP consumption, glutaminergic drive, mitochondrial dysfunction, calcium overload, free radical production and oxidative stress, permeability of the blood–brain barrier, and proinflammatory reactions.

Electroconvulsive Therapy

Its antiepileptic effects are proposed to be due to the increased presynaptic release of GABA and prolongation of the refractory period after a seizure. This is rarely used.

Cannabinoids

Cannabinoids are now used in serious refractory epilepsies. Correct dosage and sourcing can be a challenge.[28]

Epilepsy Surgery

In selected situations, mainly where there is a clearly definable radiological lesion and/or electrophysiological evidence of a focal onset, emergency surgical resection has been used as a "last-resort" treatment of SRSE. The common procedures are focal cortical resection, lobar and multilobar resection, anatomic and functional hemispherectomy, corpus callosotomy, and multiple subpial transections.

NEUROIMAGING

Most patients will get some imaging during the management of SE. A CT scan will usually not yield much and should not be done routinely. An MRI is needed to look for infective or treatable etiologies. In a study by Yoong of 80 children after suffering from SE for a mean of 31.2 days, structural abnormalities were found in 31%. Hence in the first episode of SE, an MRI is recommended, although SE itself can produce changes in the MRI and atrophy or changes of hypoxic ischemic injury may confuse the picture.[32] The neurology services get repeat MRIs which often do not add to diagnosis or management and may only show changes associated with RSE.

CONCLUSION

Status epilepticus is a common pediatric as well as critical care emergency. Attention to the timeline is essential as early cessation of seizure activity is vital. A proposed protocol for management is provided in **Table 24.2**. Long-term patient-related outcome measures (PROM) for quality of life, rather than mortality alone should be measures of treatment success.

KEY POINTS

- Status epilepticus is a common pediatric as well as critical care emergency.
- Attention to the timeline is essential as early cessation of seizure activity is vital.
- Good supportive care goes hand in hand with prompt seizure termination.
- Status epilepticus is a common pediatric as well as critical care emergency.
- Attention to the timeline is essential as early cessation of seizure activity is vital.
- Good supportive care goes hand in hand with prompt seizure termination.
- Immunotherapy needs to be considered.
- Attention to oxygenation and blood pressure will prevent further brain damage.

- Optimization of doses before adding new drugs should be attempted.
- Every unit must make its own implementable protocol within available guidelines.
- A multidisciplinary approach is needed in RSE with high level monitoring.
- There should be no hesitation to transfer if optimal care cannot be delivered.

■ REFERENCES

1. Hauptmann A. Luminal bei Epilepsie. Munchen Med Wochenschr. 1912;59:1907-9.
2. World Health Organization. (2019). WHO Global Report. [online] Available from https://www.who.int› Health topics [Last accessed December, 2021].
3. Amudhan S, Gururaj G, Satishchandra P. Epilepsy in India I: Epidemiology and public health. Ann Indian Acad Neurol. 2015;18(3):263-77.
4. Lambrechtsen FA, Buchhalter JR. Aborted and refractory status epilepticus in children: a comparative analysis. Epilepsia. 2008;49(4):615-25.
5. Sadik KC, Mishra D, Juneja M, Jhamb U. Clinico-etiological profile of pediatric refractory status epilepticus at a public hospital in India. J Epilepsy Res. 2019;9(1):36-41.
6. Gulati S, Kalra V, Ramaiah S. Status epilepticus in Indian children in a tertiary care center. Indian J Pediatr. 2005;72(2):105-8.
7. Santhanam I, Yoganathan S, Sivakumar VA, Ramakrishnamurugan R, Sathish S, Thandavarayan M. Predictors of outcome in children with status epilepticus during resuscitation in pediatric emergency department: A retrospective observational study. Ann Indian Acad Neurol. 2017;20(2):142-8.
8. Sculier C, Gaínza-Lein M, Fernández IS, Loddenkemper T. Long-term outcomes of status epilepticus: A critical assessment. Epilepsia. 2018;59(Suppl 2):155-69.
9. Wasterlain CG, Baxter CF, Baldwin RA. GABA metabolism in the substantia nigra, cortex, and hippocampus during status epilepticus. Neurochem Res. 1993;18(4):527-32.
10. Naylor DE, Liu H, Wasterlain CG. Trafficking of $GABA_A$ receptors, loss of inhibition, and a mechanism for pharmacoresistance in status epilepticus. J Neurosci. 2005;25(34):7724-33.
11. Trinka E, Cock H, Hesdorffer D, Rossetti AO, Scheffer IE, Shinnar S, et al. A definition and classification of status epilepticus—Report of the ILAE Task Force on Classification of Status Epilepticus. Epilepsia. 2015;56(10):1515-23.
12. Hocker S, Tatum WO, LaRoche S, Freeman WD. Refractory and super-refractory status epilepticus—an update. Curr Neurol Neurosci Rep. 2014;14(6):452.
13. Hanhan UA, Fiallos MR, Orlowski JP. Status epilepticus. Pediatr Clin North Am. 2001;48(3):683-94.
14. Glausser T, Shinnar S, Gloss D, Alldredge B, Arya R, Bainbridge J, et al. Evidence-based guideline: Treatment of convulsive status epilepticus in children and adults: Report of the Guideline Committee of the American Epilepsy Society. Epilepsy Curr. 2016;16(1):48-61.
15. Kapur J, Elm J, Chamberlain JM, Barsan W, Cloyd J, Lowenstein D, et al. Randomized trial of three anticonvulsant medications for status epilepticus. N Engl J Med. 2019;381(22):2103-13.
16. Chamberlain JM, Okada P, Holsti M, Mahajan P, Brown KM, Vance C, et al. Lorazepam vs diazepam for pediatric status epilepticus: a randomized clinical trial. JAMA. 2014;311(16):1652-60

17. Hvidberg EF, Dam M. Clinical pharmacokinetics of anticonvulsants. Clin Pharmacokinet. 1976;1(3):161-88.
18. Wilkes R, Tasker, RC. Intensive care treatment of uncontrolled status epilepticus in children: systematic literature search of midazolam and anesthetic therapies. Pediatr Crit Care Med. 2014;15(7):632-9.
19. Claassen J, Hirsch LJ, Emerson RG, Mayer SA. Treatment of refractory status epilepticus with pentobarbital, propofol, or midazolam: a systematic review. Epilepsia. 2002;43(2):146-53.
20. Lee WK, Liu KT, Young BW. Very-high-dose phenobarbital for childhood refractory status epilepticus. Pediatr Neurol. 2006;34(1):63-5.
21. Gaspard N, Foreman B, Judd LM, Brenton JN, Nathan BR, McCoy BM, et al. Intravenous ketamine for the treatment of refractory status epilepticus: a retrospective multicenter study. Epilepsia. 2013;54(8):1498-503.
22. Alkhachroum A, Der-Nigoghossian CA, Mathews E, Massad N, Letchinger R, Doyle K, et al. Ketamine to treat super-refractory status epilepticus. Neurology. 2020;95(16):e2286-94.
23. Redecker J, Wittstock M, Benecke R, Rösche J. Comparison of the effectiveness of four antiepileptic drugs in the treatment of status epilepticus according to four different efficacy criteria. Epilepsy Behav. 2015;49:351-3.
24. Mahmoud SH, Ho-Huang E, Buhler J. Systematic review of ketogenic diet use in adult patients with status epilepticus. Epilepsia Open. 2019;5(1):10-21.
25. Arya R, Peariso K, Gaínza-Lein M, Harvey J, Bergin A, Brenton JN, et al; Pediatric Status Epilepticus Research Group (pSERG). Efficacy and safety of ketogenic diet for treatment of pediatric convulsive refractory status epilepticus. Epilepsy Res. 2018;144:1-6.
26. Koh S, Wirrell E, Vezzani A, Nabbout R, Muscal E, Kaliakatsos M, et al. Proposal to optimize evaluation and treatment of febrile infection-related epilepsy syndrome (FIRES): A report from FIRES workshop. Epilepsia Open. 2021;6(1):62-72.
27. Kenney-Jung DL, Vezzani A, Kahoud RJ, LaFrance-Corey RG, Mai-Lan Ho, Wampler T, et al. Febrile infection-related epilepsy syndrome treated with anakinra. Ann Neurol. 2016;80(6):939-45.
28. Gofshteyn JS, Wilfong A, Devinsky O, Bluvstein J, Charuta J, Ciliberto MA, et al. Cannabidiol as a potential treatment for febrile infection-related epilepsy syndrome (FIRES) in the acute and chronic phases. J Child Neurol. 2017;32(1):35-40.
29. Strzelczyk A, Zollner PJ, Willems LM, Jost J, Paule E, Schubert-Bast S, et al. Lacosamide in status epilepticus: systematic review of current evidence. Epilepsia. 2017;58(6):938-50.
30. Perry MS, Holt PJ, Sladky JT. Topiramate loading for refractory status epilepticus in children. Epilepsia. 2006;47(6):1070-1.
31. Lehtimäki K, Långsjö JW, Ollikainen J, Heinonen H, Möttönen T, Tähtinen T, et al. Successful management of super-refractory status epilepticus with thalamic deep brain stimulation. Ann Neurol. 2017;81(1):142-6.
32. Yoong M, Madari R, Martinos M, Clark C, Chong K, Neville B, et al. The role of magnetic resonance imaging in the follow-up of children with convulsive status epilepticus. Dev Med Child Neurol. 2012;54(4):328-33.

Pediatric Surgery

CHAPTER 25

Intussusception

Praveen Mathur, Priyanka Mittal

"Agony of intussusception is borne by the child, reported by the mother, seen by the clinician, and managed by the surgeon!"

■ HISTORY

Intussusception was differentiated from other forms of intestinal obstruction about 400 years ago, but it was not until 1793 when Hunter provided the first detailed description of intussusception.[1] In 1871, Hutchinson reported the first successful operative reduction in an infant.[1] Ladd is credited with reporting the use of diagnostic imaging with bismuth enemas in 1913.[2]

■ INTRODUCTION

The word intussusception is derived from the Latin words *intus* (within) and *suscipere* (to receive). Intussusception is an indrawing of one part of bowel into another, which is usually in the direction of peristalsis, but can be otherwise too.[3] It has two parts—(1) *intussusceptum* (proximal or indrawing bowel) and (2) *intussuscipiens* (distal or recipient bowel).[4] The inner and middle layers constitute intussusceptum and outer layer forms intussuscipiens **(Fig. 25.1)**. It is one of the most common causes of acute bowel obstruction in infants and toddlers.

■ INCIDENCE

The worldwide incidence of intussusception ranges from 1 to 4 per 1,000 live births per year.[5] Males are affected more than females in a ratio of 3:2.

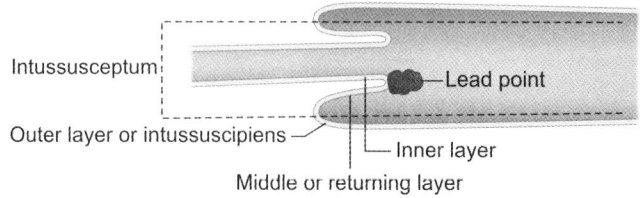

Fig. 25.1: Line diagram of an intussusception.

Male preponderance is more evident in the 6–9 months age group.[5] Intussusception can be seen in all age groups, spanning from perinatal to adulthood. However, most of the cases are reported within 3 years of age. Maximum cases are seen between 4 and 9 months of age. This pathology displays a seasonal variation and peak incidence is experienced in the spring/summer and middle of winter months correlating with the incidence of respiratory and gastrointestinal infections, respectively.[5]

ETIOPATHOGENESIS

Numerous gastrointestinal pathogens of viral origin (rotavirus, reovirus, and echovirus) are known to be causative of intussusception. This can be explained by the hypertrophy of the gut wall lymphoid tissue (which is in abundance in pediatric population) and mesenteric lymph nodes in response to the infections, which act as a *lead point*. Adenovirus infections are also known to be associated with increased incidence of childhood intussusception.[6]

Rotavirus and Intussusception

The US Food and Drug Administration (FDA) suspended tetravalent rhesus-human reassortant rotavirus vaccine (RRV-TV, RotaShield) in July 1999, in view of a strong association between the vaccine and intussusception in otherwise healthy infants.[7] However, in 2009 World Health Organization's Global Advisory Committee on Vaccine Safety recommended the use of two live oral rotavirus vaccines, RotaTeq (RV5) and Rotarix (RVl) in children <15 weeks of age, citing no increased risk of intussusception.[8] This applies truer to countries where high childhood mortality can be ascribed to diarrheal illnesses, and hence, for these countries the benefits of vaccination exceed the possible increased risk of intussusception.

Dietary Factors

The incidence of intussusception is influenced by dietary factors. Children with intussusception are generally healthy and well-nourished. Malnourished children have a lower risk, because of less prominent intestinal lymphoid tissue. Increased incidence of intussusception has also been observed at the time of weaning, i.e., between 4 and 9 months of age. This strongly suggests that change from milk to a more solid diet alters the intestinal peristalsis and hence intussusception is initiated. Second, probable explanation for this finding could be more incidences of enteric infections with the introduction of outside food. This disturbs intestinal peristalsis and leads to hypertrophy of Peyer's patches and thus setting a stage for intussusception. This also explains the occurrence of intussusception during or shortly after an attack of acute gastroenteritis.

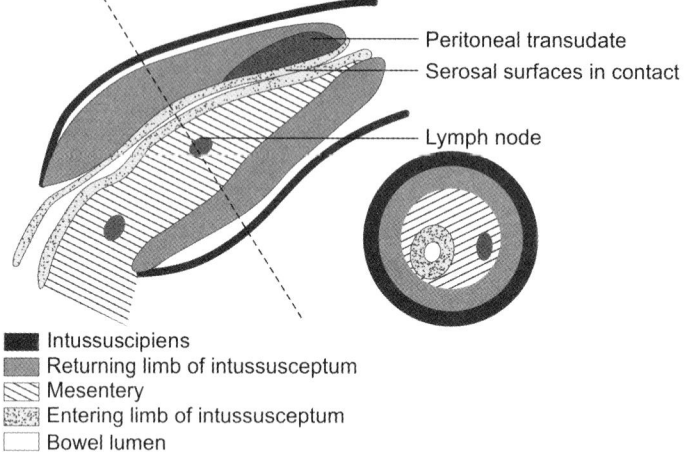

Fig. 25.2: The pathophysiology of intussusception.

An association has also been observed between food allergy and intussusception. Taking breastmilk as the reference group, infants who consumed soymilk-based formula had a much lower risk than infants who consumed cow's milk formula.[9]

■ PATHOPHYSIOLOGY

Intussusception develops with antegrade peristalsis when the proximal bowel (intussusceptum) drags along with its mesentery into the distal bowel (intussuscipiens). Compression of mesentery leads to edema of intussusceptum, causing impairment of lymphatic drainage and venous congestion and stasis; resulting in outpouring of blood and mucus giving rise to classic *red currant jelly stool*. If untreated, ischemic changes amount to bowel necrosis in the intussusceptum **(Fig. 25.2)**.

The gangrenous changes first commence at the distal end of the returning or middle layer and then extend proximally to involve inner layer. The outermost layer or intussuscipiens rarely loses its viability.

It generally takes >72 hours for ischemic changes to set in. If ischemic changes go untreated, sepsis can culminate into death.

■ CLASSIFICATION

Broadly, intussusception can be categorized as *permanent or fixed* which is common and almost always requires treatment; and *spontaneous or transient* which is less common having a short segment (<2 cm), seen in gastroenteritis, mostly ileoileal and resolves spontaneously.[4] Taking etiology into account, it can be classified into *primary or idiopathic* (95%) with hypertrophied Peyer's patches acting as lead point; and *secondary* (4–5%) associated with pathological lead points **(Table 25.1 and Fig. 25.3)**.[4]

TABLE 25.1: Common lead points for intussusception.

Lead point	Example
Mechanical	• Meckel's diverticulum • Intestinal polyps **(Fig. 25.3)** • Duplication cysts • Appendiceal mucocele • Foreign bodies (e.g., bezoars) • Lymphoma • Lymphangioma • Hemangioma • Lipoma
Hematological	• Henoch-Schönlein purpura (HSP) • Idiopathic thrombocytopenic purpura (ITP) • Leukemia • Hemolytic-uremic syndrome • Hemophilia
Miscellaneous	• Cystic fibrosis • Celiac disease • Peutz-Jeghers syndrome • Familial polyposis

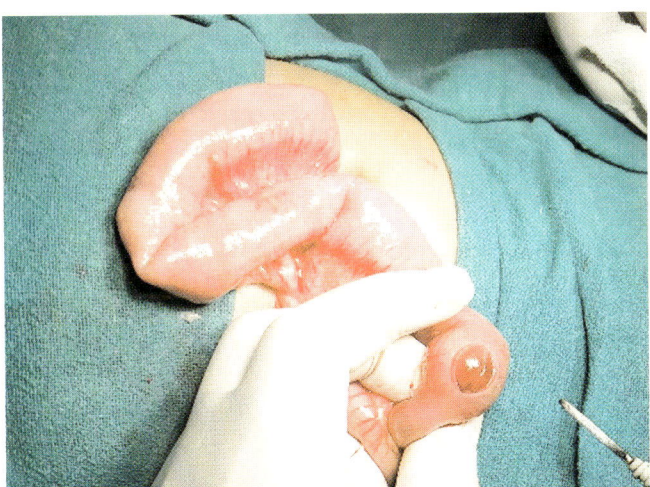

Fig. 25.3: Intestinal polyp acting as a lead point.

In most of the cases, intussusception commences just proximal to ileocecal valve (ileocolic). Less commonly it can be jejunojejunal, jejunoileal, ileoileal, appendicocolic, cecocolic, and colocolic (found in parasitic diseases in children); and can be at multiple sites too.[4]

Intussusception can also be recurrent—when after being spontaneously reduced, rediagnosed clinically and on ultrasound, later confirmed during surgery. Lead point should be suspected in such cases.[4]

■ SIGNS AND SYMPTOMS

The principal signs and symptoms of intussusception are:
- Vomiting (85%)
- Abdominal pain (83%)
- Passage of bloody mucus per rectum (53%)
- Palpable abdominal mass
- Lethargy
- Diarrhea (10–20% of cases)[5]

The classical triad of pain, vomiting, and red currant stools occurs in only about one-third of patients with intussusception.[5]

Vomiting is an early symptom. To begin with, it is reflexive in nature and hence nonbilious. Once the obstruction sets in, it becomes bilious.

The *pain* is characteristic in intussusception. It is episodic, colicky, and severe in nature. The baby manifests the pain by drawing up legs onto the abdomen, crying inconsolably, and holding the breath in a grunting manner. There is refusal to feed. After the attack subsides, the baby is quiet and turns pale and returns to normal activity for a while; to be followed by the same sequence of events. This description given by the mother is enough for the clinician to suspect intussusception even without examining the baby.

Persistent pallor, apathy, listlessness, and evidence of dehydration are described as *knocked out sign*.

The *passage of blood in stools* is seen within 24 hours of onset. It has a classical red currant (dried raisin) jelly appearance—blood and mucus mixed with stools. Fever, tachycardia, and hypotension are the signs of bacteremia. If diagnosis or the management is delayed, ischemic changes set in, leading to frank rectal bleeding. The amount of bleeding is proportional to the degree of strangulation. It is the last sign to occur and carries grave prognosis. Timely management is of utmost importance to prevent a fatal outcome.

Abdominal mass can be palpated when the patient is lying quietly in between the attacks. This finding is elicited on palpation, but sometimes can present on inspection as a visible protuberance. The pull of the mesentery on the telescoping bowel, constrains the tumor to the sausage-shaped mass with concavity toward umbilicus. This leads to emptiness of right iliac fossa (RIF), and hence the *Signe-de-Dance sign*.[5] The mass may be slightly tender on palpation. In a few cases (5%), the intussusception traverses quite distally and may be palpated on rectal examination.[10]

Conditions that may Make Mass Difficult to Palpate
- In the early stages, when the mass passes into the hepatic flexure behind the right costal region margin and under the right lobe of the liver, it evades detection.

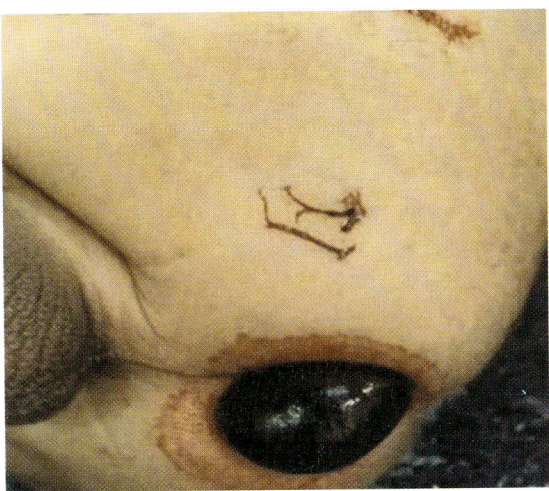

Fig. 25.4: Transanal protrusion of intussusception.

- Small bowel intussusceptions (SBIs)
- Pneumoperitoneum
- Massive abdominal distension
- Mass palpable per rectum
- Trans anal protrusion of intussusception (TAPI)—it is the protrusion of head of intussusception per anus. This accounts for 8–29% of intussusceptions.[11]
- Postoperative intussusception.

Rectal examination with bimanual palpation of abdomen is often informative. This maneuver is more important when child is either straining or abdomen is tense. In a few cases, the intussusceptum may progress so far that it can be felt in the rectum or lower sigmoid. It can protrude per anally (as in TAPI), as mentioned above and can be mistaken for rectal prolapse (Fig. 25.4).

■ DIAGNOSIS

Blood Investigations

There are no specific blood investigations that can help in the diagnostic evaluation of intussusception. However, leukocytosis and electrolyte abnormalities can set in with the onset of ischemic changes.

Radiological Investigations

If the clinical history and physical examination point toward intussusception as diagnosis; there are several imaging modalities which would aid in confirmation of the same.

Plain Abdominal Radiograph

Plain abdominal X-ray may show normal or nonspecific gas pattern in the early course of disease. However, with the progression of the disease pathology, a more obvious pattern of small bowel obstruction; with a relative paucity or absence of gas in the colon is seen. In 25–60% cases, plain abdominal radiographs demonstrate a soft tissue density that displaces air filled loops of bowel.[3]

Ultrasonography of Abdomen

Ultrasonography (USG) is considered as the gold standard investigation for confirmation of diagnosis of intussusception in the suspected cases. It is a highly accurate investigation for the diagnosis of intussusception, with sensitivity of 98–100%, specificity of 88–100%, and negative predictability value of 100%.[12] Most importantly, it can also detect lead points.

The characteristic findings are the "*target sign*" or "*doughnut sign*" or "*bull's eye sign*" on transverse view; and the "*pseudo-kidney*" or "*hayfork sign*" on longitudinal view **(Figs. 25.5A and B)**.[13] In addition to diagnosis, it can also predict the amenability of intussusception to enema reduction by commenting on diameter of hypoechoic rim. This can be further explained by the following principle—edematous tissue is echo-free and normal bowel is echogenic. Hence, more severe the obstruction, greater the edema of intussusception and hence wider the diameter of hypoechoic ring in the *target sign*. With this understanding, it has been observed that a diameter of hypoechoic rim <7.2 mm is amenable to enema reduction. However, a diameter >14 mm, trapped fluid within the intussusception, free intraperitoneal fluid, enlarged lymph nodes dragged along with mesentery, and a pathological lead point are also predictive of unsuccessful enema reduction or requirement of operative intervention.[14] However, visible wall motion on real time ultrasound observation may suggest an easy reduction. This also aids in differentiating transient intussusception from a fixed one. Transient intussusceptions are SBIs and are benign in nature and hardly require any intervention. They need only close follow up. They are of short segment (<2 cm) and have less mesenteric fat and lymph nodes.[4]

When combined with a Doppler study, signs of necrosis, i.e., absence of blood flow can be elicited. However, Doppler study is not mandatorily advised, as vascular flow does not always exclude necrotic bowel, and moreover, not all institutions have availability of Doppler facilities round the clock.

Contrast Enema

Before the wide availability of ultrasound, barium contrast enema (BE) used to be the preferred modality to diagnose or exclude intussusception. It is

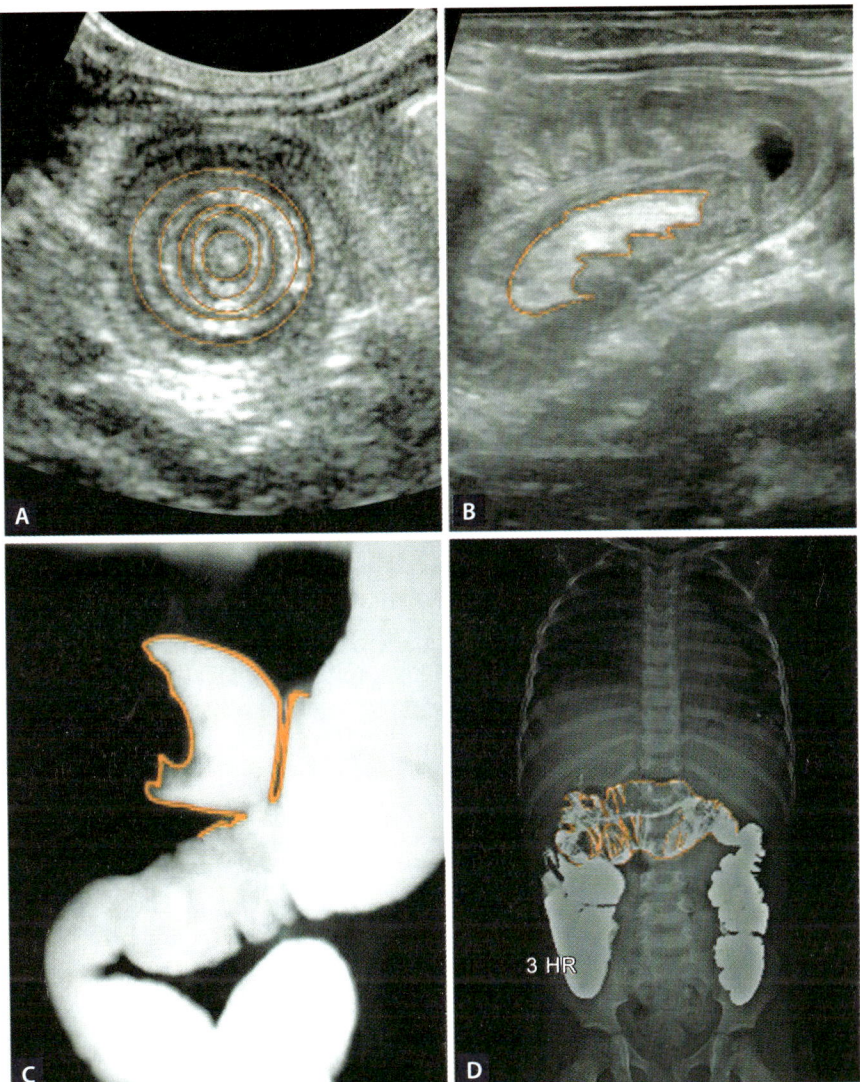

Figs. 25.5A to D: Imaging in intussusception. (A) "Target sign" on transverse view in ultrasonogram (USG) of abdomen; (B) "Pseudo-kidney sign" on longitudinal view in USG abdomen; (C) "Claw sign" appearance in barium enema study; (D) "Coiled-spring appearance" in barium enema study.

both a diagnostic and therapeutic investigation. Classical findings seen in a contrast enema are:
- *"Claw sign"*—it is formed by the rounded head of intussusception protruding into the column of contrast material **(Fig. 25.5C)**.[15] This sign is indicative of a snugly fit intussusception.
- *"Coiled spring sign"*—this is formed by the outlining of edematous mucosal folds of the returning limb of the intussusceptum by contrast

material in the lumen of the colon **(Fig. 25.5D)**.[15] This sign is found in quite loose intussusception; hence allowing seepage of contrast between the coats of intussusception.[14]

However, BE is not used these days; because of radiation exposure and chemical peritonitis in case perforation occurs during reduction attempts.

Contrast-enhanced Computed Tomography and Magnetic Resonance Imaging

They are not routinely indicated. However, it is more sensitive in picking up SBIs that may be missed on ultrasound study. Intussusception may be an incidental finding in imaging performed for other causes. The characteristic finding is again a *target sign* or *doughnut sign*. They are mainly of utility in suspected lead points; or fixed SBIs as they are more likely to associated with lead points and less amenable enema reductions.

■ DIFFERENTIAL DIAGNOSIS

- *Gastroenteritis*: It is the most common differential diagnosis. But here diarrhea, foul smelling stools and fever will be the presenting features, whereas in intussusception diarrhea will be of less severity and shorter duration.
- *Acute appendicitis*: Appendicitis is quite rare in patients under 2 years of age, which is a common age group for intussusception. Patient will present with periumbilical pain followed by tenderness in RIF; whereas an intussuscepted child will have emptiness of RIF. Ultrasound abdomen will clear the doubt.
- *Rectal prolapse*: It can masquerade as transanal protrusion of intussusception (TAPI). However, a careful examination can differentiate between the two. Apart from the absence of typical history, the anal crypts will be everted with rectal prolapse, which would not be there in the case with intussusception. Another method is insertion of finger between the mass and encircling anal opening. This would be possible in TAPI, but not in rectal prolapse.

■ TREATMENT

Treatment can be categorized into operative and nonoperative measures. The nonoperative measures are discussed first.

Nonoperative Measures (Radiological Reductions)

Nonoperative measures comprise radiological reductions which include:
- Pneumatic reduction
- Hydrostatic reduction
- Delayed repeat enema

It is imperative to streamline the patients who are suitable for radiological reduction. The indications of radiological reductions have been widened; and almost all patients are subjected to radiologic reductions before embarking upon surgery. The contraindications include the following:
- Clinical evidence of shock and peritonitis
- Radiological evidence of pneumoperitoneum
- Mass protruding per rectum.

Younger age (<6 months), bleeding per rectum and long duration of symptoms (>72 hours) which were previously considered as contraindication, now no longer hold true; and radiologic reductions can be attempted under close observation.

Steroids can also be administered before, along with and after radiological reduction. Steroids reduce bowel wall edema and lymphoid hyperplasia; but exact mechanism remains unclear.

The approach varies from one treatment center to another. Commonly used modalities are pneumatic reduction and hydrostatic reduction, either under fluoroscopic or USG guidance. The advantages of USG over fluoroscopy include:
- USG avoids radiation exposure.
- USG provides more information than fluoroscopy.
- USG has high accuracy, and reliability in monitoring the reduction process as it can visualize all components of intussusception.
- USG can more easily recognize pathologic lead points.

The disadvantages of USG are the need of more expertise and the high probability of missing a perforation.[4] The choice of technique depends on personal preference and experience, institutional set up and expertise of the radiologist. We will discuss both pneumatic and hydrostatic reduction.

Pneumatic Enema Reduction

This is the widely practiced technique these days. The air enema technique, i.e., *Shields' technique* is well described in literature.[16] The simple device consists of disposable enema tip, tubing system, hand-held pressure gauge, and insufflator. However, we use a little modification by using Foley's catheter instead of an enema tip. The advantage includes less air leak as it can be held snugly by inflating the bulb.

The baby is placed in prone position. Mild sedation and analgesia are given. The Foley's catheter is inserted within the child's rectum and bulb is inflated; and buttocks are squeezed together and taped to prevent air leakage. Air is rapidly insufflated into the colon with the insufflator. The progress is followed radiologically intermittently **(Fig. 25.6)**. Air should flow freely from cecum into the distal small bowel loops to signify complete reduction. The critical safety point is to keep the pressure till 80 mm Hg and in no

Intussusception

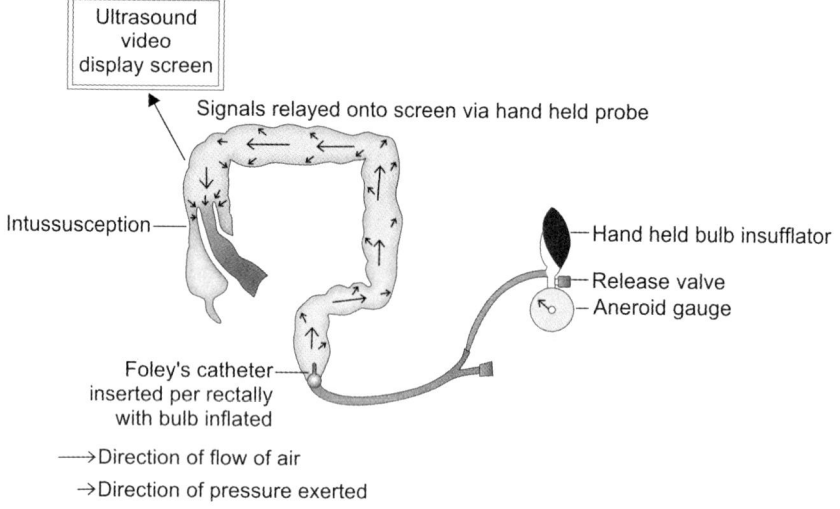

Fig. 25.6: Basic technique of pneumatic reduction.

circumstances > 120 mm Hg.[17] The pressure can be maintained if reduction is occurring. But in the absence of any progress, the attempt should not be continued for >3 minutes. A total of three attempts are made and one can reattempt after a suitable gap (6–8 hours) if the child is stable.

The advantages of this technique are smaller perforations and less peritoneal contamination.[18] Disadvantages include passage of air into the proximal bowel without complete reduction and possible tension pneumoperitoneum in case perforation occurs.[19] In the latter situation, the child should be immediately taken to the operating room.

Hydrostatic Enema Reduction

Many centers prefer hydrostatic enema reduction to pneumatic enema reduction, as monitoring with ultrasound is relatively easy. There are many disadvantages, namely larger perforations, increased peritoneal contamination, messy to use and rapid fluid shifts in case of hypertonic water-soluble agents.[4] There are many agents available like normal saline, ringer lactate, gastrografin and barium. Barium and gastrografin are no longer preferred these days because of risk of rapid fluid shifts and chemical peritonitis in case perforation occurs.[4] Hence, normal saline is the most preferred agent.

Device set up and basic methodology is the same as for pneumatic enema reduction. The pressure is routinely kept between 60 and 80 mm Hg and in no circumstances, it is >120 mm Hg. The *"rule of threes"* (three attempts, each lasting for 3 minutes, and enema can placed 3 feet above the table) is applied by the radiologists.[4] However, pressure should not be raised >80 mm Hg in the following conditions.[15]

- Duration of symptoms >48 hours
- Intussusception below splenic flexure
- Poor general condition
- Age >3 months.

The reduction may occur rapidly or slowly.

The reduction is marked complete by following findings:
- Free flow of contrast well into the small bowel
- Expulsion of flatus and feces with the contrast
- Disappearance of the sausage shaped mass per abdomen
- Improvement in the general look of the patient, who may fall into a natural sleep.

Delayed Repeat Enema

Repeat radiologic reductions can be attempted even after three failed attempts, if the patient is stable, there is no worsening of abdominal signs and if intussusception has shown partial reduction. Partial reduction and time delay allow resolution of venous congestion and bowel edema to aid in further reduction.

However, the time interval between the repeat enema and number of attempts is yet to be defined. The safest approach is to tailor it according to the condition of patient and experience of the radiologist.

Postreduction Care

The child should be monitored closely for a few hours after successful enema reduction. Once the abdomen settles and child passes flatus, clear fluids can be initiated, and oral intake can be increased as tolerated. It is imperative to titrate fluids in accordance with oral intake and urine output to maintain optimal hydration status. The preoperative gram negative and anaerobic bacterial coverage can be discontinued if the patient is afebrile and total leukocyte counts are within normal limits.

If the child is feeding well, passing motions and playful, s/he can be discharged without a repeat USG.

Repeat USG is advocated only if there is a doubt about the success of reduction or if abdominal pain recurs. In case of recurrent intussusception, choice is made between repeat enema and surgical intervention as per patient's clinical condition.

Operative Measures

This comprises surgical interventions which include:
- Exploratory laparotomy
- Laparoscopy

As a first step in hospital therapy, *nasogastric suction* should be instituted to prevent vomiting and pulmonary aspiration. Intravenous fluids and antibiotics are started. Routine hematological and biochemistry panel is obtained. Furthermore, child should be properly covered to prevent hypothermia. It is important to correct preoperative shock before taking up patient for surgery. Surgical intervention is indicated in cases of:
- Failure of enema reduction
- Persistent filling defect noted at the time of enema reduction which is suggestive of a lead point
- Signs of peritonitis
- Pneumoperitoneum on plain abdominal X-ray
- Documented lead point on radiological assessment
- All scenarios when enema reduction is contraindicated.

Decision regarding laparotomy or laparoscopy is made as per surgeon's preference, expertise, and resource settings. Standard management approach has been illustrated in **Flowchart 25.1**.

Laparotomy

After necessary optimization and resuscitation, patient is induced under general anesthesia. Nasogastric tube should be in situ. Laparotomy is performed via right supraumbilical incision. The lump (or intussusception) is palpated, and gentle manual reduction is attempted, without delivering the lump outside the peritoneal cavity; by retrograde milking known as *"taxis"*— just like squeezing toothpaste out of its tube.[4] Unnecessary bowel handling should be avoided. The crux is that distal most part of intussusceptum is pinched and finger movements are directed more toward pushing than pulling. Pathologic lead point should be ruled out.

However, in difficult reductions the lump is delivered outside the peritoneal cavity and back of the forceps or little finger can be used to create space between intussusceptum and intussuscipiens as it also drains edema fluid and aids in reduction (*modified Hutchinson maneuver*).[20] In case of failure of this maneuver, enterotomy is advised to aid in reduction and to save maximum possible length of bowel. More distal the intussusception, more difficult is manual reduction. If the reduction is incomplete, bowel should be wrapped with warm sponges and checked for viability by inspecting the color and visible peristalsis. In case of doubtful viability, surgeon should ask anesthetist to give 100% oxygen. If the color restores to normal, abdomen can be closed once the presence of lead point has been ruled out. If the color remains dusky, resection of the unhealthy part and anastomosis of the remaining bowel can be done. Diversion stoma is generally not required as the pathology is localized. However, it can be considered in case of hemodynamic instability and when multiple resections are indicated.

Flowchart 25.1: Management approach towards patient of intussusception.

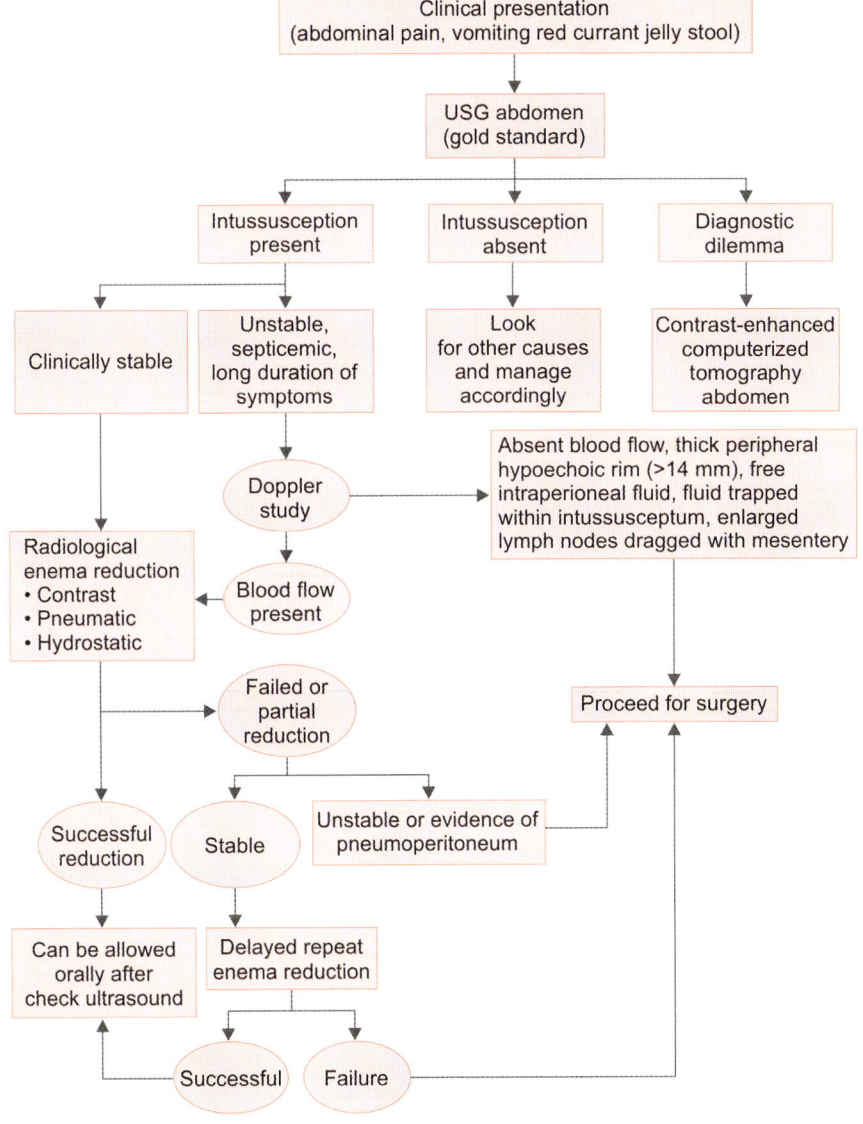

(USG: ultrasonography)

In cases, where the surgery is done for postenema reduction complications such as pneumoperitoneum, primary repair of perforation can be attempted.

Laparoscopy

Previously, the role of laparoscopy was said to be limited to confirmation of pathological lead point in cases of recurrent intussusception. But nowadays, role of laparoscopy has shifted more toward therapeutic rather than diagnostic one.

Patients presenting early (<36 hours), without signs of peritonitis or suspected incompletely reduced intussusception, are ideal candidates amenable to successful laparoscopic reduction.

Mostly, three-port technique is used—one on umbilicus (optical port) and two lateral ports (working ports); one in right lower quadrant and other in left upper quadrant.[21] Gentle pressure is applied distal to the intussusceptum with bowel graspers. Contrary to open surgery, traction should be applied proximal to intussuscipiens to achieve a successful reduction.[4] This should be followed by a careful inspection to look for gangrenous changes or any perforation, and in particular pathologic lead point.

Postoperative bowel adhesions are less with laparoscopic reduction.

■ COMPLICATIONS

Radiologic

Complications with enema reduction are extremely uncommon and reported to be <1% in most of the series.[4] Bowel perforation is the major complication. It is more common in infants <6 months of age and in patients with longer duration of symptoms. Technical factors amounting to pressure include too high pressures or rapid change in pressures.

In case perforation occurs at lower pressures, it should be presumed that it was already present and has been unmasked by partial reduction.

Surgical

Surgical complications include wound infection, fascial dehiscence, and adhesive bowel obstruction. The risk of complications is more in the cases where enterotomy or bowel resection has been performed than in the cases in which only manual reduction was done.

■ RECURRENCE

Recurrent intussusceptions can occur in up to 20% of cases and most of the recurrences occur within 6 months of the first episode.[4] Recurrences are less common after surgical reduction or bowel resections as lead point is supposed to be ruled out.

Multiple recurrences should prompt the surgeon to rule out a lead point. USG is the first investigation in these cases also, but contrast-enhanced computed tomography (CECT) of abdomen would be more informative.

■ OUTCOME

The outcome of patients with intussusception depends upon the judgment of clinician and pediatric surgeon. Taking together the clinical and radiologic assessment, diagnostic accuracy approaches almost 100%. Major improvements have been made over a period of time in radiologic enema reduction with success rate approaching up to 74% in stable patients.[22] Recurrence rate has been reported up to 20% in literature, which can be managed with repeat enema reduction in most of the cases.[4]

Mortality associated with intussusception is on steady decline and is <1% for both surgical and radiologic reduction.[4]

■ CONCLUSION

Intussusception is truly an acute surgical emergency, and it must be consistently in the mind of pediatrician who first sees the patient. The interval between onset of symptoms and institution of treatment is of paramount importance, to reduce the mortality. Therefore, the greatest emphasis must be given to the timely reference to pediatric surgeons.

■ KEY POINTS

- Intussusception develops with antegrade peristalsis when the proximal bowel (intussusceptum) drags along with its mesentery into the distal bowel (intussuscipiens).
- In most cases, intussusception commences just proximal to ileocecal valve (ileocolic).
- The classical triad of abdominal pain, vomiting, and red currant stools occurs in only about one-third of patients with intussusception.
- The characteristic findings on USG are the "target sign" or "doughnut sign" or "bull's eye sign" on transverse view; and the "pseudo-kidney" or "hayfork sign" on longitudinal view.
- Conventional nonoperative radiological reductions include pneumatic reduction, hydrostatic reduction, and delayed repeat enema.
- Contraindications for radiological reduction include clinical evidence of shock and peritonitis, radiological evidence of pneumoperitoneum and a mass protruding per rectum.
- Patients presenting within 36 hours without signs of peritonitis or suspected incompletely reduced intussusception are ideal candidates amenable to successful laparoscopic reduction.

■ REFERENCES

1. Grosfeld J. Intussusception then and now: A historical vignette. J Am Coll Surg. 2005;201(6):830-3.
2. Ladd WE. Progress in the diagnosis and treatment of intussusception. Boston Med Surg J. 1913;168:542-44.
3. Al-Salem A. Intussusception. In: Al-Salem A (Ed). An illustrated guide to Pediatric Surgery. Switzerland: Springer; 2014. pp. 167-72.
4. Scholz S, Columbani P. Intussusception. In: Coran A, Adzick N, Krummel T, Laberge J, Caldamone A, Shamberger R (Eds). Pediatric Surgery, 7th edition. Philadelphia: Elsevier; 2012. pp. 1093-110.

5. Kim J, Lam V, Arensman R. Intussusception. In: Arensman R, Bambini D, Almond P, Adolph V, Radhakrishnan J (Eds). Pediatric Surgery, 2nd edition. Texas: Landes Bioscience; 2009; pp. 90-4.
6. Minney-Smith C, Levy A, Hodge M, Jacoby P, Williams S, Carcione D, et al. Intussusception is associated with the detection of adenovirus C, enterovirus B and rotavirus in a rotavirus vaccinated population. J Clin Virol. 2014;61(4):579-84.
7. Murphi T, Gargiullo P, Massoudi M, Nelson D, Jumaan A, Okoro C, et al. Intussusception among infants given an oral rotavirus vaccine. N Engl J Med. 2001;344(8):564-72.
8. Lee P, Chen P, Huang Y, Lee C, Lu C, Chang M, et al. Recommendations for rotavirus vaccine. Pediatr Neonatol. 2013;54(6):355-9.
9. Johnson B, Gargiullo P, Murphy T, Parashar U, Patel M. Sociodemographic and dietary risk factors for natural infant intussusception in the United States. J Pediatr Gastroenterol Nutr. 2010;51(4);458-63.
10. Ravitch MM. Intussusception. In: Ravitch MM (Ed). Pediatric Surgery, 4th edition. Chicago; Year Book Medical Publishers; 1986. pp. 868-82.
11. Mathur P, Sultania S, Boipai M, Joshi V, Farooq A, Bhandari A, et al. Trans-anal protrusion of intussusception in a neonate. J Pediatr Surg Case Rep. 2020; 54:101393.
12. Verschelden P, Filiatrault D, Garel L, Grignon A, Perreault G, Boisvert J, et al. intussusception in children: reliability of US in diagnosis- a prospective study. Radiology. 1992;184(3):741-4.
13. Ramsey K, Halm B. Diagnosis of intussusception using bedside ultrasound by a pediatric resident in the emergency department. Hawaii J Med Public Health. 2014;73(2):58-60.
14. Till H, Sorantin E. Intussusception. In: Puri P, Hollwarth ME (Eds). Pediatric Surgery, 2nd edition. Berlin; Springer; 2006. pp. 279-85.
15. Pozo G, Albillos J, Tejedor D, Calero R, Rasero M, Calle U, et al. Intussusception in children: current concepts in diagnosis and enema reduction. Radiographics. 1999;19(2):299-319.
16. Shiels W, Bisset G, Kirks D. Simple device for air reduction of intussusception. Pediatric Radiol. 1990;20(6):472-4.
17. Shiels W, Maves C, Hedlung G, Kirks D. Air enema for diagnosis and reduction of intussusception: clinical experience and pressure correlates. Radiology. 1991;181(1):169-72.
18. Stringer D, Ein S. Pneumatic reduction: Advantages, risks and indications. Pediatr Radiol. 1990:20(6):475-7.
19. Murakami J, Winters W, Wienberger E, Rosenbaum D. Extensive reflux of air during enema for intussusception: case report. Can Assoc Radiol J. 1998;49(5):334-35.
20. Hase T, Kodama M, Mizukuro T, Kishida A, Shimadera S, Ohno M, et al. Manual reduction with the index finger for infantile intussusception: A modification of Hutchinson's maneuver. Pediatr Surg Int. 1998;13(2):223-5.
21. Philips JD. Intussusception treatment. In: Saxena A, Hollwarth ME (Eds). Essentials of Pediatric Endoscopic Surgery. Heidelberg: Springer; 2009. pp. 241-6.
22. Daneman A, Novarro O. Intussusception: the debate endures. Pediatr Radiol. 2004;35(1):95-6.

Child Rights, Abuse and Exploitation

CHAPTER 26: Child Neglect, Abuse and Exploitation

Rajendra Nath Srivastava

■ INTRODUCTION

In recent decades, the issues of child rights, child neglect, and abuse of children have been globally addressed. The *United Nations (UN) Convention on the Rights of the Child (CRC)* of 1990 was the precursor of this movement with definition of "child" as one who has not completed the age of 18 years.[1] Nearly 193 countries including all in Asia Pacific region ratified CRC. They have been called to take appropriate legislative, administrative, social, and educational measures to protect the child from all forms of physical or mental violence, injury or abuse, neglect or negligent treatment, maltreatment, or exploitation including sexual abuse. The document takes a "child rights" line of action to caregiving and security and broadens the limited importance on protection from death and imminent impairment to include safeguarding the child's wellbeing, growth, and progress. It emphasizes that child safety must begin with pre-emptive primary prevention and elimination of all forms of violence. The UN convention respects the worth and dignity of every child equally, regardless of race, color, gender, language, religion, opinions, origins, wealth status, or ability.

In India, the *National Charter for Children* espoused in 2004 emphasized the commitment to secure for every child, the essential right to be a child and enjoy a happy childhood. It also addresses the origin of grounds that deny their normal growth and development and sensitize the community to protect children from all forms of abuse. The *National Policy for Children, 2013* reiterates the commitment to safeguard, inform, include, support, and empower all children, and to take affirmative measures to promote child rights, especially the marginalized and disadvantaged, and ensure that all children have equal opportunities.[2] No custom, tradition, and/or cultural or religious practice should be allowed to violate or restrict child rights.

■ CHILD RIGHTS

Child rights have been explicitly spelled out in the CRC document. The *"rights-based approach"* has been adopted to address children's problems, in contrast to the *"welfare approach".*[3] Thus, whatever measures are undertaken to provide for and protect children are children's right rather than child welfare services. Of various child rights, survivals, health care, education, and protections from harm are crucial. Inability to safeguard the right to protection negatively affects all other rights of the child. Inadequate nurturing care by the parents can be due to multiple causes that include poverty, parental illiteracy, and large family size. Appropriate interventions should address these issues. Wherever required, parents should be helped by the family, proximate community, and local health authorities and empowered by the State.

Socioeconomic Influences

The affluent and educated proportion of India's population, mostly residing in cities, are vastly different from the majority who are illiterate and poor and live in the villages and underprivileged urban areas. Of the total population of India, around 30% are children below the age of 14 years and of these 14% are <6 years. Nearly 74% of those between 0 and 6 years live in rural areas. About 26 million newborns are added every year. The privileged and educated are able to look after their children. The parents with low resources and meager information lack the capability to sufficiently nurture the young child and provide for necessary inputs for care and learning. The burden of child marriage adds to this problem.

■ CHILD NEGLECT

The World Health Organization (WHO) defined child neglect as inattention or omission on the part of a caregiver to provide for the child in all spheres: health, education, nutrition, emotional development, shelter, and safe conditions in the context of resources reasonably available to the family.[4] Insufficient provision of these because of poor socioeconomic and illiteracy causes or has a high probability of causing harm to the child's physical, mental, social, or moral development. Whereas the definitions of neglect are globally approved, the needs of the child must be prioritized taking cognizance of the socioeconomic conditions in different countries. Limited resources available to most of the populations in developing countries result in deprivation of the basic needs of children such as nutrition, hygiene and cleanliness, clothing, and proper shelter. Denial of comprehensive health care and education must be regarded as the most severe form of neglect, which is largely due to parental lack of awareness and means. A loving caring environment is difficult to ensure in the presence of poverty and large family size, where both parents might be working.

Neglect of Early Childcare and Education

The components of "Early Childcare and Education (ECCE)" include the needs of the mother, perinatal care, providing nutrition, and health care to the infant and the growing child, stimulatory and safe environment, and opportunities for learning and education. Insufficient provision of these leads to physical retardation and deficient cognizant development, which can be irreversible. The parents and caregivers are often unaware of the needs of the young child who remains uncared for. The preschool child in the rural poor and underprivileged population usually remains deprived of learning opportunities and school preparedness.

Neglect during Disasters and Conflict Zones

Children are the worst sufferers during natural disasters and in conflict zones, when large populations are on the move or confined in relief camps. Often, they spend several months or years in such conditions where their education and health care remain neglected.

■ CHILD ABUSE (MALTREATMENT) AND EXPLOITATION

Intentional infliction of various forms of maltreatment of children is an issue of serious concern. The definitions, patterns, prevalence, and the magnitude of child abuse and exploitation vary in different countries. The term *"maltreatment"* is often used to describe child abuse but is seemingly too mild to include more serious forms of abuse and exploitation. The forms of violence are listed in the **Box 26.1**.

Physical Violence

Corporal Punishment

Corporal punishment is a very frequent form of violence in the day-to-day lives of children.[5] Physical and humiliating "disciplinary" measures are universally adopted in homes and schools. Hitting the child with the hand or fist or with an implement (stick, belt, whip, wooden spoon, shoe, etc.), besides being cruel and degrading, often results in serious injury, and occasional mortality. Social attitudes and long-standing traditions usually ignore or condone such punishment. Milder forms of physical punitive acts inflicted upon young children as corrective measures are common, seemingly innocuous, and

---

BOX 26.1: Forms of violence.

- Physical violence
- Corporal punishment
- Mental or emotional violence
- Torture and inhuman or degrading treatment or punishment
- Violence among children including bullying and self-harm
- Harmful cultural and child raising practices
- Violence in the media and information technology
- Sexual abuse and exploitation

culturally regarded as a way of upbringing of children. Parents, caregivers, and teachers often argue that these measures do not cause any permanent damage. Various domestic disciplinary measures are accepted as a way of life, especially in poor and illiterate households with many children. Domestic violence is not uncommon among educated societies in affluent countries where social norms are different and the incidence of domestic discords and alcohol and substance abuse is high.

Schoolteachers, especially in primary schools, express the difficulty in controlling classes having large numbers of pupils, which contrasts with the situation in affluent countries. However, the teachers need to understand these issues and ensure that no child is subjected to physical or mental harassment.[6] Under India's *Right to Education Act,* corporal punishment is prohibited in schools. Prohibition of corporal punishment must be regarded as a human rights obligation. Legal measures alone cannot stop such practice and must be supported by societal attitudinal changes. Civil society should be made aware of child rights to protection and the dangers of corporal punishment.

Nonaccidental Injuries

It is important to recognize intentional injury inflicted upon the child.[5] Unless identified and prevented, abusive acts tend to be repeated and may lead to serious injury. Pediatricians should be aware of various forms of abusive trauma. Unusual patterns of injury that cannot be explained by the history given by the caretakers should raise the suspicion of intentional trauma. A detailed explanation of the injury should be obtained from the caregiver and, if possible, from the child separately, in a sympathetic, nonjudgmental manner. The child's developmental skills should be considered when evaluating the description. The age of the child is important. Thus, injuries in an infant who is not independently mobile should raise suspicion of abuse. Infants with incessant crying, for several reasons, are often subjected to pulling, hitting, or more serious trauma. A thorough physical examination without clothes should be carried out. The injuries should be described, drawn, and their extent measured.

Bruises: Bruises are the most common form of nonaccidental injury. Their shape and location help differentiation from those sustained by falls. Thus, bruises on the face, ears, neck, upper arms, buttocks, and thighs suggest the likelihood of willful injury, while those due to falls are seen over bony prominences involving shins, knees, ankles, forehead, and elbows. Accidental bruises are rare in infants below 6 months of age and appear when the child starts to walk. A slap injury may leave outline of the hand while hitting with a stick causes linear injury. A hard blow to the ear often produces cauliflower-like swelling. The timing of the bruises, whether fresh or old, is difficult to identify since the pattern and healing are variable. The possibility of an underlying bleeding or clotting disorder should be kept in mind while evaluating these injuries.

Fractures: Fractures of posterior ribs, scapula, spinous process, and sternum are suggestive of abusive injury. Classic metaphyseal lesions occur when the infant is twisted or pulled. The presence of intracranial injury should be examined. Fractures may be multiple, bilateral, and of different ages and a skeletal survey may be required. The likelihood of metabolic and congenital disorders should be considered and excluded by appropriate investigations. Rickets, renal tubulopathies, and congenital disorders such as osteogenesis imperfecta may lead to fractures with mild trauma. Fractures are often ascribed to falls, but a careful inquiry of the incident will help to exclude that likelihood. The height from which the child is reported to have fallen, immediate events that followed, and the presence of concussion should be probed. The injury should be consistent with the explanation given by the parents.

Burns: Inflicted burn injury must be differentiated from accidental burns by a careful enquiry into the description and setting of the injury. Intentional scalds usually involve feet, legs, hands, and buttocks. Instances of burns caused by cigarettes are not uncommon forms. Burn injuries from hot metallic objects used as bonding by quacks for a variety of ailments are also occasionally seen. A detailed examination should be carried out and documented. Referral to a specialist may be necessary.

Childline

Childline India foundation is a nongovernmental organization (NGO) and the nodal agency for the Ministry of Women and Child development, which operates a telephonic helpline across the country.[7] It provides emergency services through coordination with several agencies for rescue and care and rehabilitation. The physician, or any other person, may call Childline (phone 1098) for assistance to report any form of child abuse and exploitation.

Consequences of Child Maltreatment

Many studies indicate that corporal punishment is associated with aggression and antisocial behavior in late childhood, and continues into adulthood. In recent years, a great deal of concern has been expressed over the relationship of violence and abuse in children with their long-term deleterious effects.[8,9] Development of such adverse effects is also likely to depend upon subsequent domestic and work environment and the support of family and peers.

CHILD SEXUAL ABUSE

Among the many dangers children may face, the crime of sexual offence and exploitation is most reprehensible. Child sexual abuse (CSA) has been defined as any sexual activity with a child (defined as below the age of 18 years).[10,11] This definition encompasses various forms of sexual abuse such as sexual assault (penetrative or nonpenetrative), sexual harassment, commercial sexual exploitation, sex tourism, and online exploitation. CSA is as common in developing countries as in well-off countries but less reported in the former. The prevalence rates of CSA in Asia are much higher than that in Europe and America—23.9% compared to 9–10%.[12] The reasons for nonreporting of these crimes include sociocultural practices, the ethos of secrecy, protection of family honor, and trepidation of social humiliation. Lesser forms of CSA are very often overlooked.

Sexual violence may take place in any location, whether home or outside—including schools, childcare institutions, workplaces, and in the community. The information on the prevalence and forms of CSA in India is scarce. The Ministry of Women and Child Development interviewed 125,000 children in 13 Indian states in 2007 and noted that about half of them had already experienced CSA.[13] Boys were abused as much as girls and >20% were exposed to severe forms of abuse. The National Crime Records Bureau (NCRB) had reported >10,000 cases of rape in children in India in a report published in 2015. The perpetrators were mostly persons known to the children—the neighbors, friends, relatives, and employers at workplaces, who easily lured the children by offering simple gifts.[11] Acts of CSA are often repeated over varying periods and may result in grave long-term adverse effects.

Management of Child Sexual Abuse

Every case of sexual assault should be treated as a medical emergency. Affected children should be provided with free treatment whether it is a government or private medical facility.[11,14,15] No document or precondition is necessary for providing emergency medical care.

A victim of CSA may also approach a health facility directly for treatment with a police requisition after police complaint, or with a court directive. The hospital should conduct a medical examination after obtaining an informed consent from the child or the parent/guardian (depending upon the age of the child) and provide appropriate treatment. The victim may not wish to lodge a complaint but still requires medical examination and treatment. In such cases, the doctor is required to inform the police as per law. However, the survivor cannot be forced by the police or the court to undergo medical examination without an informed consent of the child/parent/guardian.[11] Even, if the victim does not want to register a police case, a medicolegal case (MLC) must be made and an informed refusal documented. If the victim has reported with a police requisition or wishes to lodge a complaint later, the information about MLC number and police station must be recorded.[11]

Medical Evaluation of a Child Subjected to Sexual Abuse

An informed consent is obligatory for examination, collection of samples for forensic examination, treatment, and police intimation. If the child is over 12 years, consent should be obtained from the child. For those below the age of 12, consent from the parent/guardian is required. The person giving the consent should be clearly explained the purpose, expected risks, benefits, and any adverse effects of the examination and the length of time it might take. This information should be provided before the examination is conducted. CSA, whether confirmed or strongly suspected, must be reported to the appropriate authorities.[10,11,14,15]

History

The diagnosis of child sexual abuse is most often based on the history. The doctor should try to obtain a reliable history of the child's experiences. The conversation should be in a facilitative, nonjudgmental, and empathetic approach without an investigative tone similar to that of the police and courts. The psychosocial background of the family should be evaluated and the level of cognitive development of the child assessed. The complete interview should be recorded verbatim using the "words of the child" as far as possible.

It is important to note the body language, demeanor, and emotional responses of the child during the interview. Observe specially for any behaviors and physical findings that may mimic CSA. The past medical history should be enquired in detail including instances of abuse or suspicious injuries, and menstrual history. The behavior of the child, and in young children, the names the child uses for body parts especially breasts, vagina, penis, and anus should be noted. Leading and suggestive interrogations are avoided and expression of strong emotional responses such as shock or disbelief resisted. A historical review of all organ systems with a special focus on genital and anal areas such as pain, bleeding, discharge, or genital injuries is carried out. The history of CSA is ideally obtained without the presence of the parent or caregiver.

Detailed and well-documented medical records must be kept, since these are crucial in legal proceedings, which may take place after a delay of long periods. The likelihood that sexual abuse might not be an isolated incident and, in suspicious circumstances, the possibility that the child may have been trafficked should be considered. Child trafficking compounds the gravity of the offense.

Examination

Health care professionals (HCPs) generally do not receive necessary training to examine and manage a child with CSA, but it is important that they develop the required expertise. They need to know the measures that can be taken to prevent CSA and the essential components of the Protection of Children from Sexual Offences (POCSO) Act, which specifies their responsibility in the management of CSA.

The child and the parents should be explained that physical examination is usually not invasive or painful and that internal instrumentation or insertion of a speculum is carried out only, if essential. Documentation, collection of forensic evidence, and timely reporting are important tools in investigation of CSA. Avoid the presence of police personnel during examination. If the victim is a girl, the medical examination is conducted by a lady physician in the presence of the parent of the child, preferably the mother, or any other female person whom the child can trust. If such a person is not available at that time, the examination is conducted in the presence of a woman nominated by the head of the medical institution.[11,14]

The child should be calmed before examination. Proper positioning is necessary for optimal exposure of prepubertal genital structures. Anogenital area, mons pubis, labia majora and minora, clitoris, urethral meatus, hymen, posterior fourchette, and fossa navicularis are examined. Handheld magnification or colposcopy may be required. Specimens are collected for sexually transmitted disease (STD) screening and forensic evidence.

Interpretation of Observations

Physical examination in victims of CSA may not show any abnormality since many types of CSA do not cause physical injury. Mucosal tissue is elastic and may be stretched without injury, and superficial abrasions and fissures may heal within a few days. The child very often knows the perpetrators and family, and the use of physical force is rarely a major component in CSA, as in adult sexual assaults. Disclosure of CSA is often delayed for weeks or months by which time the physical evidences may be absent. The degree of harm should be clearly documented since that is taken into consideration while deciding on the severity of punishment in a court of law.

Investigations

Investigations that are routinely carried out are shown in the **Box 26.2**.[11]

Forensic Examination

Collection of Forensic Evidence

Specimens and material should be obtained, if the physical examination is being conducted within 96 hours of the sexual contact. Proper collection,

> **BOX 26.2:** Investigations to be carried out in a suspected case of child sexual abuse.
> - Gram stain of vaginal or anal discharge
> - Genital, anal, and pharyngeal culture for *Gonorrhea*
> - Genital and anal culture for *Chlamydia*
> - Serology for syphilis
> - Wet preparation of vaginal discharge for *Trichomonas vaginalis*
> - Culture of lesions for herpes virus
> - Serology for human immunodeficiency virus (HIV) (based on suspected risk)
>
> *Note:* Collection of forensic evidence employing the rape kit and urine toxicology screen (if the abuse or assault was likely to be substance-facilitated) may be required.

depending on the history of sexual violence, is decisive for medicolegal purposes. The specimens to be collected include semen, saliva, lubricant, hair, and fecal matter as well as debris (e.g., carpet fibers and cloth material that might help to identify the location). The Ministry of Health and Family Welfare, Government of India (GOI) has provided detailed instructions about collection of forensic evidence.[15] The material collected should be properly packed, sealed, labeled, and sent to the police.

Physician's Responsibility

Health care professionals are legally required to examine and provide emergency medical treatment to victims of CSA and sexual violence. For this requisition from the police or law agencies is not required. Treatment of STDs is carried out with appropriate medications. In postmenarcheal girls, the likelihood of pregnancy and the need for emergency contraception should be considered. Emotional support should be provided the child. The child may need assistance during medical procedures and traumatic interventions. Referral to a mental health specialist is often required for evaluation and treatment of acute stress reaction.

Mental Health Support and Post-traumatic Stress Disorder

Mental health professionals are of help in assisting the child and the family during examination and for complete management of CSA. Victims of CSA are exposed to psychoemotional distress and may have a tendency to self-harming behavior. Experts should counsel the child and try to help to reduce the emotional burden of trauma. Appropriate measures must be taken to prevent further abuse, trauma, and revictimization.[10,16]

Adverse mental health consequences and various manifestations of CSA are well recognized and frequently observed during adulthood.[10,17] Post-traumatic stress disorder (PTSD) is one of the mental disorders that can develop after CSA. The others are depression, anxiety, and substance use disorder. Adverse mental health consequences include feelings of guilt, excessive fear of adults, regression to infantile behavior, sexualized play with children, depression, and poor scholastic performance. Victims of CSA should be referred for psychological assessment for appropriate interventions. Such management is also necessary for the parents and caregivers to enable them to deal with emotional turmoil. The long-term impact of CSA varies depending upon the adequacy of the support systems and the attitudes of the family and the proximate community. The consequences of adverse childhood experiences (ACE) are often observed in adults.

Prevention of Child Sexual Abuse

Child sexual abuse should be considered a preventable crime.[10,16,18] The society must shed long-held traditions of silence, shame and embarrassment, and strongly act against this most reprehensible violation of child right and dignity. The parents have the main responsibility for protecting their children and they need the support from the civil society. Information about the prevalence of CSA, its occurrence in all societies, knowledge of the common perpetrators, legal aspects, and its prevention should be widely publicized. The parents should know the facts about CSA and take every care to guard the child and never leave them unsupervised. The child at 18 months can be taught the names of body parts. A child between 3 and 5 years can be explained the differences between an "okay touch" and "bad touch", and places over the body where nobody, except the mother can touch or clean. Older children can be told about different body parts including sexual, the differences between boys and girls in their sex organs, and issues of privacy. Such communication should be a continuum and is often difficult, mostly when using expressions for body parts and explaining topics like "how babies are born". Parents usually find their own methods once they understand the importance of empowering the child. Leaflets, fliers, images, and informative guides for parents are available and should be distributed widely in civil society.[10,16,18]

Adolescents require more detailed cognizance of body physiology, sexual intercourse, pregnancy, healthy relationships, and sexual violence. A group of "trained" teachers can provide this information at schools. This information may be packaged as *"health and family life skills-based comprehensive education"*, and not as "sex education". The parents should encourage the child to report any unusual behavior by adults.

Prevention of Child Sexual Abuse in Institutions, Workplaces, and Schools

It is not uncommon to receive reports of CSA from schools, children's homes, and workplaces. Independent agencies should supervise these institutions and maintain the records of inspection. Care should be taken in recruiting staff for these centers and they should be clearly told about their responsibilities and legal protective measures. Their work and actions should be scrutinized. School authorities and teachers should be informed about the problems of CSA and the need to maintain strict vigilance.

The Law on Child Sexual Abuse—Protection of Children from Sexual Offences Act

In November 2012, India adopted POCSO with the aim of provision of POCSO and assault and to safeguard the interest and wellbeing of children.[11] Amendments were made in the Act in 2019. The Act includes child-friendly mechanisms for reporting, recording of evidence, investigation, and speedy trial of offences through designated courts. Under POCSO Act, age of sexual consent is 18 years. As per the Act, sexual assault is considered *"aggravated"* when the abuse is committed by a person in a position of trust or authority vis-a-vis the child, such as a family member, police officer, teacher, or doctor.[11] The levels of punishment differ depending on the type of CSA and are more severe in cases of aggravated assault.

Mandatory Reporting

The Act calls for mandatory reporting of sexual offences so that the physician or any other HCP who has the knowledge that a child has been sexually abused is obliged to report the offence, failing which she/he may face legal punishment.[11] The mandatory reporter does not have an obligation to inform the child or her/his parents or guardian about her/his duty to report. In that report, the physician or other HCP should describe the nature of the abuse and mention all involved parties. The reporter is not expected to investigate the matter, or even know the identity of the perpetrator, which is the task for the police and other investigative agencies.

Multidisciplinary Approach

The POCSO Act envisions a multidisciplinary approach, which is favorable to medical care and delivery of justice to a sexually-abused child.[11] This requires coordination and convergence between all key stakeholders such as Juvenile Police Units, Child Welfare Committees, District Child Protection Units, HCPs, mental health professionals including psychiatrists, psychologists and counsellors, child developmental experts, medical social workers, advocates, magistrates, and other members of legal profession. The components of comprehensive health care response to sexual violence, as per Guidelines and Protocols of the Ministry of Health and Family Welfare include first aid, informed consent, history and examination, collection of forensic material, and its further handling.[16] Appropriate treatment of injuries is carried out along with management of sexually transmitted infections, HIV testing and prophylaxis, and emergency contraception, if indicated. Referral to other specialists is made, if required.

■ CHILD LABOR AND EXPLOITATION

A large proportion of children are in the workforce, while they should be in schools. Some are employed in the organized sector, but a majority is engaged in a variety of work such as roadside eateries, repair shops, and domestic help. They are denied education and often subject to physical and sexual abuse.[19-21] In India, children below 18 years comprise 41% of the population. Children between 6 and 10 years are usually not formally *employed,* but often engaged in taking care of younger siblings, begging, rag picking, and helping adults in cleaning and running errands. Older children between 10 and 18 years constitute the bulk of child workforce.

Magnitude of Child Labor

Although official reports mention that there are 11 million child workers, but estimates from nongovernmental sources suggest that 40 million children may be engaged in some form of work, forming about 13% of workforce.[19] More than 300,000 are working in the carpet industry. It is extremely difficult to find the exact numbers, given the size of the country, and regional disparities. About 80% of children work in the rural sector and 20% in the urban and semiurban areas. With rapid growth of nonorganized sector, especially in urban areas, the location of work has changed. A small proportion of children work in factories. Children are made to work long hours and are paid little, which is of economic benefit to the employer.

Hazardous Work

Work that harms health, safety, and morals is called hazardous. 70% of children are employed in such work, which is carried out in dangerous and unhealthy conditions.[22] In the agriculture sector they are often in proximity of dangerous machinery with no training in its proper working and taking safety measures. They may be exposed to pesticides and made to carry heavy loads. In workshops and small factories children often work in closed environment with poor ventilation. Adolescents between 14 and 17 years doing hazardous work constitute around 63% of the total child labor population. Of these nearly 10% work in family enterprises. Prevalence of infections (e.g., tuberculosis) and nutritional deficiencies is high. Specific injurious conditions related to the type of work include tobacco ingestion, acid burns, and inhalation of fiber in carpet and garment making. Silica dust inhalation in children working in brick making and stone quarries is another example.

Vehicle Repair Work and Roadside Eateries

Over the past several years, the cities have expanded very fast with rural to urban migration, leading to an increase in supporting services. The result is a large increase in infrastructure, vehicular transport, roadside eateries, and domestic help. Children are employed in a wide variety of work as helpers in cooking, serving, cleaning, and sundry activities.

Street Children, Rag Picking, and Organized Begging

Homeless children living on the streets are engaged in selling all kinds of objects at roadside, couriering, and rag picking. There are organized gangs who traffic or kidnap children and force them to beg. These children are subjected to all forms of abuse and addiction to tobacco, alcohol, and drugs. Substance abuse begins early, at around 9–13 years. Sexual exploitation of these children is not uncommon as they need of money for buying drugs.

Domestic Helpers

Children are often employed as domestic helpers among the well-to-do households. The conditions of work and their overall treatment differ depending on the attitudes of the employers. These children face harsh treatment and few are allowed schooling. Girls seem to be favored for domestic work with resulting maltreatment. Their nutritional and health care needs are not looked after.

Child Sex Workers

Children form >40% of sex workers in India currently. Sexual work is carried out in brothels or under the guise of massage parlors, especially at tourist circuits. Crowded localities such as railway stations and bus stations are common places of sexual exploitation. Organized groups often traffick or lure children from impoverished families in rural areas into sex work by with the promise of employment or marriage.

Modern Slavery and Bonded Labor

The term *"modern slavery"* refers to engagement of children in various forms of work since their permission is not obtained for employment. An inclusive definition would encompass forced labor and child trafficking, bonded labor or debt bondage, domestic servitude, and recruitment and use of child soldiers as combatants or other work by paramilitary or other organizations.[19,23] In India, slavery would strictly apply to children in bonded servitude and those trafficked into sexual work.

Child Trafficking

Trafficking in persons, especially in women and children for various purposes such as commercial sex exploitation, forced labor in organized industries, forced marriage, domestic servitude, adoption, and begging is an organized crime that gravely violates basic human rights.[24,25] Child trafficking is a serious problem in India and the neighboring countries. The common activities for which children undergo trafficking include couriering for drugs, explosives, and forced begging. The magnitude of trafficking in children is greater than in adults.

Missing Children

A large number of children go "missing" every year. NGOs estimate that 110,000 are missed and of these about 40% remain untraced, and are believed to be trafficked.[19,20] There exist organized gangs of recruiters, transporters, sellers, and purchasers. A recent report citing NCRB's data mentions that every 8 minutes a child goes missing in India, some of them being as young as between 7 and 15 years. Most of them are forced into various forms of child labor. Reports of bonded child workers being rescued frequently appear in the media, but these represent only the tip of the iceberg. There are serious health issues related to child labor. Whereas physical consequences are usually obvious, mental problems are often more subtle and elicited on careful enquiry.

Antihuman Trafficking Units

The legal response to human trafficking has not been very adequate and remains ineffective. Moreover, there is a lack of awareness among the police personnel about the magnitude and the seriousness of trafficking as compared to the crimes of murder, rape arson, and other law and order issues. The Ministry of Home Affairs, GOI, has set up "antihuman trafficking units (AHTUs)" in 270 districts of the country to strengthen the law enforcement response against trafficking of humans through training and capacity building.[25]

Why do Children have to Work?

A substantial proportion of population in India lives in abject poverty. Illiterate parents do not see any immediate benefits from schooling, while work in whatever capacity is of some monetary benefit.[8,12] The lack of openings and constant battles in their lives for existence in the rural areas have led to large population migration to cities, setting tremendous strain on urban infrastructure. Most migrants lack skills and education, still manage to get subsistence work but cannot obtain proper living conditions. No wonder that their children get engaged in activities with meager retributions with their education and overall development taking a nosedive.[8]

Consequences of Child Labor

Loss of Childhood, Deprivation of Education, and Health Care

Children who help in the family enterprises such as small businesses, handicrafts, may get adequate care, and education. All other forms of work in whatever settings trigger denial of a "happy childhood" resulting in loss of self-esteem and dignity. They grow up feeling different and inferior. Lack of proper education and equal opportunity impedes achievement of full potential for development and as adults they are unable to contribute to nation building in appropriate measure. Societal attitudes to treat them as "*servants*" rather than helpers are particularly despicable.

Prevention of Child Labor

The state and the civil society have a duty to ensure that children are brought up in financially stable family homes and educated in schools.[23,26,27] Multiple factors underlie persistence of poverty. Inadequate education ultimately leads to human capital of poor quality and restricts employment opportunities.

Large Family Size and Gender Discrimination

The family size among the poor and underprivileged populations in many regions continues to remain unacceptably large. The result is a great liability on the parents who cannot ensure adequate nurturing care, nutrition, health care, and education for their children. India has had a "*family planning or family welfare*" policy and a number of measures for its institution several decades, but it has achieved very limited success. Gender bias against the girl child has always existed in India and South Asia. Girls continue to be denied education, particularly beyond primary level, and compelled to help in household chores and take care of younger siblings. The large number of children in poverty-ridden families forces the parents to "get rid of the girls" by marrying them off early. Child marriages, although legally prohibited, remain frequent, and carry serious hazards to mothers and their children. Recently, the minimum age at marriage has been increased to 21 years. However, such legal stances are unlikely to beneficial until the families are empowered and the girl-provided proper education and job opportunities.

Child Exploitation

Children working in organized industries may encompass a relatively small proportion of child labor but are the worst exploited. Employers often disregard the legal measures adopted to protect children. There have been attempts to boycott manufactured goods and products from various industries that utilize child labor. Such measures are difficult to implement and may be counterproductive. Instead, the employers must be made to pay the workers their just dues, ensure proper working conditions, and provide health care and educational opportunities.

Legal Protective Measures

In 2017, India ratified all key international conventions concerning child labor, notably both International Labor Organization (ILO) convention 182 (against worst forms of child labor) and convention 138. The government amended the Child Labor Act to prohibit any child below the age of 18 years from working in hazardous occupation and processes.[27] The minimum age of work and hazardous work have been defined by several laws and regulations. Laws prohibit forced labor, child trafficking, and commercial sexual exploitation of children. The National Plan of Action for Children identifies key areas that include survival, health and nutrition, education and development, protection, and participation. It also addresses various issues in child labor and child trafficking. Some important Acts include the following:

- *The Criminal Law (amendment) Act,* 2013
- *The Bonded Labor System (Abolition) Act,* 1976
- *The Child and Adolescent Labor (Prohibition and Regulation) Act,* 1986 prohibits employment of a child below 14 years in any form of employment
- *The Juvenile Justice (JJ) (Care and Protection) Act,* 2015, makes it a crime, punishable with prison term, for anyone to keep a child in bondage for employment
- *The Immoral Traffic Prevention Act* (1956) identifies various forms of trafficking such as that for bonded labor, sexual exploitation, pornography, forced begging, removal of organs, etc.

Rehabilitation of Child Laborers

Rehabilitation of homeless child laborers and those forced in debt servitude is a mammoth task. The GOI has undertaken several measures to help children working in organized industries. These include opening of special schools, providing stipends, vocational training, and health care.[23] Many difficulties are faced when the families move from place to place to find work, where medical facilities, and schooling are deficient. Several NGOs have established homes for rescued child laborers and tried to return them to their families with limited success.

Implementation of Laws and Regulations

The responsibility for the implementation of various laws and regulations on child labor rests with the State and local administrative authorities, local police, and child welfare committees. National Human Rights Commission and National Commission for Protection of Child Rights also have well-defined roles in implementation of the policies and programmes. However, the laws are often flouted and those employing and exploiting children are seldom brought to book.

Children in Alternative Care and Institutions

Children rescued from forced employment, orphans (comprising about 4% of child population in India) and abandoned children, and need alternative care. Several NGOs have provided such care in various settings such as children's villages where all needs of children are taken care of. Efforts are made to place them in community where they can interact with their peers and families in a friendly environment. Foster care for children has been a restricted undertaking in our country because of social inhibitions. Community-based activities should be closely supervised to ensure that children are not humiliated or maltreated. Only few children are being legally adopted for which Central Adoption Resource Authority (CARA) regulates the mechanisms.

Many children where caretakers cannot be found, and those in conflict with the law, must receive institutional care. Such arrangement must be considered as the last resort and children must be kept for the shortest possible time. The standards of care provided in the institutions are variable but usually inadequate, and proper supervision is lacking. The incidence of abuse is high in childcare institutions. The longer the period of stay in the institution, the harder it becomes for children to return to the mainstream. Even a short stay may create a stigma and further marginalize them.

Child Protection Mechanisms

Protection of children from any perceived danger or risk to life is a crucial child right. Children in difficult circumstances, constituting about 40% of child population, are particularly vulnerable and need special attention. Failure to provide protection adversely impacts all other rights of the child. The National Policy for Children, 2013, reiterates the Government's commitment to safeguard, inform, include, support, and empower all children. Affirmative actions are to be taken to provide them equal opportunities and prevent inimical traditional, cultural, or religious practices that prevent or restrict child rights.[2]

Child protection is the primary responsibility of the family and the proximate community and ultimately that of the government. The family capabilities must be strengthened so that they can provide sufficient care. Where circumstances preclude that, alternative community-based care should be organized. Institutional care, although widely employed in India, should be regarded as the last resort.

Integrated Child Protection Scheme

Integrated Child Protection Scheme (ICPS), a centrally sponsored government scheme, was launched in 2009. It is aimed at building a protective environment for children in difficult circumstances, as well as other vulnerable children, through Government and Civil Society Partnership.[28] ICPS brings together various child protective schemes of the ministry and integrates additional interventions for protecting children and preventing harm. It has enhanced infrastructure for protection services, provided financial support for implementation of the JJ (Care and Protection of Children) Act, 2000 and increased investment in child protection.

Child Protection Committees (CPCs) are set up at village, district, and state level. CPCs in villages support community-based management of violence against children, exploitation, child labor, and prevention of child marriages. A multidisciplinary approach is adopted to tackle various problems. Village officials, Anganwadi workers, accredited social health activists (ASHAs), auxiliary nurse midwives (ANMs), and school teachers are explained and oriented toward these problems. Their involvement and responsibility are crucial.

Children in Conflict with the Law

Children in large cities and marginalized communities often get involved in unlawful activities, which are often minor but occasionally serious. The JJ Act provides clear instructions to the police personnel and judiciary about handling such cases.[29] This act applies to all children (below the age of 18 years), irrespective of the offences they may have been alleged to have committed.

Legal Measures

Many legal measures are in place to prevent offences against children and impose punitive actions against the perpetrators.[30] Most notable of these include the JJ (Care and Protection of Children) Act 2015, the POCSO Act Amendment 2019, the Child and Adolescent Labor (prevention and regulation) Act 1986, and the Prohibition of Child Marriage Act 2006. The JJ Act also addresses various issues concerning children in conflict with law. Implementation of these measures depends upon cooperation of the community and their surveillance of various activities. Law alone cannot counteract traditional beliefs, inimical religious practices, and actions directly consequential to poverty. The root causes must be tackled.

Health Care Infrastructure

India has a vast network of health care facilities through the Integrated Child Development Service (ICDS) program, with 14 lakhs Anganwadi centers with 1.8 lakh workers, and 30,000 primary health centers and referral services.[31]

These provide maternal and neonatal care, immunizations, nutritional supplements, treatment of illnesses, and referrals. Anganwadi workers and Accredited Social Work Activists (ASHA) perform multiple functions but need appropriate training to be able to advise the mother about nurturing care and education. They can be instructed for the importance of protection from violence and prevention of abuse and exploitation.

Societal Attitudes and Advocacy

Poverty, illiteracy, inadequate health care, large family size, children of migrant population, homeless and street children, orphans and abandoned children, and children at work present gigantic problems that seem insurmountable. Equally important is the adverse and uncaring attitude of the society at large toward the difficulties faced by most of our population. We need to sensitize teachers, police personnel, medical staff, lawyers, religious leaders, media persons and the community at large toward child rights, child protection, and child abuse and exploitation. Exploitative, abuse, or demeaning portrayal of children by any form of media must be prohibited. Government must institute the necessary measures to provide *comprehensive free health care and quality education to all children*. We need to interact with NGOs, industrial and business houses, and most of all with politicians on behalf of children and advocate for their rights, welfare, and development.

Role and Responsibilities of Pediatricians

Pediatricians have the chief responsibility of taking care of sick children and carrying out preventive and promotive work. They have played crucial roles in the management of diarrheal disorders, newborn care, infant and child nutrition, immunizations, delivery of state-of-the-art tertiary care, and a host of other problems of children. It is not surprising that about 36,000 pediatricians in the country remain engaged with management of children with various diseases. Nevertheless, pediatricians need to expand their frontiers of care and address the wider issues of the underprivileged child population in the country. Nurturing care and education must be focused on those who need it most.

Awareness of Child Rights and Children's Problems

Pediatricians should have knowledge of child rights, problems of child neglect, maltreatment and exploitation, child protection mechanisms and governmental policies, and laws that address these issues.[31] Every opportunity should be taken in their clinical practice to explain and educate the parents about upbringing care, child development, and preventive measures. Some of the pediatricians have prepared informative materials regarding positive parenting, but these are more relevant to the educated families.

Advocacy and Speaking up for Children

Pediatricians should regard themselves as custodian of children, speak up for them, and demand child rights. We cannot remain unconcerned and say that it is not our business. It must be our business and our responsibility. We need to interact with other groups, professionals, NGOs, media, religious leaders, and civil society. Corporate and industrial houses should be asked to support child welfare programs. Social media platforms can be used for sensitization and community awareness and empowerment. A concerted effort must be made to demand increased resources from the governments and adequate implementation of their existing plans and policies.

■ KEY POINTS

- Various issues concerning child rights, child neglect, and abuse have been globally recognized and specified in the UN CRC. The CRC document recommends various administrative, social, and educational measures to protect the child from maltreatment and exploitation.
- The civil society and the government must ensure that children get their rights and attain optimal development.
- Children commonly face violence during their upbringing, some in the guise of disciplinary measures, but often willfully inflicted by the caregivers.
- Pediatricians should be able to recognize nonaccidental injury and take the necessary action to protect the child.
- Child sexual abuse is a most reprehensible crime, which is very frequent in all societies, but frequently goes unreported because of the associated social stigma of shame and guilt.
- The recently introduced POCSO Act spells out forms of sexual abuse, their identification and management by the first contact physician and medicolegal requirements. The Act mandates reporting by the physician and provision of immediate treatment.
- Child labor in its various forms (domestic servitude, employment in unorganized sector, hazardous work, bonded labor, street children, and trafficking of children) is an extremely difficult problem as it is being closely related to poverty, illiteracy, and large family size.
- There are number of legal provisions for protection of child rights and prevention of abuse, but they are poorly implemented.
- Pediatricians, as the custodians of children, must recognize the CANCL issues, join hand with professionals and civil society, Act for children and demand child rights and justice for children.

■ ACKNOWLEDGMENT

Permission from the Editor-in-Chief of Indian Pediatrics, official journal of the Indian Academy of Pediatrics is gratefully acknowledged for including citations from two articles, reference no. 11 and 19.

REFERENCES

1. Convention on the Rights of the child. http://unicef.og/crc. Accessed May 17, 2021
2. National plan of action for children. WCD.nic.in/sites/default/files/National%20 Plan%20of%20Action. Accessed May 17, 2021
3. Goldhagen J, Clarke A, Dixon P, Gierreiro AI, Lansdown G, Vaghri Z. Thirtieth anniversary of the UN Convention on the Rights of the Child: advancing a child rights-based approach to child health and well-being. BMJ Paediatrics Open. 2020;4:e000589.
4. Mehnaz A. Child neglect: wider dimensions. In: Srivastava RN, Seth R, Van Niekerk J, (Eds). Child Abuse and Neglect: challenges and opportunities. New Delhi: Jaypee Brothers Medical Publishers; 2013. pp. 100-9.
5. Agrawal N. Child physical abuse. In: Srivastava RN, Seth R, Van Niekerk J (Eds). Child Abuse and Neglect: challenge and opportunities. New Delhi: Jaypee Brothers Medical Publishers; 2003. pp. 19-23.
6. Guideline for eliminating corporal punishment in schools. Ncpcr.gov.in/view_file.hp/fid=108. Accessed May 17, 2021
7. Childline. Childlineindia.org/a/about/childline-India
8. Afifi TO, Fortier J, Sareen J, Taillieu T. Associations of harsh physical punishment and child maltreatment with antisocial behaviours. JAMA Network Open. 2019;2(1):e/187374.
9. Lippard ETC, Nemeroff CB. The devastating clinical consequences of child abuse and neglect: increased disease vulnerability and poor treatment response in mood disorders. Am J Psychiatry. 2020;177:20-36.
10. Bhave S, Saxena A. Child sexual abuse in India. In: Srivastava RN, Seth R, Van Niekerk J (Eds). Child Abuse and Neglect: challenges and opportunities. New Delhi: Jaypee Brothers Medical Publishers; 2013. pp. 62-70.
11. Seth R, Srivastava RN. Child sexual abuse. Management and prevention, and Protection of Children from Sexual Offences (POCSO) Act. Indian Pediatr. 2017;54:949-53.
12. Singh MM, Parsekar SS, Nair SN. An epidemiological overview of child sexual abuse. J Family Med Prim Care. 2014;3:430-5.
13. Study on Child Abuse: India (2007). Ministry of Women and Child Development, Government of India, available from www.wcd.nic.in/childabuse.pdf. Accessed May 30, 2017
14. Finkel MA. Medical evaluation of child sexual abuse. In: Srivastava RN, Seth R, Van Niekerk J (Eds). Child Abuse and Neglect: challenges and opportunities. New Delhi: Jaypee Brothers Medical Publishers; 2013. pp. 62-70.
15. Guidelines and protocols. Medicolegal care of survivors/victims of sexual violence, 2014. [online] Available from: http://mohfw.nic.in (Last accessed December, 2021).
16. Child Sexual Abuse: Prevention and Response. Information for doctors and health care professionals (2015). UNICEF & Indian Medical Association.
17. The Protection of Children from Sexual Offences Act, 2012. [online] Available from: https://wcd.nic.in/sites/default/files/POCSO%20Act%2C%202012.pdf (Last accessed December, 2021).
18. Cashmore J, Shackel R. The long-term effects of child sexual abuse. Child Family Community Australia. 2013.

19. Srivastava RN. Children at work, child labor and modern slavery in India: An overview. Indian Pediatr. 2019;56(8):633-8.
20. Child labour in India. Available from : UNICEF.in/whatwedo/21 [Accessed 2021-5-16]21.
21. Seth R. Child labor. In: Srivastava RN, Seth R, von Niekerk J (Eds). Child Abuse and Neglect: challenges and opportunities. New Delhi: Jaypee Brothers Medical Publishers; 2013. Pp. 79-85.
22. Parker DL, Overby M. A discussion of hazardous child labor. Public Health Rep. 2005;120(6):586-8.
23. Rehman MM. Bonded labor in India. In: *A manual on identification, release, and rehabilitation*. VV Giri Labour Institute, NOIDA: Aurobindo Printing and Publishing Associate; 1997.
24. Nair PM. Child trafficking in Asian-Pacific countries. In: Srivastava RN, Seth R, von Niekerk J (Eds). Child Abuse and Neglect: challenges and opportunities. New Delhi: Jaypee Brothers Medical Publishers; 2013. pp. 71-8.
25. Anti-trafficking cell. [online] Available from mha.gov.in/division_of_mha/anti-trafficking-cell (Last accessed December, 2021).
26. Kumari V. Juvenile justice in India: challenges and the way forward. In: Srivastava RN, Seth R, Niekerk V (Eds). Child Abuse and neglect: challenges and opportunities. New Delhi: Jaypee Brothers Medical Publishers; 2013. pp. 182-90.
27. Abolition of child labor and making education a reality for every child as a right. [online] Available from NCPCR.gov.in/showfile.php?lid=2008 (Last accessed December, 2021).
28. Integrated Child Protection Scheme. https://wcd.nic.in/sites/default/files/revised%20ICPS%20scheme, Accessed May 17, 2021
29. Child labor prohibition and regulation act, 1986. [online] Available from: http://WWW.childlineindia.org.in (Last accessed December, 2021).
30. Child related legislation. F:/child%20Related%20Legislation.html. Accessed May 17, 2021
31. Anganwadi Centres. https://economictime.indiaties.com/topic/anganwadi, Accessed May 17, 2021

Dermatology

Skin Care of the Newborn

Rashmi Sarkar, Udhay Preet Sidhu

■ INTRODUCTION

Skin being the largest and outermost organ performs the functions of protection, thermoregulation, secretion, sensation, and hydration of the body. From the sterile aqueous intrauterine environment to the dry and aerobic extrauterine environment, there is a major transition for the neonate. The structural and functional development of the skin begins during embryogenesis and ends in the first year of life. The dynamic process of skin maturation starts immediately after birth for full-term newborns, whereas in preterm newborns, it is initiated at 2–3 weeks post birth.[1] The skin of the healthy term infant is well developed and competent. The skin structure is completed by 34 weeks of pregnancy as revealed by microanalysis of the tissue.[1] It is comprised of the *stratum corneum*, the viable *epidermis, dermis*, and the cells—*Langerhans cells* and *melanocytes*. Transepidermal water loss (TEWL) is a reliable indicator of epidermal barrier function. Normal TEWL is 4–8 $g/m^2/h$. The newborn skin undergoes various adaptations after birth. On the first day of life, stratum corneum (SC) hydration decreases rapidly and over the next 2 weeks, it increases, emphasizing the skin adaptability and smoothening of SC required for flexibility and prevention of cracking. Full-term neonates have a neutral pH (6.35–7.5) which reduces to 5 within the first 2 weeks of life. Acidification of SC is required for epidermal barrier maturation and repair.[2]

The skin of full-term newborn and adults differ in structure, composition, and function. This is illustrated in **Table 27.1**. This helps to understand the peculiar characteristics and challenges, and emphasizes about optimizing the skin care of the newborn. The goal of skin care of the newborn involves maintaining skin integrity, regulating fluid and electrolyte balance, preventing exposure to unwanted harmful chemicals, regulate body temperature and enrich the child–parent eternal bonding. As the newborn skin is thin, fragile and sensitive, clarity on skin care education, bathing practice, care of diaper area, and massage methodologies help the care providers to preserve the integrity of the newborn skin.

TABLE 27.1: Various differences between the full-term newborn skin and the adult skin.

	Full-term newborn skin	Adult skin
Skin structure		
Epidermis	Thinner	Thicker
Melanin content	Low	Normal
Demoepidermal junction	Flat	Undulating
Dermis	No clear transition between papillary and reticular dermis	Clear transition present
Skin composition		
pH	6.34–7.5	5–5.5
Natural moisturizing factor	Lower	Higher
Skin microbiome	Firmicutes Actinobacteria Proteobacteria Bacteroidetes	*Propionibacterium* and *Staphylococcus* (sebaceous areas), *Flavobacteriales*, *Proteobacteria* (dry area), *Staphylococcus* and *Corynebacterium* (moist areas)
Skin function		
Barrier	Weak, fragile	Strong
Absorption to topicals	High permeability	Low permeability

■ CUTANEOUS MICROFLORA

The composition of cutaneous microflora in the newborn is determined by the mode of delivery.[3] Lactobacillus is the predominant bacteria on the vaginally delivered newborn. *Staphylococcus, Streptococcus, Corynebacterium,* and *Propionibacterium* are present on the skin of cesarean delivered babies.[4] By the age of 1 month, similar bacterial colonization is seen, irrespective of the mode of delivery.[4] Owing to the hydration, the microbiome in the newborn skin resembles the microbiome of the moist areas in the adult skin. Unlike the adults, skin microbes in early life do not vary based on the anatomic locations.[4] The transmission of microbiota during vaginal delivery provides a defense mechanism for the naïve newborn skin. The difference in the skin microbial pattern in the cesarean born babies may lead to nutritional and immune function delay.[3] Fungal colonization is represented by *Malassezia restricta* and *M. globosa*, in equal ratio, pointing toward the transmission from mother to child.[5] Also, at day 30, *M. restricta* proportion is higher which is more like adults. Cutaneous microbiome is diverse and evolves with age. During the neonatal period, crucial role is played by skin microbiota in the development of immune system and skin pathologies. Dysbiosis is linked to pathogenesis of seborrheic dermatitis and atopic dermatitis.

■ VERNIX CASEOSA: NATURE'S BARRIER

The word "vernix caseosa" first appeared in the Dunglison Dictionary of Medical Sciences in 1846, wherein "vernix" implied "to varnish" and "caseous" as "cheesy".[6] The vernix is unique to the humans. It is a naturally occurring membranous structure produced partly by fetal sebaceous glands in the third trimester of pregnancy. It is a hydrophobic and proteolipid material, seen as anteroposterior and dorsoventral manner in the fetus. It consists of water in hydrated corneocytes (80%) and embedded in a matrix of proteins (10%) and lipids (10%). Triglycerides, waxes, and sterol esters are products of sebaceous lipids while ceramides and cholesterol belong to the epidermal lipids. The vernix corneocytes are 1–2 µm thick, polygonal, or ovoid and enucleated and lack the typical lamellar structure of stratum corneum.[7] It plays a significant role in lubricating the birth canal, waterproofing the fetus in utero, demonstrates antibacterial and antioxidant properties, aids in moisturizing the skin postpartum and shows wound healing properties. The World Health Organization (WHO) recommends using a clean dry cloth and thoroughly drying the baby starting within first 5 seconds of birth. It also recommends not wiping the vernix, if present.[8]

■ BATHING THE NEWBORN

The timing and technique of the first bath of the newborn is an ongoing debate. As per the WHO guidelines, first bath should be delayed up to 24 hours of birth.[9] In case of cultural reasons where this is not permissible, the baby should not be bathed until 6 hours of age.[9,10] The Neonatal Skin Care Evidence-Based Clinical Practice Guideline, developed by the Association of Women's Health, Obstetric and Neonatal Nurses (AWHONN) suggest that neonates can be bathed at 2–4 hours of age provided there is thermal and cardiorespiratory stability.[11] The guidelines by the National Institute for Health and Clinical Excellence (NICE) recommend bath to be initiated no sooner that 1 hour after birth.[12] Infants born to human immunodeficiency virus (HIV)-positive mother should be bathed as soon as possible to prevent transmission of the infection. Skin-to-skin contact (SSC) either immediately or shortly after birth is widely propagated by Baby-Friendly Hospital Initiative (BFHI), internationally. The naked baby wearing only a diaper, is placed on the bare chest of the mother. This is beneficial for the mother as well as the full-term and preterm infants. This enhances the mother–child bonding, reduces depressive symptoms in the mother, and is associated with long-term breastfeeding.[13] Delayed bathing helps in thermoregulation, prevents hypothermia, increases success of breastfeeding, and improves bonding.[14] A recent study by Gozen et al. concluded that postponing the bath to 48 hours postpartum was helpful in maintaining the body temperature and favorably affects the skin moisture level in the infant.[15] Temperature of the room should be maintained at around 26–28°C and water should be warm (37.8–8.8°C). Standard safety measures should be taken. Gloves should be worn, and the bath equipment should be clean and disinfected. Duration of first bath should be short and not exceed >5 minutes to avoid cold stress. To minimize air currents and convective heat loss, the bathroom door should be kept closed.[16] Bathing the infant once in few days or twice weekly is recommended. Different techniques of newborn bathing are sponge bathing, small tub bathing, immersion tub bathing, and swaddled tub bathing. Immersion tub bath is recommended over others. Tub bath is safe to maintain temperature stability and cord integrity, and is more pleasurable and less stressful for infants and mother.[17] Post bath, the child is immediately covered in a towel, dried thoroughly, covered after drying and rewarming measures such as SSC must be ensured.

■ NEONATAL SKIN CLEANSING

Intent of neonatal skin cleansing is to effectively clean the skin without affecting skin microbiota, pH level, and the protective function of skin. Cleansers contain active substances, consisting of alkaline soaps or non-soap-based synthetic surfactant known as *syndets*. Soaps typically have a pH of 9–10 while syndets have neutral or mildly acidic pH of 5.5–7.[18] Four main categories of cleansers are known—traditional soaps, modern soaps, syndets, and combars. They are available in different formulations such as bar or liquid cleansers. Current strong recommendation from the European Roundtable Meeting on Best Practice Healthy Infant Skin Care is that the baby skin may be cleansed with water alone or by adding an appropriately formulated liquid cleanser to water, without impairing the skin maturation process.[19] *The recommendations do not advocate that liquid cleansers "should" be used, but that they "can" be used.*[19] **Box 27.1** lists the recommendations on properties of ideal liquid cleansers, wipes, and emollients by the European Roundtable Meeting on Best Practice Healthy Infant Skin Care.[19]

■ MASSAGE OF THE NEWBORN

Massaging the newborn has been a traditional practice in India since centuries. It can be done with or without the use of a lubricant, though cultural bend is toward oil massage. Tactile and kinetic stimulation is a cost-effective technique which encourages growth pattern in preterm infants.[20] Massaging is believed to aid in good health and regularize sleep pattern in the newborn. The mother or a trained professional can administer it. To prevent regurgitation or vomiting of the feed, it should be administered an hour after the feed. A firm, moderate pressure with flat of the fingers is helpful for weight gain.[21] Local availability, cost effectivity, and safety determine

> **BOX 27.1:** Recommendation on properties of ideal liquid cleansers, wipes, and emollients.[19]
> - Cleanser should be able to maintain a pH of 5.5 on infants' skin and should not interfere with normal skin microbiota.
> - Formulation and all ingredients should undergo extensive safety testing; usage of ingredients only approved by regulators.
> - Regulator approved preservatives should be used.
> - Fragrance used should be regulator approved and should have the least probability of adverse effects.
> - High-quality clinical trials should be done to monitor safety and efficacy.
> - Emollient in a cleanser is added to exert positive effect on skin barrier.
> - Formulation should be an effective cleansing agent and to safely remove damaging substances.
> - Harsh surfactants such as sodium lauryl sulfate should not be incorporated in the formulation.
> - Formulation should not be irritating to the infant's skin and eyes.

the oil used for massage in a particular region. Owing to lower chances of allergic reactions, natural oils are favored. Coconut oil and sunflower oil are recommended.[22] Massage has multiple positive benefits. It enhances mother–child bonding, helps in weight gain, improves thermoregulation, improves skin barrier function, enhance quality of sleep and aids in better neuromotor development.[21] In preterm infants' massage with coconut and safflower oil resulted in weight gain and increased triglyceride following transcutaneous absorption of oils. Increases in vagal activity, gastric motility, and insulin-like growth factor-1 (IGF-1) are the underlying mechanisms in weight gain.[23] Sunflower seed oil has high linoleic acid concentration and benefits in prevention of atopic dermatitis in term infants. Olive oil is not favored, as applications have shown to increase TEWL and favor growth of *Malassezia* yeast species.[24]

■ DIAPER CARE

Presence of excessive moisture and irritation from urine and fecal matter leads to disruption of the skin barrier in the diaper area. Complete hygiene and appropriate cleansing are major parts of the important aspects of skin care and prevention of diaper dermatitis. Cleansing should be done with warm water and cotton wool from front to back.[25] Cotton nappies though still commonly used have the concerns of poor absorption and leakage. From the use of cotton diapers to the advent of thin super-absorbent lotioned diapers, there has been a significant change in diaper design and technology. Lotioned diapers have an inner topsheet laden with lotion, barrier ointment such as petrolatum. Traditional cleansing involved cleaning the diaper area with soap and water. Gradual change in cleaning practice has led to the increased use of disposable baby wipes. Basesheet, formulation, and packaging are the three main components of a baby wipe. A randomized study by Lavender et al. on 280 healthy term babies showed that baby wipes had an equivalent effect on skin hydration when compared with cotton wool and water.[26] Ideally, baby wipes should be hypoallergenic, mild, and efficacious and should meet the safety requirements. The surfactant fraction in the wipes would not be expected to exceed 1% by weight of the formula and, in most cases, would be below 0.3% by weight.[27] Diaper dermatitis or diaper rash has multifactorial etiology. Parents and care providers should be instructed to change diapers frequently, air the area, and to provide nappy-free time to babies. Use of barrier creams and emollients can reduce the incidence of diaper dermatitis and are used as prevention and as a first line of treatment. A thin layer prevents occlusion and helps in maintaining skin barrier function. Zinc oxide, petrolatum, cod liver oil, dimethicone, lanolin, dexpanthenol, and Burow's solution are the common ingredients used.[28] The use of emollients is discussed in the following text.

■ CARE OF THE SCALP

Infantile seborrheic dermatitis is a chronic, inflammatory, self-limiting scaly skin condition presenting as redness and greasy scales. When it involves the scalp, it is commonly referred to as *cradle cap*. The etiology is evolving, though several factors are thought to play a role, involving an interplay between sebaceous gland secretions, microflora metabolism, and individual susceptibility.[29] For mild and localized lesions, treatment includes softening with help of emollient creams, mineral, or vegetable oils (e.g., olive oil or borage oil) followed by shampooing or combing to aid in removal of scales. For extensive lesions or those not responding to initial treatment, 2% ketoconazole cream or 1% hydrocortisone cream can be used for 1–2 weeks. To suit the low sebum production, pediatric shampoos are mild cleansing agents and are nonirritating in nature. The scalp pH is 5.5 and the hair shaft pH is 3.67. "No tear shampoos" have a higher pH. They use detergents from the amphoteric group, such as the betaines.[30] This attributes to the anesthetic and low stinging effect on the eye if the shampoo accidently enters the eye, though damage to the eye can still occur.

■ CARE OF THE UMBILICAL CORD

Umbilical cord care is a vital part of newborn care. The umbilical cord is clamped after birth and cut using sterile blade and gloves. *Omphalitis* refers to the inflammation of the umbilical cord stump, a risk factor for neonatal sepsis. It begins with local inflammation and can progress to severe complications such as intraabdominal abscesses, periumbilical cellulitis, thrombophlebitis in the portal and/or umbilical veins, peritonitis, and bowel ischemia.[31,32] The WHO and the Ministry of Health and Family Welfare (MoHFW), India recommend dry cord care for newborn infants. The WHO

> **BOX 27.2:** Classification of emollients.
>
> - *Based on its origin*:
>   - *Plant derivatives*: Castor oil, jojoba oil, coco butter
>   - *Animal derivative*: Lanolin
>   - *Bioactive emollients with proven clinical efficacy*: Soline, Acovadin® HU25
> - *Based on properties of excipients*:
>   - *Dry emollients*: Decyl oleate, isopropyl palmitate, isostearyl alcohol
>   - *Fatty emollients*: Castor oil, glyceryl stearate, propylene glycol
>   - *Astringent emollients*: Cyclomethicone, dimethicone
>   - *Protective emollients*: Diisopropyl dilinoleate, isopropyl isostearate

recommends the application of chlorhexidine to the umbilical stump in the first week of life, for home births in areas with high neonatal mortality.[33] It is of paramount importance to educate the parents about the signs and symptoms of omphalitis in order to provide early and appropriate treatment and reducing the potential complications.

EMOLLIENTS

"Emollire" in Latin means to soften. Terms such as "emollient" and "moisturizer" are often used synonymously. Emollient refers to a topical compound composed of fat or oil. It is used to lubricate, soften, and hydrate the stratum corneum. Properly formulated liquid cleansing agents and emollients maintain the skin barrier and its integrity. They keep the skin free of microbial pathogens and are friendly toward the acid mantle of the skin. **Box 27.2** provides the classification of commonly used emollients.

Emollients should be applied twice a week, post-bath as a thin layer. Skin folds should be kept clean and dry. A study by Bonchak et al, which analyzed 533 unique personal baby care products concluded that most of these products for babies and children contain one or more sensitizers such as fragrances, betaines, methylchloroisothiazolinone, and lanolin.[34] Petrolatum is an inexpensive skin moisturizer, which is free from contact allergen. Owing to the geographic variation, in warmer climatic areas, oil in water emulsion (cream) is favored but in colder and dry regions water in oil emulsion (ointment) is preferred.

■ NEONATAL SKIN CONDITION SCORE

The Association of Women's Health, Obstetric and Neonatal Nurses (AWHONN) and the National Association of Neonatal Nurses (NANN) developed the Neonatal Skin Condition Score (NSCS). The score helps to evaluate the overall skin condition of the neonate. With help of this easy-to-use tool, daily neonatal assessment can be done. It serves to standardize the quality of nursing care in neonatal health care. NSCS evaluates three factors: *Dryness, erythema,* and *breakdown*. The details are provided in **Box 27.3**.

> **BOX 27.3:** The Neonatal Skin Condition Score (NSCS).[35]
> - *Dryness:*
>   1 = Normal, no sign of dry skin
>   2 = Dry skin, visible scaling
>   3 = Very dry skin, cracking/ fissures
> - *Erythema:*
>   1 = No evidence of erythema
>   2 = Visible erythema, <50% body surface
>   3 = Visible erythema, >50% body surface
> - *Breakdown or excoriation:*
>   1 = Non-evident
>   2 = Small, localized areas
>   3 = Extensive

For each the score is from 1 to 3. The final score is arrived by summing the responses of all the three parameters, ranging from 3 to 9. The perfect score is 3 and worst score is 9. The NSCS is reliable when used by single and multiple raters for assessing various neonatal skin conditions, even across weight and racial groups.[35]

■ BABY POWDERS

Traditionally talcum powder is used as a routine skin care of newborn. The use is attributed to the belief that talc reduces diaper rash.[36] Hydrated magnesium silicate is the main component. By acting as a skin lubricant, it prevents chafing of the delicate skin and maintains the integrity of the skin.[37] In addition, it aids in preventing and absorbing excessive skin moisture in the skin folds.[38] The concern regarding inhalation of talc warrants the careful use of baby powders.[39] The regular use of baby powders is not required. After bathing, the newborn should be adequately dried with absorbent towel with special attention to skin folds to prevent occlusion by moisture. In case powder is used, it should not be applied directly to the skin, instead should be applied to the hands of care provider and then put on the infant's skin. Care should be taken to keep the product away from nose and mouth to prevent accidental inhalation and choking.

■ SKIN CARE IN PRETERM INFANTS

Preterm infants have a gestational age of <37 weeks. Their skin is fragile, underdeveloped, has poor barrier function, prone for infections and allergen sensitization. Preterm infants should be bathed every fourth day, as it does not negatively affect the skin flora and helps in thermoregulation. Tub bath is preferred over sponge bath and does not lead to temperature variability.[40] Dry cord care reaps same results as with antiseptic treatment. In developing countries, use of emollients is related with lower incidence of nosocomial infections; whereas on the contrary, use of topical petrolatum was linked with higher rates of coagulase-negative Staphylococcus infection in developed countries. On a short-term basis, impermeable wraps prevent heat loss and reduce the risk of hypothermia. Later, semipermeable wraps are used to reduce transepidermal water loss.

Choice of a skin adhesive should be individualized. Natural and synthetic adhesives are available. Natural adhesives include karaya gum obtained from the Sterculia tree and water-soluble carbohydrate substances such as pectin from the peel of fruits such as citrus peels or apple pomace.[41] Synthetic adhesives include those based on polyisobutylene or other synthetic rubbers, acrylate polymers, and silicone polymers. Removal of adhesives should be done gently and patiently, with warm water and cotton ball.[42] In case reapplication of adhesive is not required mineral oil or petrolatum can be used additionally. Semipermeable and transparent adhesive dressings are preferred. Povidone iodine and 0.2% chlorhexidine gluconate are the chosen antiseptic for procedures.[43]

■ CONCLUSION

Newborn skin with its unique characteristics goes through a gradual process of adaptation to the extrauterine environment. Appropriate and scientific skin care practices facilitate this process. They aid in maintaining optimal skin functions and preventing skin diseases in the newborn. It is vital for healthcare professionals to have an in-depth knowledge about these practices, as the play an important role in well-being of a healthy as well as hospitalized newborn.

■ KEY POINTS

- The difference in the skin microbial pattern in the cesarean born babies may lead to nutritional and immune function delay.
- The WHO recommends using a clean, dry cloth and thoroughly drying the baby starting within first 5 seconds of birth and not wiping the vernix, if present.
- The baby can be given a bath 1 hour after birth, but may be delayed up to 48 hours, and after bath, the naked baby wearing only a diaper, is placed on the bare chest of the mother to improve bonding and breastfeeding.
- The baby skin may be cleansed with water alone or by adding, if necessary, an appropriately formulated liquid cleanser to water, without impairing the skin maturation process.
- Baby massaging with natural oils such as coconut oil or sunflower seed oil enhances mother–child bonding, helps in weight gain, improves thermoregulation, improves skin barrier function, enhance quality of sleep, and aids in better neuromotor development.
- Baby wipes should be hypoallergenic, mild, and efficacious and the surfactant fraction in the wipes would not be expected to exceed 1% by weight of the formula.
- Infantile seborrheic dermatitis or cradle cap is a chronic inflammatory, self-limiting scaly skin condition and treatment includes softening with help of emollient creams, mineral, or vegetable oils.

- Routine application of baby talc is recommended; it should not be applied directly to the skin of the newborn, instead should be applied to the hands of care provider and then put on the infant's skin.
- Preterm infants should be bathed every fourth day, as it does not negatively affect the skin flora and helps in thermoregulation.

■ REFERENCES

1. de-Souza IMF, Vitral GLN, Reis ZSN. Skin thickness dimensions in histological section measurement during late fetal and neonatal developmental period: A systematic review. Skin Res Technol. 2019;25(6):793-800.
2. Fluhr JW, Darlenski R, Taieb A, Hachem JP, Baudouin C, Msika P, et al. Functional skin adaptation in infancy - almost complete but not fully competent. Exp Dermatol. 2010;19(6):483-92.
3. Dominguez-Bello MG, Costello EK, Contreras M, Magris M, Hidalgo G, Fierer N, et al. Delivery mode shapes the acquisition and structure of the initial microbiota across multiple body habitats in newborns. Proc Natl Acad Sci. 2010;107(26):11971-5.
4. Chu DM, Ma J, Prince AL, Antony KM, Seferovic MD, Aagaard KM. Maturation of the infant microbiome community structure and function across multiple body sites and in relation to mode of delivery. Nat Med. 2017;23(3):314-26.
5. Nagata R, Nagano H, Ogishima D, Nakamura Y, Hiruma M, Sugita T. Transmission of the major skin microbiota, *Malassezia*, from mother to neonate. Pediatr Int. 2012;54(3):350-5.
6. Singh G, Archana G. Unraveling the mystery of vernix caseosa. Indian J Dermatol 2008;53(2):54-60.
7. Rissmann R, Groenink HW, Weerheim AM, Hoath SB, Ponec M, Bouwstra JA. New insights into ultrastructure, lipid composition and organization of vernix caseosa. J Invest Dermatol. 2006;126(8):1823-33.
8. World Health Organization. (2014). Library Cataloguing-in-Publication Data. Early Essential Newborn Care: Clinical Practice Pocket Guide. [online] Available from: https://apps.who.int/iris/bitstream/handle/10665/208158/9789290616856_eng.pdf. [Last accessed December, 2021].
9. World Health Organization. (2017). Recommendation on Newborn Health. Guidelines approved by the WHO Guidelines Review Committee. [online] Available from: https://apps.who.int/iris/handle/10665/259269. [Last accessed December, 2021].
10. World Health Organization, United Nations Population Fund, World Bank, United Nations Children's Fund (2015). Pregnancy, childbirth, postpartum and newborn care: a guide for essential practice, 3rd edition. [online] Available from: https://apps.who.int/iris/handle/10665/249580. [Last accessed December, 2021].
11. Association of Women's Health, Obstetric and Neonatal Nurses (AWHONN). Neonatal Skin Care: Evidence-based Clinical Practice Guideline, 3rd edition: Washington DC: AWHONN; 2013.
12. Demott K, Bick D, Norman R. Clinical guidelines and evidence review for post natal care: routine post natal care of recently delivered women and their babies. London, England: National Collaborating Centre for Primary Care and Royal College of General Practitioners; 2006.

13. Widström AM, Brimdyr K, Svensson K, Cadwell K, Nissen E. Skin-to-skin contact the first hour after birth, underlying implications and clinical practice. Acta Paediatr. 2019;108(7):1192-204.
14. DiCioccio HC, Ady C, Bena JF, Albert NM. Initiative to improve exclusive breastfeeding by delaying the newborn bath. J Obstet Gynecol Neonatal Nurs. 2019;48(2):189-96.
15. Gözen D, Çaka SY, Beşirik SA, Perk Y. First bathing time of newborn infants after birth: A comparative analysis. J Spec Pediatr Nurs. 2019;24(2):e12239.
16. Association of Women's Health, Obstetric and Neonatal Nurses (AWHONN). Neonatal Skin Care: Evidence-Based Clinical Practice Guideline, 4th edition: Washington DC: AWOHNN; 2018.
17. Bryanton J, Walsh D, Barrett M, Gaudet D. Tub bathing versus traditional sponge bathing for the newborn. J Obstet Gynecol Neonatal Nurs. 2004;33(6):704-12.
18. Wortzman MS. Evaluation of mild skin cleansers. Dermatol Clin. 1991;9(1):35-44.
19. Blume-Peytavi U, Lavender T, Jenerowicz D, Ryumina I, Stalder JF, Torrelo A, et al. Recommendations from a European Roundtable Meeting on Best Practice Healthy Infant Skin Care. Pediatr Dermatol. 2016;33(3):311-21.
20. Field T. Massage therapy. Med Clin North Am. 2002;86(1):168-71.
21. Kulkarni A, Kaushij JS, Gupta P, Sharma H, Agrawal RK. Massage and touch therapy in neonates : The current evidence. Indian Pediatr. 2010;47(9):771-6.
22. Dhar S, Banerjee R, Malakar R. Oil massage in babies: Indian perspectives. Indian J Paediatr Dermatol. 2013;14(1):1-3.
23. Field T, Diego M, Hernandez-Reif M. Preterm infant massage therapy research: A review. Infant Behav Dev. 2010;33(2):11524.
24. Karagounis TK, Gittler JK, Rotemberg V, Morel KD. Use of 'natural' oils for moisturization: review of olive, coconut, and sunflower seed oil. Pediatr Dermatol. 2019;36(1):9-15.
25. Sarkar R, Basu S, Aggarwal RK, Gupta P. Skin care for the newborn. Indian Pediatr. 2010;47(7):593-8.
26. Lavender T, Furber C, Campbell M, Victor S, Roberts I, Bedwell C, et al. Effect on skin hydration of using baby wipes to clean the napkin area of newborn babies: assessor-blinded randomised controlled equivalence trial. BMC Pediatr. 2012;12:59.
27. Cunningham C, Mundschau S, Seidling J, Wenzel S. Baby care In: Schlossman M, (Ed). The Chemistry and Manufacture of Cosmetics, 2nd edition, vol. 2 Chicago: Allured; 2008. pp. 1063-154.
28. Blume-Peytavi U, Kanti V. Prevention and treatment of diaper dermatitis. Pediatr Dermatol. 2018;35:19-23.
29. Ro BI, Dawson TL. The role of sebaceous gland activity and scalp microfloral metabolism in the etiology of seborrheic dermatitis and dandruff. J Invest Dermatol Symposium Proceedings. 2005;10(3):194-7.
30. Wilkinson JB, Moore RJ. Harry's Cosmetology. New York: Chemical Publishing; 1982. pp. 457-8.
31. Jayaswal S, Shah H, Kumbhar V. Analysis of factors affecting outcome in pediatric omphalitis. International Surg J. 2016 ;3(4):29-32.
32. Stewart D, Benitz W; Committee on Fetus And Newborn. Umbilical cord care in the newborn infant. Pediatrics. 2016;138(3):e20162149.

33. Dandona R, Kochar PS, Kumar GA, Dandona L. Use of antiseptic for cord care and its association with neonatal mortality in a population-based assessment in Bihar State, India. BMJ Open. 2017;7(1):e012436.
34. Bonchak JG, Prouty ME, de la Feld SF. Prevalence of contact allergens in personal care products for babies and children. Dermatitis. 2018;29(2):81-4.
35. Lund CK, Osborne JW. Validity and Reliability of the Neonatal Skin Condition Score. J Obstet Gynecol Neonat Nurs. 2004;33(3):320-7.
36. Hayden GF, Sproul GT. Baby powder use in infant skin care. Parental knowledge and determinants of powder usage. Clin Pediatr. 1984;23(3):163-5.
37. Wilkinson JB, Moore RJ. Skin products for babies. Harry's Cosmetology, 7th edition. Harlow: Longman Scientific and Technical Publishing; 1982. pp. 111-8.
38. Leyden JJ. Bacteriology of newborn skin. In: Maibach HI, Boisits EK, (Eds). Neonatal Skin. New York: Marcel Dekker;1982. pp. 167-81.
39. Mofenson HC, Caraccio TR, Okun S, Greensher J, Hazards of baby powder. Pediatrics. 1986;78(3):546-7.
40. Loring C, Gregory K, Gargan B, LeBlanc V, Lundgran D, Reilly J, et al. Tub bathing improves thermoregulation of the late preterm infant. J Obstet Gynecol Neonatal Nurs. 2012;41(2):171-9.
41. Cartlidge P, Rutter N. Karaya gum electrocardiographic electrodes for preterm infants. Arch Dis Child. 1987;62:1281-2.
42. Hoath SB, Narendran V. Adhesives and emollients in the preterm infant. Semin Neonatol. 2000;5(4):289-96.
43. Kusari A, Han AM, Virgen CA, Matiz C, Rasmussen M, Friedlander SF, et al. Evidence-based skin care in preterm infants. Pediatr Dermatol. 2019;36(1):16-23.

Index

Page numbers followed by *b* refer to box, *f* refer to figure, *fc* refer to flowchart, and *t* refer to table.

A

Abatacept 299, 325, 334
Abdomen 474
  ultrasonography of 466
Abdominal catastrophe 47
Abdominal distension 218
  massive 465
Abdominal mass 464
  palpable 464
Abdominal pain 464
Acanthosis 284
Accredited social
  health activists 494
  work activists 495
Acetaminophen 290
Acid base homeostasis, mechanisms of 250*f*
Acute respiratory distress syndrome 44
Acute-onset neuropsychiatric syndrome 146
Adalimumab 325, 327
Adenoma 318
  secretory 318
Adenosine 176, 178
  deaminase 290, 350
Adenotonsillar hypertrophy 364
Adenotonsillectomy 367, 371
Adenovirus 47
Adequate nutrition 384
Adrenal adenoma 318
Adrenal insufficiency 3, 197, 278
Agalsidase alpha 351
Agalsidase beta 351
Aggressive behavior 29
Airway 90
  clearance therapy 201
  colonization 200
  management 428
Alanine aminotransferase 208, 231, 325
Aldosterone 318
Alemtuzumab 299
Alglucosidase alpha 351
Alkaline phosphatase 319
Allergic bronchopulmonary aspergillosis 194, 205
Alphacoronavirus 41
Alpha-fetoprotein 307-310
Alphaviruses 103
Amino acid formula 220, 223
Aminoaciduria 245, 259

Aminocaproic acid 206
Amiodarone 178
Amphotericin B
  colloidal dispersion 59, 73
  deoxycholate 56, 59, 73, 74
  dosing of 75*t*
  lipid
    complex 76
    formulations of 74
    preparations 74
Anakinra 332
  adverse effects of 332
Anaphylactic reactions 29
Anaphylaxis 217, 223
Androgens 318
Anemia 291
  pernicious 278
Anganwadi workers 494, 495
Angelman syndrome 344
Angioedema 223
Angiotensin-converting enzyme 101, 147
Anidulafungin 59
Anorexia 45
Anti-B cell antibody 333
Antibiotic choices 91
Antibiotic therapy 203
Antibody
  neutralizing 108
  test 48
Anticardiolipin antibody 327
Antiepileptic drug 450
Antifungal
  agents 59
  susceptibility 60*t*
  therapy, history of 56
Antigen presenting cell 44, 334
Antihuman trafficking units 490
Anti-neutrophil cytoplasmic antibody 147, 325, 333
Anti-N-methyl-D-aspartate receptor encephalitis 142, 144*b*
Antinuclear antibody 147, 290, 301, 327
Antiphospholipid antibody syndrome 290, 300, 325, 333
Anti-rheumatic drugs, disease-modifying 324
Antisense oligonucleotides 355, 357
Antistreptolysin-O 147
Antithymocyte globulin 296
Anti-thyroid peroxidase 277

Anti-TNF therapy 328
Antituberculous therapy 329, 330
Antiviral agents 50
Aortic aneurysm dissection 29
Apnea
   central 369
   mixed 369
Appendiceal mucocele 463
Appendicitis 47
   acute 468
Apremilast 337
Arginine vasopressin 257*f*
Arrhythmia 29, 49, 177, 179
Arterial blood pressure 450
Arthritis 93
   enthesitis-related 325
Ascitic fluid 307
Asfotase alpha 351
Aspartate aminotransferase 70, 208, 232, 325
Aspartate transaminase 295
Aspergillosis 58
Aspergillus fumigatus 205
Asphyxia 3
AstraZeneca vaccine 107, 108*t*
Ataxia 252
   telangiectasia 309, 310
Atopic dermatitis 197
Atopy, severe 218
Atrial flutter 172, 177
Atrial tachycardia 177
Attention deficit hyperactivity disorder 26, 29, 400
Auditory brainstem responses 423
Auditory hazards 417
Autism spectrum disorders 346
Autoantibody, absence of 284
Autoimmune
   cerebellar syndrome 141
   diseases 290
   encephalitis 138, 139, 140*b*, 141*t*, 142*t*, 147, 147*f*, 152*f*, 154, 155, 157
   hepatitis 290
   limbic encephalitis 144
   lymphoproliferative syndrome 290, 291, 300
   panel 455*b*
Autoimmune hemolytic anemia 289, 290, 292, 295, 295*fc*, 297, 297*fc*, 298, 305
   classification of 289*t*
   mixed 305
   secondary 296
Automatic arrhythmias 177
Autonomic dysfunction 144
Autosomal dominant 344
Autosomal recessive 344
   multisystem disorder 190

Auxiliary nurse midwives 494
Azathioprine 299, 337
Azithromycin therapy, long-term 204
Azole 62
   drugs
      dosing of 66*t*
      properties of 64*t*

■ B

Baby-friendly hospital initiative 501
Bacterial colonization, eradication therapies for 204
Bacterial infections 146
Bacterial meningitis 88*t*
Baricitinib 336
Barium contrast enema 466
Bartter and Gitelman syndromes, treatment of 255
Bartter syndrome 254*f*, 255, 260
Basal bolus regimen 268
Beckwith-Wiedemann syndrome 344
Behavior audiometry evaluation 423
Behavioral change theories 401
Behçet's disease 337
Behçet's syndrome 332
Belimumab 334
Benzodiazepines 156, 444, 447
Betacoronavirus 41
Beta-D-glucan 57, 58
Beta-thalassemia 344
Bicarbonate 243
Bicarbonaturia 245
Bickerstaff encephalitis 141
Biliary obstruction 309
Biosimilars 337
Biotinidase levels 164
Birth asphyxia, severe 14
Bladder tumor 29
Blood 307
   cultures 87
   gas analysis 7
   glucose 270, 271
      control, targets of 275*t*
      premeal 270*b*
      self-monitoring of 269, 272, 275
   in stools 464
   investigations 465
   pressure 2, 5, 5*t*, 9, 11
      normal 247
   tests 150
   transfusion 298
Blood-brain barrier 81
Bloody mucus per rectum, passage of 464
Body mass index 25, 230, 236
Body surface area 428

Bonded labor 489
Bonded Labor System Act 492
Bone
    alkaline phosphatase 317
    mineralization, defective 27
    tumor 316
        angiogenesis markers 317
Bradycardia 173*f*
Brain 2
    deep 456
    development 393
    injury, traumatic 446
    magnetic resonance imaging of 145, 164
    malformation, congenital 446
    positron emission tomography 150
    tissue staining 148
    tumors 29
Brainstem
    auditory evoked response 423
    encephalitis 141
Breathing 90
    exercises 202
Bronchoalveolar lavage 47, 58, 59
Brugada syndrome 183, 184*f*, 185
Bruises 480
Bull's eye sign 466
Burkholderia cepacia 195
Burn 428, 430, 438, 481
    chemical 430
    electrical 430
    hypermetabolic phase after 439
    injuries, types of 430
    management of 428
    patient, care of 434
    specific pain anxiety scale monitors pain 436
    surface area calculation 429*f*
    transfusion in 438
    wound
        assessment 435
        care, advances in 435

C

Calcipenic rickets 258
Calcium 243, 450
Canakinumab 333
Candida cystitis 76
Candidiasis 58
Cannabinoids 457
Capillary refill time 2, 11
    delayed 5
Carbohydrate
    antigen 308, 312
    higher consumption of 26
Carbon dioxide monitoring 368

Carcinoembryonic antigen 308, 317
Carcinoid syndrome, symptoms of 316
Carcinoid tumors 316, 318
Carcinoma 318
Cardiac arrhythmias 169, 181*f*
    common 171, 177*t*
Cardiac output 8
Cardiac resynchronization therapy 181
Cardiac systolic functions, assessment of 8
Cardiology 169
Cardiometabolic biomarkers 29
    abnormal 25
Cardiomyopathy 29
Cardiopulmonary resuscitation 446
Cardiovascular disorders 419, 420
Cardiovascular dysfunction 6
Caspofungin 59, 72
Castleman disease 300
Catecholamine
    catabolism 314*f*
    role of 313, 315
Catecholaminergic polymorphic ventricular tachycardia 183, 185
Catechol-o-methyl transferase 314
Celiac disease 218, 277, 463
Central nervous system 70, 71, 83, 146, 351
    infections 86, 443, 446
    manifestations 27
Central venous
    access 9
    pressure 8, 9, 90, 450
Cephalosporins 290
Cerebellitis 141
Cerebral edema 29
Cerebral vasospasm 29
Cerebral venous sinus thrombosis 110
Cerebrospinal fluid 7, 10, 58, 65, 79, 88, 88*f*, 93, 140, 144, 145, 147, 164, 307, 455
    analysis 148
Cerliponase alpha 351
Certolizumab pegol 328
Chaperone therapy 358
Chemiluminescence enzyme immunoassays 48
Chemoprophylaxis 94
Chest
    hyperinflation 193
    physiotherapy 202
Child abuse 479
Child and Adolescent Labor (Prohibition and Regulation) Act 492
Child labor
    and exploitation 488
    consequences of 491
    prevention of 491
    rehabilitation of 492
Child neglect 477, 478

Index

Child Protection Committees 494
Child protection mechanisms 493
Child rights 477
Child sex workers 489
Child sexual abuse 482, 485*b*
    diagnosis of 483
    management of 482
    prevention of 486
Child trafficking 490
Chloride 243
    channel, calcium-dependent 191
Chlorpromazine 314
Chocolate agar culture plates 87*f*
Cholesterol ester storage disease 230
Choriocarcinoma 307, 312
Chromaffin tumors 315
Chromosomal breakage 29
Chromosomal disorders 343
Chromosomal microarray 345, 346, 347*f*
Ciprofloxacin 95, 203
Cirrhosis 309
Citrin deficiency 230
Citrullinemia 309
Claw sign 467
    appearance 467*f*
Clotrimazole 62
Coagulation disorders 93
Coagulopathy 45
Coccidioides immitis 63
Cognitive impairment 419, 420
Coiled spring sign 467
Cold agglutinin disease 301
Cold agglutinin syndrome 301, 302, 302*f*
    pathophysiology of 302
    treatment of 303
Colitis 309
Combination therapy 153
Common tubular disorders, causes of 246
Communication 35
Comparative genomic hybridization 345, 345*f*, 346
Complete blood count 7, 48, 89, 290, 297, 302, 325, 450
Congestive cardiac failure 291
Conn syndrome 318
Consciousness, altered 218
Continuous glucose monitoring system 269, 272, 276, 285
Continuous subcutaneous insulin infusion 271
Coombs test 296*b*
    direct 289, 294, 295
    false positive direct 295
Coronary thrombosis, acute 29
Coronary vasospasm 29

Coronavirus disease-2019 (COVID-19) 40, 41, 45, 46*fc*, 52, 52*fc*, 101, 104, 105, 111, 118, 118*t*, 119*t*, 331
    epidemic 53
    infection 44, 49, 111, 121
        phases of 43*f*
    pandemic 40, 332, 396, 405
    pathogenesis of 43
    pneumonia 48, 49, 50, 53
    prevention of 107
    signs of 46
    structure of 42*f*
    symptoms of 46
    types of 40*f*
    vaccine 102, 103, 106, 120, 121, 126
        effectiveness of 127
        equitable distribution of 120
        inactivated 106
        prioritization of 121
        rapid development of 102
        second-generation 129
Cortical dysplasia 145
Cortisol 318
Costimulatory pathway, inhibition of 334
Cotrimoxazole 203
Cough, chronic 193
Covaxin 106
Cow's milk 219
    protein allergy 215, 216, 218, 218*b*, 219*t*, 221*fc*, 223, 226
        diagnosis of 215
    related symptom score 219
C-reactive protein 48, 52, 89
Creatine kinase-muscle brain 10
Creatinine phosphokinase 451
Crepitations 193
Criminal Law (Amendment) Act 492
Critical care 428, 442
    pain observation tool 436
Cryopyrin-associated periodic syndrome 332
Cryptococcal meningitis 76
Cryptococcosis 58
Cryptococcus neoformans 62
Curreri junior formula 437, 438*t*
Cushing's syndrome 318
Cutaneous microflora 500
Cyclic adenosine monophosphate 337
Cyclophosphamide 155, 299
Cyclosporin 299
Cystic fibrosis 190, 193*t*, 194, 194*t*, 196*fc*, 344, 463
    diagnosis of 196
    newborn screening 198
    nutritional management of 206
Cysts, duplication 463
Cytomegalovirus 47, 146, 290, 300

D

Daily sleep duration 398
Deafness 193
Dehydration 193, 208
Dehydroepiandrosterone 233
Delinquency 29
Delta variant 125
Deltacoronavirus 41
Demyelinating diseases 141
Dendritic cells 43, 44
Dengue 46, 86
    fever 46
Dent disease 245, 246, 252, 260
Dental erosions 27, 29
Deoxyribonucleic acid 344, 345
    antibodies 290
Depression 29
Dermatology 499
Dermatophytes 57
Dermis 499
Dexamethasone 255
Diabetes
    center, monitoring at 276
    Control and Complications Trial 265
    education 282
    insipidus 91, 258*f*
Diabetes mellitus 264, 266*f*, 284
    clinical features of 264
    cystic fibrosis related 208
    diagnosis of 265, 265*b*
    management of 264, 265
    neonatal 284
    type 1 264, 285
Diabetic ketoacidosis 47, 264, 269
Diaper care 503
Diarrhea 45, 464
    persistent 218
    watery 318
Diastolic functions, assessment of 8
Differential lymphocyte count 48
Digoxin 178
Dihydroxyphenylacetic acid 314
Disasters, neglect during 479
Disseminated intravascular coagulation 16
Distal intestinal obstruction syndrome 195, 205
Dobutamine 13
Donath Landsteiner antibody 304
Dopamine 13, 313
Doughnut sign 466
Down syndrome 231
Drowning 446
Drug interactions 72
Drug therapy 185
Dry powder inhalation 202
Duchenne muscular dystrophy 314, 344, 356
Dysgerminoma 312
Dyslipidemia 29

E

Early learning
    opportunities for 385
    promote 389
Early multiple organ dysfunction syndrome 46
Eating disorders 400
Echinocandins 62, 72
Echocardiography 49
Eczema 218
Elafibranor 238
Eleclazine 186
Electroconvulsive therapy 457
Electroencephalogram 144, 147, 150, 161, 165, 368
Electrolyte imbalances 446
Electromyogram 368
Electroretinogram 166
Elevated beta-human chorionic gonadotropin, causes of 312*t*
Elevated urine catecholamine metabolites, causes of 314*b*
Elexacaftor 209
Embryonal carcinoma 312
Emollients, classification of 505*b*
Empyema 193
Encephalitis 446
    causes of 138
Encephalomyelitis, acute disseminated 156
Encephalopathy, acute necrotizing 146
Endocarditis, infective 86
Endocrinology 264
Endothelial damage 93
Enema, delayed repeat 468, 471
Energy drinks 29
    banning of 32
    harmful effects of 26
    reduce consumption of 31
Energy-dense low-nutrient density foods 20
Enteric fever 47
Enterocolitis syndrome, food protein-induced 216-218
Enteroviruses 8, 47
Environment protection agency 417
Environmental noise pollution 425
    health hazards of 416, 416*t*
Enzyme phenylethanolamine-N-methyltransferase, lack of 313
Enzyme replacement therapy 350, 351, 351*t*
    principle of 350

Enzyme-linked immunosorbent assay 48, 109, 148, 290, 294
Eosinophilic gastrointestinal syndromes 218
Epilepsy 141, 252, 442, 445
    surgery 457
    syndrome 161
        febrile infection-related 454
Epileptic spasms 161, 163, 166
Epinephrine 13, 15
Epithelial autografts, cultured 436
Epithelial sodium channels 191
Epstein-Barr virus 47, 146, 290, 300, 302
Erythrocyte sedimentation rate 48, 93, 327
Erythromycin 290
Escherichia coli 88
Estrogens 318
Etanercept 325, 326
Eteplirsen, mechanism of action of 356*f*
Etripamil 176
European Medicines Agency 354
Evans syndrome 290, 299, 300*b*
    treatment of 301
Exome sequencing 348
Extensively hydrolyzed formula 220, 222
Extracorporeal membrane oxygenation 11, 15, 49
Eye
    congestion 47
    problems 401

F

Fabry disease 351
Failure to thrive 193, 217, 218
Falling sickness 442
Familial polyposis 463
Family planning 491
Family welfare 491
Fanconi anemia 309, 311
Fanconi syndrome 243
Fanconi-Bickel syndrome 252
Fast food 19
    in schools, regulation on consumption of 28
Fatigue 291
Fats, higher consumption of 26
Fatty liver indicator, ultrasonography 236
Feminization 318
Fetomaternal bleed 3
Fever 46, 47
Fibrinogen 48
Fibroblast growth factor 260
Fibrosis score 234
Flecainide 178
Flowcytometry 148
Fluconazole 59, 62, 63, 64, 66, 71

Flucytosine 59, 62, 76
Fluid management 431
Fluid resuscitation 14, 90
Fluorescence in situ hybridization 343
Fluoroquinolone 203
Food 314
    additive sensitivity 215
    allergy 215
    aversion 215
    intolerance 215
    labeling 23, 30
    processing 21
    ultra-processed 19
Food Safety and Standards Authority 21
Forensic evidence, collection of 484
Fractures 481
Fragile X syndrome 344
Fresh frozen plasma 15, 93
Frontline healthcare workers 121
Fungal infections 146
    invasive 56
Fungi, classification of 57*f*

G

Galactomannan 59
Galactorrhea 318
Galactosemia 252
Galsulfase 351
Gamma-aminobutyric acid 443
    receptors 444*f*
Gammacoronavirus 41
Gamma-glutamyl transferase 208, 236
Gangrene 93
Gastrin 318
Gastrinoma 318
Gastroenteritis 468
Gastroenterology 215
Gastrointestinal complications, management of 207
Gastrointestinal effects 83
Gastrointestinal losses 12
Gastrointestinal symptoms 45
Gastrointestinal tract 215
Gaucher disease 344, 351
Gene therapy 352
    strategies 352*fc*
Genetic disorders
    diagnosis of 343
    treatment of 343
Genetic metabolic encephalopathies 146
Genome sequencing 348
Genotoxicity 29
Germ cell tumors 307, 310-312
    malignant 310
    non-seminomatous 309

Germinoma, pure 312
Germline gene therapy 352
Gestational trophoblastic disease 312
Giant-cell hepatitis 300
Gibson and Cooke method 197
Giemsa stain 293*f*, 302*f*
Gigantism 318
Gitelman syndrome 254*f*
Glasgow coma scale 90
Glasgow meningococcal septicemia
 prognostic score 93, 94*b*
Glioma 145
Glucagon 318
Glucagonoma 318
Glucocorticoid 337
 responsive circulatory collapse 14
Glucose-6-phosphate dehydrogenase 292
Glucosuria 245
Glutamate 443
Glutamic acid decarboxylase 138, 141
 antibody 147
Glycemic control 439
 monitoring of 274
Glycemic index 279
Glycine receptor 141
Glycogen storage disorder 197
Glycogenosis, hepatic forms of 230
Glycosylated hemoglobin 52, 265, 275
Glycosylation, congenital disorders of 230
Golimumab 328
Gram stain 88
Granulosa cell tumor 318
Graves' disease 278
Growth 376
 factor, insulin-like 317
 failure 252
 hormone 318, 438, 439
Guselkumab 335

■ H

H1N1 120
Haemophilus influenzae 88, 195
Haemorrhage 162
Hallucinations 29
Hayfork sign 466
Headache 29
Health care
 infrastructure 494
 professionals 484
Hearing
 organs of 412, 412*f*
 protectors, use of 424
 surveillance 425
Hearing loss 29, 414, 415

classification of 415, 415*b*
diagnosis of noise-induced 423
etiology of 415
hidden 417
noise-induced 411, 415, 417, 423
treatment of noise-induced 423
types of 415
Heart 2
 block, complete 173, 173*f*, 177
 disease, congenital 10, 11, 179
 electrical activity of 183
Heart rate 13
 abnormalities 4
 calculation of 170
Helicobacter pylori 300
Hemangioma 463
 infantile 309
Hematology, pediatric 289
Hematopoietic stem cell transplant 299, 306
Hemodynamic monitoring, signs of 6
Hemodynamic status 428
Hemoglobinemia 292
Hemoglobinuria 292
Hemolytic-uremic syndrome 463
Hemophagocytic histiocytosis 146
Hemophagocytic lymphohistiocytosis 336
Hemophilia 463
Hemosiderinuria 292
Henoch-Schönlein purpura 463
Hepatic steatosis 231
Hepatic tumors 309, 312
Hepatitis
 acute 309
 C 290
  virus 300
 chronic 309
Hepatoblastoma 309, 318
Hepatocellular carcinoma 309
Hepatocellular malignant neoplasm 309
Hepatology 230
Hepatoma 318
Hereditary fructose intolerance 230
Hereditary nephrogenic diabetes insipidus 197
Hereditary spherocytosis 292
Hereditary tyrosinemia 310
Herpes simplex
 encephalitis 141, 157
 virus 8, 139, 146
Herpes viruses 103
Heterozygosity, loss of 346
Histocompatibility complex, major 334
Holter evaluation 174
Homovanillic acid 313
Hormonal tumor 318
 markers 318*t*

Hormone 308, 317
　adrenocorticotropic 13, 165
　antidiuretic 255
　artificial pancreas, dual 274
　follicle stimulating 311
　high parathyroid 259
　intramuscular adrenocorticotropic 164
　luteinizing 311
　parathyroid 259*f*, 318
　serum thyroid stimulating 232
　thyroid 317
　thyroid-stimulating 277, 311
Human chorionic gonadotropin 311
　beta fraction of 307, 311
Human coronaviruses 43
Human embryonic kidney 148
Human herpes virus 146
Human immunodeficiency virus 86, 146, 231, 290, 291, 300
　infection 353
Human papillomavirus vaccine 338
Hutchinson maneuver, modified 472
Hybrid-closed loop pump 273
Hydrocortisone 16
Hydrolyzed formula 224
　partially 224
Hydrostatic enema reduction 470
Hydrostatic reduction 468
Hydroxyindolacetic acid 316
Hyperactivity 29
Hyperaldosteronism 255
Hypercalciuria 248, 252
　chronic 255
Hyperchloremic metabolic acidosis 244-246
Hyperekplexia 163
Hyperglycemia 318
　history of 284
Hyperkalemia 245, 248
Hypermetabolism 438
Hypernatremia 91
Hyperparathyroidism 260
Hypersensitivity 29
　reaction 274
Hypertension 25, 29, 144, 247, 248, 318
　monogenic disorders of 253
Hyperthermia 144
Hyperthyroidism 260, 318
Hypertonic saline 201
Hypoallergenic formula 224
Hypocalcemia 91
　severe 259
Hypoglycemia 7, 280, 281, 284, 318, 446
　management of 280*fc*
　severe 281
Hypokalemia 91, 244-246, 252, 318
　chronic 255

Hypokalemic metabolic alkalosis 247
Hypomagnesemia 91, 248, 255, 260
Hyponatremia 91, 248, 446
Hypophosphatasia 351
Hypophosphatemia 91
Hypophosphatemic rickets 259
Hypopnea 368, 369
Hypotension 2, 4, 6, 16, 29, 218, 446
　catecholamine-resistant 15
Hypothalamic diseases 231
Hypothermia 218, 456
Hypothyroidism 197, 231
Hypoventilation, sleep-related 369
Hypovolemia 3, 83
Hypoxia 45, 49, 54, 446
Hypoxic ischemic
　encephalopathy 162
　insult, acute 446
Hypsarrhythmia 164

I

Ibuprofen 290
Idiopathic thrombocytopenic purpura 463
Idursulfase
　alpha 351
　beta 351
Imidazoles 62
Imiglucerase 351
Immune
　deficiency 218
　hemolytic anemia, drug-induced 296
　mediated disorders 146
　responses, cell-mediated 105
Immunizations 101
Immunodeficiency
　common variable 290, 300
　disorders 290, 300
　severe combined 300
Immunoglobulin
　G 289
　intravenous 52, 59, 93, 153, 296, 298, 299
　M 289
　profile 290
Immunohistochemistry 86
Immunomodulation 50
Immunoreactive trypsinogen 198
Immunotherapy 455*b*
Implantable cardiac devices 181
Implantable cardioverter-defibrillators 181
Incontinentia pigmenti 344
Indigenous sweat collection system 197*f*
Infantile spams
　diagnosis of 163
　etiology of 163
　pathogenesis of 161

Index

Infection, chronic 296
Infectious bronchitis virus 40
Infectious diseases 40, 56, 79
Inflammatory disorders 146
Inflammatory inhaled nasal steroids 372
Infliximab 325, 327
Influenza vaccination 338
Inhalational injury 431
Inherited arrhythmias 183, 185
Inherited disorders 446
Insulin 318
   adverse effects of 274
   carbohydrate ratio 270*b*
   conventional 267
   delivery, modes of 271
   dosing 269
   edema 274
   inhaled 284
   injection technique 269
   neuritis 274
   newer 267
   pump 271-273
      advantages of 273
      set 271*f*
   regimen 268
   requirement, low 284
   sensitivity factor 270*b*
   therapy 266
      principles of 268
   types of 267*t*
Insulinoma 318
Integrated Child Development Services 391, 494
Integrated Child Protection Scheme 494
Intellectual disability 346
Intensive care units 50, 54, 122
Interferon gamma release assay 328, 329
Interferon genes, stimulators of 336
Interleukin inhibitors 331, 330, 335
International League Against Epilepsy Task Force 444
International Society of Pediatric and Adolescent Diabetes 278
Intestinal polyps 463
Intoxication 446
Intracranial tension 29
   raised 83, 92
Intussusception 460, 460*f*, 473*f*, 475
   pathophysiology of 462*f*
   transanal protrusion of 465*f*, 468
Invasive meningococcal disease 79, 85, 86
   prevention of 94
   prognosis of 93
Iron overload 292
Irritability 29

Isavuconazole 59, 62, 63, 65, 70, 72
Isosexual precocity 318
Isseminated intravascular coagulation 93
Itraconazole 59, 62-64, 67, 71
Ivabradine 177
Ivacaftor 209
Ixekizumab 335

J

Janus kinase 52
   signal transduction 335
Jaundice 291, 292
Junctional ectopic tachycardia, congenital 177
Junk food 19, 20
   harmful effects of 25
   reduce consumption of 28
Juvenile dermatomyositis 325, 331, 333
Juvenile idiopathic arthritis 290, 325
   pathogenesis of 324
   systemic-onset 330
Juvenile Justice (Care and Protection) Act 492

K

Kawasaki disease 46, 122, 325
Ketamine 437, 453
Ketoconazole 62
Ketogenic diet 454
Ketone testing 276
Klinefelter syndrome 284

L

Lacosamide 455
Lactate dehydrogenase 292, 297, 308, 317
Lactose intolerance 215, 218, 219*t*
Langerhans cells 499
Language dysfunction 143
Laparoscopy 473
Laparotomy 472
Laronidase 351
Latex agglutination test 87
Law on Child Sexual Abuse 487
L-dopa 314
Leber congenital amaurosis 353
Left atrial pressure 9
Lens culinaris hemagglutinin 308
Leptospirosis 46, 47, 86
Lethargy 218, 464
Leucine-rich glioma inactivated protein 141
Leukemia 300, 463
   acute 290
Leukodystrophy 148
Leukoencephalopathy, acute 146

Leukomalacia, periventricular 162
Levofloxacin 203
Levosimendan 13
Leydig cell tumor 318
Liddle syndrome 254, 255
Limb
  ischemia 93
  thick ascending 244
Limbic encephalitis 141
Lipid complex amphotericin B 59
Lipodystrophy 274
Lipoma 463
Lipo-oligosaccharide 82
Lipoprotein cholesterol
  high-density 25, 29
  low-density 25, 29
Liposomal amphotericin 59, 76
Liquid chromatography, high-performance 313
Live attenuated vaccines 103
Liver
  biopsy 234
  damage, drug-induced 309
  disease 296
    cystic fibrosis related 207
  disorders, benign 309
  fibrosis, enhanced 232, 236
  function test 236, 327, 450
Loop of Henle 253f
Low birth weight 378, 379
  extremely 3, 11
Low molecular weight
  heparin 43
  proteinuria 245
Lowe syndrome 243, 252
Lumacaftor 209
Lumbar puncture 87
Lund-Browder chart 429t
Lung injury, transfusion-associated acute 438
Lyme disease 86
Lymphangioma 463
Lymphocyte subset analysis 290
Lymphoma 29, 300, 463
Lysosomal acid lipase deficiency 351
Lysosomal storage disorders 349, 350

■ M

Macrophage activation syndrome 332
Macrovascular disease 278
Magnesium 243, 450
  fractional excretion of 262
Magnetic stimulation therapy 456
Maintenance therapy 155
Malabsorption 193
Malformations 162

Malnutrition 197
  severe 193
Marfan syndrome 344
Mass palpable per rectum 465
Maternal mental health, support 389
Matrix metalloproteinases 332
Maturity-onset diabetes of young 284
Mean arterial pressure 5, 11
Mean corpuscular volume 302
Measles virus 103
Mechanical ventilation 49
Meckel's diverticulum 463
Meconium ileus 193, 207
  equivalent 193, 207
Medical nutrition therapy 278
Medical therapy 372
Medicines and Healthcare Products
    Regulatory Agency 110
Medicolegal case 483
Medullary nephrocalcinosis 252
Medullary thyroid carcinoma 318
Melanocytes 499
Meningitis 84, 446
  belt 80
Meningococcal
  disease 79, 80, 95t
  meningitis 84, 86
  septicemia 84, 86
Meningococcemia 84, 85f
Mental health support 485
Mercuric nitrate 197f
Mesenchymal hamartoma 309
Metabolic abnormality 208
  correction of 91
Metabolic acidosis 91
Metabolic alkalosis 195, 252, 254fc
Metabolic disease 230, 446
Metabolic disorders 148
Metabolic effects 25
Metabolism, inborn error of 349, 446
Metabotropic glutamate receptor 141
Metadrenaline, free 316
Metalloproteinase, tissue inhibitor of 234
Metered dose inhaler 201
Methotrexate 337
Methylprednisolone 299
Mexiletine 185
Micafungin 59, 73
Miconazole 62
Microangiopathic hemolytic anemia 292
Microneutralization test 123
Microsporum 57
Microvascular injury 82
Midazolam 451
Middle east respiratory syndrome 40

Index

Milrinone 13
Minimal nutritional value, foods of 20
Mitochondrial inheritance 344
Mixed venous oxygen saturation 8
Modern slavery 489
Molnupiravir 53
Monoamine oxidase 314
Monoclonal antibodies 51
Monogenic disorders 343, 347, 354*t*
Motor neuron, survival of 356
Movement disorder 141, 143
Mucopolysaccharidosis 197, 350, 351
Mucormycosis 58
Multifactorial disorders 343
Multifocal leukoencephalopathy, progressive 325
Multiple daily injections 268
Multiple food allergies 218
Multiple sclerosis 325
Multisystem inflammatory syndrome 46, 52, 332
Muscle activity increase 446
Mutation analysis 197
Mycophenolate mofetil 299
Mycoplasma
    pneumonia 290, 300, 302
        infection 303
    serology 290
Myelin oligodendrocyte glycoprotein 141, 147
    antibody 147
Myelodysplasia 300
Myelodysplastic syndrome 290
Myeloid leukemia, chronic 290
Myoclonic epilepsy, progressive 446
Myopericarditis 113
Myotonic dystrophy 344

■ N

Nasal oxygen, high-flow 49
Nasal polyposis 193
Nasal potential difference 196, 198
Nasal swabs 47
Nasogastric suction 472
Nasogastric tube 207
National Centre for Disease Control 96
National Charter for Children 477
National Early Childhood Care and Education 391
National Glycohemoglobin Standardization Program 265
National Health and Nutrition Examination Survey 415
National Institute for Health and Clinical Excellence 90, 501
National Institute of Health 21, 102
National Nutrition Policy 391
National Plan of Action for Children 391
National Policy for Children 477
National Policy for Education 391
National Regulatory Agencies 106
National Regulatory Authority 106
Nausea 45
Near infrared spectroscopy 8
Neisseria meningitides, colonies of 87*f*
Neisseria meningitidis 79
Neonatal intensive care units 1
Neonatal Resuscitation Program 11
Neonatal skin condition score 505, 506*b*
Neonatology 1
Neoplasm 148
Neoplastic disorders 146
Neoplastic tissue, proteins produced by 308
Nephritis 290
Nephrocalcinosis 248, 260
    evaluation for 261*b*
Nephrogenic diabetes insipidus 257*f*
Nephrolithiasis 248, 260
    evaluation for 261*b*
Nephrology 243
Nephronophthisis 255
Nephropathy 278
Neuroblastoma 307, 313, 318
Neurofibromatosis 344
Neurogenic tumors 316
Neurologic signs 6
Neurology 138, 161
Neuromyelitis optica spectrum disorders 147
Neuron-specific enolase 313, 315
Neuropathy 278
Neuroplasticity 376
Neuropsychiatric symptoms 141
Neurosecretory proteins 315
Neutropenia 331
Neutrophil ratio 7
Newborn, massage of 502
Next generation sequencing 348
Nirmatrelvir 51
Nitric oxide, inhaled 13
N-methyl-d-aspartate 444
    receptor 138, 141, 144
        antibodies 147
Noise 414
    annoyance 419
    harmful effects of 424
    monitoring 424
    pollution 421
        areas of 416
    sensitivity 419
    sources of 416

Index

Nonaccidental injuries 480
Nonalcoholic fatty liver disease 230, 236
   clinical diagnosis of 231
   diagnosis of 231
   metabolic signature of 233
   microbiome signature of 233
Nonalcoholic steatohepatitis 230, 231
Non-auditory hazards 418
Non-Hodgkin lymphoma 290
Noninvasive management 373
Noninvasive ventilation 49
Nonrespiratory therapy 206
Nonsteroidal anti-inflammatory drugs 437
Noradrenaline 13
Norepinephrine 313
Normetadrenaline, free 316
Nucleic acid
   amplification testing 47, 53, 108
   vaccines 104
Nucleocapsid protein 124
Numerous gastrointestinal pathogens 461
Nurturing care framework 381, 393
Nusinersen, mechanism of action of 356f
Nutrient profiling 23
Nutrition 19, 437

O

Obesity 29, 284, 400
Obeticholic acid 238
Obstructed sleep disordered breathing,
   spectrum of 363f
Obstructive apnea 369
   hypopnea index 369
      score 370t
Obstructive sleep apnea 361, 364
Ofloxacin 203
Oligodendrocyte glycoprotein 138
Oliguria 83
Omicron variant 51, 126
   emergence of 51
Omphalitis 504
Oncology 307
Opsoclonus myoclonus syndrome 141
Oral food challenge 220, 222
   test 215
Oral glucose tolerance test 209, 265
Oral rehydrating solution 208, 432
Oropharyngeal swab 47
Osteoporosis 29
Otoacoustic emissions 423
Otorhinolaryngology 361
Ovarian teratoma 150
Oximetry score 367
Oxygen 49
   saturations 367

P

Packed cell volume 11
Pain 464
   management 436
   relief, paracetamol for 430
Pancreas, artificial 273
Pancreatic enzyme replacement therapy 206
Pancreatitis 47
Pandemic speed vaccines 102
Paracetamol 314, 437
Paraganglioma 315
Parathyroid hyperplasia 318
Paroxysmal cold hemoglobinuria 292, 295, 304
   treatment of 304
Paroxysmal supraventricular tachycardia 172, 176-178
Partial thromboplastin time 48
Parvovirus B19 290, 300
Patent ductus arteriosus 2, 3, 14
Pathogen-associated molecular patterns 104
Pediatric arrhythmias, pharmacologic
   therapy of 176
Pediatric autoimmune
   encephalitis 146t
   neuropsychiatric disorders 146
Pediatric cardiac arrhythmias, diagnosis of 169
Pediatric emergency departments 169
Pediatric intensive care unit 430, 434, 434t, 450
Pediatric multisystem inflammatory
   syndrome 46
Pediatric nonalcoholic fatty liver disease
   fibrosis index 234, 236
   histological score 235
Pediatric surgery 460
Penicillins 290
Perinatal hypoxic-ischemic injury 446
Personal audio device 415, 418
Peutz-Jeghers syndrome 463
Peyer's patches 462
pH 243
Phenobarbitone, high-dose 453
Pheochromocytoma 315, 318
Phosphate 243
Phosphaturia 245
Phosphodiesterase inhibitors 337
Phosphorus 450
Physical violence 479
Physician's responsibility 485
Piperacillin 290
Plaque reduction neutralization test 123, 123t
Plasma
   catecholamines 313
   exchange 153
   glucose 265
Plasmapheresis 153

Plasminogen activator inhibitor 83, 238
Pneumatic enema reduction 469
Pneumatic reduction 468
Pneumococcal vaccination 338
Pneumocystis jirovecii 57
    infection 155
Pneumonia 44, 45
    persistent 193
Pneumoperitoneum 465
Pneumothorax 193, 206
Poisoning 446
Polyamines, free 317
Polychromatic cells 293*f*
Polyenes 62, 73
Polymerase chain reaction 57, 58
    tests 8
Polymorphic ventricular tachycardia 185*f*
Polysomnogram 365
Polysomnography 365
Polysymptomatic encephalopathy 141
Polyuria 248, 255, 256
Pompe disease 350, 351
Posaconazole 59, 62, 63, 65, 69, 71
Positive airway pressure 370
    therapy 372
Positive expiratory pressure 202
    devices 202
Post-infectious encephalopathy 146
Poststatus epilepticus 145
Post-stem cell transplantation 300
Post-traumatic stress disorder 485
Potassium 243
Poxviruses 103
Prader-Willi syndrome 344, 362
Prandial insulin 270*b*
Precocious puberty 318
Prednisolone 299
Propofol 451
Propranolol 178
Prostaglandin 11
    E1 11
Protection of Children from Sexual Offences
    Act 484, 487
Prothrombin time 48, 450
Prothromboplastin time, active 50
Proton
    density fat fraction 235
    pump inhibitors 65
    secretion of 243
Proximal tubule 244
Pseudo-kidney 466
    sign 467*f*
Pseudomonas 191, 203
    aeruginosa 195, 204
    infection 203

Psoriatic arthritis 325
Psychiatric disorders 146
Psychiatric disturbances 27
Psychological behaviour, abnormal 26
Psychological disorders 29, 401
Psychosocial aspects 283
Public education 424
Pulmonary complications 205
Pulmonary effects 83
Pulmonary exacerbations
    management of 202
    prevention of 204
Pulmonary hypertension, persistent 13, 14
Pulmonary involvement 45
Pulmonology 190
Pulse oximetry 366
Purpura fulminans 85*f*

Q

QRS complex 170
QT prolongation 29
QT syndrome, long 185
Quantitative fluorescence polymerase chain
    reaction 345

R

Radiofrequency ablation 179
Radioimmunoassay 148
Rag picking 489
Randomized control trial 50
Rapid antigen test 47, 53
Rapid maxillary expansion 371
Rash 46
Rashtriya Bal Surakhsha Karyakram 392
Reactions, systemic 218
Receptor-binding domain 101
Rectal prolapse 193, 468
Red blood cell 289
Red currant jelly stool 462
Red flag signs 218*b*
Refractory autoimmune hemolytic anemia 298
Refractory rickets 258
Relapses 156
Remdesivir 53
Renal carcinoma 318
Renal diseases 255
Renal disorders 296
Renal dysplasia 255
Renal impairment 83
Renal signs 6
Renal tubular
    acidosis 244, 250*f*, 251, 259*f*
    disorders 243

Index

Respiratory effort-related arousal 369
Respiratory inductance plethysmography 368
Respiratory management 201
Respiratory signs 6
Responsive caregiving 386, 389
Resuscitation, endpoints of 432
Reticulocytopenia 295
Reticulocytosis 304
Retinopathy 278
Reverse transcription polymerase chain reaction 47, 52, 53
Rhesus 289
Rhesus-human reassortant rotavirus vaccine 461
Rheumatic disorders, pediatric 324, 325*t*
Rheumatoid arthritis 300
Rheumatological disorders 300
Rheumatology 324
Rhinosinusitis 362
Ribonucleic acid 355
   aptamers 355
   messenger 356, 357
   small interfering 355
   therapeutics 355
   vaccines 104
Rice-based feeds 224
Rickettsiosis 86
Right iliac fossa, emptiness of 464
Right to Education Act 480
Rilonacept 333
Ringer's lactate 90
Risdiplam 358
Ritonavir 51
Rituximab 154, 155, 299, 303, 325, 333
Rotavirus 461
Rubella 290
Rule of Nines 429
Russell-Silver syndrome 344
Ruxolitinib 336

■ S

Salicylate 215
Salt craving 193
Salty taste 193
Sawtooth appearance 173*f*
Scalp, care of 504
Scarlet fever 46
Scleroderma 331
Sclerosing cholangitis, primary 290
Sclerosing panencephalitis, subacute 150
Scrub typhus 46
Sebelipase alpha 351
Secukinumab 335
Seizures 29, 92, 143, 155
Selonsertib 238

Seminoma 312
Sensor augmented pump 273
Sensorineural deafness 252
Sensorineural hearing loss 417
Sensorium, altered 29
Septicemia 84
Sertoli cell tumor 318
Sertoli-Leydig cell 318
   tumors 309
Serum
   and urinary catecholamines 307
   creatine phosphokinase 232
   sodium 243
   uric acid 232
Severe acute respiratory distress syndrome 40, 101
Severe acute respiratory syndrome-related coronavirus
   infection 40, 45
   structure 42*f*
   vaccine 101, 112
   variants 125*f*
Sexual abuse 483
Sexually transmitted disease 484
Shields technique 469
Shigella dysentery 218
Shock 1, 2, 4, 7, 14, 47, 84, 89
   compensated 9
   in transitional circulation 12
   neonatal 1, 9*t*, 10*t*
   pathophysiology of neonatal 3*t*
   septic 3, 6, 14, 47
   septicemia with 86
   septicemia without 83
   time sensitive management of 11*fc*
   types of 10
Shunts, intracardiac 3
Sick day management
   education 283
   guidelines 283*b*
Sigmoidoscopy 220
Signe-de-dance sign 464
Single nucleotide polymorphism 345, 346
   chromosomal microarray 346*f*
Sinus
   bradycardia 173
   rhythm 171
Sinusitis, recurrent 193
Sirolimus 299
Skin
   care 499, 506
      neonatal 501
   cleansing, neonatal 502
   composition 500
   function 500
   prick test 219

rashes 193
structure 500
Sleep 400
   disordered breathing 361
   disturbance 143
      and insomnia 419
   endoscopy, drug-induced 370
   pattern, disturbed 29
Small bowel intussusceptions 465
Small molecule therapy 358
Snorers, primary 363
Social cognitive theory 401
Sodium
   and chloride ions, absorption of 253*f*
   bicarbonate cotransporter 250
   channels, voltage-gated 455
Somatic gene therapy 352
Sotalol 178
Sotrovimab 51
Sound 411
   assessment of 411
   frequencies 413
Soy protein formula 224
Spasms, infantile 161, 162, 166
Spirometry 200
Splenectomy 299
Split mix regimen 268
Sporothrix schenckii 74
Sputnik light 114
Staphylococcus 191
   aureus 195, 205
Status epilepticus 141, 445, 450, 457
   febrile infection-related 146
   generalized 442
   management of 442
   nonconvulsive 443, 451
   refractory 143, 442, 445, 450, 454
   super-refractory 445, 450
Steatohepatitis 231
Stem cell transplant 58
Steroids 15, 49, 92, 153, 469
   inhaled 202
Stratum corneum 499
Street children 489
Streptococcal infections 146
Streptococcus pneumoniae 88
Streptomyces nodosus 73
Stroke 29, 148, 162
Substrate reduction therapy 358
Subunit vaccines 104
Sudden cardiac death 29
Sudden infant death syndrome 184
Sugar-sweetened beverages 30
Suicidal tendencies 29
Supraventricular tachycardia 175*f*
Sweat chloride estimation 196

Symptomatic disease 130
Symptomatic status epilepticus, acute 446
Syndrome of inappropriate antidiuretic
      hormone secretion 156
Syndromic epilepsies 446
Systemic antifungal
   agents 59
   therapy 56
Systemic autoimmune disorders 146
Systemic disorders 45
Systemic fungal infections 57
   diagnosis of 57, 58*t*
Systemic inflammatory response syndrome 10
Systemic lupus erythematosus 47, 141, 146,
      296, 300, 302, 325, 327
Systemic mycoses 57*f*
Systemic sclerosis 325
Systemic vascular resistance 4, 9, 13

T

Tachycardia 4, 29, 144, 172*f*
Taliglucerase alpha 351
Target sign 466
Teratoma 309, 312
   benign 312
Testis 318
Testosterone 438
Tetracycline 290
Tezacaftor 209
Theophylline 314
Therapeutic drug monitoring 70
Therapeutic plasma exchange 153
Thrombotic thrombocytopenia, vaccine
      induced 109
Thyrocalcitonin 318
Thyroid
   adenoma 318
   peroxidase antibodies 147
Thyroiditis 290
Tinnitus 417
Tissue
   hypoxia, measurement of 8
   perfusion, inadequate 2
   transglutaminase antibodies 147
Tocilizumab 154, 325, 330
Tofacitinib 336
Topiramate 456
Toxic encephalopathies 146
Toxic shock syndrome 46
Toxicity 75, 76
Tranexamic acid 206
Transaminitis 331
Transcription activator-like effector
      nuclease 353
Transcription inhibitors, activation of 335

Transepidermal water loss 499
Transepithelial sodium chloride absorption 253*f*
Trans-fatty acids 20
Trauma 446
Tremors 29
Triazoles 62
Triglycerides 25
Triiodothyronine 317
Triplet repeat disorders 344
Troponin 48
Tubercular meningitis 86
Tuberculin skin test 328, 329
Tuberculosis 325, 328, 329
Tuberous sclerosis complex 162
Tubular disorders 243, 261
Tubular dysfunction, patterns of 244
Tubular reabsorption 243
Tubulopathy 252
Tumbler test 86
Tumor 318
    markers 307, 308, 317
    necrosis factor 317, 324, 329, 438
    screening 150
    tissue 307
Turner syndrome 231, 284
Tyrosinemia 252, 309

U

Umbilical cord, care of 504
Upper airway resistance syndrome 363
Urinary catecholamines 313
Urine organic acids 164
Ursodeoxycholic acid 208, 237
Urticaria 29, 223
Ustekinumab 335

V

Vaccine
    efficacy 117
    inactivated 103
    platforms 103
Vagal nerve stimulation 456
Valsalva maneuver 176
Valvular pulmonic stenosis, severe 173*f*
Vanillylmandelic acid 313
Varicella 290
Vascular endothelial growth factor 317, 357
Vasculitis 93, 325, 333
Vasoactive intestinal
    peptide 318
    polypeptide 316
Vasopressin 13
Velaglucerase alpha 351

Vena cava
    inferior 8
    superior 14
Verapamil 178
Vernix caseosa 501
Vesicular stomatitis virus 103
Vestronidase 351
Viable epidermis 499
Vigabatrin 166
Violence, forms of 479*b*
Vipoma 318
Viral infection 146, 204
Viral myocarditis 47, 173*f*
Viral prodrome 141
Viral transmission 42
Viral vectored vaccines 103
Vitamin
    D 223
        deficiency 193
        dependent rickets 258
        excess 260
    deficiency 193
Vitiligo 278
Volume resuscitation 11
Vomiting 45, 464
Voriconazole 59, 62-64, 67, 71

W

Warm autoimmune hemolytic anemia 292, 293*f*, 299*b*
    treatment of 296
West syndrome 161
Wheezing, recurrent 193
White blood cell 93
Whole exome sequencing 164, 348
Whole genome sequencing 348
Wilms tumor 309, 310, 316, 318
Wilson disease 252
Wolff-Parkinson-White syndrome 174, 174*f*, 178
Wound management 434

X

X-linked dominant 344
X-linked hypophosphatemic rickets 344

Y

Y-aminobutyric acid-B receptor 141
Yolk sac tumor 309, 310

Z

Zero fluoroscopy procedures 180
Zinc-finger nuclease 353
Zollinger-Ellison syndrome 318
Z-score 193